T0183085

Lecture Notes
in Business Information Processing 202

Series Editors

Wil van der Aalst
Eindhoven Technical University, Eindhoven, The Netherlands

John Mylopoulos
University of Trento, Povo, Italy

Michael Rosemann
Queensland University of Technology, Brisbane, QLD, Australia

Michael J. Shaw
University of Illinois, Urbana-Champaign, IL, USA

Clemens Szyperski
Microsoft Research, Redmond, WA, USA

More information about this series at http://www.springer.com/series/7911

Fabiana Fournier · Jan Mendling (Eds.)

Business Process Management Workshops

BPM 2014 International Workshops, Eindhoven
The Netherlands, September 7–8, 2014
Revised Papers

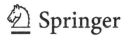 Springer

Editors
Fabiana Fournier
IBM Research – Haifa
Haifa
Israel

Jan Mendling
Vienna University of Economics
    and Business
Vienna
Austria

ISSN 1865-1348   ISSN 1865-1356   (electronic)
Lecture Notes in Business Information Processing
ISBN 978-3-319-15894-5   ISBN 978-3-319-15895-2   (eBook)
DOI 10.1007/978-3-319-15895-2

Library of Congress Control Number: 2015932973

Springer Cham Heidelberg New York Dordrecht London

Printed on acid-free paper

Springer International Publishing AG Switzerland is part of Springer Science+Business Media
(www.springer.com)

Preface

Business process management (BPM) is an established research domain for computer science, information systems, and management scholars. The International Conference on Business Process Management (BPM 2014) was the 12th conference in a series that provided the most distinguished and specialized forum for researchers and practitioners in BPM. The conference has a record of attracting innovative research of the highest quality related to all aspects of BPM, including theory, frameworks, methods, techniques, architectures, and empirical findings.

It is a tradition that topical workshops accompany the main BPM conference in order to allow groups to coalesce around new research topics, to present emerging research issues, or focus in-depth on a particular area of research. BPM 2014 was accompanied by ten workshops – some new, some well-established ones. In addition, a doctoral consortium took place at which young researchers could present and further develop their doctoral research lines. The workshops attracted 84 submissions, out of which the respective Program Committees selected 38 as full papers. This made a full paper acceptance rate of 45 %. In addition to these full papers, the proceedings for the LNBIP volume also included short papers, invited papers of key notes and tutorials, and the position papers of the doctoral consortium.

The following workshops of the BPM 2014 conference were held on September 8, 2014 on the campus of the Technical University of Eindhoven, The Netherlands:

- The 7th International Workshop on Process-oriented Information Systems in Healthcare (ProHealth 2014)
- The 3rd Workshop on Security in Business Processes (SBP 2014)
- The 4th International Workshop on Process Model Collections: Management and Reuse (PMC-MR 2014)
- The 1st International Workshop on Business Processes in Collective Adaptive Systems (BPCAS 2014)
- The 3rd International Workshop on Data- and Artifact- centric BPM (DAB 2014)
- The 10th International Workshop on Business Process Intelligence (BPI 2014)
- The 2nd InternationalWorkshop on Business Process Management in the Cloud (BPMC 2014)
- The 3rd International Workshop on Theory and Applications of Process Visualization (TaProViz 2014)
- The 7th Workshop on Business Process Management and Social Software (BPMS2 2014)
- The 2nd Decision Mining and Modeling for Business Processes (DeMiMoP 2014)
- In addition, the Doctoral Consortium was held on September 7, 2014 in the city center of Eindhoven.

We would like to express our sincere gratitude to the organizers of each workshop and of the doctoral consortium for arranging entertaining, high-quality programs that were well received by all attendees. We are grateful to the service of the countless reviewers who supported the Workshop Chairs and provided valuable feedback to the authors. Several workshops had invited keynote presentations that framed the presented research papers and we would like to thank the keynote speakers for their contribution to the Workshop Program. We would like to thank Ralf Gerstner, Viktoria Meyer, and the team at Springer for their support in the publication of this LNBIP volume.

December 2014   Fabiana Fournier
                                                          Jan Mendling

Preface to the 7th International Workshop on Process-Oriented Information Systems in Healthcare (Prohealth 2014)

Richard Lenz[1], Mor Peleg[2], and Manfred Reichert[3]

[1] Department Informatik, Friedrich-Alexander Universität Erlangen-Nürnberg, Germany
richard.lenz@fau.de
[2] Department of Information Systems, University of Haifa, Israel
morpeleg@is.haifa.ac.il
[3] Institute of Databases and Information Systems, Ulm University, Germany
manfred.reichert@uni-ulm.de

Introduction

Healthcare organizations and providers are facing the challenge of delivering high-quality services to their patients, at affordable costs. High degree of specialization of medical disciplines, prolonged medical care for the aging population, increased costs for dealing with chronic diseases, and the need for personalized healthcare are prevalent trends in this information-intensive domain. The emerging situation necessitates a change in the way healthcare is delivered to the patients and healthcare processes are managed.

BPM technology provides a key to implement these changes. Though patient-centered process support becomes increasingly crucial in healthcare, BPM technology has not yet been broadly used in healthcare environments. This workshop elaborates both the potential and the limitations of IT support for healthcare processes. It further provides a forum wherein challenges, paradigms, and tools for optimized process support in healthcare can be debated.

We bring together researchers and practitioners from different communities (e.g., BPM, Information Systems, Medical Informatics, E-Health), who share an interest in both healthcare processes and BPM technologies.

The first ProHealth workshop took place in the context of the 5th Int'l Conference on Business Process Management (BPM) in 2007. The next three ProHealth Workshops were also held in conjunction with BPM conferences (BPM 2008, BPM 2009, and BPM 2011). The next two ProHealth workshops brought together researchers from the BPM and the Medical Informatics communities, as joint ProHealth/Knowledge Representation for Healthcare (KR4HC) workshops held in 2012 and 2013. The success of the previous six ProHealth Workshops demonstrated the potential of such an interdisciplinary forum to improve the understanding of domain-specific requirements, methods and theories, tools and techniques, and the gaps between IT support and healthcare processes that are yet to be closed.

The ProHealth 2014 workshop focused on IT support of high-quality healthcare processes. It addressed topics including modeling and enactment of clinical guidelines and healthcare processes.

The workshop received nine papers from Germany (3), Israel (1), Italy (1), Chile (1), and the UK (1), a paper by authors from Israel, Italy, The Netherlands and Spain, and a paper by authors from Canada and Poland (1). Papers had to clearly establish their research contribution as well as their relation to healthcare processes. Five full papers and one position paper were selected to be presented at the workshop according to their relevance, quality, and originality.

In his keynote paper "On Measuring, Modeling and Analyzing Healthcare Systems in Real-Time: From Small Measurements through Big Data to Analytics," Prof. Avishai Mandelbaum from the Faculty of Industrial Engineering and Management at the Technion – Israel Institute of Technology discusses his platform for real-time creation of data-based models – simulation and analytical, which is based on modeling a service system as a processing network from event logs, and inferring model primitives, structure, and protocols.

The following three papers focus on modeling.

The paper "Modeling and Monitoring Variability in Hospital Treatments: A Scenario using CMMN" by Herzberg et al. addresses the problem of how to transfer a hospital-specific clinical pathway modeled in BPMN to another hospital. The authors use a questionnaire to capture practices in other hospitals and derive a generally valid case plan.

The paper "Recommendations for Medical Treatment Processes: The PIGS Approach" by Marcin Hewelt et al. introduces a BPMN-based knowledge management approach for multi-morbid patients. The authors formally introduce the concept of Treatment Cases (TCs) and explain how recommendations for the next treatment steps within a TC can be derived from multiple BPMN process models.

The paper "Modeling and Implementation of Correct by Construction Healthcare Workflows" by Papapanagiotou and Fleuriot proposes an approach for constructing healthcare workflows based on the "proofs-as-processes paradigm." The generated workflows have a number of guaranteed properties such as type correctness and freedom of deadlocks and livelocks.

The next three papers focus on execution.

The paper "MET4: Supporting Workflow Execution for Interdisciplinary Healthcare Teams" by Wilk et al. describes an agent-based approach for maintaining a healthcare team. In particular, the paper focuses on the specific support for the team leadership, team maintenance, and patient participation features.

The position paper "Enhancing Guideline-based Decision Support with Distributed Computation through Local Mobile Application" by Shalom et al. introduces the need for a distributed guideline-based decision support (DSS) process, describes its characteristics, and explains how this process was implemented within the European Union's MobiGuide project (www.mobiguide-project.eu).

The paper "Storlet Engine for Executing Biomedical Processes within the Storage System" by Rabinovici-Cohen et al. proposes expanding the storage system from only storing biomedical data to directly producing value from the data by executing computational modules — storlets — close to where the data is stored. Their paper describes the Storlet Engine, an engine to support computations in secure sandboxes within the storage system.

We would like to thank the invited speaker as well as the members of the Program Committee and the reviewers for their efforts in selecting the papers. They helped us to compile a high-quality program for the ProHealth 2014 workshop. We would also like to acknowledge the splendid support of the local organization and the BPM 2014 Workshop Chairs.

We hope you will find the papers of the ProHealth 2014 workshop interesting and stimulating, and look forward to seeing you at the next ProHealth workshop.

Organizers

Richard Lenz	University of Erlangen-Nuremberg, Germany
Mor Peleg	University of Haifa, Israel
Manfred Reichert	University of Ulm, Germany

Program Committee

Nachman Ash	Israel
Yaron Denekamp	Israel
Arturo Gonzalez-Ferrer	Spain
Adela Grando	USA
Stefan Jablonski	Germany
Wendy MacCaull	Canada
Ronny Mans	The Netherlands
Silvia Miksch	Austria
Bela Mutschler	Germany
Øystein Nytrø	Norway
Leon Osterweil	USA
Yardena Peres	Israel
Hajo Reijers	The Netherlands
David Riano	Spain
Shazia Sadiq	Australia
Danielle Sent	The Netherlands
Yuval Shahar	Israel
Annette ten Teije	The Netherlands
Lucineia Thom	Brazil
Dongwen Wang	USA
Barbara Weber	Austria

Preface to the 3rd International Workshop on Security in Business Processes (SBP 2014)

Raimundas Matulevičius[1], Rafael Accorsi[2], and Jason Crampton[3]

[1] University of Tartu, Estonia
rma@ut.ee
[2] University of Freiburg, Germany
rafael.accorsi@iig.uni-freiburg.de
[3] University of London, UK
Jason.Crampton@rhul.ac.uk

Introduction

Despite the growing demand for business processes that comply with security policies, security and privacy incidents caused by erroneous workflow specifications are regrettably common. The third edition of the Workshop on Security in Business Processes (SBP 2014) seeks to bring together researchers and practitioners interested in the management and modeling of secure business processes in process-aware information systems. The major goal is to obtain a deeper understanding of a rapidly maturing, yet still largely under-investigated field of business process security, audit and control, including both thorough security requirements formalization, secure process modeling, and mechanisms for verification, monitoring, and auditing. Besides the "technical" intent to substantially advance the current state of the art, SBP 2014 aims to identify active research areas in academia and industry, current approaches in industry, and existing tool-support; encourage approaches and techniques that combine formal foundations with industrial applicability; and highlight new research directions and challenges.

The SBP 2014 program included one keynote, one long and two short papers, and a tutorial. The keynote speech by van Geffen gave the audience a coherent view on the importance of the process mining and its influence on the security solutions. The second presentation given by Lu *et al*, considers conformance checking and more specifically on the use of the partially ordered traces and partially ordered alignments. In the first short paper presentation by van der Werf and Verbeek, online compliance monitoring is analyzed. The authors suggest using some golden configuration to discover process inconsistencies from the process logs. The second short paper presentation by Guanciale and Gurov considers how privacy is preserved in the virtual enterprises. The authors illustrate how to implement privacy preserving fusion of business processes using bounded Petri nets. In the tutorial presentation, based on the running example, Matulevičius has illustrated how to elicit security requirements from the business process models using security risk management method.

We wish to thank all those who contributed to making SBP a success: the authors who submitted papers, the members of the Program Committee who carefully reviewed and discussed the submissions, and the speakers who presented their work at the workshop. In particular, we thank the keynote speaker for their enthusiastic and insightful presentation. We also express our gratitude to the BPM 2014 Workshop Chairs for their support in preparing the workshop.

Organizers

Honorary PC Chair

Wil van der Aalst   Eindhoven University of Technology,
                                     The Netherlands

Program Committee Chairs

Raimundas Matulevičius   University of Tartu, Estonia
Rafael Accorsi   University of Freiburg, Germany
Jason Crampton   University of London, UK

Publicity Chair

Giovanni Livraga   University of Milan, Italy

Program Committee

Anne Baumgraß   University of Potsdam, Germany
Achim D. Brucker   SAP Labs, Germany
Khaled Gaaloul   CRP Henri Tudor, Luxembourg
Aditya Ghose   University of Wollongong, Australia
Mati Golani   ORT Braude College, Israel
Anat Goldstein   Ben-Gurion University of the Negev, Israel
Hejiao Huang   Harbin Institute of Technology, China
Michael Huth   Imperial College, UK
Fuyuki Ishikawa   National Institute of Informatics Tokyo, Japan
Jan Jürjens   Technical University of Dortmund, Germany
Dimka Karastoyanova   University of Stuttgart, Germany
Günter Karjoth   Lucerne University of Applied Sciences and Arts,
                                     Switzerland
Seok-Won Lee   Ajou University, Korea
Lin Liu   Tsinghua University, China
Heiko Ludwig   IBM Research, USA
Nicolas Mayer   CRP Henri Tudor, Luxembourg
Per Håkon Meland   SINTEF ICT, Norway
Marco Montali   Free University of Bozen-Bolzano, Italy
Haralambos Mouratidis   University of Brighton, UK
Andreas Opdahl   University of Bergen, Norway
Günther Pernul   University of Regensburg, Germany
Silvio Ranise   FBK-IRST, Italy
Stefanie Rinderle-Ma   University of Vienna, Austria

David G. Rosado	University of Castilla-La Mancha, Spain
Shazia Sadiq	University of Queensland, Australia
Guttorm Sindre	Norwegian University of Science and Technology, Norway
Pnina Soffer	University of Haifa, Israel
Mark Strembeck	Vienna University of Economics and Business, Austria
Arnon Sturm	Ben-Gurion University of the Negev, Israel
Matthias Weidlich	Imperial College, UK
Jan Martijn van der Werf	Utrecht University, The Netherlands
Nicola Zannone	Eindhoven University of Technology, The Netherlands

Security Requirements Elicitation
from Business Processes
(Extended Abstract)

Raimundas Matulevičius

University of Tartu, Estonia
rma@ut.ee

Nowadays, *information systems* (IS) are the cornerstones upon which the vast majority of mission-critical *business processes* are executed in modern organizations. Because of their mission-criticality, ensuring *security* is a central concern during IS development. Organizations strive for confidentiality, integrity, and availability of their vital business information. However, security concerns are commonly overlooked when working with business process management. The reason is that while business analysts are expert in their own domains, they have limited knowledge about the security domain.

In this tutorial we discuss how security risk management process could help to understand and elicit security requirements from the business processes. We base our presentation on the domain model for *information systems security risk management* [1]. This domain model defines security risk management concepts at three interrelated levels. *Asset-related* concepts (i.e., *business assets*, *IS assets*, and *security criterion*) explain the organization and business values that need to be protected. The needed protection level is defined as the security needs, typically in terms of confidentiality, availability, and integrity. *Risk-related* concepts (i.e., *risk, impact, event, vulnerability, threat, attack method*, and *threat agent*) define the risk itself and its components. Risk is a combination of threat with one or more vulnerabilities, which leads to a negative impact, harming some assets. An impact shows the negative consequence of a risk on an asset if the threat is accomplished. A vulnerability is a weakness or flaw of one or more IS assets. An attack method is a standard means by which a threat agent executes a threat. *Risk treatment-related* concepts (i.e., *risk treatment decision, security requirement*, and *control*) describe how to treat the identified risks. A risk treatment leads to security requirements mitigating the risk, implemented as security controls.

Based on the running example, this tutorial illustrates how to define the security-oriented context and assets from the business models and how to systematically introduce and reason for security requirements. Once one determines security objectives (e.g., confidentiality, integrity, and availability), the risk analysis and assessment results in potential risks and their impacts. After risk assessment, risk treatment decision should be taken. This would result in security requirements definition. Security requirements should potentially be implemented into security controls. Such a risk management process is iterative, because new security controls suggested for securing business processes might open the possibility for new (not yet determined) security risks.

Systematic security requirements elicitation from the business processes, potentially, might envision the security threats, their consequences, and countermeasures, before developing software systems to support these business processes. Therefore in collaboration with the business analyst, security analysts could identify and discard alternative design solutions that do not offer a sufficient security level or even re-scope or cancel a project if the cost of treating security risks is too high. Potentially, security requirements discovered from the business processes can help business analysts to understand security trade-off within the business context.

Reference

1. Dubois E., Heymans P., Mayer N., Matulevičius R.: A systematic approach to define the domain of information system security risk management. In: Nurcan, S., Salinesi, C., Souveyet, C., Ralytė, J. (eds.) Intentional Perspectives on Information Systems Engineering, pp. 289–306. Springer, Heidelberg (2010)

From Early Experiments to a Company-Wide Process Mining Success (Extended Abstract)

Frank van Geffen

Rabobank, The Netherlands
F.Geffen@rn.rabobank.nl

One of the main challenges nowadays is to match and satisfy the customer needs of tomorrow. The speed and complexity of today's changes require a different approach to process improvement. Process mining, or automated business process discovery, is a BMP technique that helps in gaining insight into how processes are actually performed, how systems are used, and how people work together. Through the explosive growth of data and significant advances in analysis and visualization technology it is possible to unlock valuable process information by analyzing transaction data. The use of automated business process discovery techniques yields new valuable insights. Process analysis done this way becomes fact based, full, for real, and fast.

This keynote speech presented the experience with introducing the process mining technology and highlighted its value at Rabobank. The main focus was placed on the trade-off between rapid and continuous innovation and security aspects of processes.

Preface to the 4th International Workshop on Process Model Collections: Management and Reuse

Lucinéia Heloisa Thom[1], Marcelo Fantinato[2],
Marcello La Rosa[3], and Remco Dijkman[4]

[1] Federal University of Rio Grande do Sul, Brazil
lucineia@inf.ufrgs.br
[2] University of São Paulo, Brazil
fantinato@outlook.com
[3] Queensland University of Technology, Australia
m.larosa AT qut.edu.au
[4] Eindhoven University of Technology, The Netherlands
r.m.dijkman@tue.nl

Introduction

Nowadays, as organizations reach higher levels of Business Process Management maturity, they tend to collect and actively use large numbers of business process models. It is quite common that such collections of industry-strength business process models include thousands of activities and related business objects such as data, applications, risks, etc. These models are used for a variety of business needs, including requirements analysis, communication, automation, and compliance.

Such large collections of process models introduce both new challenges and opportunities to the area of business process management. On the one hand, it may not come as a surprise that many organizations struggle to manage such volumes of complex process models. This problem is exacerbated by overlapping content across models, poor version management, process models that are used simultaneously for different purposes, the use of different modeling notations such as EPCs, BPMN, etc. On the other hand, the process models in the collection provide a valuable source of information, which can be reused to facilitate the development of new process models. This reuse will lead to more efficient development of models that are of higher quality and better integrated with the existing models in the collection.

Against this backdrop, the aim of the workshop is to discuss novel research in the area of business process model collections, their management, and reuse. To this end, four papers were selected for presentation and a keynote speaker was invited.

Organizers

Lucinéia Heloisa Thom	Federal University of Rio Grande do Sul, Brazil
Marcelo Fantinato	University of São Paulo, Brazil
Marcello La Rosa	Queensland University of Technology, Australia
Remco Dijkman	Eindhoven University of Technology, The Netherlands

Program Committee

Agnes Koschmider	Karlsruhe Institute of Technology, Germany
Akhil Kumar	Penn State University, USA
Artem Polyvyanyy	Queensland University of Technology, Australia
Barbara Weber	University of Innsbruck, Austria
Christoph Bussler	Tropo, Inc., USA
Claudia Cappelli	Federal University of Rio de Janeiro State, Brazil
Fernanda A. Baião	Federal University of Rio de Janeiro State, Brazil
Flávia M. Santoro	Federal University of Rio de Janeiro State, Brazil
Hajo A. Reijers	Eindhoven University of Technology, The Netherlands
Jan Mendling	Wirtshaftsuniversitaet Wien, Austria
Jianmin Wang	Tsinghua University, China
João Porto de Albuquerque	University of São Paulo, Brazil
Luciano A. Digiampietri	University of São Paulo, Brazil
Luciano García-Bañuelos	University of Tartu, Estonia
Manfred Reichert	University of Ulm, Germany
Mathias Weske	University of Potsdam, Germany
Matthias Kunze	University of Potsdam, Germany
Matthias Weidlich	Imperial College London, UK
Minseok Song	Ulsan National Institute of Science and Technology, South Korea
Paulo F. Pires	Federal University of Rio Grande do Norte, Brazil
Shazia Sadiq	University of Queensland, Australia
Sherif Sakr	The University of New South Wales, Australia
Souvik Barat	Tata Consultancy Services, India
Stefanie Rinderle-Ma	University of Ulm, Germany
Uwe Zdun	University of Vienna, Austria
Vinay Kulkarni	Tata Consultancy Services, India
Xiaodong Liu	Edinburgh Napier University, UK
Zhiqiang Yan	Tsinghua University, China

Preface to the First International Workshop on Business Processes in Collective Adaptive Systems

Anna Lavygina[1], Naranker Dulay[1], Antonio Bucchiarone[2], Muhammad Adnan Tariq[3], and Dimka Karastoyanova[3]

[1] Imperial College London
{ a.lavygina,n.dulay} @imperial.ac.uk
[2] Fondazione Bruno Kessler, Trento
bucchiarone@fbk.eu
[3] University of Stuttgart
adnan.tariq@ipvs.uni-stuttgart.de,
karastoyanova@iaas.uni-stuttgart.de

Introduction to Business Processes in Collective Adaptive Systems

Collective Adaptive Systems (CAS) are heterogeneous collections of autonomous task-oriented systems that cooperate on common goals forming a collective system. To be robust, each constituent system must be able to dynamically adapt its behavior to changes in the environment while trying to reach their goals. At the same time, the different system adaptations must not be controlled centrally but rather administrated in a decentralized fashion among the systems. These aspects, collectiveness, adaptability, and decentralization are particularly relevant in businesses that wish to develop and deploy context-aware mobile applications that need to interact with pervasive and mobile technologies as well as cloud services.

BPCAS aims to provide a forum for researchers to discuss the challenges and results in the theory, design, implementation, and evaluation of collective adaptive systems.

The workshop was sponsored by the EU's Fundamentals of Collective Adaptive Systems program initiative (http://focas.eu/about-focas/) that aims to integrate, coordinate, and help increase visibility for research in all fields related to collective adaptive systems.

We want to thank Manfred Reichert from University of Ulm for giving an informative and interesting keynote talk titled: "Collective Adaptive Process-Aware Systems: Challenges, Scenarios, Techniques." We also want to thank the members of the Program Committee for very constructive reviews, which helped authors in improving their papers.

Organizers

Anna Lavygina	Imperial College London, UK
Naranker Dulay	Imperial College London, UK
Antonio Bucchiarone	Fondazione Bruno Kessler, Italy
Muhammad Adnan Tariq	University of Stuttgart, Germany
Dimka Karastoyanova	University of Stuttgart, Germany

Program Committee

Vasilios Andrikopoulos	University of Stuttgart, Germany
Salima Benbernou	L'Université Paris Descartes, France
Marina Bitsaki	University of Crete, Greece
Alexei Lapouchnian	University of Toronto, Canada
Kim Larsen	Aalborg University, Denmark
Lior Limonad	IBM Haifa, Israel
Christos Nikolaou	University of Crete, Greece
Francisco Pereira	SMART-MIT, Singapore
Marco Pistore	Fondazione Bruno Kessler, Italy
Manfred Reichert	University of Ulm, Germany
Kurt Rothermel	University of Stuttgart, Germany
Alessandra Russo	Imperial College London, UK
Nikola Šerbedžija	Fraunhofer FIRST, Germany
Pnina Soffer	University of Haifa, Israel
Arnon Sturm	Ben-Gurion University of the Negev, Israel
Yury Tsoy	Institut Pasteur Korea, South Korea
Ingo Weber	NICTA, Australia

3rd International Workshop on Data- and Artifact-Centric BPM (DAB 2014)

Dirk Fahland[1], Lior Limonad[2], and Roman Vaculín[3]

[1] Eindhoven University of Technology, The Netherlands
d.fahland@tue.nl
[2] IBM Haifa Research Lab, Carmel Mountain, Haifa, Israel
[3] IBM T.J. Watson Research Center, Yorktown Heights, NY, USA

Introduction to DAB 2014

The DAB workshop is aimed at bringing together researchers and practitioners whose common interests and experiences are the study and development of *data-* and *artifact-centric approaches* to Business Processes Management. Traditionally, both researchers and practitioners in the BPM community have studied data and control flow aspects of business processes, more or less in isolation. Such separation of concerns between the data and control perspectives turned out to be very fruitful and led to significant advances in both data and process management fields.

However, now that techniques and tools in both perspectives have matured, the *integration of data* and *control* is receiving increasing attention. In recent years, various approaches have emerged that emphasize integration of data and control as key aspects of flexible and rich business processes specification. These approaches range from *making classical BPM approaches data-driven* to more advanced approaches where the classical separation between process and data disappears, as for instance in *case management* or *artifact-centric BPM* to name a few prominent examples. From the scientific as well as the practical point of view it is critical to study the fundamental relationships, characteristics, and properties of the integrated perspective where data and process are considered together.

We invited researchers from the BPM field as well as from the related fields to submit papers that *investigate the tight interplay between data and control flow aspects of BPM*. We received 10 submissions with authors from 10 different countries. The peer-reviewing process with at least three reviews per paper selected five papers for presentation. The accepted papers were presented on September 8, 2014 in Eindhoven, The Netherlands.

Organizers

Dirk Fahland	Eindhoven University of Technology, The Netherlands *(DAB 2014 Co-chair and Local Organizer)*
Lior Limonad	IBM Haifa Research Laboratory, Carmel Mountain, Haifa, Israel *(DAB 2014 Co-chair)*

Roman Vaculín   IBM T.J. Watson Research Center, Yorktown
                                  Heights, New York, USA *(DAB 2014
                                  Co-chair)*
Felix Mannhardt   Eindhoven University of Technology,
                                  The Netherlands *(Local Organizer)*

Program Committee

Alessio Lomuscio   Imperial College London, UK
Alex Blekhman   Technion, Israel
Assaf Marron   Weizmann Institute of Science, Israel
Barbara Weber   University of Innsbruck, Austria
Dragan Gasevic   Athabasca University, Canada
Fabio Patrizi   Sapienza University of Rome, Italy
Fabrizio M. Maggi   University of Tartu, Estonia
Farouk Toumani   LIMOS - Blaise Pascal University, France
Hajo A. Reijers   Vrije Universiteit Amsterdam, The Netherlands
Karsten Wolf   Univerity of Rostock, Germany
Lijie Wen   Tsinghua University, China
Mathias Weske   HPI Potsdam, Germany
Rik Eshuis   Eindhoven University of Technology,
                                  The Netherlands
Shahar Maoz   Tel Aviv University, Israel
Thomas Hildebrandt   IT University of Copenhagen, Denmark
Victor Vianu   University of California, San Diego, USA

No external reviewers have been asked for reviews. We thank Program Committee for their careful and constructive reviews.

Preface to the 10th International Workshop on Business Process Intelligence (BPI 2014)

Barbara Weber[1], Boudewijn van Dongen[2], Diogo R. Ferreira[3], and Jochen De Weerdt[4]

[1] Institut für Informatik, Universität Innsbruck, Austria
[2] Eindhoven University of Technology, The Netherlands
[3] Instituto Superior Técnico, University of Lisbon, Portugal
[4] Faculty of Economics and Business, KU Leuven, Belgium

Business Process Intelligence (BPI) is a growing area both in industry and academia. BPI refers to the application of data- and process-mining techniques to the field of Business Process Management. In practice, BPI is embodied in tools for managing process execution by offering several features such as analysis, prediction, monitoring, control, and optimization.

The main goal of this workshop is to promote the use and development of new techniques to support the analysis of business processes based on run-time data about the past executions of such processes. We aim at bringing together practitioners and researchers from different communities, e.g., Business Process Management, Information Systems, Database Systems, Business Administration, Software Engineering, Artificial Intelligence, and Data Mining, who share an interest in the analysis and optimization of business processes and process-aware information systems. The workshop aims at discussing the current state of ongoing research and sharing practical experiences, exchanging ideas, and setting up future research directions that better respond to real needs. In a nutshell, it serves as a forum for shaping the BPI area.

The 10th edition of this workshop attracted 23 international submissions. Each paper was reviewed by at least three members of the Program Committee. From these submissions, the top nine were accepted as full papers for presentation at the workshop.

The papers presented at the workshop provided a mix of novel research ideas, evaluations of existing process mining techniques, as well as new tool support. *Botezatu*, *Voelzer*, and *Dijkman* use the information recorded in event logs to improve the scheduling of workflow activities according to resource load and performance. *Verbeek* and *van der Aalst* introduce a decomposition framework that speeds up process discovery and replay by doing them on separate clusters. *Pufahl*, *Bazhenova*, and *Weske* use queueing theory to study the cost advantage of executing certain activities in batch mode rather than separately for each process instance. *Van Eck*, *Buijs*, and *van Dongen* improve the genetic mining algorithm by working with a population of models that are aligned with the actual behavior in the event log. *Leemans*, *Fahland*, and *van der Aalst* discuss the features that process mining tools should possess in order to facilitate user exploration of process models and deviations. *Pizarro* and *Sepúlveda* present an approach for the interactive discovery of event data using multiple perspectives and levels of granularity, inspired by OLAP techniques. *Raichelson* and *Soffer* describe an approach for merging separate but related event logs, where there may be many-to-many relationships between the cases in those logs. *Depaire* focuses on the problem of whether a discovered model is likely to be the true model given that there might be an amount of unobserved behavior in the event log. Finally, *Wakup* and *Desel* use process mining techniques to analyze and discover a network protocol from the TCP/IP packets exchanged between a server and a client application.

As with previous editions of the workshop, we hope that the reader will find this selection of papers useful to keep track of the latest advances in the BPI area, and we are looking forward to keep bringing new advances in future editions of the BPI workshop.

Organizers

Barbara Weber — Institut für Informatik, Universität Innsbruck, Austria

Boudewijn van Dongen — Eindhoven University of Technology, The Netherlands

Diogo R. Ferreira — Instituto Superior Técnico, University of Lisbon, Portugal

Jochen De Weerdt — Faculty of Economics and Business, Katholieke Universiteit Leuven, Belgium

Program Committee

Boualem Benatallah — University of New South Wales, Australia
Walid Gaaloul — Télécom SudParis, France
Gianluigi Greco — University of Calabria, Italy
Daniela Grigori — Laboratoire LAMSADE, Université Paris-Dauphine, France
Antonella Guzzo — University of Calabria, Italy
Michael Leyer — Frankfurt School of Finance & Management, Germany
Ana Karla Medeiros — Capgemini Consulting, The Netherlands
Jan Mendling — Wirtschaftsuniversität Wien, Austria
Viara Popova — University of Tartu, Estonia
Manfred Reichert — University of Ulm, Germany
Michael Rosemann — Queensland University of Technology, Australia
Anne Rozinat — Fluxicon, The Netherlands
Domenico Saccà — University of Calabria, Italy
Pnina Soffer — University of Haifa, Israel
Alessandro Sperduti — University of Padua, Italy

Wil van der Aalst   Eindhoven University of Technology,
                                     The Netherlands
Eric Verbeek   Eindhoven University of Technology,
                                     The Netherlands
Hans Weigand   Tilburg University, The Netherlands

Preface for the 2nd International Workshop on Business Process Management in the Cloud (BPMC)

Ingo Weber[1,2], Christian Janiesch[3], and Stefan Schulte[4]

[1] NICTA, Sydney, Australia
[2] University of New South Wales, Sydney, Australia
[3] University of Würzburg, Germany
[4] Vienna University of Technology, Austria
ingo.weber@nicta.com.au
christian.janiesch@uni-wuerzburg.de
s.schulte@infosys.tuwien.ac.at

Introduction

Cloud computing is a paradigm for the on-demand delivery of infrastructure, platform, or software as a service. Cloud computing enables network access to a shared pool of configurable computing and storage resources as well as applications that can be tailored to the consumer's needs. Cloud resources can be rapidly provisioned and released, and are billed based on actual use, thus reducing up-front investment costs. Not only can individual services be hosted on virtual infrastructures but also complete process platforms. Further, besides benefits to run-time Business Process Management (BPM), cloud-based services can enable collaboration between geographically dispersed teams during design-time and assist the design process in general – amongst others, process modeling as a service removes the need for installation of software, and is thus more attractive for the occasional user.

A cloud-based architecture for BPM may provide important benefits:

- Elasticity: process engines or process tasks can scale up/out or down/in depending on the actual load to reduce investment cost and manage load peaks.
- Flexibility: processes can be assembled with more flexibility as service selection can not only include the software but also the platform or infrastructure for it to run on.
- Measurement: as service applications in the cloud are individually metered, detailed measurement data is available and can be used to provide additional services such as process monitoring.

The research directions of core interest to the 2nd International Workshop on Business Process Management in the Cloud (BPMC 2014) are summarized by three questions:

- How can BPM benefit from the cloud?
- What should BPM in the cloud look like?
- What can BPM bring to cloud computing practices?

Among a number of challenges, there is a lack of conceptualization and theory on BPM with respect to cloud computing. For the most part, the topic of cloud computing has only been implicitly regarded in BPM research when discussing design-time tools. Few works have addressed workflow enactment in the cloud to date. However, a detailed research agenda which covers theory, design-time, run-time, and use cases is missing. The goal of the 2nd International Workshop on Business Process Management in the Cloud is to lay the foundation for such a research agenda.

Submissions from the scientific community were invited for the above-mentioned problem domain as well as related issues. Hence, the main areas of interest to the workshop were

- Cloud and BPM: concepts and theory
- Design-time BPM in the cloud
- Run-time BPM in the cloud
- Use cases for BPM in the cloud

Unfortunately only few papers were submitted this year, out of which only one was accepted after review based on quality, relevance, and originality. The paper is titled "YAWL in the Cloud: Supporting Process Sharing and Variability." It describes an approach and tool for collaborative BPM in the cloud: using configurable process models to support the variations of processes, as encountered in different Dutch municipalities. The paper highlights the benefits of using a cloud-based approach at different stages of the BPM lifecycle, introduces the approach and tool, and presents a proof-of-concept scenario.

Furthermore, Gero Decker from Signavio gave an inspiring keynote talk at the workshop. The title of the talk and the corresponding paper is "BPM in the Cloud – Trends and Challenges." Gero Decker is a co-founder and co-CEO of Signavio, a BPM vendor and BPM Software as a Service provider. In his keynote, he discussed the differences between cloud-based and traditional BPM solutions and their respective clientele, and structured the space of BPM in the cloud.

The keynote sparked a lively debate which was moderated by Ingo Weber. He took up some of the aspects mentioned in the keynote and combined them with prevalent topics of the upcoming BPM conference as well as observations from the general mind shift toward a more service-oriented, cloud-based environment not only for BPM. The discussion continued long after the workshop. The result is the following list of open topics:

- *Process Mining in the Cloud.* Process Mining is a very hot topic in BPM, yet there are few approaches to take this success to the cloud. What would be required to achieve this, and for which parts of process mining is that a sensible approach? As it stands, process mining is an expert method, and even tools with a streamlined user experience require deep understanding of background concepts. But are there aspects of process mining that are of interest for large-scale adoption, and hence should be moved to the cloud?
- *Fragmentation.* The complexity that comes with the fragmentation of using many small, focused cloud offerings poses a challenge to traditional IT management. How can this fragmentation be managed effectively? Can BPM contribute, or is that solely a task for enterprise architecture?

- *Continuous BPM Deployment.* New cloud-based approaches that enable less specialized users to create (executable) process models will drastically reduce cycle times and frequencies. Just as with the software engineering advances of continuous integration (CI) and continuous deployment (CD), the time for designing a changed model and deploying it to production will shorten, and the frequency will increase sharply. In software engineering, release frequency has been reduced from a few times a year to many times per day. If BPM takes a similar turn, this leads to several challenges:

  - *Process model testing.* Automatic testing of process models should become prevalent. The area seems heavily underdeveloped, compared to its likely future importance, since works on process model testing are few and far between.
  - *Process model drift.* High frequency of deployments will lead to drift in process model collections: there will be many versions of each model, and the management and storage of these becomes more challenging. A particular issue is that of tracing interacting processes in the face of drift: Which versions of models A and B are integrated with version X of process C?

- *Cloud services governance.* One trend in the cloud is that individual teams start using cloud services, often without governance through their organization, and pay for it out of their team budget. A question for the BPM, services, and compliance communities is: How can targeted, mass-scale governance over cloud service usage be implemented, without imposing massive overheads?
- *Technical questions* include:

  - *Client-side data processing.* Cloud applications often implement a different data handling paradigm, where data is kept at the source and computation is moved to the data. How can BPMSs pick up this development? For instance, should process execution move in part to the UI, such as a browser interface, to process data stored locally on a user's machine directly?
  - *Open APIs.* Many cloud applications offer and use open APIs over the web. Is there enough support from BPM for this trend, both from the ease-of-use side and from the API offering side? Is lightweight integration sufficiently supported by BPMSs, will it be, or will that be a competing technology?
  - *Mobile & BPM.* Do BPMSs offer mobile access to analytics and to control over process execution?

Although only few papers were submitted, a strong audience at the conference confirmed the interest of the community in the topic. The cloud is a huge trend, and the BPM field cannot afford to miss it. In addition to the above list, a summary of the state of the art and challenges in Elastic Business Process Management authored by Schulte, Janiesch, Venugopal, Weber, and Hoenisch is currently in press at Future Generation Computer Systems. We hope the collective set of open questions will help to stimulate and guide more research in this area.

Organizers

Ingo Weber   NICTA and University of New South Wales,
                            Sydney, Australia
Christian Janiesch   University of Würzburg, Germany
Stefan Schulte   Vienna University of Technology, Austria

Program Committee

Arun Anandasivam   IBM Global Business Services, Germany
Soeren Balko   Queensland University of Technology, Australia
Gero Decker   Signavio, Germany
Schahram Dustdar   Vienna University of Technology, Austria
Dimka Karastoyanova   University of Stuttgart, Germany
Ulrich Lampe   Technische Universität Darmstadt, Germany
Jan Mendling   Wirtschaftsuniversität Wien, Austria
Hajo Reijers   Eindhoven University of Technology,
                            The Netherlands
Stefanie Rinderle-Ma   University of Vienna, Austria
Ralf Steinmetz   Technische Universität Darmstadt, Germany
Stefan Tai   Karlsruhe Institute of Technology, Germany
Srikumar Venugopal   University of New South Wales, Australia
Yi Wei   Microsoft, USA
Matthias Weidlich   Imperial College London, UK
Xiwei (Sherry) Xu   NICTA, Australia

BPM in the Cloud – Trends and Challenges (Extended Abstract)

Gero Decker, Signavio

Abstract. The cloud is the future and has an impact on IT support for business processes. This leads to an increased importance of BPM. On the other hand, BPM software in the cloud (like cloud-based modeling tools, integration platforms, and workflow products) brings new possibilities in the areas of collaboration, mobile access, and integration.

IT is getting more and more "cloudy": Gartner predicts that by 2016 cloud computing will be the bulk of new IT spend. IDC forecasts that cloud services will have an annual growth rate of 23.5% until 2017, five times that of the IT industry as a whole. Given this trend, it is interesting to investigate how cloud computing impacts the area of Business Process Management (BPM).

At first glance, it might seem that cloud services are simply alternative deployment options for the same old software from the on-premise world. Especially, web-based systems with a client/server architecture can be offered both in a classic on-premise model as well as in a Software-as-a-Service (SaaS) / Platform-as-a-Service (PaaS) model. However, it is interesting to observe that vendors with successful on-premise offerings often have a hard time catching up with the new breed of cloud-native vendors entering the same market segment. With cheap and well-understood hosting infrastructure available, it cannot be the pure delivery over the Internet that makes the difference. Obviously, there must be more to "the cloud". So what is different now?

Three major topics can be observed in the cloud age: collaboration, ease-of-use, and simplicity. Due to their technical architecture, cloud services are inherently more accessible to more people, enabling them to work together more easily. Also, as software users are more and more used to great-looking and intuitive applications from their private life, they rather pick and choose those applications they love to use. This has a heavy impact on how products are built, delivered, and sold. Finally, the relationship between customer and vendor has changed quite significantly: Rather than asking for the full attention of the software vendor and expecting a highly individual solution, customers are more and more interested in a fast delivery cycle for the best practices derived from the user community of the cloud service.

These observations apply to cloud services in general, but which impact does "cloud" have on BPM in particular?

Here, we have to distinguish between (i) the impact of cloud for business processes on the one hand and (ii) cloud software directly supporting BPM activities ("BPM software") on the other.

(i) Cloud is one of the disruptive trends in enterprise IT these days. Together with new possibilities of mobile computing, adoption of cloud services can lead to even faster change and innovation of business processes. Long implementation and upgrade cycles of on-premise applications are replaced by "consumerization" of IT: business users choose appropriate cloud services themselves, often introducing major changes to processes on-the-fly. Process design and implementation become more and more decentralized. Offering the right guidance and governance from a process and IT perspective becomes a major challenge in this age of democratization.

An interesting side effect of cloud computing is the increasing fragmentation of IT portfolios. While previously, many companies tried to consolidate around big on-premise installations/vendors (e.g., SAP), the cloud comes with many fine-grained, special purpose services used for individual tasks or process fragments. This in turn increases the need for integration when aiming for ideal process support. Therefore, iPaaS and bpmPaaS offerings (see below) are even more interesting than classical Enterprise Application Integration platforms from the on-premise world.

(ii) BPM software: Cloud-based offerings for process analysis, modeling, governance, execution, monitoring, and so on are gaining more and more momentum in the market. Apart from the general impact of cloud, what does this mean for each area and which are the main challenges?

• Cloud-based modeling tools (e.g., IBM Blueworks, Signavio) allow for easier collaboration. Also, they lower the entry barrier to BPM by adopting a self-service paradigm rather than promoting extensive user training. This helps to reach a broader adoption of process-oriented thinking within organizations and creates bigger involvement in process initiatives than previously observed. This also makes process modeling tools applicable to smaller organizations.

Making process modeling self-explanatory is probably the biggest challenge. Speeding up the graphical modeling is only a small part of the story. This can be easily achieved by avoiding typical tool "glitches" and providing shortcuts for typical usage patterns. The bigger challenge is to guide people in process modeling. What is the right level of documentation? Which processes do I need to focus on? What is the fastest way to reach a shared understanding of a process? Not all of these questions can be solved by a tool alone but maximum effort should be undertaken to turn process modeling tools from pure content-structuring to something that really empowers users to reach improved processes.

• Cloud-based integration platforms (iPaaS, covering "system workflows", e.g., Boomi, IFTTT) enjoy huge uptake in the market. The reason behind that is quite simple: Why would I connect cloud applications through an on-premise integration platform? Especially, lightweight services like IFTTT make it extremely easy to set up simple point-to-point connections, even without coding. A main enabler for this is the fact that cloud services typically come with relatively simple to use APIs, most often following REST principles. Cloud integration platforms then provide connectors to hundreds or thousands of these services, considering not only the individual data structures but also the authentication mechanisms required.

The challenge for cloud integration is the huge number of APIs to be covered and interconnected. Smart matchmaking of data structures (e.g., done through schema matching) can be enhanced by taking the process context into account. Also, the question of data governance and quality moves into the center of attention. If data is spread over multiple cloud services, how can I make sure there is consistent data available in my process context?

• Cloud-based process workflow frameworks (Gartner calls this "bpmPaaS", e.g., RunMyProcess, Effektif) are becoming more and more popular, too. Here, the typical pattern is to enable non-technical users to build their own "process apps", combining human tasks, simple data collection, and prebuilt system connectors.

Partly, these cloud workflow platforms have a similar challenge like cloud integration platforms. For the long tail of APIs out there, simple cloud integration platforms like IFTTT are sometimes leveraged for larger process settings. In terms of connecting multiple cloud services, an additional challenge arises from the fact that integration not only happens in the form of automatic tasks ("service tasks" in BPMN). Other forms of integration become relevant, too: for instance, "virtual objects" with smart caching behavior replace the old data copying paradigm. Most prominently, integrations on the user interface level are desired as well. A simple example would be to display and edit a Google doc inside of a task. Or imagine a form field for a customer name, which fetches additional contact info about this customer from the CRM system when hovering over it.

• Cloud-based process analytics frameworks are on the rise, too. They typically provide process-oriented performance dashboards to management staff. Again, a major benefit of a cloud solution in this area is mobile access to dashboards. Off-the-shelf apps are provided that connect to the cloud service over the Internet – without having to set up a VPN connection to some internal system behind the firewall.

To sum up, the cloud comes with a range of new possibilities, e.g., regarding collaboration, mobile access, and integration. Especially, the fragmentation that comes with the rise of cloud increases the value proposition and adoption of BPM out there.

Gero Decker is co-founder and co-CEO of Signavio, a Germany and USA-based BPM vendor. Signavio is also a majority shareholder in Effektif. Before starting Signavio, he worked as BPM consultant and completed his PhD in Business Process Management at the Hasso-Plattner-Institute in Potsdam, Germany.

Preface to the 3rd International Workshop on Theory and Applications of Process Visualization

Ross Brown[1], Simone Kriglstein[2], and Stefanie Rinderle-Ma[3]

[1] Queensland University of Technology, Brisbane, Australia
r.brown@qut.edu.au
[2] Faculty of Informatics, Vienna University of Technology, Vienna, Austria
kriglstein@cvast.tuwien.ac.at
[3] Faculty of Computer Science, University of Vienna, Vienna, Austria
stefanie.rinderle-ma@univie.ac.at

Introduction

This is the third TAProViz workshop being run at BPM. The intention this year is to consolidate on the results of the previous successful workshops by further developing this important topic, identifying the key research topics of interest to the BPM visualization community. We note this year the continuing interest in the visualization of process mining data and resultant process models.

Submitted papers were evaluated by at least three Program Committee members, in a double blind manner, on the basis of significance, originality, technical quality, and exposition. Three full and one position papers were accepted for presentation at the workshop. In addition, we invited a keynote speaker, Dafna Levy, a process mining practitioner from Nool, an Israeli process mining initiative. The papers address a number of topics in the area of process model visualization, in particular:

- Visualizing Differences between Process Models
- User Friendly Visualization of Process Models
- Dynamic Visualization of Process Movies in Process Mining
- Process Model Syntactical Sonification

The keynote *Intelligent Process Management and Visualization Technologies*, by Dafna Levy, was a presentation of a live process mining demonstration with real-life scenarios showing how various process analysis and monitoring techniques can be applied to process mining projects, and what kind of insights and added value can be gained with the visual deliverables generated.

Carsten Cordes, Thomas Vogelgesang, and Hans-Jürgen Appelrath presented their full paper, *A Generic Approach for Calculating and Visualizing Differences between Process Models in Multidimensional Process Mining*. This paper presents the challenges of differencing process models in multi-dimensional process mining and proposes a generic approach to deal with these challenges.

Markus Hipp, Achim Strauss, Bernd Michelberger, Bela Mutschler, and Manfred Reichert presented their full paper, *Enabling a User-Friendly Visualization of Business Process Models*. This paper presents four different concepts aiming at a user-friendly

visualization of large-scale process models to deal with problems of model comprehensibility and aesthetics.

Andrea Burattin, Marta Cimitile, and Fabrizio Maria Maggi, presented in their full
paper, *Lights, Camera, Action! Business Process Movies for Online Process
Discovery*, a method for the graphical visualization of the evolution of a process
model over time. They described a graphical visualizer for process models extracted
from an event stream through a declarative process discovery approach they have
previously developed.

In his position paper, *Toward a generalized notion of audio as part of the
concrete syntax of business process modeling languages*, Jens Gulden presented
preliminary work seeking to establish how to include audio, and other sensual
impressions, into the concrete syntax of modeling languages. Part of this work is a
reconceptualization of concrete process syntax as an interaction process between a
tool and a user.

Organizers

Ross Brown	Queensland University of Technology, Australia
Simone Kriglstein	Vienna University of Technology, Austria
Stefanie Rinderle-Ma	University of Vienna, Austria

Program Committee

Ralph Bobrik	Switzerland
Michael Burch	Germany
Massimiliano De Leoni	The Netherlands
Remco Dijkman	The Netherlands
Phillip Effinger	Germany
Kathrin Figl	Austria
Hans-Georg Fill	Austria
Thomas Hermann	Germany
Sonja Kabicher-Fuchs	Austria
Jens Kolb	Germany
Agnes Koschmider	Germany
Maya Lincoln	Israel
Wendy Lucas	USA
Jürgen Mangler	Austria
Silvia Miksch	Austria
Margit Pohl	Austria
Rune Rasmussen	Australia
Manfred Reichert	Germany
Pnina Soffer	Israel
Irene Vanderfeesten	The Netherlands

Eric Verbeek	The Netherlands
Günter Wallner	Austria
Avi Wasser	Israel

External Reviewer

| Markus Hipp | Germany |

Intelligent Process Management
and Visualization Technologies
(Extended Abstract)

Dafna Levy

NooL- Integrating People & Solutions, 99835 Srigim, Israel
dafnal@nool.co.il

Abstract. While process visualizations are perceived by many as very cool technologies, companies are not yet willing to embrace them as warmly and quickly as expected. Managers still demand more convincing and significant added value. Another issue might be with offering process visualization technologies as somewhat detached solutions, or not taking into account Business Intelligence solutions which might already exist in the company. The keynote aims to demonstrate how process and data visualization tools can be combined and applied to various business domains in order to increase process awareness which will lead to *intelligent process management*.

Keywords: Process mining, visualization technologies, intelligent process management

Summary

In the keynote, a live demo with real-life scenarios will show how various process analysis and monitoring techniques can be applied, and what kind of insights and added value can be gained with the visual deliverables generated.

The use cases discussed will cover analysis and monitoring of running processes (e.g., purchasing, service calls, warehouse management), inspection and fine-tuning of a new ERP implementation, discovery of work orders flow among machines on the production floor and extending Business Intelligence (BI) to Process Intelligence (PI). Insights will be shared about process visualization topics such as: who are the "beholders" (users vs. customers), the challenges in "deciphering" visual deliverables, offering tools versus services, integration with IT systems versus stand-alone solutions, the roles of the software providers, how to handle rejections and barriers and ideas for future developments and extensions.

Background

In many organizations, business performance is measured in terms of financial data such as revenue, profits, cash flow, etc. However, it is not generally possible to manipulate the values of these financial indices directly; rather, they reflect the results of operational activities derived from the organization's standard business processes. Hence, addressing financial data only, without considering current business processes, significantly impairs an organization's ability to improve their business performance.

Process intelligence essentially combines automatic process discovery (APD) with advanced business discovery technology. Briefly, automatic process discovery looks at historical event log data and analyzes these data to generate visual models of an organization's business processes and establish patterns linking external and internal events. The results of these analyses can be used to improve operational efficiency. In parallel, business discovery technology allows management to monitor operations and key performance indicators in real-time and alerts management of any anomalies.

Advanced process discovery analyzes log data captured by existing IT systems and provides answers to specific questions such as: Where are the bottlenecks in this process, when and why do people deviate from the defined process, are all requirements (e.g., SLA terms) being met, why does performance vary from one employee/department to the next, which business rules and alerts are actually in use, what are the actual costs of this process?

The analysis yields deliverables such as: operational data (throughput time, costs, quantities)**,** **visual** models and animation of the actual processes, discovery of anomalies, performance benchmarking, and deviation from business rules (times, quantities).

Significant benefits of advanced process discovery for a company are gaining a multidimensional and objective view of how their organization was performing in the analyzed period, and defining or refining their operational goals.

In order to keep track of how these goals are achieved, as a process is being executed, process dashboards can be used. These dashboards enable managers to proactively and continuously adjust business processes for optimal performance at a very fine resolution, instead of taking action only after a problem has been discovered. Adding gauges to process dashboards can visually alert about deviations from desired goals. In order to reveal and analyze the possible root causes for such deviations, a process discovery tool can be used. Data of the process in question are exported directly from the dashboard in the requested format.

Some benefits of such solutions are: maintaining and managing the process data in the BI database, enriching process data (i.e., event logs) with business data for an extended analysis, fine-tuning goals and KPIs, and, last but not least, creating a common language among business and process managers who can share the visual deliverables and gain better insights in a collaborative manner.

All these benefits help a company to replace "crisis-management" with a proactive approach and achieve intelligent process management.

Preface to the Seventh International Workshop on Business Process Management and Social Software (BPMS2 2014)

Rainer Schmidt[1] and Selmin Nurcan[2,3]

[1] Munich University of Applied Sciences
Faculty of Computer Science and Mathematics
Lothstrasse 64, 80335 München
Rainer.Schmidt@hm.edu
[2] Sorbonne Graduate Business School, France
[3] CRI, University Paris 1 Panthéon Sorbonne, France

Introduction

Social software is a new paradigm that is spreading quickly in society, organizations, and economics. It enables social business that has created a multitude of success stories. More and more enterprises use social software to improve their business processes and create new business models. Social software is used both in internal and external business processes. Using social software, the communication with the customer is increasingly bidirectional. For example, companies integrate customers into product development to capture ideas for new products and features. Social software also creates new possibilities to enhance internal business processes by improving the exchange of knowledge and information, to speed up decisions, etc.

Social software is based on four principles: weak ties, social production, egalitarianism, and mutual service provisioning.

• Weak ties

Weakties are spontaneously established contacts between individuals that create new views and allow combining competencies. Social software supports the creation of weak ties by supporting to create contacts in impulse between non-predetermined individuals.

• Social Production

Social Production is the creation of artifacts, by combining the input from independent contributors without predetermining the way to do this. By this means it is possible to integrate new and innovative contributions not identified or planned in advance. Reputation-based mechanisms assure quality following an a posteriori approach.

• Egalitarianism

Egalitarianism is the attitude of handling individuals equally. Social software highly relies on egalitarianism and therefore strives for giving all participants the same rights to contribute. This is done with the intention to encourage a maximum of contributors and to get the best solution fusioning a high number of contributions, thus enabling the wisdom of the crowds. Social software realizes egalitarianism by abolishing hierarchical structures, merging the roles of contributors and consumers, and introducing a culture of trust.

• Mutual Service Provisioning

Social software abolishes the separation of service provider and consumer by introducing the idea that service provisioning is a mutual process of service exchange. Thus both service provider and consumer (or better prosumer) provide services to one another in order to cocreate value. This mutual service provisioning contrasts to the idea of industrial service provisioning, where services are produced in separation from the customer to achieve scaling effects.

Up to now, the interaction of social software and its underlying paradigms with business processes have not been investigated in-depth. Therefore, the objective of the workshop is to explore how social software interacts with business process management, how business process management has to change to comply with weak ties, social production, egalitarianism and mutual service, and how business processes may profit from these principles.

The workshop will discuss three topics. Social Business Process Management, Social Business, and Big Data in Social Business. Social Business Process Management is the use of social software to support one or multiple phases of the business process life cycle.

1. Social Business Process Management (SBPM)

- Which phases of the BPM lifecycle (Design, Deployment, Operation, and Evaluation) can profit the most by social software?
- Do we need new BPM methods and/or paradigms to cope with social software?
- Is there an influence of weak ties, social production, egalitarianism, and mutual service provisioning on BPM methods themselves?
- How are trust and reputation established in business processes using social software?
- How do weak ties, social production, egalitarianism, and mutual service provisioning influence the design of business processes?
- How does social software interact with WFMS or other business process support systems?
- What is the impact on conceptual models for those categories of business processes which are not well-defined ?

2. Social Business: Social software supporting business processes

- Which new possibilities for the support of business processes are created by social software?
- Are there business processes which require sociality, especially when they are not predictable (as production workflows) but collaborative or ad hoc?
- How can we use Wikis, Blogs, etc., to support business processes?
- Which types of social software can be used in which phases of the BPM lifecycle?
- What new kinds of business knowledge representation are offered by social production?

3. Big Data in Social Business

- Which data created with social software can be used to support business processes?
- Which categories of business processes can profit from big data ?
- Are there any similarities or relationships with process mining techniques and also with workflow control and role patterns?

Based on the successful BPMS2 2008, BPMS2 2009, BPMS2 2010, BPMS2 2011, BPMS2 2012, and BPMS2 2013 workshops, the goal of the workshop is to promote the integration of business process management with social software and to enlarge the community pursuing the theme.

Five papers have been accepted for presentation.

In their paper "Tagging Model for Enhancing Knowledge Transfer and Usage during Business Process Execution," Reuven Karni and Meira Levy present two tagging models. The first one combines structured, automatically generated metadata, with manually inserted unstructured tagging labels. It facilitates the annotation of content and thus enhances knowledge transfer and usage. The second tagging model describes a tagged knowledge cycle. It allows process performers to create and tag their knowledge and experiences during process execution.

David Gruenert, Elke Brucker-Kley, and Thomas Keller introduce with Opportunistic Business Process Modeling (oBPM) a new paradigm for modeling and executing business processes that is both user- and document-centric, adequate for bottom-up modeling, agile process modification, opportunistic task scheduling, and process mining.

Rainer Schmidt, Alfred Zimmermann, Michael Möhring, Dierk Jugel, Florian Baer, and Christian Schweda show in their paper "Social-Software-based Support for Enterprise Architecture Management Processes" the application of social-software-based support for enterprise architecture management processes. A cockpit provides interactive functions and visualization methods to cope with complexity and enable the practical use of social software in enterprise architecture management processes.

Nick Russell and Alistair Barros review in their paper "Business Processes in Connected Communities" the implications of digital connectedness between human actors in a process-oriented context, surveys potential community archetypes, and outlines core characteristics of connected communities and their significance in a broader BPM context.

Michael Möhring, Rainer Schmidt, Ralf Härting, Florian Baer, and Alfred Zimmermann provide in their paper "Classification Framework for Context Data from Business Processes" a foundation for the methodical exploitation of context data. Context data consists of two base classes intrinsic and extrinsic data. The paper gives a foundation to leverage context data for business process management.

We wish to thank all authors for having shared their work with us, as well as the members of the BPMS2 2014 Program Committee and the Workshop Organizers of BPM 2014 for their help with the organization of the workshop.

Organizers

Selmin Nurcan	Université de Paris 1 Panthéon-Sorbonne, France
Rainer Schmidt	Munich University of Applied Sciences, Germany

Workshop Program Committee

Renata Araujo	Department of Applied Informatics, UNIRIO
Ofer Arazy	Technion – Israel Institute of Technology, Israel
Ilia Bider	Stockholm University/IbisSoft, Sweden
Jan Bosch	Chalmers University of Technology, Sweden
Marco Brambilla	Politecnico di Milano, Italy
Chihab Hanachi	Toulouse 1 University Capitole, France
Monique Janneck	Fachhochschule Lübeck, Germany
Ralf Klamma	RWTH Aachen University, Germany
Sai Peck Lee	University of Malaya, Malaysia
Myriam Lewkowicz	University of Technology of Troyes, France
Bela Mutschler	University of Applied Sciences Ravensburg-Weingarten, Germany
Gustaf Neumann	Wirtschaftsuniversität Wien, Austria
Selmin Nurcan	Université de Paris 1 Panthéon-Sorbonne, France
Andreas Oberweis	Universität Karlsruhe, Germany
Henderik A. Proper	Public Research Centre Henri Tudor, Luxembourg
Rainer Schmidt	Munich University of Applied Sciences, Germany
Miguel-Angel Sicilia	University of Alcalá, Spain
Pnina Soffer	University of Haifa, Israel
Karsten Wendland	Hochschule Aalen, Germany

Preface to the Second International Workshop on Decision Mining and Modeling for Business Processes (DeMiMoP 2014)

Jan Vanthienen[1], Bart Baesens[2], Guoqing Chen[3], and Qiang Wei[4]

[1] Department of Decision Sciences and Information Management,
Katholieke Universiteit Leuven
Naamsestraat 69, 3000 Leuven, Belgium
jan.vanthienen@kuleuven.be

[2] Department of Decision Sciences and Information Management,
Katholieke Universiteit Leuven
Naamsestraat 69, 3000 Leuven, Belgium
bart.baesens@kuleuven.be

[3] School of Economics and Management (SEM), Tsinghua University
30 双清路, Haidian, Beijing, China
chengq@sem.tsinghua.edu.cn

[4] School of Economics and Management (SEM), Tsinghua University
30 双清路, Haidian, Beijing, China
weiq@sem.tsinghua.edu.cn

Introduction

Most processes and business process models incorporate decisions of some kind. Decisions are typically based upon a number of business (decision) rules that describe the premises and possible outcomes of a specific situation. Since these decisions guide the activities and workflows of all process stakeholders (participants, owners), they should be regarded as first-class citizens in Business Process Management. Sometimes, the entire decision can be included as a decision activity or as a service (a decision service). Typical decisions are: creditworthiness of the customer in a financial process, claim acceptance in an insurance process, eligibility decision in social security, etc. The process then handles a number of steps, shows the appropriate decision points, and represents the path to follow for each of the alternatives.

Business decisions are important, but are often hidden in process flows, process activities, or in the head of employees (tacit knowledge), so that they need to be discovered using state-of-the-art intelligent techniques. Decisions can be straightforward, based on a number of simple rules, or can be the result of complex analytics (decision mining). Moreover, in a large number of cases, a particular business process does not just contain decisions, but the entire process is about making a decision. The major purpose of a loan process, e.g., or an insurance claim process, etc., is to prepare and make a final decision. The process shows different steps, models the communication between parties, records the decision, and returns the result.

It is not considered good practice to model the detailed decision paths in the business process model. Separating rules and decisions from the process simplifies the process model (separation of concerns). The aim of the workshop is to examine the relationship between decisions and processes, including models not only to model the process, but also to model the decisions, to enhance decision mining based on process data, and to find a good integration between decision modeling and process modeling.

Organizers

Jan Vanthienen	Katholieke Universiteit Leuven, Belgium
Bart Baesens	Katholieke Universiteit Leuven, Belgium
Guoqing Chen	Tsinghua University, China
Qiang Wei	Tsinghua University, China

Program Committee

Guoqing Chen	Tsinghua University, China
Qiang Wei	Tsinghua University, China
Jae-Yoon Jung	Kyung Hee University, South Korea
Dimitris Karagiannis	Universität Wien, Austria
Xunhua Guo	Tsinghua University, China
Hajo A. Reijers	Eindhoven University of Technology, The Netherlands
Robert Golan	DBmind Technologies, USA
Markus Helfert	Dublin City University, Ireland
Leszek Maciaszek	Wrocław University of Economics, Poland
Pericles Loucopoulos	Loughborough University, UK
Josep Carmona	Universitat Politècnica de Catalunya, Spain
Jochen De Weerdt	Queensland University of Technology, Australia
Seppe vanden Broucke	Katholieke Universiteit Leuven, Belgium
Filip Caron	Katholieke Universiteit Leuven, Belgium

Doctoral Consortium of the 12th International Conference on Business Process Management (BPM-DC 2014)

Dirk Fahland[1] and Stefanie Rinderle-Ma[2]

[1] Eindhoven University of Technology, The Netherlands
d.fahland@tue.nl
[2] University of Vienna, Austria
stefanie.rinderle-ma@univie.ac.at

Introduction to BPM-DC 2014

The Doctoral Consortium (DC) of the BPM conference provides a venue specifically open for young researchers in the domain of business process management, who are working on their doctoral research projects. PhD students are offered a forum to present their entire project to a larger expert audience outside of their home universities. The aim of the DC is

- to provide valuable feedback on students' research methods and plans;
- to provide helpful guidance on students' research directions and topics;
- to promote the development of a community of scholars that will help students in their future careers; and
- to provide students with opportunities to meet and interact with other researchers (senior and junior) in the area of BPM.

The DC received 9 submissions out of which 6 were accepted for presentation on September 7, 2014 in Eindhoven, The Netherlands. The submissions covered a wide range of topics from classical BPM topics, such as process model matching and process mining, to highly relevant topics that are currently less in focus of the main conferences, such as adoption of BPM in practice and handling data inaccuracies.

Organizers

Dirk Fahland	Eindhoven University of Technology, The Netherlands (*BPM-DC Co-chair and Reviewer*)
Stefanie Rinderle-Ma	University of Vienna, Austria (*BPM-DC Co-chair and Reviewer*)
Sander Leemans	Eindhoven University of Technology, The Netherlands (*Local Organizer*)

Experts Participating in BPM-DC 2014

The following senior researchers of the BPM community attended the Doctoral Consortium as shepherds participating in the discussions and providing feedback to the students.

Avigdor Gal	Technion – Israel Institute of Technology, Haifa, Israel
Raimundas Matulevicius	University of Tartu, Estonia
Jan Mendling	Vienna University of Economics and Business, Austria
Hajo A. Reijers	Vrije Universiteit Amsterdam, The Netherlands
Pnina Soffer	University of Haifa, Israel
Barbara Weber	University of Innsbruck, Austria

We thank the shepherds for the rich discussions and feedback provided during the Doctoral Consortium.

Contents

ProHealth 2014

Modeling and Monitoring Variability in Hospital Treatments:
A Scenario Using CMMN 3
Nico Herzberg, Kathrin Kirchner, and Mathias Weske

Recommendations for Medical Treatment Processes: The PIGS Approach . . . 16
Marcin Hewelt, Aaron Kunde, Mathias Weske, and Christoph Meinel

Modelling and Implementation of Correct by Construction Healthcare
Workflows. 28
Petros Papapanagiotou and Jacques Fleuriot

MET4: Supporting Workflow Execution for Interdisciplinary Healthcare
Teams 40
Szymon Wilk, Davood Astaraky, Wojtek Michalowski, Daniel Amyot,
Runzhuo Li, Craig Kuziemsky, and Pavel Andreev

Enhancing Guideline-Based Decision Support with Distributed Computation
Through Local Mobile Application (Short Paper) 53
Erez Shalom, Yuval Shahar, Ayelet Goldstein, Elior Ariel,
Silvana Quaglini, Lucia Sacchi, Nick Fung, Valerie Jones,
Tom Broens, Gema García-Sáez, and Elena Hernando

Storlet Engine for Executing Biomedical Processes Within the Storage
System 59
Simona Rabinovici-Cohen, Ealan Henis, John Marberg, and Kenneth Nagin

SBP 2014

Conformance Checking Based on Partially Ordered Event Data 75
Xixi Lu, Dirk Fahland, and Wil M.P. van der Aalst

Online Compliance Monitoring of Service Landscapes (Short Paper). 89
J.M.E.M. van der Werf and H.M.W. Verbeek

Privacy Preserving Business Process Fusion (Short Paper) 96
Roberto Guanciale and Dilian Gurov

PMC-MR 2014

Configuring Configurable Process Models Made Easier: An Automated
Approach.. 105
  D.M.M. Schunselaar, Henrik Leopold, H.M.W. Verbeek,
  Wil M.P. van der Aalst, and Hajo A. Reijers

When Language Meets Language: Anti Patterns Resulting from Mixing
Natural and Modeling Language................................... 118
  Fabian Pittke, Henrik Leopold, and Jan Mendling

vrBPMN* and FM: An Approach to Model Business Process Line........ 130
  Geraldo Landre, Edilson Palma, Débora Maria Paiva,
  Elisa Yumi Nakagawa, and Maria Istela Cagnin

BPCAS 2014

Context-Aware Programming for Hybrid and Diversity-Aware Collective
Adaptive Systems.. 145
  Hong-Linh Truong and Schahram Dustdar

Towards Cognitive BPM as the Next Generation BPM Platform
for Analytics-Driven Business Processes (Short Paper).............. 158
  Hamid R. Motahari Nezhad and Rama Akkiraju

Towards Ensuring High Availability in Collective Adaptive Systems
(Short Paper)... 165
  David Richard Schäfer, Santiago Gómez Sáez, Thomas Bach,
  Vasilios Andrikopoulos, and Muhammad Adnan Tariq

DAB 2014

Analytics Process Management: A New Challenge for the BPM
Community.. 175
  Fenno F. (Terry) Heath III and Richard Hull

Towards Location-Aware Process Modeling and Execution 186
  Xinwei Zhu, Guobin Zhu, Seppe K.L.M. Vanden Broucke,
  Jan Vanthienen, and Bart Baesens

Extending CPN Tools with Ontologies to Support the Management
of Context-Adaptive Business Processes.......................... 198
  Estefanía Serral, Johannes De Smedt, and Jan Vanthienen

Using Data-Object Flow Relations to Derive Control Flow Variants
in Configurable Business Processes.............................. 210
  Riccardo Cognini, Flavio Corradini, Andrea Polini, and Barbara Re

The BE^2 Model: When Business Events Meet Business Entities   222
Fabiana Fournier and Lior Limonad

Extending Process Logs with Events from Supplementary Sources   235
Felix Mannhardt, Massimiliano de Leoni, and Hajo A. Reijers

BPI 2014

A Case Study in Workflow Scheduling Driven by Log Data   251
Mirela Botezatu, Hagen Völzer, and Remco Dijkman

Decomposed Process Mining: The ILP Case.   264
H.M.W. Verbeek and Wil M.P. van der Aalst

Evaluating the Performance of a Batch Activity in Process Models   277
Luise Pufahl, Ekaterina Bazhenova, and Mathias Weske

Genetic Process Mining: Alignment-Based Process Model Mutation   291
M.L. van Eck, J.C.A.M. Buijs, and B.F. van Dongen

Exploring Processes and Deviations.   304
Sander J.J. Leemans, Dirk Fahland, and Wil M.P. van der Aalst

Experimenting with an OLAP Approach for Interactive Discovery
in Process Mining.   317
Gustavo Pizarro and Marcos Sepúlveda

Merging Event Logs with Many to Many Relationships.   330
Lihi Raichelson and Pnina Soffer

Process Model Realism: Measuring Implicit Realism.   342
Benoît Depaire

Analyzing a TCP/IP-Protocol with Process Mining Techniques.   353
Christian Wakup and Jörg Desel

BPMC 2014

YAWL in the Cloud: Supporting Process Sharing and Variability   367
*D.M.M. Schunselaar, H.M.W. Verbeek, H.A. Reijers,
and Wil M.P. van der Aalst*

TaProViz 2014

A Generic Approach for Calculating and Visualizing Differences
Between Process Models in Multidimensional Process Mining   383
Carsten Cordes, Thomas Vogelgesang, and Hans-Jürgen Appelrath

Enabling a User-Friendly Visualization of Business Process Models   395
Markus Hipp, Achim Strauss, Bernd Michelberger, Bela Mutschler,
and Manfred Reichert

Lights, Camera, Action! Business Process Movies for Online Process
Discovery.   408
Andrea Burattin, Marta Cimitile, and Fabrizio Maria Maggi

Towards a Generalized Notion of Audio as Part of the Concrete Syntax
of Business Process Modeling Languages (Short Paper).   420
Jens Gulden

BPMS2 2014

Tagging Model for Enhancing Knowledge Transfer and Usage during
Business Process Execution   429
Reuven Karni and Meira Levy

Classification Framework for Context Data from Business Processes
(Short Paper)   440
Michael Möhring, Rainer Schmidt, Ralf-Christian Härting, Florian Bär,
and Alfred Zimmermann

Business Processes in Connected Communities (Short Paper)   446
Nick Russell and Alistair Barros

Social-Software-Based Support for Enterprise Architecture Management
Processes.   452
Rainer Schmidt, Alfred Zimmermann, Michael Möhring, Dierk Jugel,
Florian Bär, and Christian M. Schweda

oBPM – An Opportunistic Approach to Business Process Modeling
and Execution.   463
David Grünert, Elke Brucker-Kley, and Thomas Keller

DeMiMoP 2014

Constructing Probabilistic Process Models Based on Hidden Markov
Models for Resource Allocation   477
Berny Carrera and Jae-Yoon Jung

Business Rules: From SBVR to Information Systems   489
Jandisson Soares de Jesus and Ana Cristina Vieira de Melo

Integration of Business Processes with Visual Decision Modeling.
Presentation of the HaDEs Toolchain.   504
Krzysztof Kluza, Krzysztof Kaczor, and Grzegorz J. Nalepa

Generating Business Process Recommendations with a Population-Based
Meta-Heuristic   516
  Steven Mertens, Frederik Gailly, and Geert Poels

Bidimensional Process Discovery for Mining BPMN Models   529
  Jochen De Weerdt, Seppe K.L.M. vanden Broucke, and Filip Caron

Designing and Evaluating an Interpretable Predictive Modeling Technique
for Business Processes.   541
  Dominic Breuker, Patrick Delfmann, Martin Matzner, and Jörg Becker

Doctoral Consortium at BPM 2014

Detecting, Assessing, and Mitigating Data Inaccuracy-Related Risks
in Business Processes (Short Paper).   557
  Arava Tsoury, Soffer Pnina, and Iris Reinhartz-Berger

Adaptation of Business Process Management to Requirements of Small
and Medium-Sized Enterprises in the Context of Strategic Flexibility
(Short Paper)   561
  Felix Reher

A Language for Process Map Design (Short Paper)   567
  Monika Malinova

Graph-Based Process Model Matching (Short Paper)   573
  Christina Tsagkani

Service Analysis and Simulation in Process Mining (Short Paper)   578
  Arik Senderovich

Process Discovery and Exploration (Short Paper)   582
  Sander J.J. Leemans

Author Index   587

ProHealth 2014

Modeling and Monitoring Variability in Hospital Treatments: A Scenario Using CMMN

Nico Herzberg[1]([✉]), Kathrin Kirchner[2], and Mathias Weske[1]

[1] Hasso Plattner Institute at the University of Potsdam,
Prof.-Dr.-Helmert-Straße 2-3, 14482 Potsdam, Germany
{Nico.Herzberg,Mathias.Weske}@hpi.uni-potsdam.de
[2] University Hospital Jena, Bachstrasse 18, 07743 Jena, Germany
kathrin.kirchner@med.uni-jena.de

Abstract. Healthcare faces the challenge to deliver high treatment quality and patient satisfaction while being cost efficient which is tackled by introducing clinical pathways to standardize the treatment processes. At the Jena University Hospital, the clinical pathway for living donor liver transplantation was modeled using Business Process Model and Notation. A survey based on that model investigates on the transferability of this pathway to other hospitals and lists the requirements for a general model including the need for flexibility caused by differences in treatments in various hospitals. In this paper, we show an approach to tackle the requirements for such a flexible process by using the Case Management Model and Notation standard. Further, we show how case monitoring and analysis can be established by using an approach combining event processing and case management. The holistic approach is exemplified by using a scenario of the evaluation of living liver donors.

Keywords: Flexible healthcare processes · Process monitoring · CMMN

1 Introduction

Nowadays, healthcare faces the challenge to deliver high treatment quality and patient satisfaction while being cost and resource efficient. This challenge is tackled by introducing clinical pathways. A clinical pathway is a structured, multidisciplinary care plan that defines the steps of patient care for a certain disease in a specific hospital [22]. It is usually built upon a clinical guideline that provides a generic recommendation for a particular disease. Clinical pathways can improve the quality of patient care through efficient use of resources and clear responsibilities [20].

Compared to processes in industry, clinical pathways are more flexible as a treatment process varies for each individual patient. Additional therapies might be necessary and the sequence of treatment steps might change due to interpreting patient-specific data. Furthermore, treatment processes can vary for the same disease for every hospital, although they generally follow a clinical guideline.

In [13], we provided a life cycle approach for process intelligence in an hospital environment, which consists of four phases. First, the treatment process has to

© Springer International Publishing Switzerland 2015
F. Fournier and J. Mendling (Eds.): BPM 2014 Workshops, LNBIP 202, pp. 3–15, 2015.
DOI: 10.1007/978-3-319-15895-2_1

be (re)designed in the form of a process model and event monitoring points have to be defined. In a second phase, the monitoring system is configured. In the third phase, data have to be gathered according to the defined event monitoring points and the process execution is monitored accordingly. In the fourth phase, the process monitoring results are analyzed, i.e., conformance between recorded data and the designed process model is checked.

The elicitation and modeling of a clinical pathway in phase one involves physicians and nurses and is usually time consuming. Transferring and adopting a clinical pathway from one hospital to another would reduce this time tremendously. Especially, when a clinical guideline exits, the treatment process is done in a similar way, but deviations based on medical expert knowledge and specific departmental situations exist and require flexibility. Further flexibility is required by the fact, that the clinical pathway execution depends on the health state of the patient and therefore, needs to be adopted dynamically by medical doctors and nurses. This flexibility complicates the other phases of the mentioned life cycle [13] and challenges the monitoring of such flexible processes.

In this paper, we present an approach for modeling clinical pathways by applying the concept of case management and utilizing Case Management Model and Notation (CMMN) – an OMG modeling standard for case modeling [17] – to tackle the need for flexibility and transferability of clinical pathways between hospitals. We discuss the application of CMMN in healthcare and show specific challenges during modeling. Further, we show the monitoring and analysis of cases and how these results can be visualized, e.g., for identifying case improvements. Therewith, we provide an holistic view on applying case management in healthcare based on the life cycle we introduced in [13].

The paper is structured as follows. Section 2 gives an overview of related work. Section 3 describes the scenario for living liver donor evaluation which is used in the subsequent sections of this paper. In Sect. 4, we provide a means of modeling flexible clinical pathways by applying CMMN and discuss the experiences we made. We describe an approach for case monitoring in Sect. 5 and conclude the paper including a brief outlook on future work in Sect. 6.

2   Related Work

In this Section, we will provide related work about concept, methods, and techniques for flexibility in clinical pathway modeling and for process monitoring.

2.1   Flexibility in Clinical Pathway Modeling

Especially in emergency cases, but also in their daily work, physicians and nurses need to be free to react and make their own decisions based on the health state of the patient. Thus, clinical pathways are influenced by medical knowledge and the information collected about the patient. Thus, deviations from pre-planned treatment processes are frequent. An IT-supported clinical pathway cannot restrict medical staff in their daily work [19]. The task of designing and executing flexible processes has led to several research initiatives [23].

The ADEPT system offers the functionality of making dynamic changes during the execution time of a pathway. Running process instances can be migrated to new process model versions [5]. Based on ADEPT, MinAdept provides techniques for mining flexible processes [14]. Till now, the ADEPT concept does not include a concept for monitoring flexible processes. With CarePlan, the adaption of clinical pathways is based on a semantic framework [1]. In [4], a system to evaluate the conformance is proposed that checks whether the pathway execution follows a clinical guideline and suggests possible reconfigurations.

Declarative process modeling is activity-centered [18]. Constraints are used to prevent certain behavior. During run-time, only allowed activities are shown to the user, and he decides about next activity to be executed. Derived form the the Event-driven Process Chain (EPC) modeling language, [21] proposes Configurable EPCs that allows the explicit specification of configurations in reference process models. The Provop approach provides flexible processes by managing variants. A particular process variant can be configured by applying a set of well-defined change operations to a reference process model [9].

In the case handling approach, activities can be executed based on data dependencies [25]. For example, if an activity is still running but produced already data necessary to execute the next step, the following activity can start already. In the same vein the concept of Proclets targets which allows the division of a process into several process parts. This snippets can be executed one after the other or interactively. Late binding provides a flexible process execution [24].

Case management requires modeling that can express the flexibility of a knowledge worker during run-time while selecting and executing tasks for a specific case. This is covered by CMMN [17]. Tasks are modeled and can be specified as either mandatory or discretionary (additional possible tasks) during design-time and serve as recommendation during run-time.

2.2 Process Monitoring

Besides prediction, control, and optimization, process monitoring and analysis are features of Business Process Intelligence (BPI) to enable quality management for process executions [8]. Business process execution data capturing and storage is discussed numerously in literature [2, 8]. However, most of these approaches assume that every process step is observable and thus, the recorded event log is complete, which is not the fact in manual executing process environments such as in healthcare. Mutschler et al. [15] introduces a reference architecture for BPI, describing three layers, i.e., integration, function, and visualization. The approach in this paper targets in particular on integration and functionality for process monitoring and analysis of cases by accessing and processing required data. Further, we sketch a visualization for process monitoring and analysis results.

For monitoring and analyzing cases, techniques and methods from Business Activity Monitoring (BAM) can be adopted. Dahanayake et al. [6] gives an overview of BAM and classifies BAM systems into four classes: pure BAM, discovery-oriented BAM, simulation-oriented BAM, and reporting-oriented BAM. All of them could be adopted to case management, as the presented approach delivers high-quality events for these systems. With regard to business process evaluation, the concept of Process Performance Indicators (PPI), the process-related form of key performance indicators, is introduced in Business Process Management (BPM) to measure process execution performance, such as time, costs, and occurrences [7]. In this paper, we show a concept for case execution performance.

3   Scenario

As scenario, we selected the clinical pathway for living donors in liver transplantation. Living Donor Liver Transplantation (LDLT) has emerged in recent decades as a critical surgical option for patients with end stage liver disease. This process is not yet described in a medical guideline. Nevertheless, a common understanding of which investigations need to be undertaken is existing and discussed in the literature, e.g., [16]. In Jena University Hospital, we modeled the process of the adult living donor transplantation using Business Process Model and Notation (BPMN). A business process model, e.g., a BPMN model, specifies related activities and their dependencies to reach a business goal.

A person that is considering to donate a part of her liver has to be medically evaluated to ensure that she can undergo the surgery. While some of the investigations can be done in the hospital ambulance, others are done during an in-patient stay. The sub-process of the in-patient evaluation is shown in Fig. 1. As shown in the model, a potential donor has to undergo some mandatory investigations, i.e., *blood analysis*, *psychological evaluation*, *med/tech investigations*, and *mandatory referrals*. Based on results, additional investigations might be necessary. A potential donor can be considered as non-suitable already in early stages of the evaluation, or later at the end of the in-patient evaluation.

In order to compare our pathway with the processes carried out in other hospitals and to evaluate the transferability of our pathway to other hospitals,

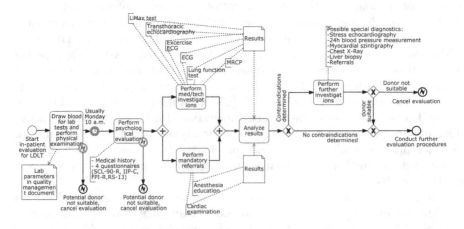

Fig. 1. BPMN process model of the adult living donor.

a questionnaire was developed within a doctoral thesis and sent round to all 14 centers in Germany that perform LDLT. To the questions about the steps performed during the LDLT with the adult donor, nine centers answered. From the evaluation of the results, we found out that several examinations are the same in all hospitals, but other steps are only performed if certain conditions (e.g., donor age or previous health problems) are held. A common treatment process for all centers might be possible in case these variations are included.

4   Case Modeling

In the following, we will show how the scenario described in Section 3 is modeled using CMMN. Into that model, results from our questionnaire that investigates the transferability of the LDLT pathway from Jena University Hospital to other hospitals, are integrated. Concluding this Section, we discuss some advantages and disadvantage of modeling a clinical pathway with CMMN.

4.1   The Case Plan Model

In the life cycle approach for process intelligence in a hospital environment [13], first, the treatment process has to be designed as a process model. Based on the model for living liver donor evaluation, described in Sect. 3, and the results from the related questionnaire, we defined a case plan model using CMMN. A case plan model specifies the behavior of cases, i.e., by describing tasks that can be or must be executed to reach a business goal. The case plan model is shown in Fig. 2. We kept the modeling on a single level and did not introduce case tasks – the call of another case described by another case plan model – as the initial process model does not use the concept of sub-processes. Thus, all stages and tasks are arranged within the outer-most stage describing the case plan model for handling the evaluation of a donor in the LDLT treatment.

Each evaluation case needs to be started with performing the required task of *Draw blood for lab tests and perform physical examination*. Afterwards, *Perform psychological evaluation* must be performed before the milestone *Initial examination performed* is reached. Reaching that milestone enables the execution of two stages *Med/Tech investigations* and *Mandatory referrals*.

In the stage of *Med/Tech investigations*, we modeled investigations that are performed in all hospitals as tasks: *Perform abdominal ultrasound, Perform ECG*, and *Perform CT*. Examinations that are performed in some hospitals only are modeled as discretionary tasks, e.g., *Perform MRI* or *Perform lung function test*. These tasks can be planned during case execution by the knowledge worker, i.e., the doctor, according the medical requirements and the individual hospital pathway. Further discretionary tasks, *Perform MRCP* and *Perform exercise ECG*, are dependent on patients' condition, i.e., *Status for MRCP met* and *Medical history and CVRF necessitate exercise ECG*. These conditions are modeled as milestones. Stage *Mandatory referrals* consists of two required tasks that can be conducted in arbitrary order.

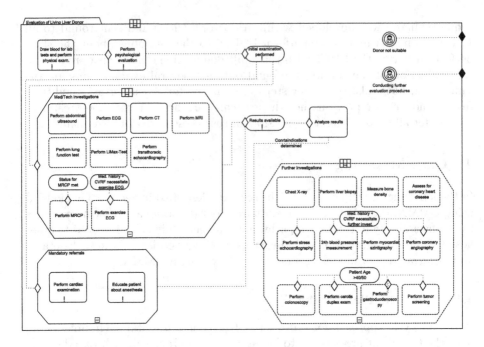

Fig. 2. Case plan model (CMMN [17]) of the adult living liver donor evaluation.

Both stages are prerequisites for the milestone *Results available*. Reaching this milestone allows for the task of *Analyze Results*. When this analysis results in the determination of contraindications, further investigations can be conducted, cf. stage *Further Investigations*. In this stage, all tasks are discretionary and can be planned according to their need during case execution. Some of these tasks are dependent on medical situations, i.e., *Medical history and CVRF necessitate further investigations*, or patients' criteria, i.e., *Patient age is above 40/50*.

At any time, the knowledge worker, i.e., the doctor, can decide about the suitability of the donor and the continuation of the evaluation procedures. In case the donor is not suitable the user event *Donor not suitable* can be triggered, otherwise the user event *Conducting further evaluation procedures*.

4.2   Discussion

During the presented research work, we discussed our case plan model with medical staff from the University Hospital Jena. From these discussions, we identified some advantages and disadvantages for the usage of CMMN. These are compared to the usage of BPMN in the following.

Modeling a general process valid for several hospitals. With CMMN it is possible to describe a treatment for several hospitals, even if they work differently, by using the concept of tasks and discretionary tasks and their setting to be required. Nonetheless, it is difficult to express tasks that are mandatory in only one hospital. In Fig. 2, the tasks that are done in all hospitals are modeled as tasks resp. required tasks. This does not mean that in a particular hospital a certain task is not obligatory, e.g., at Jena University Hospital *Perform MRI* is done in every donor evaluation, but it is modeled as an discretionary task as it is performed on request only in other hospitals. The doctor needs to know these hospital specific rules or it is specified in a hospital-specific best practice guideline existing in parallel to the case plan model. To fulfill this requirement in BPMN would be even harder, as the different variants have to be modeled by using gateways, which will increase the complexity of the diagram.

Explicit modeling of roles not supported. Seeing who is responsible for the execution of a task is very valuable for the reader of a process model in general, however, this is not supported by CMMN. The CMMN standard allows the assignment of roles to a case and the specification of human tasks in the related case plan model. However, role information is not shown in the model explicitly and targets only on human tasks. In contrast, in BPMN this requirement is fulfilled by the concept of pools and lanes. To express the information more explicitly in CMMN, one can introduce a case hierarchy consisting of one case referring to several sub-cases each described by its own case plan model and more fine-grained role set, but this will increase model complexity.

Explicit modeling of locations not supported. Information about the location is a very important information not only in the healthcare domain, but cannot be expressed in CMMN. The same holds for BPMN, but there the grouping element can be used for expressing the location. In CMMN, this information could be made more explicitly by split up the model into several stages.

A central question is, in which way a case plan model as it is described in Sect. 4.1 should be used. As already sketched, it can be used as it is and a hospital-specific best practice document can be introduced in parallel, describing which aspects need to be followed in the particular hospital. A second possibility would be to use the case plan model as a template and adopt it according to the procedure of the respective hospital. This would mainly result in turning discretionary tasks into required ones. A third way to gain value of the case plan model is using it as inspiration to model the clinical pathway from scratch, e.g., by using another modeling language like BPMN.

5   Case Monitoring

In the following, we briefly introduce some requirements to case monitoring and provide analysis questions for our scenario. Afterwards, we show how our concept for process monitoring and analysis based on BPMN [13] is adopted to CMMN. In the third part, a potential case management monitoring solution is sketched.

5.1   Requirements for Monitoring Cases

Monitoring and analysis of cases require the evaluation of time aspects, cost-related details, and domain resp. case-specific questions. A detailed list of requirements and their evaluation in the domain of healthcare is given in [3]. For our scenario, we discussed possible case-related monitoring and analysis questions together with the surgeons:

- How many potential living liver donors are considered for one recipient?
- How many of these potential donors undergo a transplant operation later?
- How many of potential donors are considered as not suitable for transplantation already during the out-patient evaluation procedure for transplantation?
- How many transplantation operations needed to be canceled?
- How many liver donors are under evaluation and in which phase are they?

From a time perspective, it is very valuable to get insights into the handling time in each of the steps, i.e., tasks. An interesting question posed by the surgeons was: How long has a potential donor to stay in hospital for the in-patient part of evaluation procedure? To support the monitoring and analysis of such required questions for single cases, we adopted an established approach based on BPMN to case management.

5.2   Approach to Monitoring Cases

In [10] an approach is introduced that describes the utilization of data about process executions, namely events, in connection with the knowledge from process models to leverage process monitoring and analysis. An event is a real-world happening occurring in a particular *point in time*, at a particular *location*, in a certain *context*. Context data, describing the context in which the event happens, is used for correlating the process execution information and the processes.

We refer to events that are recorded in an IT system as *raw events*, as the form of this data is not generally specified (lower part in Fig. 3). Raw events build the very basis for our process monitoring and analysis approach. According to [10], raw event data need to be normalized for structuring the event data in a common format for further processing. The structure as well as the binding – the specification where the event data are stored in the IT system landscape – are defined in the corresponding normalized event type during design-time. By setting the normalized events into the process context during run-time, so-called process events are created that could be used for process monitoring and analysis applications [12]. The detailed instructions how the normalized event is correlated to the matching process instance(s) – a particular process execution following a process model – is defined in the corresponding process event type during design-time. The assignment of process events to particular places within a process model is reached by implementing Process Event Monitoring Points (PEMP) [13]. A PEMP is bound to a state transition of a process model's node, i.e., activity, gateway or event, during design-time. Node states and their transitions are described by the corresponding node life cycles. This configuration enables the assignment of a process event to a process model node instance to indicate its corresponding state transition during run-time.

The correlation to a case that is specified by its respective case plan model could be established in a similar way. The life cycles of CMMN elements are

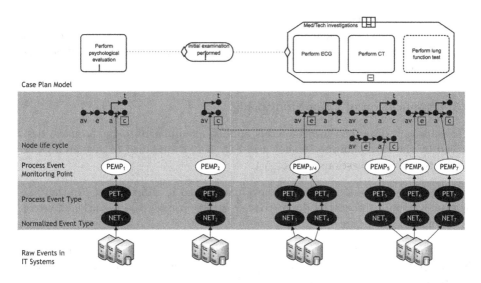

Fig. 3. Detail of a case plan model with assigned life cycles (simplified) for tasks, stages and milestones and the corresponding defined and placed PEMPs. Each PEMP is associated with process event types that describe process events that are created by utilizing normalized events, specified by normalized event types, during run-time.

described in the specification [17] and supported by our approach, however, in this paper, we refer to simplified life cycles for visibility reasons. The simplified life cycle for a task consists of the states (av)ailable, (e)nabled, (a)ctive, (c)ompleted, and (t)erminated and their corresponding state transitions in between. The simplified life cycle for stages is similar and consists of the states (av)ailable, (e)nabled, (a)ctive, and (c)ompleted and their corresponding state transitions. The states (av)ailable, (c)ompleted, and (t)erminated and their corresponding state transitions describe the simplified life cycle for milestones. To the specified state transitions in the life cycles mentioned above, a PEMP is defined during design-time (upper part of Fig. 3). To such a PEMP, process event types can be bound. These configurations are used during run-time, to assign process events that have a certain type to the corresponding case plan model node instance to indicate its corresponding state transition. Referring to our example shown in Fig. 3, the occurrence of a process event of process event type PET_1 correlating to a particular case instance indicates that the task *Perform psychological evaluation* was performed and transitioned to the state *completed*. A case instance is a particular case execution following a case plan model. Further, recognizing a correlated event of the process event type PET_2 indicates that the milestone *Initial examination performed* is met and transitioned to state *completed*.

Having process knowledge described by the case plan model allows further monitoring of a case without considering further events, i.e., the state of a case plan model node instance can be derived from the states of other nodes. For example, it is possible to derive the enablement of a node, e.g., a stage, based on the information that a required node, e.g., a task, was completed. Referring to our example, the enablement of stage *Med/Tech investigations* can be derived from the information about completing the milestone *Initial examination performed*, shown as dashed arrow in Fig. 3.

5.3 Application of Case Monitoring

The approach described in Sect. 5.2 is applied exemplarily to the scenario described by the case plan model shown in Fig. 4. It is intended to give an answer to the two raised questions in Sect. 5.1:

- How many liver donors are under evaluation and in which phase are they?
- How long has a potential donor to stay in hospital for the in-patient part of evaluation procedure?

A solution proposal for a monitoring application is shown in Fig. 4. In the cycles in the upper right corner it is shown how many patients are currently treated in the particular task. In the rectangle in the lower right corner the average time the task takes is shown. This data is calculated by including all cases.

For example, currently there are three patients treated in the task of *Draw blood for lab tests and perform physical examination*. This task takes in average two hours and 18 min. In *Perform psychological evaluation* two patients are treated who need to assume that this task will take one hour and 25 min. Many treatment steps are not performed at the moment – that is indicated by the

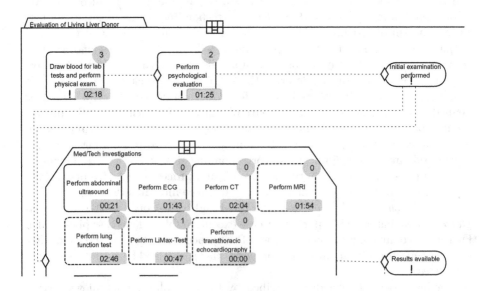

Fig. 4. Mock-Up for a monitoring component to analyze how many living liver donors are in treatment and at which stage, and how long the single tasks took in average in the context of a case plan model (excerpt).

zero in the upper right corner of every task – however, their average processing time is shown to enable case analysis to identify points for improvement. Task *Perform transthoracic echocardiography* shows a processing time of zero. This is caused by the fact that in the particular hospital this task was not performed to at least one patient.

This view on case executions is inspired by the results of our research project PIGE – process intelligence in healthcare[1] [12]. It shows a mock up to demonstrate the application of monitoring case executions in context of case plan' models. Such a view can be integrated into a process cockpit as proposed by [3]. A process cockpit also allows further functionality for filtering, sorting etc. to break down the monitoring results to such details that are required for answering a certain analysis question. At Jena University Hospital, with the analysis of data, evaluation investigations could be rearranged and therefore the hospital stay could be reduced [11]. Thereby, case monitoring relies on the data quality in the underlying IT-Systems, i.e., clinical information systems. The better the data quality and quantity the better and precise case monitoring results are possible.

6 Conclusion

Providing a common description for a clinical treatment process for different hospitals as a model requires even more flexibility than the necessity for adaption of clinical pathways during run-time depending on the patients' health state. In this paper, we showed the application of the CMMN standard in healthcare by bringing a clinical pathway modeled in BPMN based on results of a questionnaire about the practices in other hospitals to a case plan model that is valid for all hospitals. Further, we discussed our experiences and the advantages and disadvantages we see in the application of CMMN. Inspired by the life cycle approach for process intelligence we introduced in [13], we showed how process monitoring and analysis based on the case specification can be established by utilizing events during run-time. Therefore, after specifying the case in CMMN, PEMPs are defined together with medical personnel to measure interesting aspects during case execution. With this information the cases can be analyzed to ensure higher quality and transparency of treatment processes. The whole approach is shown with the scenario of the evaluation of living liver donors.

In the future, we will evaluate the created case plan model with medical staff and apply CMMN modeling to other healthcare processes. We will evaluate the usage of CMMN in hospitals in a more general view and work on best practices for using CMMN in healthcare. Further, we will elaborate on the usage of case plan models and their occurring events during run-time to provide system support for case execution and deliver decision guidance.

---

[1] http://www.pige-projekt.de.

Acknowledgment. The authors thank Anita Francke, PhD student at University Hospital Jena, for revising the LDLT pathway, developing the questionnaire and collecting answers from living liver transplantation centers as part of her dissertation work.

References

1. Abidi, S.S.R., Chen, H.: Adaptable personalized care planning via a semantic web framework. In: 20th International Congress of the European Federation for Medical Informatics (2006)
2. Azvine, B., Cui, Z., Nauck, D.D., Majeed, B.: Real time business intelligence for the adaptive enterprise. In: CEC/EEE, p. 29. IEEE (2006)
3. Böhme, R.: Prozessanalyse & -monitoring - Entwurf und Evaluation eines prozessorientierten User Interface Cockpits. Masters thesis, University of Potsdam (2013)
4. Bottrighi, A., Chesani, F., Mello, P., Molino, G., Montali, M., Montani, S., Storari, S., Terenziani, P., Torchio, M.: A hybrid approach to clinical guideline and to basic medical knowledge conformance. In: Combi, C., Shahar, Y., Abu-Hanna, A. (eds.) AIME 2009. LNCS, vol. 5651, pp. 91–95. Springer, Heidelberg (2009)
5. Dadam, P., Reichert, M.: The ADEPT Project: a decade of research and development for robust and flexible process support. Comput. Sci. Res. Dev. **23**(2), 81–97 (2009)
6. Dahanayake, A., Welke, R.J., Cavalheiro, G.: Improving the understanding of BAM technology for real-time decision support. Int. J. Bus. Inf. Syst. **7**, 1–26 (2011)
7. del-Río-Ortega, A., Resinas, M., Ruiz-Cortés, A.: Defining process performance indicators: an ontological approach. In: Meersman, R., Dillon, T.S., Herrero, P. (eds.) OTM 2010. LNCS, vol. 6426, pp. 555–572. Springer, Heidelberg (2010)
8. Grigori, D., Casati, F., Castellanos, M., Dayal, U., Sayal, M., Shan, M.: Business process intelligence. Comput. Ind. **53**(3), 321–343 (2004)
9. Hallerbach, A., Bauer, T., Reichert, M.: Capturing variability in business process models: the provop approach. J. Softw. Maint. Evol.: Res. Pract. **22**(6–7), 519–546 (2010)
10. Herzberg, N., Meyer, A., Weske, M.: An event processing platform for business process management. In: EDOC, Vancouver, pp. 107–116. IEEE (2013)
11. Kirchner, K., Malessa, C., Bauschke, A., Settmacher, U.: Utilizing a clinical pathway for liver transplantation: first lessons learnt. Transpl. Int. **26**(sup. 1), 49 (2013)
12. Kirchner, K., Malessa, C., Herzberg, N., Krumnow, S., Habrecht, O., Scheuerlein, H., Bauschke, A., Settmacher, U.: Supporting liver transplantation by clinical pathway intelligence. Transpl. Proc. **45**(5), 1981–1982 (2013)
13. Kirchner, K., Herzberg, N., Rogge-Solti, A., Weske, M.: Embedding conformance checking in a process intelligence system in hospital environments. In: Lenz, R., Miksch, S., Peleg, M., Reichert, M., Riaño, D., ten Teije, A. (eds.) ProHealth 2012 and KR4HC 2012. LNCS, vol. 7738, pp. 126–139. Springer, Heidelberg (2013)
14. Li, C., Reichert, M., Wombacher, A.: The MinAdept clustering approach for discovering reference process models out of process variants. Int. J. Coop. Inf. Syst. **19**(03n04), 159–203 (2010)
15. Mutschler, B., Bumiller, J., Reichert, M.: An approach to quantify the costs of business process intelligence. In: EMISA, pp. 152–163 (2005)
16. Neumann, U.P., Neuhaus, P., Schmeding, M.: Lebendspende-Lebertransplantation beim Erwachsenen. Der Chirurg **81**(9), 804–812 (2010)
17. OMG. Case Management Model and Notation (CMMN) Version 1.0, May 2014

18. Pesic, M., van der Aalst, W.M.P.: A declarative approach for flexible business processes management. In: Eder, J., Dustdar, S. (eds.) BPM Workshops 2006. LNCS, vol. 4103, pp. 169–180. Springer, Heidelberg (2006)
19. Reichert, M.: What BPM technology can do for healthcare process support. In: Peleg, M., Lavrač, N., Combi, C. (eds.) AIME 2011. LNCS, vol. 6747, pp. 2–13. Springer, Heidelberg (2011)
20. Ronellenfitsch, U., Vargas Hein, O., Uerlich, M., Dahmen, A., Tuschy, S., Schwarzbach, M.: Klinische Pfade als Instrument zur Qualitätsverbesserung in der perioperativen Medizin. Periop. Med. 1(3), 164–172 (2009)
21. Rosemann, M., van der Aalst, W.M.P.: A configurable reference modelling language. Inf. Syst. 32(1), 1–23 (2007)
22. Rotter, Th., Kinsman, L., James, E., Machotta, A., Gothe, H., Willis, J., Snow, P., et al.: Clinical pathways: effects on professional practice, patient outcomes, length of stay and hospital costs. Cochrane Database Syst. Rev. 3(3) (2010). doi:10.1002/14651858.CD006632.pub2
23. Schonenberg, H., Mans, R., Russell, N., Mulyar, N., van der Aalst, W.: Process flexibility: a survey of contemporary approaches. In: Dietz, J.L.G., Albani, A., Barjis, J. (eds.) CIAO! 2008 and EOMAS 2008. LNBIP, vol. 10, pp. 16–30. Springer, Heidelberg (2008)
24. van der Aalst, W.M.P., Barthelmess, P., Ellis, C.A., Wainer, J.: Proclets: a framework for lightweight interacting workflow processes. Int. J. Coop. Inf. Syst. 10(04), 443–481 (2001)
25. van der Aalst, W.M.P., Weske, M., Grünbauer, D.: Case handling: a new paradigm for business process support. Data Knowl. Eng. 53(2), 129–162 (2005)

Recommendations for Medical Treatment Processes: The PIGS Approach

Marcin Hewelt[(⊠)], Aaron Kunde, Mathias Weske, and Christoph Meinel

Hasso Plattner Institute at the University of Potsdam, Potsdam, Germany
{marcin.hewelt,aaron.kunde,mathias.weske,christoph.meinel}@hpi.de

Abstract. Medical treatment processes in hospitals are complex inter-actions of various actors, in the course of which treatment decisions have to be made.Clinical practice guidelines and clinical pathways provide guidance for practicioners for certain diseases. Especially for multi-morbid patients several guidelines and pathways might apply. Current process-oriented IT support in hospitals, however, does not consider multiple models for treatment recommendations.

In this contribution we define Treatment Cases (TCs) and give an operational semantics for their evolution based on Business Process Model and Notation (BPMN) models, which we use to model guidelines, pathways and standard operating procedures. This work is part of the Process Information and Guidance System (PIGS) approach, which aims at providing an overview of treatment history and give recommendations based on the current treatment state and multiple process models.

1 Introduction

The treatment of a patient in the hospital is a complex interaction of medical actors in different departments, involving both organizational and medical activities, e.g. scheduling of radiology appointments and prescription of drugs. Business Process Management (BPM) has been devised to deal with exactly this kind of interaction [1]. Decisions about the next treatment steps have to be made, based on the current patient condition and the treatment history. To support these decisions, Clinical Practice Guidelines (CPGs) were introduced as sets of evidence-based best practices for diagnosis and treatment of certain diseases, published by medical societies and updated regularly [2]. Since CPGs consist of free form text with some flow charts, their formalization in so called Computer Interpretable Guidelines (CIGs) has been thoroughly researched, leading to a variety of different formalisms, e.g. PRO*forma* [3], GLIF3 [4] or GUIDE [5]. Based on these CIGs clinical decision support tools have been proposed to guide practitioners through diagnosis and treatment of a disease, e.g. *Tallis*[1]. Because CPGs only cover medical aspects of a treatment, they need to be adapted to concrete hospital settings and enriched with organizational aspects, resulting in Clinical Pathways (CPs), which depict the complete path of a patient through a

---

[1] http://www.cossac.org/tallis, built on PRO*forma*.

© Springer International Publishing Switzerland 2015
F. Fournier and J. Mendling (Eds.): BPM 2014 Workshops, LNBIP 202, pp. 16–27, 2015.
DOI: 10.1007/978-3-319-15895-2_2

specific institution [6]. Only then can the path be supported by IT systems. For certain, often-occuring or critical activities hospitals implement implement Standard Operating Proceduress (SOPs), which in detail describe the order of steps to take, e.g. for the reanimation of a patient. SOPs can be seen as the building blocks of CPs.

Hence, in reality several process models govern the treatment of a patient and inform treatment decisions. A special case are multi-morbid patients, whose treatment relies on multiple CPGs, which can contradict or prescribe redundant medical procedures. We approach this multi-model problem by extending the usual semantics of BPMN, which are defined in [7], to allow the integrated execution of multiple process models at the same time. To this end we formally define Treatment Cases (TCs) that where introduced in [8] to capture the complete treatment history of a patient, and propose an operational semantics based on partially ordered events. This allows us to recommend treatment steps based on the current treatment state taking into account multiple process models, which we assume to be modeled using BPMN. Medical actors interact with the TC, e.g. by adding recommended steps or skipping respectively executing certain activities, thus progressing the state of the treatment. This contribution details central aspects of the PIGS approach introduced in [8], which aims at process-oriented IT support for organizational and treatment processes in the hospital. We exemplify our approach with an usecase.

2 Related Work

Milla-Millán et al. [9] and Sánchez-Garzón et al. [10] use a multi-agent planning approach to deal with the generation of a personalized treatment plan for co-morbid patients. The CPGs are modeled in HTN Planning Domain Language (HPDL) which is an extension of Planning Domain Definition Language (PDDL) for Hierarchical Task Networks (HTNs). In contrast, we want to use BPMN in order to include business processes, which have already been modeled.

Alexandrou et al. [11] describe the challenge of personalizing CP to a specific patient. To this end, a software environment (SEMPATH) is presented, which adapts multiple CPs during execution time and creates a personalized CP for the patient on the fly. A CP is defined as a peculiar case of business process, which means, it can be modeled with BPMN. However, it is not described, if CPGs are modeled and used as well.

Pryss et al. [12] investigate four ward rounds in different clinical departments to determine requirements for tasks management during these ward rounds. The ward rounds have been modeled as BPMN processes to ease discussion with the doctors and identify workflows. That shows, that BPMN is sufficient to model healthcare processes.

3 Usecase

This section introduces a clinical treatment scenario, exemplifying the process-oriented support of medical treatment processes within the PIGS approach.

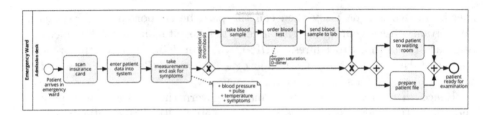

Fig. 1. Patient admission process

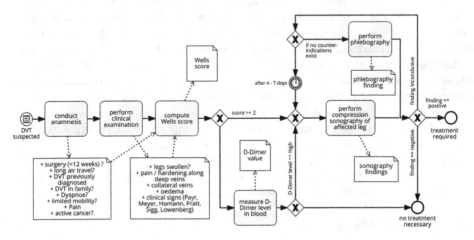

Fig. 2. Diagnosis of Thrombosis

The patient in our scenario is a 65 year old woman, who is transfered from her general practicioner with thrombosis suspicion and overall indisposition.

Figures 1, 2, 3 and 4 show a number of process models of a hospital. The patient admission process in Fig. 1 captures the organizational process of admitting a patient to the hospital, starting with the arrival of the patient in the emergency ward. Figure 2 shows the diagnostic part of the German S2 guideline for deep vein thrombosis (DVT), modeled with BPMN. It is activated when thrombosis is suspected. Based on information acquired during anamnesis and clinical examination, the Wells score needs to be computed to determine the likelihood of thrombosis. If the score value is below two, a blood test for D-dimers is performed, which due to its high specificity is adequate to exclude the possibility of thrombosis with high probability. If the test yields a high D-value or the Wells score was greater than one, a sonography of the affected leg is conducted by an experienced doctor to make the conclusive diagnosis of DVT. Figure 3 displays the guideline for treatment of DVT, which is triggered when the thrombosis diagnosis has been made. It consists of three different therapies, two of which are started immediately. Prior to vitamin K antagonist treatment, however, a gastroscopy is performed to determine the risk of stomach bleeding. The option

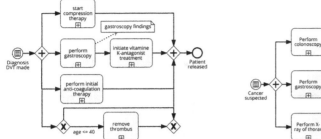

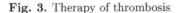

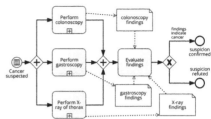

Fig. 3. Therapy of thrombosis   **Fig. 4.** SOP for cancer elimination

of removing the thrombus is only considered for patients below the age of 40 (the real condition is more complicated). To save space, the therapies are modeled as subprocesses. Figure 4 shows a hospital-specific SOP used to exclude cancer, which is triggered when the doctor suspects cancer as reason for the patient's condition. During anamnesis the doctor asks for the patient's overal condition (appetite, nausea, weight change, etc.) per default and based on the answers might suspect a cancer illness, which often acts as the originator of thrombosis, especially in elderly people. Together these process models form the model level of a PIGS.

We now turn to the execution level, on which the TC for one patient is located. Initially the TC is empty. When a patient arrives, the condition of the admission process becomes true and its start event 'patient arrived' is added to the TC. The first activity is added as recommendation to the TC, yielding the state displayed in Fig. 5.

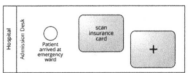

Fig. 5. Initial TC

A later state of the TC is displayed in Fig. 6. At this point in time, already several examinations have been performed, the diagnosis of DVT was confirmed, and therapy started with a Heparin injection and compression of the leg. The patient also was transfered from the emergency ward to a stationary ward of the hospital. Because of the cancer suspicion that arised during the anamnesis the SOP for cancer exclusion is active, as can be seen by the event 'cancer suspected' in Fig. 6. Therefore the three activities 'perform gastroscopy', 'perform colonoscopy', 'order X-ray of thorax' from the cancer exclusion SOP are recommended. However, the activity 'perform gastroscopy' is also part of the DVT treatment CPG, and thus executing it progresses both process models. Figure 6 displays a possible visualization of treatment history and recommendations. Data objects are used to denote the outcome of examinations. The lane construct of BPMN is used to illustrate who performed which task. Lanes are a good starting point to define role-specific views on the TC, i.e. a medical actor would only see the lane of her role or could filter out specific lanes. Furthermore, process

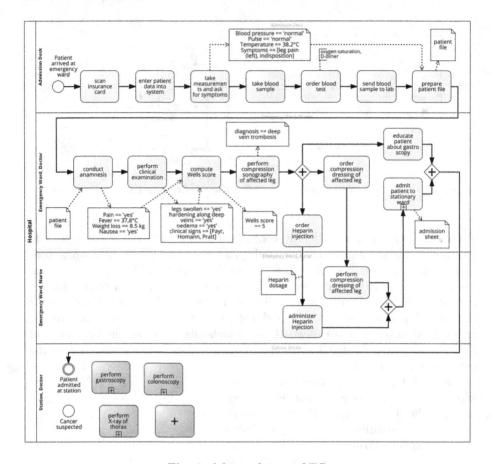

Fig. 6. Advanced state of TC

model abstraction could be used to reduce the number of displayed activities, by summarizing a set of activities into a collapsed subprocess. This is indicated by the collapsed subprocess 'admit patient to stationary ward', as well as by the recommended activities, which are also subprocesses. An additional task with the label '+' is shown in Figs. 5 and 6. This modeling element represents an arbitrary activity that can be added to the treatment case. It thus allows medical users to add activities that are not part of a process model.

4   Formalizing Treatment Cases

As was described in the usecase in Sect. 3 several process models and rules govern the recommended behavior of hospital actors during patient treatment. The PIGS approach distinguishes between the model level, where all these models reside, and the execution level, which contains the TC. We first give a formalization of the model level and then turn to how those process models contribute to the actual TC.

4.1   The Model Level

Although CIGs, CPs, SOPs all have a different scope, our approach treats them alike and assumes that they are represented with BPMN. Therefore, we refer to all these different models on model level simply as process models. For this contribution we restrain ourselves to a small subset of BPMN constructs, leaving out timer events, exception handling, complex gateways among others. As the goal of the PIGS approach is to support hospital actors by providing an overview of and guiding them through the treatment process, we need to represent these processes formally in a computer system. A process model is a directed graph consisting of activity, event, gateway and data object nodes, connected by (control and data) flow edges.

Definition 1 (Process Model). A *process model P* is a tuple $(A, E, G, D, F, \varepsilon)$ where A is a set of activities, E a set of events, $G = G^{\wedge} \cup G^{\times}$ is a set of parallel resp. exclusive gateways, D is a set of data objects used in the model, $F \subseteq (A \times D) \cup (D \times A) \cup (A \cup E \cup G)^2$ is the flow relation, and ε is a partial function that assigns an expression to some activities and events.

Data objects are connected to activities by the flow relation F, which also connects activities, events and gateways with each other. The set of predecessors resp. successors is denoted by $\bullet N$ resp. $N\bullet$ for $N \in A \cup E \cup G$; the set of data preconditions resp. postconditions is denoted by $\blacksquare N$ resp. $N\blacksquare$ for $N \in A$. We assume that activities have at most one predecessor ($\bullet A \leq 1$) and at most one successor ($A\bullet \leq 1$). Furthermore, if a gateway has multiple successors it can only have one predecessor and vice versa. In the first case the gateway is called a split gateway (denoted $G^<$), in the latter case it is called a join gateway (denoted $G^>$). Expressions are used to specify conditions for activities and events, e.g. $\varepsilon(\text{'remove thrombus'}) = \text{"}age >= 40\text{"}$ in Fig. 2, stating that 'remove thrombus' activity can only be performed if the patient is younger than 40 years old. In the same way the start event of the admission process in Fig. 1 can only occur, when a patient arrives at the emergency ward. We leave the formal specification of the expression language for future work and just state here that expression terms can be formed over patient data and event of TCs.

Definition 2 (Model Level). The *model level* of a PIGS consists of set of process models $\mathcal{P}$ and an universe for activities $\mathcal{A}$, events $\mathcal{E}$, and data objects $\mathcal{D}$, such that $\forall P_i \in \mathcal{P} : A_i \in \mathcal{A}, E_i \in \mathcal{E}, D_i \in \mathcal{D}$.

The universes hence encompass all activities, events, and data objects that occur in the process models. However, $\mathcal{A}$ can contain additional activities that can be added manually to the TC by medical actors. The above definition allows for process models to share activities, events, and data objects, e.g. in our usecase the activity 'perform gastroscopy' is used both in the cancer exclusion SOP and the DVT treatment CPG.

In BPMN, activities and gateways are not atomic, but rather have internal states, e.g. they can be **running** or **terminated** [1]. These states are necessary to faithfully capture the progress of the activities' execution and to define an operational semantics for process models. For example, an activity can only terminate if it is in state **running**. These fine-grained activity states are formalized as transition system called *lifecycle*, which depicts possible states an activity can be in and viable state transitions. We use a simplified lifecycle, similar to the one stated in [1], which can be seen as an abstraction of what is used in actual process engines, like jBPM[2] (described in Chap. 7.4 of [13]). Lifecycles are represented graphically with dots (states) and arrows (state transitions); state transitions are annotated with the event that triggers the transition. The lifecycle of an activity is shown in Fig. 7a and the one for gateways in Fig. 7b.

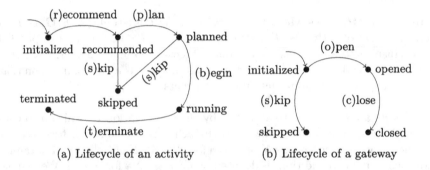

(a) Lifecycle of an activity   (b) Lifecycle of a gateway

Fig. 7. Lifecycles of activities and gateways

After creation, an activity is in the state **initialized**. Once the PIGS determines the activity's preconditions are fulfilled, the system puts the activity into the state **recommended**, meaning that it is displayed to the medical user. Now the user can either add it to the TC, leading to state **planned** or skip its execution (state **skipped**). A planned activity can begin execution, resulting in state **running**. The final state **terminated** indicates that the activity finished execution. States **recommended** and **planned** replace the state **enabled** usually used in activity lifecycle [1]. This allows to distinguish between activities recommended by the system and planned for execution by the medical user. Gateways are initialized in the beginning and can transition to state **opened**. From there they can transition to state **closed** or be skipped. The rules governing the transitions are described in Sect. 5.

4.2   The Execution Level

The central artefact on the execution level is the TC, which represents the running treatment process for one specific patient. Contrary to a process instance in BPMN, a TC does not belong to a single process model, but to a set of

---

[2] http://jbpm.jboss.org.

models on the model level, that contributed some treatment steps to this particular TC. Whenever an activity or gateway transitions to a new lifecycle state, the occurence of that transition is captured in the TC by adding an corresponding event to E_c and extending the order $<_c$. Hence, the TC records the history of one patient's treatment. Formally, the TC can be defined as follows.

Definition 3 (TC). A *TC* c is a tuple $(E_c, <_c)$, where E_c is a set of events corresponding to occurences of lifecycle transitions of activities, gateways, and BPMN events; and $<_c$ is a partial order on E_c, representing causal dependencies of events and respecting activity and gateway lifecycles.

$<_c^\circ := \{x \in E_c \mid \neg \exists y \in E_c : (x, y) \in <_c\}$ denotes the set of maximal elements of the partial order.

While a TC c represents the whole treatment history, the set $<_c^\circ$ of maximal elements represents the current state, i.e. only the last events that occured. Figure 8b shows a TC for the BPMN model in Fig. 8a. We use the shorthand notation $X.y$ to denote the event that activity X performed the transition y. $D := 7$ represents the event that A produced the data object D with the result 7. Therefore, $\varepsilon(B) = $ "$D \geq 5$" was satisfied and B recommended, as well as C, which has no attached expression. This particular TC displays the state after C has been planned. At the same time B is skipped and the gateway is closed. `Init` transitions are not displayed.

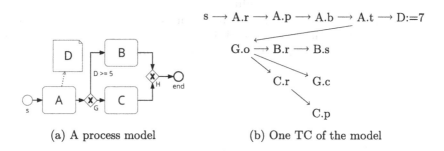

(a) A process model   (b) One TC of the model

Fig. 8. Example of a process model and a possible TC

5   Generating Treatment Recommendations

Having introduced the model level and TCs, we now turn to explaining how the PIGS approach recommends treatment steps. We approach this problem by giving an operational semantics to TCs, which formally specifies how they evolve. Thus, recommendation of treatment steps reduces to determining those activities from active process models, for which the preconditions are fulfilled. In the case of one active process model this coincides with the usual execution semantics of

BPMN, given by Weske [1] through event diagrams. This contribution formalizes and extends the usual semantics for the case of multiple active process models.

The semantics is defined as a set of inference rules (antecedent $\Rightarrow$ consequent), which are applied by the recommendation algorithm to the current treatment state, thus progressing the TC. The antecedent of a rule is to be read as follows: $X.y$ is a shorthand notation for $X.y \in <_c^\circ$, i.e. the event y of activity or gateway X belongs to the maximal elements of the partial order of the TC. Therefore, the evolution of a TC depends only on the current state of the TC as given by $<_c^\circ$. When the antecedent of a rule is fulfilled its consequent alters the TC by adding events. A consequent $W.z$ is shorthand for $E_c' = E_c \cup \{W.z\}$ and in addition $<_c' = <_c \cup \{(X.y, W.z)\}$ if $X.y$ has been given in the antecedent. We now discuss the rules in detail, and afterwards discuss decisions.

Activation Rules. Initially the TC for a patient is empty. A process model is activated, if the condition of its start event is fulfilled. The start event is added to the TC and all elements of the respective process model get initialized as stated by rule *Init*. During the course of a treatment, other process models can become activated, resulting in their start events being added to the TC.

The rule *Rec* specifies the conditions for activities to be recommended. An activity must be initialized, its predecessor in one of the process models must have terminated, and the expression attached to the activity must be fulfilled. Since several process models might be active and therefore many activities can be recommended, the system recommends only single activities rather than a sequence of activities, to avoid confusion. However, each recommendation is linked to the process model it is derived from, thus allowing to check the further course of action. The initialization condition $X.i$ prevents the recommendation of activities that succeed manually added activities Table 1 (using rule *Manu* in Table 2).

Table 1. Activation of process models and recommendations

Init	$s \in E_i \wedge \varepsilon(s) \Rightarrow s \wedge \forall X \in G_i \cup A_i : X.i$
Rec	$X.i \wedge Y.t \wedge (Y, X) \in F_i$ for some $i \wedge \varepsilon(X) \Rightarrow X.r$

Lifecycle Rules. The rules in Table 2 describe the (straightforward) progress of activities according to the lifecycle in Fig. 7a. The *Plan* rule states that an activity in state recommended can transition via the plan action into state planned. In this case the event $X.p$ is added to the TC event set E_c and the arc $(X.r, X.p)$ is added to the partial order $<_c$. This is analogous for the rules *Skip* and *Begin*. The rule *Term* states that when an activity terminates,

Table 2. Lifecycle transition rules

Plan	$X.r \Rightarrow$	$X.p$
Skip	$X.r \Rightarrow$	$X.s$
Start	$X.p \Rightarrow$	$X.b$
Term	$X.b \Rightarrow$	$X.t \wedge D := val$
Manu	$\Rightarrow$	$X.p$

it can produces a data event when it has data postconditions, i.e. $X.\blacksquare \neq \emptyset$. This data event refers to a data object and records its value. In the partial order it is connected to $X.b$. Finally, the *Manu* rule states that users can add arbitrary activities from $\mathcal{A}$ to the TC, corresponding to the blank activity labeled with '+' discussed in Sect. 3.

The state transitions are triggered by the user of PIGS. For activities that can be executed automatically without the intervention of a medical user the states **planned**, **running**, and even **terminated** might coincide, e.g. for an activity 'send release letter to general practitioner'.

Gateway Rules. The rules in Table 3 describe how gateways are opened and closed. The first rule, *Open*, states that initialized gateways are opened when their predecessor terminates (or one of their predecessors in case of a join). The second rule, $Rec^<$, states that open split gateways recommend all of their succeeding activities, the conditions of which are fulfilled. However, only one of those activities can be choosen by the medical user, because they are exclusive. This is ensured by the rule $SClose^\times$, which skips all other successors of a XOR split when one activity transitions to state **planned**. The third rule, $Rec^>$, states that join gateways recommend their only successor unconditionally when they close. The following four rules define closing of gateways. AND splits $(SClose^\wedge)$ close when no successor was skipped or is still recommended, while XOR splits $(SClose^\times)$ close when one successor is added to the TC, simultaneously skipping all other successors. AND joins $(JClose^\wedge)$ close when all predecessors terminated, while for XOR joins $(JClose^\times)$ one terminated predecessor suffices to close.

Table 3. Gateway transition rules

Open	$G.i$	$\wedge$	$X.t$	$\wedge$	$X \in \bullet G$		$\Rightarrow G.o$	
Rec$^<$	$G^<.o \wedge$		$X \in G^< \bullet$	$\wedge$	$\varepsilon(X)$		$\Rightarrow X.r$	
Rec$^>$			$G^>.t$	$\wedge$	$X \in G^> \bullet$		$\Rightarrow X.r$	
SClose$^\times$			$G^\times.o$	$\wedge$	$\exists! Y_k \in G^\times \bullet : Y_k.p$		$\Rightarrow G^\times.c$	$\wedge \forall_{l \neq k} Y_l.s$
SClose$^\wedge$			$G^\wedge.o$	$\wedge$	$\forall X_k \in G^\wedge \bullet : \neg(X_k.r \vee X_k.s)$		$\Rightarrow G^\wedge.c$	
JClose$^\times$			$G^\times.o$	$\wedge$	$\exists X \in \bullet G^\times : X.t$		$\Rightarrow G^\times.c$	
JClose$^\wedge$			$G^\wedge.o$	$\wedge$	$\forall X \in \bullet G^\wedge : X.t$		$\Rightarrow G^\wedge.c$	

Decisions. In general, activities have three different types of preconditions: control flow, i.e. another activity has to have happened before; data flow, i.e. a certain data object needs to be present in a particular state; and decision conditions. Decisions, which are part of all process modeling approaches, describe which of several activities to choose depending on data. A simple example would be to administer a blood thinner if the blood pressure of a patient is above a certain threshold. Such decisions are specified by attaching conditions to the successor nodes of a XOR gateway using the ε function.

The rules capture control flow conditions by referring to the flow relation F_i of process models. For data preconditions and the simple decisions described above, the rules refer to the function ε defined in Definition 1, mapping activities to an expression. The condition $\varepsilon(X)$ is part some rules' antecedent, which thus is only fulfilled if the expression evaluates to true for X. However, this evaluation is outside the scope of this contribution.

In many cases decisions are more complex and have several options on which to decide, and every option has a set of supporting and opposing arguments, the evaluation of which leads to a ranking of options. In such cases the outcome of evaluating $\varepsilon(X)$ is not boolean, but rather a numerical value, quantifying the support for an option. Technically, all options above a certain threshold should be recommended, weighted by their support. This would require to add the confidence of recommendations to the TC formalism and will be part of future work.

6   Conclusion

In this contribution we presented further details of the PIGS approach for process-oriented IT support of medical and organizational processes in hospitals. A set of BPMN process models capturing CPGs, CPs, SOPs and organizational processes is used to derive recommendations for treatment steps based on the current state of a TC. Therefore, we extended the usual lifecycle of an BPMN activity by an additional state. We gave a formal definition of a TC and a set of inference rules, which specify the evolution of the TC. Redundant and conflicting execution of activities can thus be avoided, since the treatment history is available to the user and the system. Since we only work with atomic tasks in the sense of BPMN in the Treatment Case, subprocesses in the model are handled by unfolding its internal to an atomic level. One limitation is the strict interpretation of process models, i.e. if activities from one guideline are performed in a different order or are skipped, the user "leaves" the process and therfore the guideline. This means she gets no further support for this model. A less strict interpretation should be considered in the future, especially if a step was skipped, because it has already been done in the nearer past or it would contradict to another recommendation. Another aspect, we haven't considered yet are tasks, which have to be scheduled at a specific point in time or that occur repetitively. Data-binding is out of scope in this work, but a data model (or ontology) has to be specified, when we implement the system. For now, we assume a simple key-value-store for the process models and treatment cases, which then has to be mapped to a specific ontology.

References

1. Weske, M.: Business Process Management: Concepts, Languages, Architectures, 2nd edn. Springer, Heidelberg (2012)
2. Grimshaw, J.M., Russel, I.T.: Effect of clinical guidelines on medical practice: a systematic review of rigorous evaluations. Lancet **342**(8883), 1317–1322 (1993)
3. Sutton, D.R., Fox, J.: The syntax and semantics of the PROforma guideline modeling language. J. Am. Med. Inform. Assoc. **10**(5), 433–443 (2003)

4. Boxwala, A.A., Peleg, M., Tu, S., Ogunyemi, O., Zeng, Q.T., Wang, D., Patel, V.L., Greenes, R.A., Shortliffe, E.H.: GLIF3: a representation format for sharable computer-interpretable CPGs. J. Biomed. Inform. **37**(3), 147–161 (2004)
5. Quaglini, S., Stefanelli, M., Cavallini, A., Micieli, G., Fassino, C., Mossa, C.: Guideline-based careflow systems. Artif. Intell. Med. **20**(1), 5–22 (2000)
6. Scheuerlein, H., Rauchfuss, F., Dittmar, Y., Molle, R., Lehmann, T., Pienkos, N., Settmacher, U.: New methods for clinical pathways - business process modeling notation (BPMN) and tangible business process modeling (t.BPM). Langenbecks. Arch. Surg. **397**(5), 755–761 (2012)
7. ISO/IEC: Information technology - object management group business process model and notation. Technical Report 19510, ISO/IEC, July 2013
8. Hewelt, M.: Process information and guidance systems in the hospital. In: KR4HC 2014 workshop proceedings (2014)
9. Milla-Millán, G., Fdez-Olivares, J., Sánchez-Garzón, I.: A common-recipe and conflict-solving MAP approach for care planning in comorbid patients. In: Bielza, C., Salmerón, A., Alonso-Betanzos, A., Hidalgo, J.I., Martínez, L., Troncoso, A., Corchado, E., Corchado, J.M. (eds.) CAEPIA 2013. LNCS, vol. 8109, pp. 178–187. Springer, Heidelberg (2013)
10. Sánchez-Garzón, I., Fdez-Olivares, J., Onaindía, E., Milla, G., Jordán, J., Castejón, P.: A multi-agent planning approach for the generation of personalized treatment plans of comorbid patients. In: Peek, N., Marín Morales, R., Peleg, M. (eds.) AIME 2013. LNCS, vol. 7885, pp. 23–27. Springer, Heidelberg (2013)
11. Alexandrou, D.A., Skitsas, I.E., Mentzas, G.N.: A Holistic Environment for the Design and Execution of Self-Adaptive Clinical Pathways. IEEE Trans. Inform. Technol. Biomed. **15**(1), 108–118 (2011)
12. Pryss, R., Langer, D., Reichert, M., Hallerbach, A.: Mobile task management for medical ward rounds – the MEDo approach. In: La Rosa, M., Soffer, P. (eds.) BPM Workshops 2012. LNBIP, vol. 132, pp. 43–54. Springer, Heidelberg (2013)
13. jBPM team, T.J.: jBPM Documentation - User Guide. jboss.org. 6.0.1.Final edn., November 2013

Modelling and Implementation of Correct by Construction Healthcare Workflows

Petros Papapanagiotou$^{(\boxtimes)}$ and Jacques Fleuriot

School of Informatics, University of Edinburgh,
10 Crichton Street, Edinburgh EH8 9AB, UK
{ppapapan,jdf}@inf.ed.ac.uk

Abstract. We present a rigorous methodology for the modelling and implementation of correct by construction healthcare workflows. It relies on the theoretical concept of proofs-as-processes that draws a connection between logical proofs and process workflows. Based on this, our methodology offers an increased level of trust through mathematical guarantees of correctness for the constructed workflows, including type correctness, systematic resource management, and deadlock and livelock freedom. Workflows are modelled as compositions of abstract processes and can be deployed as executable code automatically. We demonstrate the benefits of our approach through a prototype system involving workflows for assignment and delegation of clinical services while tracking responsibility and accountability explicitly.

Keywords: Process modelling in healthcare · Formal verification · Workflow automation · Healthcare process integration

1 Introduction

The primary aim of our research is to combine and use the rich theory of proofs-as-processes [1] and a rigorous, logical engine to develop a pragmatic methodology for the development of trustworthy, correct by construction healthcare workflows. This allows the combination of the benefits from both Business Process Modelling (BPM) and formal methods, so that in addition to the flexibility, scalability, maintainability, and separation of concerns offered by process modelling, we can obtain an added level of trust of the correctness and consistency with regards to the modelled workflows.

In particular, our efforts focus on the management of information and resources in clinical and administrative procedures involving health and social care providers. We provide a framework that allows a high level modelling of such procedures that can lead to the reduction of redundancies and process repetitions, better enforcement of policies and continuity and consistency of practice, while abstracting from the complex clinical decision making. Ultimately, this could improve patient safety and reduce costs and the time spent by carers in their effort to adhere to guidelines.

© Springer International Publishing Switzerland 2015
F. Fournier and J. Mendling (Eds.): BPM 2014 Workshops, LNBIP 202, pp. 28–39, 2015.
DOI: 10.1007/978-3-319-15895-2_3

Our methodology allows the construction of workflows as process compositions. Component processes can be specified abstractly based on their inputs, outputs, preconditions and effects. Our framework offers mathematical guarantees of correctness with respect to the information flow, resource management, typing, and deadlock and livelock freedom. Most importantly, our correct by construction workflows can be automatically deployed as executable code.

We begin the analysis of our approach by describing the core theoretical background in Sect. 2, followed by a breakdown of the methodology in Sect. 3. We analyse the added benefits of our formal approach in Sect. 4, whereas Sect. 5 describes the kind of healthcare processes that our approach is tailored to. We then demonstrate our methodology in a practical healthcare application, with emphasis on the deployment stage, in Sect. 6. We conclude with an overview of lessons learned with respect to the application of our methodology in healthcare in Sect. 7, brief comparison to related work in Sect. 8, and our plans for future work in Sect. 9.

2   Theoretical Background

Our approach involves validating that a system is correct in the sense that it is mathematically guaranteed to give the expected result based on its specification. Such guarantees of correctness are particularly important in healthcare systems, where maintaining safety and policy adherence is crucial and a bug in the code may have severe implications to patients' lives. For the purpose of formally verifying healthcare workflows, as already mentioned, we make use of the proofs-as-processes paradigm, which involves a mapping between logical proofs and processes described in process calculus terms.

Essentially, we can construct logical specifications of processes and process workflows using Classical Linear Logic (CLL) [5], which emphasizes formulas that represent resources. Assumptions cannot be ignored or copied so no resources can duplicate or vanish. CLL allows the construction of logical specifications of processes with respect to the types of their inputs, outputs, preconditions, and effects (IOPEs). Moreover, CLL allows the specification of IOPEs that are either parallel (simultaneous) or optional. Optional IOPEs can be used, for example, to express the possibility of a process throwing an exception instead of producing the expected result (e.g. when an unexpected obstacle occurs during an operation). It is worth mentioning that most process composition methodologies do not give explicit considerations to exceptions.

In order to abstract from the complicated underlying CLL specifications, we have devised an intuitive, diagrammatic representation [15], where processes are boxes with solid edges for parallel IOPEs and dashed edges for optional ones.

For instance, consider a possible specification for the process describing a blood test. In order to perform the test, we require the patient details, a referral, a scheduled time, and a blood sample. The blood test results can be either conclusive or inconclusive (in which *exceptional* case there may be a decision for repeating the blood test at a later date). This process can be specified in CLL and represented diagrammatically as shown in Fig. 1.

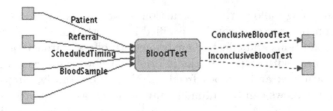

Fig. 1. Diagrammatic specification of the blood test process.

Using the proofs-as-processes paradigm, CLL workflow specifications can be translated to executable terms in the π-calculus [10], which is a formalism aimed at the description of concurrent processes as independent, atomic entities. These communicate asynchronously by message passing. Over the years, the π-calculus has inspired a variety of process algebras as well as BPM languages such as BPEL, and has been used as the means to formalise their semantics [8].

The combination of CLL and the π-calculus forms the basis for a formal semantics and rigorous workflow design, thus leading to workflow systems that are *correct by construction*, based on the methodology described next.

3   Methodology

Our methodology has been developed within the following set of assumptions:

1. We assume a set of atomic healthcare processes that can interface a variety of services, including Electronic Medical Records (EMRs), medical equipment and instruments, and Human Provided Services (HPSs) through the use of electronic forms. Each of these can be described using a type specification of their inputs, outputs, preconditions, and effects (IOPEs).
2. The methodology is agnostic to the inner working of the available processes, which are treated as 'black boxes'. We assume the processes are well behaved and always satisfy their type specification.
3. We assume all of the available processes always terminate.

Based on these assumptions, our methodology follows a standard process modelling approach. We consult with a variety of stakeholders, including healthcare practitioners, administrators, policy makers, and patients to breakdown the selected task into a number of individual but interdependent steps. The consultation is most commonly in the form of contextual interviews, shadowing, questionnaires, and frequent communication.

We then proceed to construct specifications of these steps as processes by identifying their IOPEs and formalising them using our logic based system. The system allows the combination of these processes to construct composite workflows. More specifically, processes can be combined in sequence, in parallel, and conditionally. Each process combination is formally verified by our underlying logic engine which performs the necessary inference steps automatically.

Once the composition stage is complete, the system provides a complete, executable, concurrent π-calculus specification for the constructed workflow. This allows the user to perform visual simulations using a built-in tool and empirically verify the behaviour of the workflow before deploying it as a live system.

Our system also provides advanced deployment functionality that allows the user to export executable Scala [13] code for a constructed workflow automatically. This is accomplished through our implemented extension of Scala's PiLib library [3] which allows a direct translation of π-calculus terms into Scala code.

The roadmap for our deployment procedure is shown in Fig. 2. Since we assume available processes are 'black boxes', the deployed code represents those as partially abstract classes (also known as *traits*) which need to be implemented as a concrete instance. The code of the Scala class responsible for the workflow execution and associated information flow is generated automatically.

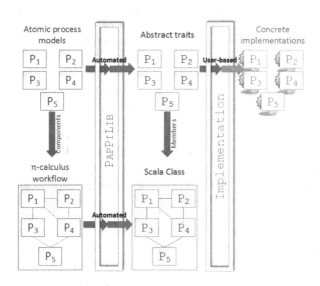

Fig. 2. The general roadmap of the workflow deployment procedure.

Scala allows a seamless integration with any available Java library, which makes the deployed system flexible with respect to integrating modern tools, such as EMRs, e-form technologies, healthcare devices etc.

The deployed code coordinates the available processes according to the corresponding formally verified workflow. It executes concurrently and asynchronously while remaining free of deadlocks and livelocks.

4   Benefits Through Proofs-as-processes

The mathematical core of the proofs-as-processes approach combines the properties of CLL with the concurrent computation of the π-calculus. We have embedded this theory in a logic-based engine called HOL Light [7]. The resulting framework allows the user to perform formally verified inference and construct process models, based on the methodology described above, while providing the following unique benefits with respect to the stated assumptions:

1. **Explicit, verified information/resource flow:** The constructed models aim to make the information and resource flow between existing atomic processes (Assumption 1) explicit and consistent. This includes enforcing the resource dependencies between the processes as introduced by the user, and allowing fine grained control of the process execution order as well as which processes should execute in which cases. This minimizes unnecessary clinical procedures and guarantees that all the necessary information (test results, patient records, clinical assessments, etc.) and resources (drugs, samples, equipment, etc.) will be available before any procedure is initiated.

2. **Systematic resource management:** As already mentioned, the properties of CLL disallow any *implicit* duplication or consumption (vanishing) of resources. This greatly facilitates resource accounting during composition so that the user does not need to manually keep track of resources, especially when there is a large number of them at a given stage. Limited resources, such as reusable results from costly, lengthy, or invasive medical tests, can not "magically" appear or disappear. Moreover, all possible outcomes (including exceptions that are often forgotten about), as defined by the IOPEs of the involved processes (Assumption 1) must be handled explicitly.

3. **Concurrent execution and deadlock and livelock freedom:** The composed workflow is executed concurrently in order to maximize efficiency. This allows for independent clinical procedures to be performed simultaneously, thus saving time, without the user having to explicitly state this (unless there is an explicit or implicit dependency, processes will run in parallel by default). At the same time, if each component process always terminates (Assumption 3), the theoretical background of our methodology guarantees that termination is preserved in the composed workflow and no deadlocks or livelocks are introduced during composition. This prevents, for example, the workflow being blocked by 2 clinicians waiting for feedback from each other.

4. **Type correctness during composition:** The logical engine guarantees the correct matching of the user-defined types (Assumption 1) as processes are being composed and eventually leads to executable code that is typechecked in advance. This allows deployment in untyped programming languages as well as integration of heterogeneous components. It also provides a degree of consistency and continuity in the workflow in the sense that it guarantees that the involved resource types do not mutate during execution.

5. **Automated workflow deployment:** The result of our composition is immediately translatable to executable code that can be used both for simulation purposes and in a production setting (e.g. a hospital). This minimizes the time and cost of workflow deployment which is particularly important, especially in cases of maintenance where minor updates in the process models or the corresponding healthcare policies can take a considerable amount of time

to be implemented in practice. In our case, this happens with the click of a button. Moreover, the abstraction from the inner working of each process (Assumption 2) allows our workflows to integrate with existing technologies, including medical devices, EMRs, mobile devices etc.

It is worth mentioning that our diagrammatic interface [15] hides the underlying reasoning engine so that little to no logic expertise is required to use our framework. The user applies mouse gestures to compose processes diagrammatically, with all logical inference steps taken care of automatically in the background. The resulting diagram depicts the information flow in the composite model so that it can be understood by a variety of stakeholders, including health carers, policy makers, and IT developers (see Fig. 3 for an example).

5   Healthcare Processes

The approach is tailored towards the modelling of everyday practices of care providers. These are governed by finite processes that repeat for every individual case, but are most commonly informal and require considerable amounts of time and effort from the carers, including the effort to track individual patient pathways daily by memory.

As previously mentioned, we focus on the exchange of resources and information in such processes, and we aim to provide automated coordination through verified workflow modelling. We, therefore, model individual, finite, terminating processes (that exclude iterative or feedback processes), which may involve the provision of healthcare services, administrative or documentation procedures, as well as interfacing with electronic systems such as medical devices and EMRs.

More specifically, our CLL based formalism, caters for abstract, high level process specifications and does not allow loops (but can include finite iterations). Although this level of expressivity may appear relatively simple in comparison to other workflow languages, and, moreover, introducing deadlock and livelock freedom in a language without loops may be viewed as less challenging, our recent experience in real-world healthcare modelling indicates that our framework fits well within the current needs of healthcare stakeholders (see Sect. 7).

We proceed to demonstrate our methodology in more detail through a working example involving collaboration patterns in healthcare.

6   Formal Verification of Collaboration Patterns in Healthcare

In our primary example, we use our formally verified process modelling methodology to model and deploy patterns of collaborative work in healthcare, originally described in recent work by Grando et al. [6]. Modelling aspects of this work have been described in detail in previous papers [14,16], whereas in the current work we concentrate on workflow automation.

We focus our investigation on basic collaboration scenarios in healthcare that involve two agents, also known as *actors*. These may correspond to any member of the medical staff, including doctors and nurses. We are particularly interested in two patterns or skeletal plans that differentiate between the types of collaboration through *assignment* and *delegation* of clinical services. In these, one of the two actors, the *requester*, asks for a particular clinical service (e.g. specialized diagnosis or treatment, administration of a drug, etc.) from the other, the *provider*. In order for a contract to be signed between the requester and the provider, it must be ensured that the provider is competent to perform the service. Moreover, depending on whether the service is assigned or delegated, responsibility and accountability is either transferred to the provider (assignment) or maintained by the requester (delegation). We proceed to explain the approach in more detail in the next few sections.

6.1 Process Modelling

The first stage of our BPM-inspired methodology involves the breakdown of the individual steps. Clinical services are broken down to a series of individual tasks and goals, also known as *keystones*, that each of the actors must perform in order to complete the service. These include tasks that must be performed in exceptional cases and unexpected situations. Each keystone has preconditions that must be met for it to be achieved, and success conditions that describe the achieved effects upon its successful completion. We give a brief description of the modelled keystones for the our healthcare collaboration patterns next:

- The `ServiceASSGRequest` and `ServiceDELGRequest` keystones initiate a request for an assignment and a delegation of a patient respectively.
- The `CollabDecision` keystone corresponds to the decision of whether there is a competent actor available to provide the service of a requested contract.
- Once a contract has been accepted by a competent provider the requester can finalize the agreement in the `ContractAwarded` keystone.
- The `ServiceProvide` keystone corresponds to the task of executing a requested clinical service that is currently pending. The service may either be completed successfully or an obstacle may occur preventing its completion.
- The `OutcomeCheck` keystone corresponds to the goal of checking the outcome of the provided service by the responsible actor. For simplicity we assume this goal is always successful.
- The `AssgResponsible` and `DelegResponsible` keystones correspond to automated procedures that determine the responsible actor in the cases of an assignment and a delegation respectively.

We proceed to compose these keystones/processes in 2 complete workflows that fully describe the patterns of assignment and delegation and enforce the responsibility and accountability constraints. Due to space limitations we only present the assignment workflow in Fig. 3, although, for those interested, both diagrams can be found in a previous paper [16].

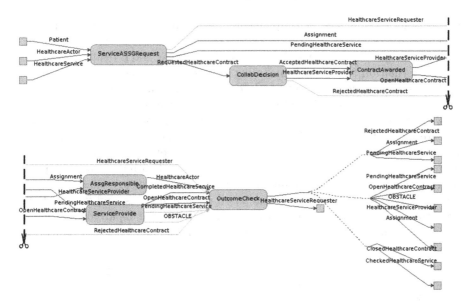

Fig. 3. Diagram of the *assignment* pattern as a verified process composition. Note that the pattern has been split into 2 parts at the indicated point for it to fit within the page.

6.2 Workflow Automation

We now come to the crux of the current paper: once the healthcare collaboration patterns have been modelled as formally verified workflows using our logic-based framework, our system allows the automatic deployment of Scala code in order to achieve computer-based coordination of the assignment and delegation procedures. The only requisite in order to produce a fully functioning system is the implementation of the keystones/processes, which can then be integrated directly in the deployed coordinator.

In order to demonstrate the functionality of such a deployment, we have developed a web-based system that emulates part of a hospital environment. We will simply refer to this system as the *DigiHealth* (Digital Healthcare) prototype.

DigiHealth includes a minimal relational database with dummy data about patients, medical staff, clinical services, handover contracts, and potential obstacles. Each keystone/process is implemented as an interaction with *DigiHealth*'s API. The order in which the API calls (process invocations) are made and the involved information is exchanged are both dictated by the formally verified workflow as opposed to some hardcoded solution. In this way, we obtain a full transition from a information/resource flow diagram (see Fig. 3) to the coordination of actual administrative procedures for the assignment and delegation of patients, with *all* the properties provided by our logic-based framework (see Sect. 4). Additional workflows can be defined on top of the same available processes, so that different guidelines, cf. the patient delegation case in the previous section, can be implemented while reusing the existing process implementations.

The user interface is accessible by any mobile device, and provides all the necessary information to the user, including available contracts, pending requests, pending services, and the ability to initiate new assignments or delegations of patients. A sample screenshot of the interface is shown in Fig. 4.

It is worth noting that the user is only shown information and processes that are relevant to them. They are relieved from the burden of keeping track of patients, monitoring the state of the assignment or delegation taking place (or more generally the state of the patient flow), coordinating the next steps, or ensuring the information is communicated to all the necessary clinical collaborators. Using simple selections, e-form based point and clicks, and standard gestures, the users only perform their own part, while the the the deployed coordinator takes care of the workflow based on the diagrammatic, logic-based specification.

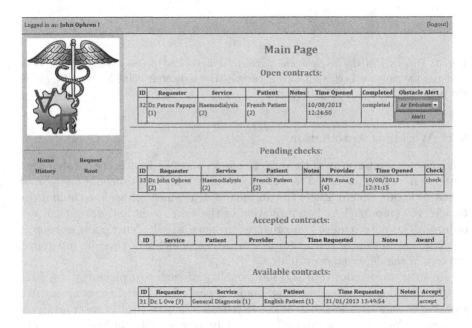

Fig. 4. Sample screenshot from the prototype DigiHealth system.

7   Lessons Learned

Our formally verified process modelling is currently being applied to real-world projects involving (distinct groups of) UK clinicians interested in aspects such intra-hospital patient transfers and integrated care pathways. For example, we are collaborating with leading HIV clinicians in Glasgow and Edinburgh in an ongoing effort for the automation of Integrated Care Pathways for HIV patients in Scotland. Our preliminary models include the first three months of care for HIV patients, including assessment and consultation. Based on these collaborations, we believe that our methodology is particularly applicable to healthcare for the following reasons:

1. In real world healthcare scenarios, there is a very large number of resources being exchanged at every stage as well as many conditional and exceptional situations, and it often becomes cumbersome to keep track of or record them in a formalised healthcare procedure. Our framework greatly facilitates this task, thanks to its resource accounting mechanisms.
2. The task of tracking information and resources itself is deemed of high importance in healthcare, because it affects the efficiency, time, and cost of every day care provision and, more importantly, patient safety, since, for example, patient drop outs due to neglected pathways are common.
3. It is often challenging to communicate the technicalities of workflows to healthcare practitioners. Experience has shown that our diagrammatic models are easily understandable by clinical collaborators and allow them to reflect upon their practices. The prospect of automated deployment is also very attractive to carers, who spend a large fraction of their valuable time tracking, memorizing, and documenting pathways.
4. The mathematical core of our framework provides guarantees that enable all stakeholders to trust that the modelled workflow will behave correctly.
5. The formal underpinnings of the used languages, namely CLL and the π-calculus, in combination with the abstract level of the process specifications open the doors to further analysis and verification, including the possibility to integrate with other workflow, simulation, and verification technologies.

To summarize, despite the relative simplicity of our process specifications, our methodology seems to fit well for the particular purpose of formalising healthcare procedures such as integrated care pathways as workflows to improve every day practices of healthcare providers.

8   Related Work

The current research is inspired by recent work by Grando et al. [6]. In this, they proposed logic-based, pen-and-paper specifications of reusable patterns for specifying assignment and delegation of tasks and goals during collaborative work and sketched proofs that desirable properties, known as *safety principles*, related to accountability, responsibility, and competence could be ensured.

Workflow-based approaches are often used in healthcare informatics to provide automated IT support for practitioners. Tallis [17], for example, is one of the leading tools for the specification and enactment of clinical applications. Such tools are most commonly used in an effort to support decision making in diagnosis and treatment. In our case, though, we are closer to a business process oriented approach that abstracts from these procedures and focuses on improving the operational support and automating some of the organizational aspects of patient care by, for instance, alleviating the need to communicate the same information to multiple people separately, automatically documenting repetitive information, and detaching social conventions from the healthcare workflow.

A related approach focusing on organisational workflows in healthcare with the aim of minimizing medical errors is presented by Malhotra et al. [9]. They focus on building a cognitive model of the workflow in order to identify error-prone regions. TESTMED [2] is another related project aimed towards providing operational support in hospital wards through multimodal interfaces.

The main advantage of our approach compared to others is the formal verification of the constructed patterns and the automated extraction of an executable model. The end-product is a system whose correctness is mechanically verified with associated guarantees regarding the enforcement of modelled conditions and policies, thereby allowing a high level of trust in the implemented workflow.

9   Conclusion and Future Work

In this work, we presented a formal verification approach to the modelling and implementation of healthcare workflows. Our methodology takes advantage of the proofs-as-processes paradigm, a theory that connects logical proofs with process workflows, in order to generate correct by construction process compositions. In particular, we provide mathematical guarantees of properties for the generated workflows, including a verified information flow, systematic resource management, type correctness, and deadlock and livelock freedom. Workflows are modelled as compositions of abstract processes, specified by their inputs, outputs, preconditions, and effects. The verified models can be automatically deployed as executable Scala code, thus greatly facilitating workflow automation and maintenance. The deployed systems support integration and interoperability with existing infrastructure and may be accessed by mobile devices.

We demonstrate the value our methodology adds to traditional process models through the prototype system *DigiHealth*. Patterns of collaboration in healthcare involving *assignment* and *delegation* of clinical services are formalised and deployed on *DigiHealth*, allowing for the automation of the corresponding procedures based on a verified protocol. The stakeholders can work their way through the two workflows using the web interface, without the need to keep track of the progress themselves, and with the added trust our rigorous framework provides.

Our plans for future work involve a variety of optimisations on the generated code, including distributed execution (for deployment on the Cloud) and tracking of workflow analytics. In addition, we plan to explore connections and mappings to existing technologies such as the Business Process Model and Notation (BPMN) [12], the Business Process Execution Language (BPEL) [11], and RESTful web services [4]. Finally, we are looking to pursue further collaborations with healthcare providers and policy makers to investigate other potential uses of our methodology for the formalisation of healthcare procedures.

Acknowledgments. This research was supported by an EPSRC doctoral scholarship, by EPSRC grant EP/J001058/1, and by a grant from the College of Sciences and Engineering of the University of Edinburgh. We would like to thank the reviewers for their constructive comments.

References

1. Bellin, G., Scott, P.: On the π-calculus and linear logic. Theoretical Computer Science **135**(1), 11–65 (1994)
2. Cossu, F., Marrella, A., Mecella, M., Russo, A., Bertazzoni, G., Suppa, M., Grasso, F.: Improving operational support in hospital wards through vocal interfaces and process-awareness. In: 2012 25th International Symposium on Computer-Based Medical Systems (CBMS), pp. 1–6. IEEE (2012)
3. Cremet, V., Odersky, M.: PiLib: a hosted language for Pi-Calculus style concurrency. In: Lengauer, C., Batory, D., Blum, A., Odersky, M. (eds.) Domain-Specific Program Generation. LNCS, vol. 3016, pp. 180–195. Springer, Heidelberg (2004)
4. Elkstein, M.: Learn REST: A tutorial, February 2008. http://rest.elkstein.org/
5. Girard, J.Y.: Linear logic: its syntax and semantics. In: Girard, J.Y., Lafont, Y., Regnier, L. (eds.) Advances in Linear Logic. London Mathematical Society Lecture Notes Series, vol. 222. Cambridge University Press, Cambridge (1995). http://iml.univ-mrs.fr/girard/Synsem.pdf.gz
6. Grando, M.A., Peleg, M., Cuggia, M., Glasspool, D.: Patterns for collaborative work in health care teams. AI in Med. **53**(3), 139–160 (2011)
7. Harrison, J.: HOL Light: A tutorial introduction. In: Srivas, M., Camilleri, A. (eds.) FMCAD 1996. LNCS, vol. 1166, pp. 265–269. Springer, Heidelberg (1996)
8. Lucchi, R., Mazzara, M.: A pi-calculus based semantics for WS-BPEL. J. logic algebraic program. **70**(1), 96–118 (2007)
9. Malhotra, S., Jordan, D., Shortliffe, E., Patel, V.L.: Workflow modeling in critical care: Piecing together your own puzzle. J. of Biomedical Informatics **40**(2), 81–92 (2007). http://dx.doi.org/10.1016/j.jbi.2006.06.002
10. Milner, R.: Communicating and mobile systems: the π-calculus. Cambridge Univ Presss, Cambridge (1999)
11. OASIS: Web Services Business Process Execution Language, version 2.0, OASIS Standard (2007). http://docs.oasis-open.org/wsbpel/2.0/OS/
12. Object Management Group: Business Process Model and Notation (BPMN), version 2.0 (2011). http://www.omg.org/spec/BPMN/2.0/PDF
13. Odersky, M.: The Scala language specification, version 2.8. Programming Methods Laboratory, EPFL Lausanne, Switzerland, October 2013
14. Papapanagiotou, P., Fleuriot, J., Grando, A.: Rigorous process-based modelling of patterns for collaborative work in healthcare teams. In: 2012 25th International Symposium on Computer-Based Medical Systems (CBMS), pp. 1–6. IEEE (2012)
15. Papapanagiotou, P., Fleuriot, J., Wilson, S.: Diagrammatically-driven formal verification of web-services composition. In: Cox, P., Plimmer, B., Rodgers, P. (eds.) Diagrams 2012. LNCS, vol. 7352, pp. 241–255. Springer, Heidelberg (2012)
16. Papapanagiotou, P., Fleuriot, J.D.: Formal verification of collaboration patterns in healthcare. Behaviour & Information Technology (2013)
17. Tallis: The tallis toolset (2011). http://archive.cossac.org/tallis/

MET4: Supporting Workflow Execution for Interdisciplinary Healthcare Teams

Szymon Wilk[1]([⊠]), Davood Astaraky[2], Wojtek Michalowski[2], Daniel Amyot[3], Runzhuo Li[3], Craig Kuziemsky[2], and Pavel Andreev[2]

[1] Institute of Computing Science, Poznan University of Technology, Poznań, Poland
szymon.wilk@cs.put.poznan.pl
[2] Telfer School of Management, University of Ottawa, Ottawa, Canada
[3] School of Electrical Engineering and Computer Science,
University of Ottawa, Ottawa, Canada

Abstract. This paper describes MET4, a multi-agent system that supports interdisciplinary healthcare teams (IHTs) in executing patient care workflows. Using the concept of capability, the system facilitates the maintenance of an IHT and assignment of workflow tasks to the most appropriate team members. Moreover, following the principles of participatory medicine, MET4 facilitates involving the patient and her preferences in the management process. We describe conceptual foundations of the system and present the system design combining multi-agent and ontology-driven paradigms. Finally, we present a prototype implementation of MET4 and illustrate operations of the prototype using an example involving chronic pain management in palliative care.

1 Introduction

An interdisciplinary healthcare team (IHT) includes healthcare practitioners from different domains/specialties, who work together to achieve a common goal of providing evidence-based care to a patient [14]. In clinical practice, team-based approach is used to manage complex medical cases – this practice has been shown to reduce patient management costs and time, improve service provision and enhance patient satisfaction [2].

Very often patient management by an IHT follows a patient care workflow that is generally defined as a sequence of steps corresponding to clinical tasks and decisions [8]. While executing these tasks, members of an IHT collaborate, communicate by exchanging information about the patient's state and care provided (directly, or through an electronic health record – EHR), and coordinate their activities [15].

The overall goal of our research is to build MET4 – a system to support an IHT in executing a patient care workflow and to operationalize principles of participatory medicine that posit patient's active involvement in a care process. This general goal is decomposed into specific goals that are addressed in this paper, namely (1) developing a conceptual model to facilitate our understanding of the problem at hand, (2) developing a formal design of an agent-based system

© Springer International Publishing Switzerland 2015
F. Fournier and J. Mendling (Eds.): BPM 2014 Workshops, LNBIP 202, pp. 40–52, 2015.
DOI: 10.1007/978-3-319-15895-2_4

and (3) implementing a prototype version of the designed system to support execution of the chronic pain management workflow. We build on our earlier research on designing and developing multi-agent clinical decision support systems (CDSSs) [1,18]. Specifically, we expand the results published in [1] by extending the conceptual foundations of the system to include the concepts of *team leadership* and *patient participation* in the management process and by revising how workflows are represented. We also describe a prototype implementation of MET4 and present its operations.

2   Related Work

Challenges of collaboration and coordination in healthcare and other domains produced intensive research in the area of computer-supported cooperative work (CSCW) [17]. The multi-agent paradigm has shown to be suitable for modeling CSCW because of the inherent cooperative nature of agents, as demonstrated in two projects aimed at designing and developing assisted living applications – K4CARE [10] and CASIS [11].

K4CARE's main objective was to create, implement, and validate a knowledge-based healthcare model (based on patient care workflows) of professional assistance to senior patients at home. While K4CARE supports IHTs, it provides relatively basic support for team management, as the team members have to be explicitly associated with workflow tasks they are capable to execute. CASIS, on the other hand, is an event-driven, service-oriented and multi-agent frame work, whose main goal is to provide context-aware healthcare services to elderly residents.

In the area of diagnosis, CDSSs often need the integration of different sources of data and involve the collaboration of different members of a team. The multi-agent paradigm in such a context was successfully used in the OHDS [16] system. OHDS supports physician in establishing a diagnosis using information pertinent to each patient and leveraging bio-medical data contained in various external databases. The system uses agents and ontologies to organize unstructured bio-medical data into structured disease information.

A common challenge faced when developing a CDSS is related to integration of patient data with the CDSS engine, as this requires interoperability between existing systems and medical devices. The MobiGuide [7] project aims to address this challenge by providing guideline-based clinical decision support integrated with a personal health record.

3   Conceptual Model of MET4

In this section, we present the conceptual model of MET4 as a description of assumptions, concepts and relations between these concepts. The goal of this model is to facilitate our understanding of workflow execution by an IHT and to lay foundations for the system design.

We assume that an IHT manages a patient according to a presentation-specific workflow (where by presentation we mean a disease, a specific type of trauma, etc.). The team is formed when the patient management needs to start (e.g., at the time of hospital admission after preliminary diagnosis has been made), and it is disbanded when the execution of the workflow is completed.

The team has a *leader* responsible for overseeing the execution of a workflow, for handling exceptional situations and for delegating workflow tasks to suitable team members (i.e., members who are qualified to perform these tasks) – in this sense the leader plays a role very similar to the role of the *most responsible physician* [3]. Moreover, following the principles of *participatory medicine* [9], the leader can consult with the patient before making any relevant decisions, such as selecting a therapy or selecting a team member. While there can be only one team leader at a time, she can change during workflow execution (e.g., at one point a surgeon leads a team, while at some other time she is replaced by an anesthesiologist) – this is similar to what has been proposed in [12].

In the conceptual model we employ a *hybrid team formation* that combines static and dynamic approaches (see [10] for their detailed description). The leader is selected when the workflow starts, and stays with an IHT until the workflow is competed, or the need for a new leader is explicitly indicated by the workflow (static approach). Other team members are recruited dynamically to execute tasks from the workflow and released from the team afterwards. Specifically, a new member is recruited only if the leader is not able to perform the task at hand. Such simplicity is the major advantage of the hybrid approach – there is no need for scheduling or thorough analysis of the workflow. At the same time, it is also a disadvantage, as it is impossible to form a team in a more efficient manner (e.g., to re-use team members for different tasks).

We distinguish between normal and urgent workflow tasks (we assume such information is given as part of the task description) – the former can be temporary suspended, while the latter have to be executed with no delay. If a practitioner qualified to perform an urgent task is busy with a normal task, then execution of this normal task is suspended and the practitioner is recruited for the urgent task.

In order to provide fine-grained characteristics of a practitioner and a task, we introduce the concept of *capability*, which is defined as an ability to perform a certain clinical task [6]. A capability is additionally annotated with a *capability level* that indicates the level of competency in performing this task. Generally, the capability level should be expressed using some ordinal scale – it could be a simple numerical score or a qualitative value. For simplicity, we assume that capability levels are given in the former form.

A practitioner may have multiple capabilities – we refer to these capabilities as *possessed capabilities*. On the other hand, capabilities associated with workflow tasks are called *required capabilities*. A practitioner is able to perform a certain task if she possesses all the required capabilities, and the levels of possessed capabilities at least meet the levels of required capabilities.

Obviously, there may be many practitioners capable to perform a given task. In such situation, a team leader should consult the patient in order to evaluate and rank possible candidates. If the patient does not have preferences, or there is a tie between the candidates, then additional criteria need to be employed. For example, the leader can select the practitioner with the best capabilities (i.e., capabilities with the highest levels), or take the one with the lowest workload.

The concept of required capability is also used for defining requirements that need to be satisfied by a team leader. Specifically, we assume a patient care workflow starts with a leader appointment task that is associated with the capabilities required from the leader. Unlike the selection of a team member, the leader selection relies solely on capabilities possessed by the practitioners considered for this position, and patient preferences are not taken into account. Moreover, if a workflow invokes another workflow, and this invoked workflow involves appointment of a new leader, then the previous leader is temporary suspended, and then restored when the invoked workflow terminates.

In order to fully conform to principles of participatory medicine that advocate integration and equal participation of IHT members and patients or family members [9], we introduce the concept of *patient representative* that complements the concept of *patient*. A patient is a passive receiver of care and a "provider" of clinical data, whereas a patient representative represents a patient and actively participates in all decision-making activities that affect patient care. While in most cases the patient and the patient representative are the same person, there are situations where such distinction is necessary, e.g., during the management of a pediatric patient when the parent or legal guardian become a representative. Also we assume that there is a single patient representative associated with the patient and the team.   .

4   Design and Implementation of MET4

In this section we show how the conceptual model of MET4 has been formalized into the system's design, and how the design has been implemented as a prototype system. The design was created using Organization-based Multi-agent System Engineering (O-MaSE) – a flexible methodology for analyzing and designing multi-agent systems (MASs) [5]. O-MaSE starts with system specifications (conceptual model in our case) and iteratively translates them into a number of models (domain model, goal model, agent class model, protocol model, plan models) that describe various aspects of a MAS and that drive subsequent implementation.

Due to the space limit, we present below only the domain and agent class models – the remaining models present hierarchy and dependencies between goals to be achieved by the system (goal model), communication protocols employed by agents (protocol models), and plans and algorithms employed by the agents to achieve goals (plan models). A detailed description of O-MaSE and its clinical application (designing a CDSS for patient management in the emergency department) is given in [18].

4.1 Domain Model

The domain model provides an ontology (Fig. 1) formalizing the system's domain knowledge. This ontology should be considered as a schema to construct ontological models that represent specific workflows, practitioners and patients. The ontology is divided into three areas that define concepts and relations associated with patients, teams and workflows. These areas overlap – in particular the concepts of capability and presentation are shared between the areas.

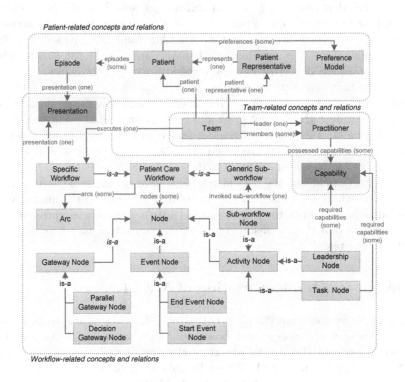

Fig. 1. Domain ontology

Most of the patient- and team-related concepts have been described in Sect. 3. A new concept here is *preference model*, which captures patient's preferences with regards to a specific type of decision (for example, a patient may have one preference model for evaluating a therapy and another for evaluating interventions). We assume preference models are represented using various formats (functional, relational and rule-based) and they are employed by a patient representative.

The workflow-related part of the domain ontology is inspired by the Business Process Model and Notation (BPMN), and it has been tailored to address the particularities of IHTs (we could not directly use BPMN because it does not allow for representing capabilities). The central concept is *patient care workflow*, specialized into *specific workflow* and *generic sub-workflow*. The former represents a "top-level" patient care workflow that is associated with a specific presentation. The latter is a generic workflow (i.e., not associated with any presentation) that can be shared and re-used (i.e., invoked by other workflows).

Each patient care workflow is composed of *arcs* and *nodes*, so it can be represented as a directed graph. The node concept is specialized into *gateway node*, *event node* and *activity node*, depending on its purpose. Gateway node is further specialized into *decision gateway node* and *parallel gateway node*, which allow for conditional branching and parallel paths, respectively. Event nodes are used to indicate starting and ending points in a workflow (by *start event node* and *end event node*). Finally, activity node is specialized into *task node*, *sub-workflow node* and *leadership node* corresponding to three types of basic activities in a workflow – executing a clinical task, invoking a sub-workflow and appointing a team leader, respectively.

4.2 Agent Class Model

An agent class model defines what types of agents are needed to achieve the goals, and it shows interactions between the agents and actors (users, external systems and other entities, such as repositories or databases). The agent class model derived for MET4 is given in Fig. 2. We need to note that several goals associated in the conceptual model with a leader (e.g., supporting team maintenance and overseeing workflow execution) have been offloaded to autonomous agents classes (*team manager* and *workflow executor*) in order to minimize the practitioner's workload associated with the leadership activities.

Most of the agent classes introduced for MET4 have been already described in detail in [1,18], therefore, we focus here on new or expanded ones. The *patient representative* agent class has been introduced to act on behalf of the patient or guardian, it manages a set of patient's preference models and uses them to evaluate possible decision choices. The *practitioner assistant* class has been extended to achieve the goals associated with consulting decision choices with a patient representative whenever necessary. Finally, the *team manager* class has been modified to support leaders' management (i.e., maintaining lists of active and temporarily suspended leaders, identifying practitioner assistant agents, who can be team leaders, informing selected agents about appointment, and informing leaders about their status). It uses information from *yellow pages* – a shared directory where agents from the *practitioner assistant* class register their possessed capabilities and availability (i.e., free, busy with a normal task, busy with an urgent task).

4.3 Prototype Implementation

The prototype of MET4 has been implemented using *Workflows and Agent Development Environment* (WADE, http://jade.tilab.com/wade). WADE allows for developing, deploying and running multi-agent systems, where agents cooperate and coordinate their activities according to a set of workflows. It provides

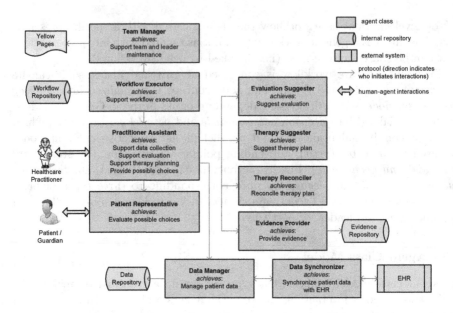

Fig. 2. Agent class model for MET4

Java programming libraries, visual workflow development tools and an execution environment acting as a middleware for developed systems.

The domain model (see Fig. 1) has been implemented and stored in Protégé (http://protege.stanford.edu). Protégé is also used as a knowledge base to store ontological models representing specific workflows, specific practitioners and patient data collected using MET4.

Finally, as indicated in Fig. 2, we assume MET4 interacts with an EHR available in a given healthcare organization to exchange patient data. For the prototype implementation, we used the OpenMRS system [19], an open-source and web-based EHR. OpenMRS and MET4 (specifically the *data synchronizer* agent) communicate using REST web services and JSON for encoding exchanged information. Data integration is achieved through the mechanism of concept maps that allow associating data concepts used in OpenMRS with concepts employed in other systems.

5   Illustrative Example

5.1   Chronic Pain Management in Palliative Care

Palliative care aims at improving the quality of life of the patient, who suffers from terminal diseases, by managing symptoms (e.g., pain, nausea or fatigue), coordinating care, and providing emotional and spiritual support [13]. Chronic pain management is a significant component of any palliative care management protocol, as it is estimated that 70 % of advanced cancer patients experience pain [4]. The complexity of chronic pain management in terminal patients necessitates that care delivery is provided by a team of practitioners from different specialties (e.g., physicians, psychologists, and physiotherapists, nurses, and occupational therapists).

Building on existing pain management guidelines and consulting with the domain experts, we created a set of workflows to structure all activities associated with assessing, diagnosing, and managing pain for a palliative care patient. These workflows were implemented in WADE, and the top-level workflow and selected sub-workflows are illustrated in Fig. 3. This figure also presents required capabilities associated with the leadership and task nodes.

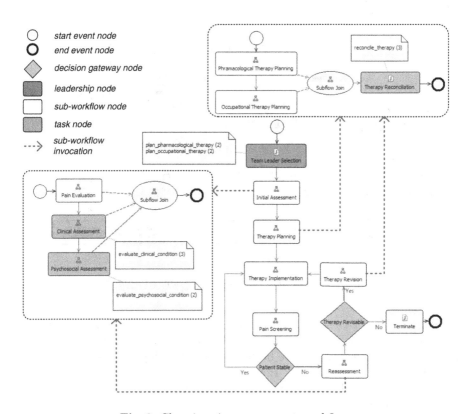

Fig. 3. Chronic pain management workflow

The workflows in Fig. 3 contain no parallel paths (and thus no parallel gateway nodes), because such paths are not directly supported by WADE. Fortunately, they can be easily simulated as a sequence of asynchronous activity nodes. Such a sequence requires a *subflow join* node that is WADE-specific and therefore has not been considered in the domain model (it may become unnecessary if we use another workflow-related technology). For example, *pain evaluation*, *clinical assessment* and *psychosocial assessment* in the initial assessment sub-workflow are actually all executed in parallel, although it is not evident from the WADE-specific representation.

5.2 Supporting Chronic Pain Management by MET4

To illustrate operations of MET4 we use three scenarios: team leader selection, team maintenance and therapy reconciliation. In all these scenarios we assume a configuration of the MET4 system presented in Fig. 4, where we use *"label : agent class"* as a notation to describe specific agents. For the sake of readability, the figure does not show the decision support agents (they are irrelevant in the considered scenarios).

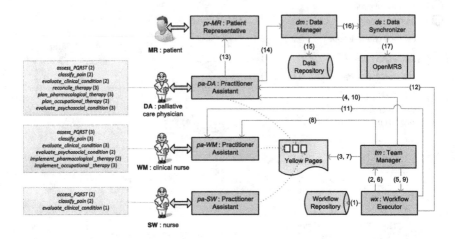

Fig. 4. Sample configuration of MET4 for chronic pain management

Figure 4 also shows interactions in the system occurring in the considered scenarios. Patterns associated with selected interactions (e.g., between the *tm* agent and the *yellow pages*) have been established during the design phase and are embedded in agents' plans. However, the overall sequence of interactions depends on a particular workflow and available practitioners, thus it is established during run-time.

For simplicity we limit the set of available practitioners to three, identified in Fig. 4 as *DA*, *WM* and *SW*. They are further described with possessed capabilities, and each has a corresponding practitioner assistant agent (*pa-DA*, *pa-WM* and *pa-SW*, respectively) described with the same capabilities as its human owner and registered in the *yellow pages*.

Finally, we assume a patient (*MR*), who has a *patient representative* agent (*pr-MR*) with a preference model for evaluating therapies – so this is a situation, where a patient and a patient representative is one person. The preference model is realized as a value function that computes an overall score for possible therapeutic options. The patient has no other preference model, which means he is indifferent to choices and options associated with other decisions, including selection of team members.

Team Leader Selection Scenario. Once the *MR* patient has been admitted, the *wx* agent retrieves from the *workflow repository* the patient care workflow for managing chronic pain ((1) in Fig. 4). The first activity node involves appointing a leader. In order to do this, the *wx* agent sends a request to the *tm* agent to find a practitioner assistant agent that possesses the capabilities required for leading the IHT (2), so the corresponding practitioner may become the leader. The *tm* agent consults the *yellow pages* for the information about available agents and their capabilities (3). The only agent that possesses the required capabilities is *pa-DA*, therefore, it is notified about being selected (4), and this choice is reported to the *wx* agent (5).

Team Maintenance Scenario. Here, the *wx* agent proceeds to the next activity node in the workflow, which is the initial assessment. Execution of this activity involves invoking a sub-workflow. One activity in this sub-workflow is *pain evaluation*, which we assume has been already completed during previous visit, and the results have been recorded in OpenMRS. The other two tasks nodes (*clinical assessment* and *psycho-social assessment*) need to be executed in parallel (see Fig. 3).

First, the *wx* agent sends a request to the *tm* agent to find two practitioner assistant agents that could perform the above tasks (6). According to the capability-based selection procedure, *pa-DA*, who is already the team leader, qualifies for *psychosocial assessment*. However, for the *clinical assessment* task node, the *tm* agent has to search for a qualified candidate in the *yellow pages*, where *pa-WM* is identified as potential team member (7). Then, *tm* asks *pa-WM* to confirm that it agrees to be part of the team (8). Assuming that practitioner *WM* accepts this request, the information about these two agents is sent back to *wx* by *tm* (9). Then, *pa-DA* and *pa-WM* are sent requests to complete the two tasks discussed here (10 and 11, in any order) and these agents through user interface (see Fig. 5) prompt practitioners *DA* and *WM* to collect patient data.

Therapy Reconciliation Scenario. Here, we assume that the *pa-DA* agent has already been selected for the *therapy reconciliation* task. First, the *wx* agent sends a request to *pa-DA* to perform this task ((12) in Fig. 4). In response, *pa-DA* checks for possible interactions between pharmacological and occupational therapies derived earlier and constructs possible combined therapies. Then, it communicates with the *pr-MR* agent to learn about patient's preferred combined therapy (13). This is accomplished by applying the preference model to possible therapies and reporting resulting scores. The *pa-DA* agent selects the therapy with the highest score and reports this choice to the *dm* agent (14). The *dm* agent stores the selected combined therapy in the *data repository* (15) and notifies the *ds* agent (16), which in turn notifies OpenMRS about the update (17).

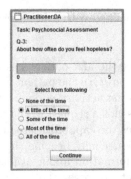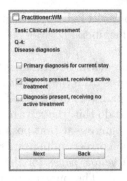

Fig. 5. Sample user interface presented to practitioners *DA* and *WM*

6   Discussion

We have presented conceptual foundations, design, implementation and operations of the MET4 system that supports an IHT in executing a patient care workflow. MET4 maintains a team and its leader and assigns workflow tasks to the most qualified team members. This is accomplished by employing capabilities to characterize practitioners and workflow tasks and by following a hybrid strategy to maintain the team.

MET4 also implements the principles of participatory medicine by introducing the concept of a patient representative and a corresponding agent class. Such solution allows for including patient preferences in the management process. Moreover, in order to support communication and awareness of practitioners, the system manages data collected during management and synchronizes it with an EHR (OpenMRS).

As part of future research we plan to enrich the team maintenance strategy by accounting for situations where a group of practitioners has to manage multiple patients at the same time – in such case the global allocation of practitioners has to be considered. Moreover, we are going to develop more sophisticated plans for the practitioner assistant agent that will allow handling exceptional and ad-hoc situations in automatic or semi-automatic manner. We are also working on considering patient preferences to modify the structure of a workflow. Finally, to ensure data security and privacy, we plan to adopt access control techniques described in [12] and to combine them with the team maintenance strategy.

References

1. Astaraky, D., Wilk, S., Michalowski, W., Andreev, P., Kuziemsky, C., Hadjiyannakis, S.: A multiagent system to support an interdisciplinary healthcare team: a case study of clinical obesity management in children. In: Proceedings of the VIII Workshop on Agents Applied in Health Care, Murcia, Spain, pp. 69–80 (2013)

2. Borrill, C., Carletta, J., Carter, A., Dawson, J., Garrod, S., Rees, A., Richards, A., Shapiro, D., West, M.: The effectiveness of health care teams in the National Health Service. University of Aston, Birmingham (2001)

3. Capen, K.: When patient care is shared, who is the most responsible physician? CMAJ **154**(6), 885–886 (1996)

4. Franks, P.J., Salisbury, C., Bosanquet, N., Wilkinson, E.K., Kite, S., Naysmith, A., Higginson, I.J.: The level of need for palliative care: a systematic review of the literature. Palliat. Med. **14**(2), 93–104 (2000)

5. Garcia-Ojeda, J.C., DeLoach, S.A., Oyenan, R.W.H., Valenzuela, J.L.: O-MaSE: a customizable approach to developing multiagent development processes. In: Luck, M., Padgham, L. (eds.) AOSE 2007. LNCS, vol. 4951, pp. 1–15. Springer, Heidelberg (2008)

6. Gardner, A., Hase, S., Gardner, G., Dunn, S.V., Carryer, J.: From competence to capability: a study of nurse practitioners in clinical practice. J. Clin. Nurs. **17**(2), 250–258 (2008)

7. González-Ferrer, A., Peleg, M., Verhees, B., Verlinden, J.-M., Marcos, C.: Data integration for clinical decision support based on openEHR archetypes and HL7 virtual medical record. In: Lenz, R., Miksch, S., Peleg, M., Reichert, M., Riaño, D., ten Teije, A. (eds.) ProHealth 2012 and KR4HC 2012. LNCS, vol. 7738, pp. 71–84. Springer, Heidelberg (2013)

8. Grando, M.A., Peleg, M., Cuggia, M., Glasspool, D.: Patterns for collaborative work in health care teams. Artif. Intel. Med. **53**(3), 139–160 (2011)

9. Hood, L., Auffray, C.: Participatory medicine: a driving force for revolutionizing healthcare. Genome Med. **5**(12), 110 (2013)

10. Isern, D., Moreno, A., Snchez, D., Hajnal, A., Pedone, G., Varga, L.Z.: Agent-based execution of personalised home care treatments. Appl. Intell. **34**(2), 155–180 (2011)

11. Jih, W., Hsu, J.Y., Tsai, T.: Context-aware service integration for elderly care in a smart environment. In: Proceedings of the 2006 AAAI Workshop on Modeling and Retrieval of Context Retrieval of Context, pp. 44–48. AAAI Press, Menlo Park (2006)

12. Le, X., Doll, T., Barbosu, M., Luque, A., Wang, D.: An enhancement of the role-based access control model to facilitate information access management in context of team collaboration and workflow. J. Biomed. Inform. **45**(6), 1084–1107 (2012)

13. Morrison, L.J., Morrison, R.S.: Palliative care and pain management. Med. Clin. North. Am. **90**(5), 983–1004 (2006)

14. Oandasan, I., D'Amour, D., Zwarenstein, M., Barker, K., Purden, M., Beaulieu, M., Reeves, S., Nasmith, L., Bosco, C., Ginsburg, L.: Interdisciplinary education for collaborative, patient-centred practice: research and findings report. Health Canada, Ottawa (2004)

15. Ruan, J., MacCaull, W., Jewers, H.: Enhancing patient-centered palliative care with collaborative agents. In: Proceedings of the 2010 IEEE/WIC/ACM International Conference on Web Intelligence and Intelligent Agent Technology (WI-IAT), vol. 3, pp. 356–360. IEEE (2010)

16. Ulieru, M., Hadzic, M., Chang, E.: Soft computing agents for e-health in application to the research and control of unknown diseases. Inform. Sci. **176**(9), 1190–1214 (2006)

17. Weerakkody, G., Ray, P.: CSCW-based system development methodology for health-care information systems. Telemed. J. E Health. **9**(3), 273–282 (2003)

18. Wilk, S., Michalowski, W., O'Sullivan, D., Farion, K., Sayyad-Shirabad, J., Kuziemsky, C., Kukawka, B.: A task-based support architecture for developing point-of-care clinical decision support systems for the emergency department. Meth. Inf. Med. **52**, 18–32 (2013)
19. Wolfe, B.A., Mamlin, B.W., Biondich, P.G., Fraser, H.S., Jazayeri, D., Allen, C., Miranda, J., Tierney, W.M.: The OpenMRS system: collaborating toward an open source EMR for developing countries. AMIA Annual Symposium Proceedings, p. 1146 (2006)

Enhancing Guideline-Based Decision Support with Distributed Computation Through Local Mobile Application

Erez Shalom[1]([⊠]), Yuval Shahar[1], Ayelet Goldstein[1], Elior Ariel[1],
Silvana Quaglini[2], Lucia Sacchi[2], Nick Fung[3], Valerie Jones[3],
Tom Broens[4], Gema García-Sáez[5,6], and Elena Hernando[5,6]

[1] Department of Information System Engineering, The Medical Informatics
Research Center, Ben Gurion University of the Negev, Beersheba, Israel
{erezsh,yshahar,gayelet,eliorar}@bgu.ac.il
[2] Dipartimento di Ingegneria Industriale e dell'Informazione,
University of Pavia, Pavia, Italy
{silvana.quaglini,lucia.sacchi}@unipv.it
[3] University of Twente, Enschede, The Netherlands
{l.s.n.fung,V.M.Jones}@ewi.utwente.nl
[4] Mobihealth BV, Enschede, The Netherlands
t.h.broens@amc.uva.nl
[5] Bioengineering and Telemedicine Centre, Universidad Politécnica de Madrid,
Madrid, Spain
{ggarcia,elena}@gbt.tfo.upm.es
[6] CIBER-BBN: Networking Research Centre for Bioengineering,
Biomaterials and Nanomedicine, Madrid, Spain

Abstract. We introduce the need for a distributed guideline-based decision support (DSS) process, describe its characteristics, and explain how we implemented this process within the European Union's MobiGuide project. In particular, we have developed a mechanism of sequential, piecemeal *projection*, i.e., 'downloading' small portions of the guideline from the central DSS server, to the local DSS in the patient's mobile device, which then applies that portion, using the mobile device's local resources. The mobile device sends a *callback* to the central DSS when it encounters a triggering pattern predefined in the projected module, which leads to an appropriate predefined action by the central DSS, including sending a new projected module, or directly controlling the rest of the workflow. We suggest that such a distributed architecture that explicitly defines a dialog between a central DSS server and a local DSS module, better balances the computational load and exploits the relative advantages of the central server and of the local mobile device.

Keywords: Clinical guidelines · Decision support · Distributed computing

1 Introduction – The Need for Distributed Decision Support

Traditional guideline-based decision-support systems (DSS) mainly target physicians at the point of care. Physicians, however, are not the only potential recipients of advice;

© Springer International Publishing Switzerland 2015
F. Fournier and J. Mendling (Eds.): BPM 2014 Workshops, LNBIP 202, pp. 53–58, 2015.
DOI: 10.1007/978-3-319-15895-2_5

patients can also be empowered to manage their own disease, especially through the use of applications running on personal mobile devices. Nevertheless, mobile-based applications might miss critical recommendations based on clinical guidelines [1], if they are not connected to a guideline server.

Thus, the main goal of the MobiGuide project [2] is to develop a distributed patient guidance system that integrates hospital and monitoring data into a Personal Health Record (PHR) accessible by patients and physicians and that provides personalized, secure, clinical-guideline-based guidance both inside and outside standard clinical environments. The distributed model of such a framework might be implemented as service oriented architecture [3], which might be more suitable for distributing a process inside a hospital. However, in the case of the MobiGuide project, we have chosen to split the architecture into two main components: a back-end DSS (BE-DSS) residing on a server system (this could be a cloud server, or, as in our case, on-premise servers in hospitals), and a mobile DSS (mDSS) residing on the patient's mobile device. The local mDSS components are necessary to distribute computationally intensive monitoring and decision-making processes, with respect to data and knowledge requirements, at the local device level.

1.1   The Factors for Decision-Support Distribution

Consider a process of monitoring each patient's high-frequency ECG sensor signals by means of patient-worn biosensors, linked via bluetooth to the mobile device, and detecting a pattern of Atrial Fibrillation (AF) that can be abstracted from these signals by the mDSS, and sent to the central PHR to support a guideline-based recommendation to the patient and/or physician by the BE-DSS: such a distribution of labor, in which the AF detection for each patient is done by the mDSS is natural, and prevents an over burdening of the central BE-DSS server. Furthermore, the local mDSS is also essential for continuity of care when for some reason there is no internet connection to the central DSS; we would still want the patient to be provided with alerts relevant to the latest guideline by which she was being managed. However, not all decisions can be made locally on the mobile (despite ever increasing processing power and storage). Some decisions require the full historical (longitudinal) patient data, which should not reside on the mobile device. In some cases the decision to be made is a part of a long-term plan in the complete clinical guideline knowledge base (which is continuously maintained by medical domain experts) and in other cases broader medical declarative (interpretation) knowledge may be needed in order to switch to another branch in the guideline, or even to a completely different guideline; such knowledge resides only on the central knowledge-base server. In such cases, we want the mDSS, when encountering certain local predefined (temporal) patterns, to send a *callback* message to the BE-DSS, asking for further instructions, resulting in a BE-DSS recommendation, and even a completely new projected guideline or guideline branch.

We adopted a distribution policy based on a number of factors in order to determine whether various decisions and actions should be applied at the BE-DSS level or at the mDSS level. These factors are: who is the actor of the decision (patient or physician); the temporal horizon of future recommendations e.g. immediate alerts by the mobile device when some value is out of range, versus longer-term guideline-based decisions at the server); the data and knowledge resources needed for the decision; the need for PHR access, and a consideration of where a potential personalization of the guideline should reside. These principles need to be considered by the knowledge engineer and expert physicians during the knowledge specification phase. However, once it is decided that the decision can be applied by the mDSS, i.e., can support the patient when he/she is not with the physician, the mDSS needs the relevant guideline knowledge. Therefore, there is a need to *project* ('download') small portions of the guideline, referred as *projections*, from the BE-DSS to the mDSS, and applies it using the mobile's local resources.

2   The Knowledge Projection Model Methodology

As the projection relates to *knowledge* and not to data, we refer to it as a *knowledge projection*, or *projection* for short. Each portion of the guideline which can be identified as a self-contained executable knowledge package to be potentially projected and applied in the mDSS, is called a *projection*. It is identified (tagged) as a *projection point* ("projection point" is a point in the guideline in which the designer made the decision to project a part of the guideline to the mobile device.). Only parts of the guideline that are applicable to the current state of the patient are projected. Hence, the projected knowledge includes implicitly also knowledge about the current state of the patient. The main challenge in designing the projection process during the guideline specification time is to choose at which level (mDSS or BE-DSS) the plans and decisions should be placed, and which patterns should trigger callbacks to the central server. When choosing these projection-points in the guideline, consideration should be given to not only to technical analysis methodologies, but also to clinical properties, such as whether the decision could be taken by the patient alone, supported by the mobile device (in that case, it could be delegated to the mDSS) or whether it should be taken by the physician using the patient's full historical record and the complete guideline knowledge (should be performed on the BE-DSS). To facilitate the process of identifying projection points, we enhanced our current guideline-specification methodology: The first phase in this methodology is to create a local consensus of the guideline. The local consensus is a structured document that describes schematically the interpretation of the guideline agreed upon by both the expert physicians and the knowledge engineers, and includes the clinical directives of the guideline and the semantic logic of the specification language [4]. After creating the local consensus, the elicitation phase splits into two parallel branches: The first branch is the "traditional" one and is directed at the care professional; the second branch includes conceptually a parallel part of the process that focuses on the patient's behavior and is added to the mobile-customized guideline. Thus, we refer to the resulting specification as the *Parallel Workflow* [5]. Each parallel workflow includes parts of the guideline that might be potentially projected. After this process, the knowledge engineer might use the characteristics listed in the previous section to determine the projection points. Currently, this process is done manually by setting as "True" a special property called "is Projected" that we added to the knowledge schema. However, based on our experience, we have started the process of designing an automatic broker that will suggest a set of projection points within the guideline, during the specification, or following phase. Figure 1 shows an example of the projection workflow: After the physician starts the Gestational Diabetes Mellitus (GDM) guideline, the plan "monitoring blood pressure twice a week", previously tagged as a projection point is downloaded to the mDSS and applied by the mobile device [6]. When the mDSS encounters the triggering pattern "abnormal blood pressure", a callback message is sent to BE-DSS, which reacts with a new projection "monitoring the blood pressure daily". Via the back-end, the physician can inspect and explore data collected from the patient mobile, or respond to recommendations.

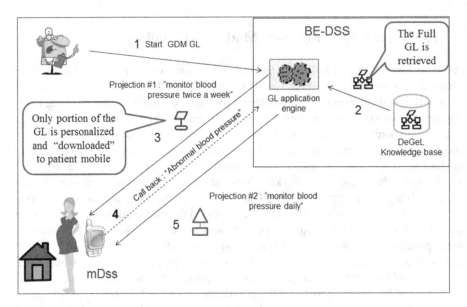

Fig. 1. An example of a projection workflow for the "monitoring blood pressure" plan, and the tagging of the "blood pressure" plan as a projection.

3 The Projection Schema and Support of Personalization

There are three principles that we suggest should be followed when defining the projection schema:

1. *Separation of declarative and procedural knowledge:* One of the principles of defining the projection schema was to benefit from using the DeGeL [7] knowledge schema which supports the separation between declarative and procedural knowledge. Therefore, the knowledge projection model is separated into two types: (1) a Declarative projection model – including concepts (raw data and simple abstractions), and personal (patient-specific) events that induce predefined customized contexts in the guideline, within which the guideline's actions might be

modified (e.g., a personal *Wedding* event might induce for a particular patient the predefined *"high carbohydrate intake"* customized context mentioned in the guideline), and (2) a Procedural projection model– including plans for general treatments, or for specific personal contexts treatments.

2. *Support of Personalization:* The personal events are sent to the mDSS before starting the guideline application session because the mDSS has to initialize the patient (mobile) interface. For example, the mDSS sends to the patient interface the list of personal events that were selected during the initial registration session as inducing certain predefined contexts in the customized guideline. These personal events will be shown to the patient at the start of the application so that he or she can choose the current personal event (e.g. "holiday", "work", "regular" or "wedding"). For example, after choosing the personal event "work" and starting the guideline application, when setting a new personal event, e.g., "holiday", a second additional procedural projection might be sent to the mDSS with different monitoring scheduling.

3. *Definition of appropriate callbacks* – When a certain predefined pattern is detected at the mobile-device end by the mDSS, it triggers the mDSS to send a message to the BE-DSS to "take control" and continue the application of the GL. One example is a pattern of several consecutive days of high fasting blood glucose levels, signifying that the patient is not well controlled. This message is called a "callback", and is predefined in the projection. A callback might lead to the sending of a new projection to the mobile. Thus, the projections and callbacks support a continuous dialog between the BE-DSS and the mDSS. In any case, the BE-DSS continues to apply the GL and to send the appropriate personalized projections to the mDSS when necessary.

4   Discussion

The projection and callback mechanism that we are implementing supports a continuous dialog between the BE-DSS and the mDSS, and exploits the relative advantages of the different computational architectures and their respective access to clinical data and medical knowledge. We believe that the principles underlying this two-tiered architecture are rather general and support both functional (e.g., scalability) and non-functional (e.g., efficiency, security) requirements.

Initially, the architecture included decision support (to both patients and clinicians) provided only by the BE-DSS. That, however, did not easily cater to multiple local monitoring actions and reminders or to the robustness of the system with respect to connectivity; thus, we added the projection and callback mechanisms, splitting the decision-support tasks between the BE-DSS and the mDSS. Currently, we are in year 3 of a 4-year project. We have implemented the distributed projection process in the case of the GDM and AF guidelines: In the case of the GDM guideline, 39 projection points were tagged, and in the case of the AF guideline, 20. Most of the projection points were cyclical plans for measurements (e.g. blood glucose), and callback messages which can significantly reduce the computational load on the BE–DSS. In the coming year, we will perform a pilot study to test the feasibility of using a distributed DSS architecture to manage patients managed under one of two guidelines: The GDM guideline in the case of the Sabadell Hospital in Barcelona, Spain, and the AF guideline in the case of the Fondazione Salvatore Maugeri, Pavia, Italy.

Acknowledgements. The MobiGuide project (http://www.mobiguide-project.eu/) has received funding from the EU's Seventh Framework Programme for research, technological development and demonstration under grant agreement no. 287811.

References

1. Chomutare, T., Fernandez-Luque, L., Arsand, E., Hartvigsen, G.: Features of mobile diabetes applications: review of the literature and analysis of current applications compared against evidence-based guidelines. J. Med. Internet Res. **13**(3), e65 (2011). doi:10.2196/jmir.1874
2. Peleg, M., Shahar, Y., Quaglini, S.: Making healthcare more accessible, better, faster, and cheaper: the MobiGuide project. Eur. J. ePractice Issue Mob. eHealth **20**, 5–20 (2014)
3. Besana, P., Barker, A.: Towards decentralised clinical decision support systems. In: Brahnam, S., Jain, L.C. (eds.) Advanced Computational Intelligence Paradigms in Healthcare 5. SCI, vol. 326, pp. 27–44. Springer, Heidelberg (2010)
4. Shalom, E., Shahar, Y., Taieb-Maimon, M., Lunenfeld, E., Bar, G., Yarkoni, A., Young, O., Martins, S.B., Vaszar, L.T., Goldstein, M.K., Liel, Y., Leibowitz, A., Marom, T., Lunenfeld, E.: A quantitative evaluation of a methodology for collaborative specification of clinical guidelines at multiple representation levels. J. BioMed. Inform. **41**(6), 889–903 (2008)
5. Sacchi, L., Fux, A., Napolitano, C., Panzarasaa, S., Peleg, M., Quaglini, S., Shalom, E., Soffer, P., Tormene, P.: Patient-tailored workflow patterns from clinical practice guidelines recommendations. In: Medinfo 2013 (2013)
6. García-Sáez, G., Rigla, M., Martínez-Sarriegui, I., Shalom, E., Peleg, M., Broens, T., Pons, B., Caballero-Ruíz, E., Gómez, E.J., Hernando, M.E.: Patient-oriented computerized clinical guidelines for mobile decision support in gestational diabetes. J. Diabetes Sci. Technol. (2014). doi:10.1177/1932296814526492
7. Shahar, Y., Young, O., Shalom, E., Galperin, M., Mayaffit, A., Moskovitch, R., et al.: A framework for a distributed, hybrid, multiple-ontology clinical-guideline library, and automated guideline-support tools. J. Biomed. Inform. **37**(5), 325–344 (2004)

Storlet Engine for Executing Biomedical Processes Within the Storage System

Simona Rabinovici-Cohen[✉], Ealan Henis, John Marberg,
and Kenneth Nagin

IBM Research – Haifa, Mount Carmel, 31905 Haifa, Israel
{simona,ealan,marberg,nagin}@il.ibm.com

Abstract. The increase in large biomedical data objects stored in long term archives that continuously need to be processed and analyzed requires new storage paradigms. We propose expanding the storage system from only storing biomedical data to directly producing value from the data by executing computational modules - storlets - close to where the data is stored. This paper describes the Storlet Engine, an engine to support computations in secure sandboxes within the storage system. We describe its architecture and security model as well as the programming model for storlets. We experimented with several data sets and storlets including de-identification storlet to de-identify sensitive medical records, image transformation storlet to transform images to sustainable formats, and various medical imaging analytics storlets to study pathology images. We also provide a performance study of the Storlet Engine prototype for OpenStack Swift object storage.

1 Introduction

Two trends are emerging in the context of storage for large biomedical data objects. The amount of biomedical data objects generated by various biomedical devices such as diagnostic imaging equipment, medical sensors, wearable devices and genomic sequencers, is increasingly growing both in the number of objects and in the size of each object. Additionally, these large data sets which may be stored in geographically dispersed archives over many years, need to be continuously maintained, processed and analyzed to reveal new insights. A second trend is the arising of new highly available, distributed object/blob stores that can serve lots of data efficiently, safely, and cheaply from anywhere over the Wide Area Network (WAN). Unlike traditional storage systems that have special purpose servers optimized for I/O throughput with low compute power, these new object stores are built from commoditized off-the-shelf hardware with powerful CPUs.

We propose to marriage these two trends and leverage the new storage system processing capabilities to execute computations. We define *Storlets* as dynamically uploadable computational modules running in a sandbox within the storage, and propose them for biomedical processes. While with traditional storage systems, analyzing biomedical data requires moving the data objects from the

© Springer International Publishing Switzerland 2015
F. Fournier and J. Mendling (Eds.): BPM 2014 Workshops, LNBIP 202, pp. 59–71, 2015.
DOI: 10.1007/978-3-319-15895-2_6

storage system to the compute system, we propose to upload data-intensive bio-medical storlets to the storage system and execute the processing close to the data residency.

For example in the pathology department, a tissue block is cut off into thin slices and mounted on glass slides. The thin slices may then be stained with different stains, e.g. HER2, PR, ER, and images are taken for the original and the stained slices. These images may be very large up to 200 K over 200 K pixels and can consume about 5–10 GB storage. Later on, business processes may be initiated to mine and analyze those large pathology images. Here are some examples:

- **ROI Extraction.** The pathologist wants to extract a region of interest (ROI) from several images taken from the same tissue block. In the traditional flow of this business process, all the many images of the tissue block are downloaded from the hospital storage infrastructure to the pathologist machine. He then applies on his machine an *Image Alignment* module to align the various images. Next, he selects a few images and apply *ROI Extraction* module to extract the relevant box from them. Afterwords, a *Format Transformation* module may also be applied to transform the data from its propriety format to a standardized one that can be rendered on the pathologist machine. With storlets technology, we can substantially improve the efficiency of this business process. The pathologist will trigger the *Image Alignment Storlet, ROI Extraction Storlet*, and *Format Transformation Storlet* to run within the storage infrastructure. Only the final result of the transformed ROI image will be downloaded to the pathologist machine.
- **Cell Detection.** In continuation to the previous flow, the oncologist now wants to analyze the ROI images created by the pathologist. The oncologist gets the ROI images and applies *Cell Detection* module to detect what are the cells, their shapes and count in the image. The *Cell Detection* module is based on heavy computer vision algorithms that require a lot of CPU, memory and even special hardware (GPU). The oncologist machine may be too weak to execute this module, and thus fails to produce the result. With storlets technology, the *Cell Detection Storlet* will run in the cluster of machines within the storage. Only the final result will be successfully displayed in the oncologist machine. Moreover, when the *Cell Detection* module is updated, e.g., due to new computer vision algorithms, we just need to upload the updated storlet to the storage infrastructure which is much less effort than downlaoding all the images to the oncologist machine again.
- **Cohort Identification.** A researcher would like to get a cohort of images with similar features from as multiple patients as possible. In the traditional business process, an hospital assistant would need to download all images from the storage infrastructure to a staging compute system. Then, the assistant would apply *Image Similarity* module to create a cohort, followed by a *De-identification* module to comply with HIPAA. Finally, the de-identified cohort is sent to the researcher. With storlets technology, the *Image Similarity Storlet* will run in the cluster of machines within the storage. Then, the

De-identification Storlet will de-identify the data within the storage and send to the researcher. This is more secure than the traditional method as it spares the need to move clear data to the staging system.

To summarize, the benefits of using storlets are:

1. **Reduce bandwidth** – reduce the number of bytes transfered over the WAN. Instead of moving the data over the WAN to the computational module, we move the computational module to the storage close to the data. Generally, the computational module has much smaller byte size than the data itself.
2. **Enhance security** – reduce exposure of sensitive data. Instead of moving data with Personally Identifiable Information (PII) outside its residence, perform the deidentification and anonymization in the storage and thereby lower the exposure of PII. This provides additional guard to the data and enables security enforcement at the storage level.
3. **Save costs** – consolidate generic functions that can be used by many applications while saving infrastructure at the client side. Instead of multiple applications writing similar code, storlets can consolidate and centralize generic logic with complex processing.
4. **Support compliance** – monitor and document the changes to the objects and improve provenance tracking. Instead of external tracking of the objects transformations over time, storlets can track provenance internally where the changes happen.

To enable the use of storlets, the storage system need to be augmented with a *Storlet Engine* that provides the capability to run storlets in a sandbox that insulates the storlet from the rest of the system and other storlets. The Storlet Engine expands the storage system's capability from only storing data to directly producing value from the data.

The concept of storlets was first introduced in our paper [1], where storlets were used to offload data-intensive computations to the Preservation DataStores (PDS). It was afterwards investigated in the VISION Cloud project[1]. Our main contribution is the introduction of storlets for biomedical processes and the definition of the Storlet Engine for OpenStack Object Storage (code-named Swift)[2]. We describe the architecture of the Storlet Engine as well as the programming model for storlets. The security model of the Storlet Engine supports storlets multi-tenancy and various types of sandboxes. We also provide a performance study of the Storlet Engine prototype.

The Storlet Engine was developed as part of PDS Cloud [2] that provides storage infrastructure for European Union ENSURE[3] and ForgetIT[4] projects. The Storlet Engine is used to process archived data sets in medical, financial, personal and organizational use cases. Various data sets and storlets were examined for the projects; some described in the above example business processes.

---

[1] http://www.visioncloud.eu.

[2] https://wiki.openstack.org/wiki/Swift.

[3] http://ensure-fp7.eu.

[4] http://www.forgetit-project.eu.

2   Storlet Engine Architecture

The Storlet Engine provides the storage system with a capability to upload storlets and run them in a sandbox close to the data. Figure 1 illustrates the Storlet Engine architecture that is generic with respect to the object storage used. It includes two main services:

– **Extension Service** – connects to the data-path of the storage system and evaluates whether a storlet should be triggered and in which storage node.
– **Execution Service** – deploys and executes storlets in a secure manner.

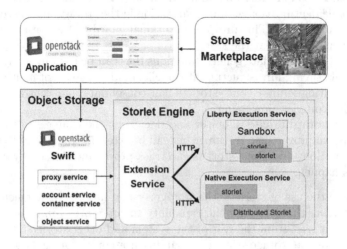

Fig. 1. Storlet engine architecture

The extension service is tied to the storage system at intercept points and identifies requests for storlets by examining the information fields (e.g., HTTP headers, HTTP query string) in the request and by evaluating predefined rules. The extension service then performs a RESTful call to one of the execution services that executes the storlet in a sandbox according to the client request and its credentials. The extension service needs to adapt the hooks into the object storage and may need for that either the source code or an open interface to internally connect to the storage system. We prototyped the Storlet Engine for OpenStack Swift Storage that is open source.

The Storlet Engine supports multiple execution services and multiple programming languages for storlets. It supports execution of Java storlets in an execution service based on IBM Websphere Liberty Profile product that is a web container with small footprint and startup time. We also support native execution service for storlets written in Python or other languages that are wrapped in a Docker[5] container, which is open source software to pack, ship and run an

---

[5] https://www.docker.io.

application as a lightweight Linux container. A storlet may call other storlets; even if the other storlet is in a different execution service.

The Storlet Engine can reside in the storage interface node (e.g. proxy node in Swift), and in the storage local node (e.g. object node in Swift). We implemented the ability to run storlets either in the interface proxy servers or in the local object servers to take advantages of each node underutilized resources. The performance study in Sect. 4 shows that it's preferable to run data-intensive storlets in the local object node. Yet, for storlets that are compute intensive or access several objects in different object servers, it may be preferable to execute them in the interface proxy node.

A Storlets Maketplace can be used as a repository of storlets from different vendors. An application on top of the storage can mashup and use different storlets from the marketplace for creating its functionality. For example, an HMO can create in the Marketplace a deidentification storlet that complies with HIPAA. A PACS provider can create in the Marketplace an imaging analytics storlet. Then, another application can use the two storlets from different vendors to analyze deidentified medical images and correlate them with deidentified medical records.

2.1 Storlet Development

A storlet is a data object in the object store that includes executable code. The storlet code is based on the standard Java servlet technology; thus the storlet developer may use the extensive existing development tools for servlets. The storlet includes three aspects:

- **Lifecycle management** – includes operations such as storlet deployment, storlet configuration and initialization, processes and threads management, storlet execution, inter-storlet communication. Lifecycle management is provided by the Storlet Engine.
- **Business logic** – the actual functionality of the storlet. This is provided by the client or application that creates the storlet.
- **Services invocation** – calls performed by the storlet to the Storlet Engine for external functionality e.g. to access additional objects, call other storlets, perform integrity check.

2.2 Services Storlets

The Storlet Engine provides special services storlets that can be used either by external clients or called by other running storlets. One such service storlet is the Distributed Storlet. The Distributed Storlet is a compound service storlet that executes multiple storlets in a pre-defined flow. It is a compound storlet in the sense that it calls other storlets and consumes their results. It is a service storlet as it is provided by the Storlet Engine itself, and not by external developers. This storlet is intended for analytics processes where distributed data-intensive processing on multiple objects is required.

The input parameters to the Distributed Storlet include the *resources* data objects to process, the *split* storlets to activate on the resources and the *merge* storlets that combine the results. We have used the Distributed Storlet to perform cells detection in pathology images. The Cell Detection storlet includes a complex time-consuming algorithm. Thus, the Distributed Storlet activates multiple Cell Detection storlets in parallel on each data object at its residence. Then, it waits for all split storlets' results and calls the merge storlet to combine the detected cells to one image.

Conceptually, the Distributed Storlet has similarity to MapReduce programs that transform lists of input data elements into lists of output data elements [3]. However, the Distributed Storlet is specialized for distributed processing within the storage system, sparing the data transfer to the compute nodes.

Another service storlet is the Sequence Storlet which is a compound service storlet that executes multiple storlets one after the other. The output of one storlet is the input to the next storlet in the sequence. The output of the final storlet is returned to the user. The Sequence Storlet is provided by the Storlet Engine as all services storlets.

Those services storlets are written in Python and run in the native execution service.

2.3   Rules Mechanism

The goal of the rules mechanism is to allow implicit storlet activation via predefined conditionals, thereby enabling automatic conditional activation of storlets. The storlets implicitly invoked by rules are in addition to the explicit storlet activation. Normally explicit storlet activation, if requested, takes priority and overrides implicit storlet activation. However, rules are also used to enforce access control related actions by marking the request with a specially marked flag. For such requests passing through the rules mechanism is mandatory. For example, mandatory de-identification storlet on sensitive data is enforced for requests having limited access credentials.

The rules mechanism is implemented via a rules handler that implements the rules logic (per stored rules), in combination with the user and system parameters. The rules handler is part of the extension service in each one of the Swift nodes that includes the Storlet Engine.

Typical inputs of the rules handler include request parameters, system metadata (e.g., content-type), user metadata (e.g., role, tenant), and the stored rules set. The output of the rules handler includes a full specification of the objects, parameters and REST request headers required for invoking a storlet.

Examples of executing storlets on the basis of predefined rules and various input parameters include: (a) de-identification storlet (depending on the role attribute of the user in the request), (b) content transformation for the entire container (depending on the content type of the object provided in the request).

3   Security Model

The Storlet Engine is an extension of the storage system. As such, it needs to adhere to the following security requirements.

- Storlets should execute in a protected environment where users (clients) do not over-reach their privileges. Specifically, access to data (e.g., Swift objects) from within a storlet should be allowed according to the user's permissions.
- In a multi-tenant storage environment, full isolation among tenants is a fundamental concept. This must be extended into the storlet's environment. Storlet requests coming from a given tenant should not be exposed to any aspect of requests coming from a different tenant (including data, state, etc.).
- Storlets originate from different sources. The code is not always fully verifiable for safety and consistency. The storlet engine must guard against malicious storlets, as well as intruding requests wanting to abuse the storlets.
- Multiple storlets serving multiple clients co-exist in the storage system. The storlet environment should support scalability. Storlets must not consume excessive resources (cpu, memory, etc.) that might degrade the performance of the system to an unacceptable level.

3.1   Sandboxes

When a storlet is deployed, it is placed in a "sandbox", that controls and limits the capabilities and actions of the code. A sandbox typically can block undesirable actions, such as direct access to cloud storage, or communication outside the local machine. It can also restrict access to the local filesystem and to local ports.

Currently two types of sandboxes are available, associating different levels of trust with different storlets:

- **Admin Sandbox:** the storlet is fully trusted, has no restrictions, and can perform all actions.
- **User Sandbox:** the storlet is less trusted, and therefore restricted from performing certain actions, such as writing to the filesystem except in designated work areas, reading from areas of the filesystem that are irrelevant to the storlet, making arbitrary network connections, or issuing sensitive system calls.

3.2   Implementing Multi-tenancy and Sandboxes

We implement a lightweight sandbox mechanism, leveraging capabilities of the underlying operating system. It does not rely on unique properties of a given storlet execution environment, and can potentially be applied in multiple different storlet execution environments in the same system. The only assumption is that the operating system is of the Linux type.

In Liberty Profile, each web server executes in a separate single Linux process. Each running process has an effective UID (Linux user identifier) and GID (Linux group identifier), as well as a real UID and GID. Consequently, all the storlets deployed in a given web server have the same UID and GID.

In our implementation, a web server provides a single type of sandbox for all storlets that are deployed in that server. In addition, we restrict each server to be engaged on behalf of a single tenant. A given storlet can be deployed independently in multiple servers, thus separate instances of the same storlet can be made available in each sandbox for each tenant.

Each tenant/sandbox pair is associated "permanently" with a unique UID and GID. In particular, different sandbox types of the same tenant have different UIDs/GIDs. All servers run as non-privileged (non-root) processes. The UIDs/GIDs are leveraged to support filesystem permissions, firewall policies, and tenant isolation. Each tenant/sandbox pair is also associated with a unique port number – on which the server listens for storlet requests.

An effect of the unique UID/GID approach is that a well behaved server and its storlets can be protected from some types of intrusion. More importantly, a storlet in one server cannot cause damage to another server, since in Linux a non-privileged process cannot assume another UID/GID.

3.3   Access Control

Each storlet request is performed on behalf of a specific userid in the storage cloud. If the invocation is on the data path of the storage system (e.g. get or put of an object), the userid is the one issuing the original data request. If the request is not on the data path (e.g. an internal request, possibly event driven), an internal userid can be used.

Access control concerns authentication and authorization to perform certain actions. In the context of the Storlet Engine, there are two aspects of permission:

– *Permission to run the storlet* on a given request on behalf of a given userid. This can be approached in several ways. It may be user/role based. Data objects specified in the request may be associated with a set of rules determining what users and/or storlets are allowed to operate on the object. In fact, when the storlet itself is maintained as an object, the rules of the storlet object can be used.
– *Permission to access an object* in the storage system (get, put, etc.). A storlet should be permitted to access only the objects that the client originating the request is allowed to access. Access rights to objects are enforced by the security mechanisms of the storage system. On access to an object, a storlet needs to present some credentials, usually obtained as a parameter. For example, a token or userid/password in Swift.

Permission to run a storlet must be enforced before the storlet is invoked. Once the storlet starts handling a request, it is assumed that the storlet is authorized for the request. A typical storlet is performed on the data path of the client's original request to the storage system. The storlet is invoked after the storage system has already authenticated and authorized the client's request.

4 Performance Study

4.1 Test Goals

The performance study attempts to answer the following questions:

1. *What performance benefits can be derived by wrapping a function as a storlet?*
   To answer this question we compare the performance of alternative storlet
   wrappings against their performance when equivalent functions are run outside of the storage system. The comparison are taken while a fixed workload
   is running concurrently in the background to simulate the environment in
   which storlets will run.
2. *How storlets affect system performance?* To answer this question we change
   our view point and examine the workload's performance when running concurrently with storlets or equivalent functions running outside of the storage
   system.
3. *What is the performance implications of running storlets on the storage system's interface nodes as oppose to running them on the local storage nodes?*
4. *What host resources are most affected by storlet?* To answer this question we
   examine host memory utilization, load, cpu utilization and swap utilization.
5. *Do the performance issues (described above) change when the storage system
   is a private cloud accessed over a high speed internal network or a public
   cloud accessed over the WAN?* To answer this question we created a Swift
   test bed with a 10 GB network to simulate a private cloud and add delays
   to the incoming packets on the client host running the storlets or equivalent
   function to simulate WAN access.

4.2 Fixity Test Set Results Overview

This subsection compares the performance of alternative fixity storlet wrappings with its counterpart equivalent application. We denote by *treatments* the
various alternative storlet wrappings or equivalent functions. The fixity test
set includes treatments that calculate a data object's digest, using MD5 and
SHA256, and returns the results to the client. We chose fixity as the subject of
the performance test since it allowed us to easily compare an eqivalent function
running inside and outside the storage system while varying the object size and
number of concurrent threads. The different treatments are described below:

- *fixityStorletAtInterfaceNode:* FixityStorlet run on interface node
- *fixityStorletAtLocalNode:* FixityStorlet run on local node
- *fixityAppWithStorletInfrastructure:* The fixity application runs on the treatment engine where it calculates the data object's digest. Even though the
  fixity application is not a storlet it is run while the storlet infrastructure is
  installed in the storage system.
- *fixityAppWithOutStorletInfrastructure:* The fixity application runs on treatment engine, but the storage system is in its native form without the storlet
  infrastructure. This treatment is included so we can evaluate the additional

overhead associated with the storlet infrastructure and compare it with the native storage system performance.

Figure 2 illustrates the relationships between the different fixity treatments' response times. We observe that the fixityStorletAtLocalNode's response time is consistently better than the two fixityApp treatments' response time. While the fixityStorletAtInterfaceNode response time is the worst. When we compare fixityAppWithStorletInfrastructure against the fixityAppWithoutStorletInfrastructure treatment we also observe that there is overhead associated with the storlet infrastructure but that it is not significant.

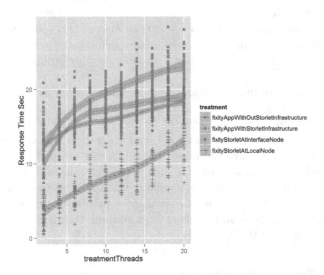

Fig. 2. Fixity treatments for MB size objects response time with less than one millisecond latency between treatment host and interface node.

4.3 Fixity Test Conclusions

1. *What performance benefits can be derived by wrapping a function as a storlet?* The test demonstrates that storlets that run on the local node and process megabyte size objects perform better than the equivalent functions running outside of the storage system.
2. *How storlets affect system performance?* The test demonstrates workloads that overlap storlets that run on the local node and process megabyte size objects perform better than those that overlap equivalent functions running outside of the storage system.
3. *What is the performance implications of running storlets on the storage system's interface nodes as oppose to running them on the their local storage nodes?* storlets that run on the interface node and process megabyte size data perform worse than storlets that run on the local node. Using the interface node to run storlets is only recommended when the storlet does not require much data handle as is the case of the Distributed Storlet.

4. *What host resources are most affected by storlet?* There is a correlation between memory utilization and load at the interface node and the resulting performance.

5. *Do the performance issues (described above) change when the storage system is a private cloud accessed over a high speed internal network or a public cloud accessed over the WAN?* The performance improvements attributed to storlets that run on the local nodes is amplified as the latency increases between the client host and storage system's interface node.

More details of the performance study can be found in the expanded version of this work [4].

5 Discussion and Conclusions

5.1 Related Work

Discovering new insights from the vast amount of the existing biomedical data is an on-going goal [5]. Challenges towards that goal include efficient processing of large biomedical data sets [6] and privacy issues [7]. The Storlet Engine can support these two challenges by processing data within the storage.

Stored procedures and active databases are at a high level analogous to storlets in object storage. However, object storage is meant for large blobs and provides eventual data consistency while databases are meant for tabular data and provides strong data consistency. Consequently, the Storlet Engine need to confront with different challenges and solve them with distinct approaches.

Efficient execution of data-intensive applications was investgated for many years e.g. [8]. As the data objects become larger and distant, there is an increasing focus on performing computations close to the data. Ceph [9] is a free software storage platform designed to present object, block, and file storage from a single distributed computer cluster. Ceph has the ability to add class methods which enables computations in the storage. However, these class methods cannot run in a sandbox for now. In contrast, our Storlet Engine runs code within a sandbox, which provides better security.

OpenStack Savanna [10] attempts to enable users to easily provision and manage Hadoop clusters on OpenStack. A similar technology is Amazon Elastic MapReduce (EMR) service that provides elastic Hadoop cluster on Amazon cloud. In both technologies, the data is still transferred from the object storage to the compute nodes, unlike our Storlet Engine that performs the compute in the object nodes of the cloud object storage.

ZeroVM [11] provides a virtual server system that can run close to your data. It is an open source lightweight virtualization platform based on the Chromium Native Client (NaCl) project. It claims to be fast, secure and disposable but the use of NaCl requires customized versions of the GNU tool-chain, specifically gcc and binutils. Consequently, existing code need to be recompiled for the NaCl tool-chain which is sometimes non-trivial. In contrast, in our Storlet Engine recompilation is not required, and existing code can be executed unaltered.

5.2   Conclusions and Future Work

The paper presented Storlet Engine, an environment supporting computations within storage system. The idea is to extend the traditional role of object storage as a repository for data, by exploiting the computing resources of storage nodes to run computation modules – storlets – on the data close to where it resides.

We described the architecture and key features of the system, and discussed the implementation of storlets for biomedical processes such as ROI Extraction, Cell Detection, Cohort Identification. Some storlets for these business processes were implemented in the context of the ENSURE and ForgetIT EU projects. We also conducted a performance study, evaluating the Storlet Engine within OpenStack Swift prototype.

There are multiple opportunities for further work and research. Our future plans include exploring the usage of storlets for genomic workflows and for medical imaging analytics of various modalities such as ultrasound, mammography, CT. Some open questions in this area include: what computations in biomedical processes should be executed as storlets? What parameters influence this decision? Can the decision be taken transparently to the business process developer and user? Exploring the merit of a storlets marketplace is a another direction, and in particular identifying biomedical use cases and applications. Finally, for this evolving methodology, a standardization effort is a long term goal.

Acknowledgments. The research leading to these results has received funding from the European Community's Seventh Framework Programme (FP7/2007–2013) under grant agreement 270000 and under grant agreement 600826.

References

1. Factor, M., Naor, D., Rabinovici-Cohen, S., Ramati, L., Reshef, P., Satran, J., Giaretta, D.: Preservation DataStores: architecture for preservation aware storage. In: MSST 2007, Proceedings of the 24th IEEE Conference on Mass Storage Systems and Technologies, San Diego, CA, pp. 3–15, September 2007
2. Rabinovici-Cohen, S., Marberg, J., Nagin, K., Pease, D.: PDS Cloud: Long term digital preservation in the cloud. In: IC2E 2013, Proceedings of the IEEE International Conference on Cloud Engineering, San Francisco, CA, March 2013
3. Rajaraman, A., Ullman, J.: Mining of Massive Datasets. Lecture Notes for Stanford CS345A Web Mining (2011)
4. Rabinovici-Cohen, S., Henis, E., Marberg, J., Nagin, K.: Storlet engine: performing computations in cloud storage. Technical report H-0320, IBM Research - Haifa, August 2014
5. Shahar, Y.: The elicitation, representation, application, and automated discovery of time-oriented declarative clinical knowledge. In: Lenz, R., Miksch, S., Peleg, M., Reichert, M., Riaño, D., ten Teije, A. (eds.) ProHealth 2012 and KR4HC 2012. LNCS, vol. 7738, pp. 1–29. Springer, Heidelberg (2013)
6. Cooper, L., Carter, A., Farris, A., Wang, F., Kong, J., Gutman, D., Widener, P., Pan, T., Cholleti, S., Sharma, A., Kurç, T., Brat, D., Saltz, J.: Digital pathology: data-intensive frontier in medical imaging. Proc. IEEE **100**(4), 317–323 (2012)

7. Le, X., Wang, D.: Neuroimage data sets: rethinking privacy policies. In: HealthSec (2012)
8. Rabinovici-Cohen, S., Wolfson, O.: Why a single parallelization strategy is not enough in knowledge bases. J. Comput. Syst. Sci. **47**(1), 2–44 (1993)
9. Weil, S., Brandt, S., Miller, E., Long, D., Maltzahn, C.: Ceph: A scalable, high-performance distributed file system. In: OSDI 2006, Proceedings of the USENIX Symposium on Operating Systems Design and Implementation (2006)
10. OpenStack Savanna. https://wiki.openstack.org/wiki/Savanna
11. ZeroVM. http://zerovm.org

SBP 2014

Conformance Checking Based on Partially Ordered Event Data

Xixi Lu$^{(\boxtimes)}$, Dirk Fahland, and Wil M.P. van der Aalst

Department of Mathematics and Computer Science,
Eindhoven University of Technology,
P.O. Box 513, 5600 MB Eindhoven, The Netherlands
{x.lu,d.fahland,w.m.p.v.d.aalst}@tue.nl

Abstract. Conformance checking is becoming more important for the analysis of business processes. While the diagnosed results of conformance checking techniques are used in diverse context such as enabling auditing and performance analysis, the quality and reliability of the conformance checking techniques themselves have not been analyzed rigorously. As the existing conformance checking techniques heavily rely on the total ordering of events, their diagnostics are unreliable and often even misleading when the timestamps of events are coarse or incorrect. This paper presents an approach to incorporate flexibility, uncertainty, concurrency and explicit orderings between events in the input as well as in the output of conformance checking using *partially ordered traces* and *partially ordered alignments*, respectively. The paper also illustrates various ways to acquire partially ordered traces from existing logs. In addition, a quantitative-based quality metric is introduced to objectively compare the results of conformance checking. The approach is implemented in ProM plugins and has been evaluated using artificial logs.

1 Introduction

Models are increasingly used to describe business processes, to automate process executions, to communicate with stakeholders, and to evaluate designs. However, process mining research shows that process executions in reality often deviate from documented process models, potentially violating security and compliance policies. As models enable various analysis techniques ranging from verification to simulation, it is essential to provide *diagnostic information about the conformance of process models with respects to event logs recording the real behavior* [1]. This information can be further used to identify and measure deviations, enable auditing and compliance analysis [2,3]. Moreover, the relationships between models and logs obtained from aligning them can be used to analyze performance and repair process models [4,5].

Dozens of approaches [1,2,4,6,7] have been proposed to check conformance between a given model and a sequence of events (a so-called *trace*) from an event log, but all of these approaches assume that the events in a trace are totally ordered (e.g. based on precise timestamps). The state-of-the-art technique in

© Springer International Publishing Switzerland 2015
F. Fournier and J. Mendling (Eds.): BPM 2014 Workshops, LNBIP 202, pp. 75–88, 2015.
DOI: 10.1007/978-3-319-15895-2_7

conformance checking is the *alignment* approach proposed in [6,7], which relates behavior observed in a sequential trace (i.e. events) to behavior documented in a model (i.e. activities) and identifies deviations between them. Alignments with the least number of deviations are considered to be optimal.

One of the limitations of computing optimal alignments for sequential traces is that current approaches heavily rely on the total ordering of events in a trace. In cases where the timestamps are too coarse (e.g. only the dates are recorded and the order of the events on the same day is unknown) or incorrect (e.g. due to manual recording), using a non-trustworthy total ordering of these events for computing alignment may result in classifying abnormal behavior as conforming and normal behavior as deviating. Moreover, sequential traces are unable to describe concurrent events (e.g. events happening at the same time or events of which we known that there is no causal dependency between then). Furthermore, the dependencies between events in the resulting alignments may be misleading because of ordering problems.

To overcome these limitations, we propose to use partially ordered events rather than totally ordered events. This way we can express causal dependencies, uncertainty, and concurrency in a better way. Moreover, we also argue that computing partially ordered alignments based on partial orders provides more precise diagnostic results for conformance checking.

In this paper, we introduce *partially ordered traces* and use these as input to compute *partially ordered alignments* with respect to a given model. An overview of our approach is shown in Fig. 1. We discuss our approach in two parts:

(1) Given a partially ordered trace and a process model, we show how to compute a partially ordered alignment.
(2) Given a log, we show how to obtain partially ordered traces which are used as input for the first part.

In the first part, we discuss a generic approach which extends the sequential alignment approach [7] to computing optimal partially ordered alignments. In addition, we also introduce a quantitative-based *alignment quality metric*

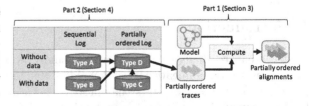

Fig. 1. An overview of our approach.

to measure and to compare the quality of alignments and to evaluate our approach.

In the second part, we discuss ways to derive the input of the first part, i.e. partially ordered traces, from a given log. More specifically, we categorize input logs into four types: sequential logs without data (Type A), sequential logs with data (Type B), partially ordered logs with data (Type C) and partially ordered logs without data (Type D). For each type, we discuss an example of computing partially ordered traces. In addition, we will demonstrate shortcomings of totally ordered alignments that can be overcome by partially ordered alignments.

The remainder of this paper is structured as follows. We first introduce some basic concepts in Sect. 2. Section 3 defines partially ordered traces and alignments, describes our approach based on computing partially ordered alignments, and introduces a novel alignment quality metric. Section 4 discusses ways to acquire partially ordered traces from classical sequential traces and shows examples where partially ordered alignments perform better than existing conformance checking approaches. Section 5 presents results of experiments we conducted. Section 6 discusses the related work, and Sect. 7 concludes the paper.

2 Preliminaries

In this section, we first introduce a running example and use the running example to recall some preliminaries related to event logs and alignments.

Running Example. Figure 2 shows a simplified process in a hospital. The process starts with a patient having an appointment (A). Next, a doctor can check the patient history (C) while the patient is scheduled for radiology (R) and followed by a lab test (L). The doctor evaluates (E) the result of these tests and determines whether to operate (O) or to send patient home for home treatment (H). Operated patients require nursing (N). Finally, the patient might be re-evaluated (V) to determine whether she has to be operated on again.

Case, Events, Traces, Logs. A *case* is a process instance, i.e. an execution of a process. An *activity* is a well-defined task in a process model (e.g. blue rectangles in Fig. 2). Executing an activity for a case results in an *event* recorded in the trace of this case. Each event includes a set of data attributes describing the event. In the classical setting of process mining, a *trace* is thus a totally ordered sequence of events of a case. We use *s-trace* to denote such a *sequential trace*. A *log* is a collection of traces that belong to the same process model. In the running example, a *case* is a patient going through this process. Figure 3(a) shows a s-trace consisting of seven events, each of which has four data attributes: the case id, the event id, the activity name and the timestamp.

Alignments. A *sequential alignment* (abbreviated to *s-alignments*) between a trace and a process model is defined as a sequence of *moves*, each of which

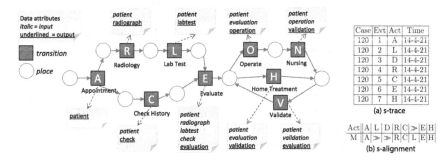

Fig. 2. An example of a simplified process in a hospital.

Fig. 3. An s-trace and its s-alignment.

relates an event in the trace to an activity in the model. A "good" move is a so-called *synchronous move*, which is an event observed in the trace and allowed according to the documented behavior (i.e. an activity to which the event can be related). Deviations are indicated by so-called *log moves* and *model moves*: a *log move* is an observed event not allowed by the modeled behavior; a *model move* is an event that should have been observed according to the modeled behavior but missed in the trace. A *cost function* assigns to each possible move a cost. An s-alignment with lowest cost according to the cost function is an *optimal s-alignment*. For the technical details, we refer to [7]. In the rest of this paper, we use the *standard cost function* which assigns to each log move and model move the same cost of 1 and to each synchronous move a cost of 0. For example, the optimal s-alignment shown in Fig. 3(b) between the s-trace in Fig. 3(a) and the model in Fig. 2 consists of four synchronous moves, two log moves $\frac{L}{\gg}$ and $\frac{D}{\gg}$ and one model move $\frac{\gg}{L}$.

Partial Orders. A *partial order* over a set V is a binary relation which is irreflexive, antisymmetric, and transitive. A *directed acyclic graph (DAG)* $G = (V, \rightarrow)$ defines a partial order $\prec$ over V, i.e. for all $v_1, v_2 \in V$, if there is a *path* from v_1 to v_2, then $v_1 \prec v_2$. The transitive reduction of a DAG and its corresponding partial order is unique [8].

3 Partially Ordered Alignment

In this section, we define the notion of partially ordered traces and alignments. Moreover, we describe our approach to compute an optimal partially ordered alignment if a partially ordered trace is given. In addition, we also define an alignment quality metric to compare two partially ordered alignments.

Definitions. Given a case with its set of events, a *partially ordered trace (p-trace)* is a directed acyclic graph (which defines a partial order) over the set of events. Each *dependency (dep.)* in p-trace from an event e_i to another event e_j indicates that event e_i has led to the execution of e_j. For example, the p-trace shown in Fig. 4 has the same events as the case of Fig. 3(a). The partial order in Fig. 4 shows that events R, L, H and D directly depend on event A, while R, L, H and D are *concurrent* to each other (i.e. in no particular order).

Correspondingly, a *partially ordered alignment (p-alignment)* between a p-trace and a process model is a directed acyclic graph (which defines a partial order) over the set of moves between them. A *move* comprises an event in the p-trace and an activity in the model to which the event is related, similar to moves in s-alignments. There are three types of moves: *synchronous moves*, *log moves* and *model moves*. The ordering of moves (i.e. dependencies between the moves) in a p-alignment respects the ordering of their events in the p-trace or the ordering of their activities in the model. For instance, Fig. 5 exemplifies a p-alignment between the p-trace shown in Fig. 4 and the model shown in Fig. 2. The p-alignment shown in Fig. 5 has five synchronous moves (denoted by green five-sided polygons, e.g. A), two log moves (denoted by yellow triangles, e.g. D) and one model move (denoted by blue rectangle, e.g. E).

Dependencies between moves originate either from dependencies between log events (yellow), between moves (blue), or from both (green), see Fig. 5. A dependency between two moves is a *direct dependency (d-dependency or d-dep.)* if and only if there is no other path between the two moves. The *minimal p-alignment* of a p-alignment is the transitive reduction of the p-alignment and only consists of d-dependencies.

An *optimal p-alignment* is a p-alignment with lowest cost according to the cost function. We also introduce the notion of the *ideal p-alignment* γ_* of a case, which is the only true p-alignment of the case, i.e. both the diagnosed moves and dependencies of γ_* are correct. The p-alignment shown in Fig. 5 is for example assumed to be the ideal p-alignment for the case shown in Fig. 3(a).

Approach. Our method extends the approach of [7] to compute an optimal p-alignment between a given p-trace and a model. We first convert the p-trace into a so-called *event net*, which is a Petri net that represents the behavior of the given p-trace. More precisely, each event in the p-trace is represented by a transition in the event net, and each dependency found between two events is converted into a place between their corresponding transitions in the event net. To complete the event net, for each event that has no predecessor or no successor, we add an input place or an output place, respectively.

After computing the event net, we join the event net with the process model to obtain a *product net* which consist three types of transition representing the three types of move (i.e. log moves, model moves, and synchronous moves). For further detail, we refer to [7]. Figure 6 exemplifies the product net between the p-trace shown in Fig. 4 and the process shown in Fig. 2.

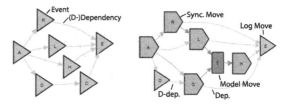

Fig. 4. A p-trace for the case in Fig. 3.

Fig. 5. An optimal p-alignment for the p-trace in Fig. 4.

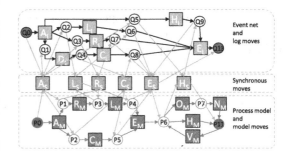

Fig. 6. A product net between the p-trace in Fig. 4 and the process model in Fig. 2.

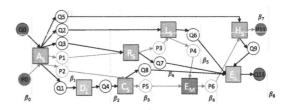

Fig. 7. The partially ordered alignment net of the p-alignment in Fig. 5.

Next, we compute a firing sequence with a lowest cost (according to the standard cost function) from the initial marking to the final marking using the A^*-approach proposed in [7]. Then, we replay the firing sequence on the product net. We only retain the places visited, the transitions fired and the arcs between them. We call the retained net an *optimal alignment net*. For example, Fig. 7 shows an optimal alignment net of the product net in Fig. 6. Finally, we convert an optimal alignment net into an optimal p-alignment by replacing the places between transitions with dependencies. Figure 5 shows the optimal p-alignment converted from the optimal alignment net shown in Fig. 7.

Table 1. Compare s-alignments and p-alignments using quality metrics.

	Sync. Move			Log Move			Model Move			d-dependencies		
	TP	FP	FN	TP	FP	FN	TP	FP	FN	TP	FP	FN
Ideal	5	0	0	2	0	0	1	0	0	8	0	0
Seq.	4	1	1	1	1	1	0	1	1	2	5	6
Type A	5	1	0	1	0	1	0	0	1	5	1	3
Type B	5	1	0	1	0	1	0	0	1	7	0	1

Alignment Quality Metrics. To compare two p-alignments, we define the true positives, false positives, and false negatives for synchronous moves, log moves, model moves, and d-dependencies. Assuming the ideal p-alignment γ_* is known for a given case, we can compute a p-trace and compare an (optimal) p-alignment γ' of the p-trace to the ideal p-alignment as follows.

- For each synchronous move $m_s \in \gamma'$, if m_s is also found in the ideal p-alignment γ_*, the synchronous move m_s is *True Positive (TP)*; if m_s not found in γ_*, m_s is *False Positive (FP)*. The same for each log move, model move and d-dependency found in γ'.
- For each synchronous move m_{s*} found in the ideal p-alignment γ_* but not in γ', m_{s*} is considered to be a *False Negative (FN)*. The same for each log move, model move and d-dependency found in γ_*.

As additional quality metric, we can compute the F1-score $F1 = (2 \times TP)/(2 \times TP + FP + FN)$ for the moves and dependencies identified, which is the harmonic mean of recall and precision [9].

Note that by definition, an s-alignment is also a p-alignment and thus can be compared to an ideal p-alignment. For example, we can convert the s-alignment in Fig. 3(b) into the p-alignment shown in Fig. 8. Assuming Fig. 5 shows the ideal p-alignment of the same case in Fig. 3(a), the first row and the second row in Table 1 respectively show the quality metrices for the ideal p-alignment and the s-alignment (compared to the ideal p-alignment). For instance, in the s-alignment we found one FP synchronous move E (i.e. the five-sided polygon E), which is a log move in the ideal p-alignment (i.e. a FN log move) in Fig. 5. This example shows that the s-alignment approach may classify abnormal behavior as conforming. Furthermore, the FP log move L found in the s-alignment is classified as a synchronous move in the ideal alignment: the s-alignment approach may claim conforming behavior as deviating.

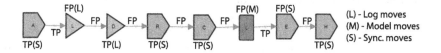

Fig. 8. A p-alignment which visualizes the s-alignment in Fig. 3(b).

4 Conversion and Comparison

In Sect. 3, we explained our approach for computing an optimal p-alignment when given a p-trace. In this section, we discuss ways to compute p-traces. Recall the four types of log defined in the introduction, if a log (with or without data) is already partially ordered, i.e. Type C and D, we can simply consider its p-traces and neglect the data attributes. For sequential logs with or without data attributes (i.e., type B and A, respectively), we illustrate for each type an example to compute partially ordered traces. In addition, we motivate p-alignments by using these examples and compare the results based on our alignment quality metrics.

4.1 Type A - Sequential Logs Without Data

Type A denotes sequential event logs without data. Each log of this type is a collection of s-traces in which each event has only the basic attributes: the event identifier, the activity name and the timestamp. For this type of log, there are various situations in which we can compute p-traces and use the p-traces to obtain p-alignments. One of the possible situations is when the timestamps of events are coarse, and the ordering of events are unreliable. For instance, for each event only the date is recorded which may lead to multiple events having the same timestamp, exemplified by the trace in Fig. 3 in which all seven events occurred on the same day.

A simple approach to compute p-traces in this situation is to consider the events having the same timestamp to be concurrent. This approach adds flexibility when computing alignments and removes false positive log moves and model moves. Figure 9 shows the p-trace computed for the s-trace shown in Fig. 3 using

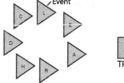

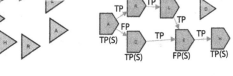

Fig. 9. A p-trace for Fig. 3(a) derived based on timestamps.

Fig. 10. An optimal p-alignment for the p-trace in Fig. 9.

this approach. Since all seven events have the same timestamp, they are considered to be concurrent, i.e. no dependency between them as shown in Fig. 9. Therefore, the events could have happened at any order, resulting in the p-alignment shown by Fig. 10.

Computing the quality metric of the p-alignment shown in Fig. 10 with respect to the ideal alignment shown in Fig. 5, we obtain the result shown by the third entry in Table 1. Compared to the s-alignment shown in Fig. 8 of the same case, there are no FP log moves or FP model moves in the p-alignment, and only one FP d-dependency. Moreover, we find 2.5 times more TP d-dependencies.

4.2   Type B - Sequential Logs Annotated with Data

In this section, we first define data annotated logs and then discuss how to use this type of log to compute p-traces.

Definition. We use the term *Data Annotated Log* (DAL) to denote a specific type of event log, in which each event has a set of clearly annotated input attributes and of output attributes, i.e. in addition to the name and the value of an attribute, we also have a meta data for each attribute which indicates whether the attribute is an input or an output of the event. *Input attributes* of an event are attributes that already existed and are *read* when executing the activity that results in the event. Similarly, *output attributes* of an event are attributes that are *written* (created or updated) by the event. In addition, we assume that if the value of a data attribute d_1 depends on the value of another data attribute d_2, there exists an event that reads d_1 and writes d_2.

Figure 11 shows an s-trace of the same case as in Fig. 3 but with data. Each event has additional data attributes that are annotated as inputs (written in italics) or outputs (underlined). The column names denote the abbreviated identifier of attributes defined in the process model shown in Fig. 2.

Obtaining DAL. One may argue that this type of log is difficult to obtain. However, there are simple heuristics to convert a log enriched with data attributes but without annotations to a DAL. Given a log in which each event has a set of data attributes, if a specification of the input and output attributes of each activity is available (e.g. given by a domain expert or documented as shown in Fig. 2), we can use this specification to annotate the data attributes of events in a log. Otherwise, we can determine for each event in a trace and each of its data attributes whether it is an input or an output using the following heuristics:

1. When a data attribute appears the first time in an event in the trace, the event has output the data (e.g. attribute p of event 1 and attribute e of event 6 in Fig. 11);
2. Every time the data attribute with the same data attribute name appears in a succeeding event, if the value of this attribute has changed compared to the previous appearance, then the event has output the data (e.g. attribute e of

event 7 in Fig. 11 has a different value compared to the previous event E that has attribute e, therefore, attribute e of event 7 is annotated as output (i.e. underlined));

3. Otherwise, the data is an input of the event (e.g. attribute p in events $2 - 6$ is considered as input because the value of p is not changed).

Thus, Fig. 11 also exemplifies a trace annotated using this simple heuristic. We have illustrated a simple heuristic approach to show that it is possible to obtain DALs without any specification. Finding better heuristics is a relevant topics, but out of scope of this paper. In the following, we assume that DALs are available for computing p-traces.

Computing Partially Ordered Traces. After obtaining a data annotated sequential log, the data dependencies between the input and output attributes of events can be used to derive dependencies and concurrency between events. When two events e_i and e_j in a trace with $i < j$ accessed a common data attribute, we assume that there is a dependency between the two events. Based on this assumption, we derive two rules: (1) when two events both read (or write) the same data attribute with the same value, then they are concurrent; (2) otherwise, there is a dependency between them.

For example, shown in Figs. 11 and 12, events D (event 3) and R (event 4) (only) have data element p in common but both have read the same value for p which indicates there is no dependency between D and R, whereas events D (event 3) and C (event 5) have data element p and d in common and since D writes d and C read d, we add a dependency from D to C.

Using the p-trace shown in Fig. 12 as input, we compute an optimal p-alignment shown in Fig. 13. The fourth entry in Table 1 shows the measurement of this p-alignment. Compared to the s-alignment, the p-alignment in Fig. 13 shows the same improvements as the p-alignment in Fig. 10. Moreover, the p-alignment computed using data dependencies is able to locate the log move D more precisely than the other two alignments, increasing the true positive d-dependencies to 7.

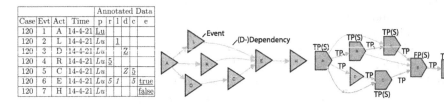

Case	Evt	Act	Time	p	r	l	d	c	e
120	1	A	14-4-21	Lu					
120	2	L	14-4-21	Lu	1				
120	3	D	14-4-21	Lu			Z		
120	4	R	14-4-21	Lu	5				
120	5	C	14-4-21	Lu			Z	5	
120	6	E	14-4-21	Lu	5	1		5	true
120	7	H	14-4-21	Lu					false

Fig. 11. An s-trace with annotated attributes.

Fig. 12. A p-trace for Fig. 11 derived based on data dependencies.

Fig. 13. An optimal p-alignment for the p-trace in Fig. 12.

5 Experimental Results

We implemented our p-alignment approach described in Sects. 3 and 4 in the *PartialOrderReplayer* package of the process mining toolkit ProM. The package provides the plug-in named *Partial Aware Replayer*. To evaluate our approach, we designed the hospital model shown in Fig. 2 in a tool called CPN Tools and randomly simulated an event log of 1000 traces with in total 6590 events[1]; each trace with 6 to 12 events. All events have the *same* timestamp, and each has 1 to 5 data attributes as specified in Fig. 2. We performed four small experiments[2]. For each experiment, we computed three types of optimal alignments using three approaches: (1) s-alignments using the approach in [7]; (2) p-alignments using the p-traces converted based on the approach for Type A logs described in Sect. 4.1; (3) p-alignments of the p-traces obtained using the approach for Type B logs (with data attributes already annotated) described in Sect. 4.2. The quality of each optimal alignment is measured with respect to the ideal alignment, which is known since the log is generated artificially.

- **Experiment 1.** In this experiment, the input is the perfectly generated sequential log in which all events are correctly ordered.
- **Experiment 2 with shuffled events.** The perfectly generated event log is used but the events in a trace are randomly shuffled. Thus the ordering of events is unreliable.
- **Experiment 3.** The input is the generated sequential log with deviations added as follows. For each trace, two events are added, and two are removed from the trace. For each event added, a predecessor and a successor are randomly chosen which ensure the true direct causal dependencies (for obtaining ideal alignments only). Each added event is then inserted between the range of its predecessor and successor and has the same timestamps as other events. Each added event reads a data attribute produced by its predecessor and writes an output data attribute being an input to it successor.
- **Experiment 4 with shuffled events.** For this experiment, we randomly shuffled the events of each trace in the log obtained in experiment 3.

Discussion. Table 2 shows the average quality measurements per optimal p-alignment (rounded in two decimals) of ten random executions of each experiment. In addition, we added the average F1-scores of moves (column 12) and of d-dependencies (column 16). The difference between the scores of the three types of p-alignments is significant for experiments 2 to 4 (see Footnote 1). Figure 14 illustrates the confidence intervals of the TP synchronous move rates of experiment 3 and 4 (i.e. the last 6 entries in column 3 of Table 2).

---

[1] The files can be downloaded at https://svn.win.tue.nl/repos/prom/Documentation/PartialOrderReplayer/SBP2014.zip.

[2] The implementation of the experiments can be found in the same package of ProM (i.e. the class *ExperimentSBP*).

Table 2. The average results of 10 runs of the four experiments.

| | | Moves | | | | | | | | | d-dependencies | | | |
| | | Sync. Moves | | | Log Moves | | | Model Moves | | | | | | | |
		TP	FP	FN	TP	FP	FN	TP	FP	FN	F1	TP	FP	FN	F1
Exp 1.	Seq.	6.59	0	0	0	0	0	0	0	0	1*	4.28	1.31	2.31	0.70
	A	6.59	0	0	0	0	0	0	0	0	1*	6.54	0.05	0.05	<u>0.99</u>
	B	6.59	0	0	0	0	0	0	0	0	1*	6.59	0	0	<u>1.00</u>
Exp 2.	Seq.	3.61	0	2.98	0	2.98	0	0	2.64	0	0.71*	3.07	5.16	3.52	0.41
shuffled	A	<u>6.59</u>	0	0	0	<u>0</u>	0	0	<u>0</u>	0	<u>1*</u>	6.48	0.11	0.11	<u>0.98</u>
	B	<u>4.09</u>	0	2.50	0	<u>2.50</u>	0	0	<u>2.29</u>	0	<u>0.77*</u>	5.72	3.44	0.87	<u>0.73</u>
Exp 3.	Seq.	**4.21**	0.60	0.38	1.40	0.38	0.60	1.64	0.08	0.36	0.84	3.92	3.39	5.68	0.46
	A	**3.94**	<u>1.23</u>	0.65	0.77	0.65	1.23	1.39	0.02	0.61	<u>0.69</u>	5.40	1.18	4.20	<u>0.67</u>
	B	**4.03**	<u>0.92</u>	0.56	1.08	0.56	0.92	1.53	0.06	0.47	<u>0.76</u>	6.60	1.96	3.00	<u>0.73</u>
Exp 4.	Seq.	**2.43**	0.84	2.16	1.16	2.16	0.84	1.48	1.51	0.52	0.55	2.93	5.65	6.67	0.32
shuffled	A	**3.93**	<u>1.24</u>	0.66	0.77	<u>0.66</u>	1.24	1.39	<u>0.02</u>	<u>0.61</u>	0.69	5.28	1.29	4.32	<u>0.65</u>
	B	**2.67**	<u>1.04</u>	1.92	0.96	<u>1.92</u>	1.04	1.46	<u>1.19</u>	<u>0.54</u>	0.55	5.23	4.42	4.37	<u>0.54</u>

* denotes F1 scores of synchronous moves. The discussed results are underlined.

As can be seen in the last four columns of Table 2, in all four experiments, the TP, FP and FN scores of d-dependencies of the p-alignments are improved compared to the s-alignments, identifying 1.5 to 3.4 TP d-dependencies more and 1.2 to 5 FP d-dependencies less per alignment on average compared to the s-alignments. An increase of 40 % to 130 % percent of the F1-scores of the d-dependencies in the p-alignments confirms this observation.

The results also show that when the ordering of events is unreliable, i.e. in Exp. 2 and Exp. 4, the two p-alignment approaches identify more TP synchronous moves and less FP log moves and FP model moves than the s-alignment approach, which suggest that the p-alignment approaches are more flexible. However, this flexibility also leads to identifying more FP synchronous moves (in Exp. 3 and 4). The average F1-scores of moves also show that the p-alignment approaches perform at least as good as the s-alignment approach except in situations when the ordering of events is reliable and traces contain noise as in Exp. 3.

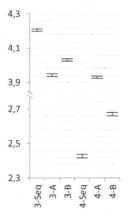

Fig. 14. The CIs of TP Sync. moves of Exp.3 and 4.

Based on the results of the experiments, we have shown that we can obtain better results using the p-alignment approach, especially in unreliable and flexible settings. In addition, the difference between the quality metrics of the two p-alignment approaches indicates that the quality of p-alignments also depends on the quality of derived p-traces.

6   Related Work

Various techniques have been proposed to check conformance between the modeled and observed behavior. The token-based replay approach proposed by Rozinat and Van der Aalst [1] measures the number of remaining tokens and of missing tokens in the process model when replaying the log to provide diagnotics about the quality of the model and deviations in the log. The state-of-art technique in conformance checking is the alignment approach proposed by Adriansyah et al. [2,6,7] which can handle complex constructs such as invisible transitions and duplicated transitions while providing detail information on deviations. The resulting diagnostics of these techniques have been applied in various context. For example, it is used to assess the quality of a model with respect to the reality [10], to repair or simplify models based on diagnosed deviations [5,11], to perform auditing and compliance analysis [2,3,12], to find decision points in processes [13], to conduct root cause analysis [14] and performance analysis [4].

While using the result of conformance checking in various applications, much less literature are found in investigating the quality of the input of conformance checking as well as the quality of its results. Bose et al. [15] discussed various quality issues found in event logs. The alignment approach assumes that with assigning the right cost to moves the "ideal alignment" can be found in optimal alignments [4,6] without considering that the log may have quality problems.

In comparison to existing conformance checking techniques, the approach presented in this paper used partially ordered traces and alignments to provide a way to incorporate flexibility, uncertainty, concurrency and explicit dependencies in inputs as well as in outputs of conformance checking to improve the quality of results. Partially ordered traces and runs have been defined and discussed in diverse other settings. Lorenz et al. define partially ordered runs of Petri nets in order to analyze properties of Petri nets [16]. Lassen et al. presented an approach to convert basic message sequence charts into p-traces and used these explicit casual dependencies to improve the process discovery result [17]. Fahland and Van der Aalst used partially ordered runs to simplify process models [11].

7   Conclusion

In this paper, we presented a generic approach for computing partially ordered alignments using partially ordered traces. In addition, we illustrated two ways to obtain partially ordered traces as input for computing p-alignments from given sequential event logs. Furthermore, we introduced a quantitative quality metric to compare alignments with respect to the ideal alignments. The evaluation results show that the quality of p-alignments is improved compared to s-alignments especially in unreliable settings. Our approach provided a first step towards improving the quality of conformance checking in more realistic circumstances.

Future research aims at incorporating probabilistic data to find better p-alignments. In addition, we are also interested in approaches to compute the ideal partially ordered trace. Moreover, partially ordered alignments can be used to analyze data flows or to compute alignments in a distributed manner.

Acknowledgments. This research is supported by the Dutch Cyber Security program in the context of the PriCE project. We thank Boudewijn van Dongen for his support in this work.

References

1. Rozinat, A., van der Aalst, W.M.P.: Conformance checking of processes based on monitoring real behavior. Inf. Syst. **33**(1), 64–95 (2008)
2. Adriansyah, A., van Dongen, B.F., Zannone, N.: Controlling break-the-glass through alignment. In: 2013 International Conference on Social Computing, pp. 606–611. IEEE (2013)
3. Ramezani, E., Fahland, D., van der Aalst, W.M.P.: Where did i misbehave? diagnostic information in compliance checking. In: Barros, A., Gal, A., Kindler, E. (eds.) BPM 2012. LNCS, vol. 7481, pp. 262–278. Springer, Heidelberg (2012)
4. van der Aalst, W.M.P., Adriansyah, A., van Dongen, B.: Replaying history on process models for conformance checking and performance analysis. Wiley Interdisc. Rev. Data Min. Knowl. Disc. **2**(2), 182–192 (2012)
5. Fahland, D., van der Aalst, W.M.P.: Model repair - aligning process models to reality. Inf. Syst. **47**, 220–243 (2015). doi:10.1016/j.is.2013.12.007
6. Adriansyah, A., van Dongen, B.F., van der Aalst, W.M.P.: Conformance checking using cost-based fitness analysis. In: 2011 15th IEEE International Enterprise Distributed Object Computing Conference (EDOC), pp. 55–64. IEEE (2011)
7. Adriansyah, A., van Dongen, B.F., van der Aalst, W.M.P.: Memory-efficient alignment of observed and modeled behavior. BPMcenter.org, Technical report (2013)
8. Aho, A.V., Garey, M.R., Ullman, J.D.: The transitive reduction of a directed graph. SIAM J. Comput. **1**(2), 131–137 (1972)
9. Manning, C.D., Raghavan, P., Schütze, H.: Introduction to Information Retrieval, vol. 1. Cambridge University Press, Cambridge (2008)
10. Buijs, J.C.A.M., van Dongen, B.F., van der Aalst, W.M.P.: On the role of fitness, precision, generalization and simplicity in process discovery. In: Meersman, R., Panetto, H., Dillon, T., Rinderle-Ma, S., Dadam, P., Zhou, X., Pearson, S., Ferscha, A., Bergamaschi, S., Cruz, I.F. (eds.) OTM 2012, Part I. LNCS, vol. 7565, pp. 305–322. Springer, Heidelberg (2012)
11. Fahland, D., van der Aalst, W.M.P.: Simplifying discovered process models in a controlled manner. Inf. Syst. **38**(4), 585–605 (2013)
12. Cederquist, J.G., Corin, R., Dekker, M.A.C., Etalle, S., den Hartog, J.I., Lenzini, G.: Audit-based compliance control. Int. J. Inf. Secur. **6**(2–3), 133–151 (2007)
13. de Leoni, M., Dumas, M., García-Bañuelos, L.: Discovering branching conditions from business process execution logs. In: Cortellessa, V., Varró, D. (eds.) FASE 2013 (ETAPS 2013). LNCS, vol. 7793, pp. 114–129. Springer, Heidelberg (2013)
14. Suriadi, S., Ouyang, C., van der Aalst, W.M.P., ter Hofstede, A.H.M.: Root cause analysis with enriched process logs. In: La Rosa, M., Soffer, P. (eds.) BPM Workshops 2012. LNBIP, vol. 132, pp. 174–186. Springer, Heidelberg (2013)
15. Bose, R.P.J.C., Mans, R.S., van der Aalst, W.M.P.: Wanna improve process mining results? In: 2013 IEEE Symposium on Computational Intelligence and Data Mining (CIDM), pp. 127–134. IEEE (2013)

16. Lorenz, R., Desel, J., Juhás, G.: Models from scenarios. In: Jensen, K., van der Aalst, W.M.P., Balbo, G., Koutny, M., Wolf, K. (eds.) Transactions on Petri Nets and Other Models of Concurrency VII. LNCS, vol. 7480, pp. 314–371. Springer, Heidelberg (2013)
17. Lassen, K.B., van Dongen, B.F.: Translating message sequence charts to other process languages using process mining. In: Jensen, K., van der Aalst, W.M.P., Billington, J. (eds.) Transactions on Petri Nets and Other Models of Concurrency I. LNCS, vol. 5100, pp. 71–85. Springer, Heidelberg (2008)

Online Compliance Monitoring
of Service Landscapes

J.M.E.M. van der Werf[1]($^{(\boxtimes)}$) and H.M.W. Verbeek[2]

[1] Department of Information and Computing Science,
University of Utrecht, Utrecht, The Netherlands
`j.m.e.m.vanderwerf@uu.nl`
[2] Department of Mathematics and Computer Science,
Eindhoven University of Technology, Eindhoven, The Netherlands
`h.m.w.verbeek@tue.nl`

Abstract. Today, it is a challenging task to keep a service application running over the internet safe and secure. Based on a collection of security requirements, a so-called *golden configuration* can be created for such an application. When the application has been configured according to this golden configuration, it is assumed that it satisfies these requirements, that is, that it is safe and secure. This assumption is based on the best practices that were used for creating the golden configuration, and on assumptions like that nothing out-of-the-ordinary occurs. Whether the requirements are actually violated, can be checked on the traces that are left behind by the configured service application. Today's applications typically log an enormous amount of data to keep track of everything that has happened. As such, such an event log can be regarded as the ground truth for the entire application: A security requirement is violated if and only if it shows in the event log. This paper introduces the ProMSecCo tool, which has been built to check whether the security requirements that have been used to create the golden configuration are violated by the event log as generated by the configured service application.

1 Introduction

The introduction of new internet architectures like Service Oriented Architectures and Software as a Service, allows organisations to cooperate via the internet. Organisations deliver their businesses by offering services. These services may be delivered by the organisation itself, or may be composed out of services offered by other suppliers. Consequently, the service landscape of organisations become more diffuse and hence, more complex.

The service provider has to show that it fulfills its obligations to its clients. For this, many certifications and procedures exist, such as the ISO standards 27001 and 17799 [7]. Auditing is the task of checking whether all agreed obligations are adhered to. The main task within an audit is to validate whether the service landscape is configured correctly, i.e., whether all obligations have been translated into safety and security requirements, and whether these requirements have been implemented correctly. Different approaches to validate correctness exist.

© Springer International Publishing Switzerland 2015
F. Fournier and J. Mendling (Eds.): BPM 2014 Workshops, LNBIP 202, pp. 89–95, 2015.
DOI: 10.1007/978-3-319-15895-2_8

For example, the requirements can be embedded in the development process [11], or the process of configuring the service landscape can be automated, as proposed in [4,5], resulting in a *golden configuration*.

The golden configuration defines an ideal set of configurations that complies with all security requirements and that implements these in a cost-efficient way. This golden configuration is used to derive the actual service landscape configuration. The actual configuration of the service landscape is then stored in a configuration management system (CMS).

In the PoSecCo project[1], the chain of defining high-level business agreements to the creation of the appropriate configuration files for a service landscape has been automated [6]. Typically, these configuration files concern controls that implement and monitor the safety and security constraints. Implementing controls is however not always feasible, nor is it guaranteed that the configuration files have been changed between two audits. To overcome this, we propose in the PoSecCo project not only to automate the creation of the golden configuration, but to complement the approach with the ProMSecCo tool, that analyzes *execution data* generated by the running service landscape.

During its execution, a service landscape produces execution data that records its usage, such as users that logged in and the actions performed by the different components on the landscape. This omnipresence of execution data, coupled with process mining techniques enable a new form of auditing: *continuous auditing* [3,14], in which the execution data is used to monitor and detect compliance violations.

The remainder of this paper is organized as follows. Section 2 explains how semantic process mining techniques can support audits in a service landscape. In Sect. 3 we present the ProMSecCo tool, and its integration in service landscapes. Section 4 concludes the paper.

2   Semantic Process Mining

Process mining [1] analyzes execution data in the form of event logs. As proposed in [2,3,8,9], process mining can support the auditor towards continuous auditing.

Most of the security requirements are expressed in high-level terms, on the level of the business services, whereas the execution data resides on the lowest level, at the infrastructure. In order to automatically check such high-level requirements, we need to bridge the gap between the different layers of abstraction. To do so, we need to relate elements in the event logs to concepts at higher levels of abstractions. For this, we combine techniques from the semantic web, like ontologies with process mining techniques. Semantic process mining defines *annotation rules* that relate elements from the event log with elements from other sources [14].

To use process mining techniques for checking compliance of a service landscape, its execution data has to be transformed into event logs. Then, based on

---

[1] European FP7 project on POlicy and SECurity COnfiguration management, see http://www.posecco.eu/.

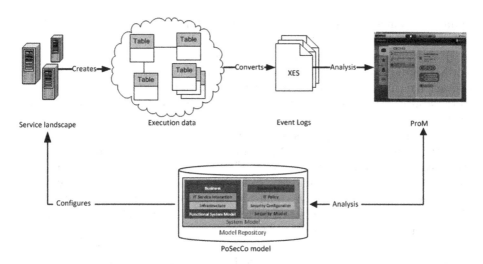

Fig. 1. Relation between configuration, execution data and process mining

the model that is used to configure the service landscape, called the PoSecCo model, the event logs can be analyzed to check compliance. Figure 1 depicts the central idea of using process mining in service landscapes.

As an example, consider a Segregation-of-Duty (SoD) constraint that, in short, specifies that a single user should not hold both an application administrator role and a database administrator role. These aspects are part of the PoSecCo model, together with the golden configuration of the service landscape. From this model we obtain information which files should be monitored, such as configuration files. During the execution of the service landscape, user access to these files is monitored and regularly exported for analysis of the constraint.

Assume that we obtained system execution data in the form of an event log[2] from the actual service landscape, and that Table 1 represents this event log. The event log depicted in Table 1 consists of 4 cases, with events for two activities,

Table 1. Partial event log from system landscape

Case	Activity	User
1	Edit /etc/tomcat6/server.xml	frank
1	Edit /etc/my.cnf	gerard
2	Edit /etc/tomcat6/server.xml	frank
3	Edit /etc/my.cnf	gerard
4	Edit /etc/my.cnf	gerard
4	Edit /etc/tomcat6/server.xml	hank

---

[2] The event log and other files used can be downloaded from http://www.promtools.org/prom6/PoSecCo.

"Edit /etc/tomcat6/server.xml" and "Edit /etc/my.cnf". There are three users that executed these events: "frank", "gerard" and "hank".

In a straightforward way, we can check the SoD constraint on an event log. The assumptions made on the event log are that it contains (1) a trace for every relevant file (like "/etc/tomcat6/server.xml") and (2) an event for every access to these files, where (3) the user who has accessed the file is recorded by the event.

Based on these assumptions, we can relate the elements of the event log to elements in the PoSecCo model. As each trace contains events of a file, we map the traces to the concept "File". A "File" has a "filename", which is stored in the event log as the trace attribute "concept:name". Each event indicates a file update or file read by some user. Thus, we can use the "org:resource" attribute of the event to indicate whether a user read or writes a file. This results in a set of additional annotation rules, including:

AR 1 (User accesses a file) Inverse of "File accessed by user" rule

source	`//event/string[@key='org:resource']`
relation	`http://www.posecco.eu/ontologies/landscape/file.owl#accesses`
target	`ancestor::trace`

AR 2 (File "/etc/my.cnf" configures DB) This file is a configuration file of the DB.

source	`//trace[./string[@key='concept:name' and @value='/etc/my.cnf']]`
relation	
target	`http://www.posecco.eu/ontologies/landscape/file.owl#DB`

Using all annotation rules on the event log, we can check the SoD-constraint by checking the following query on the ontology:

$$\text{User } \textbf{and } (\text{accesses } \textbf{some } DB) \textbf{ and } (\text{accesses } \textbf{some } APP)$$

Clearly, any non-empty result of the defined query violates the SoD constraint, as no user should be able to do so.

3   ProMSecCo

The approach has been implemented in the tool ProMSecCo[3], which has been implemented in ProM 6 [13] as a coherent collection of packages, among which the PoSecCo package. The tool has been developed in the context of the PoSecCo project to support semantic process mining, as introduced in [12,14]. The tool extends the functionality of ProM by reading and writing context models in the form of ontologies, relating these context models with the data elements in event logs, and analyzing these enriched event logs on conformance and compliance.

---

[3] ProMSecCo can be downloaded from http://www.promtools.org/prom6/PoSecCo/.

Service landscape

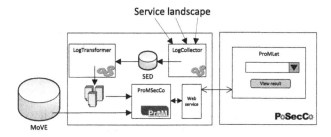

Fig. 2. ProM Deployment in PoSecCo environment

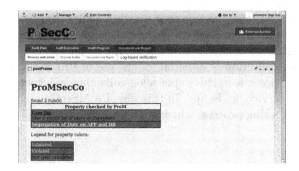

Fig. 3. Inspection of the results of the automated checking of the SoD constraint.

In the context of PoSecCo, ProMSecCo has been integrated into a log-collecting architecture, as introduced in [3,10]. This architecture can support the knowledge user (in this project this would be the auditor) by (partly) automating frequently occurring tasks, such as checking whether certain constraints are not violated. The log-collecting architecture assists in the following tasks:

1. regularly download system execution data from the service landscape;
2. generate event logs for the different properties; and
3. calculate the results of each of the properties.

The proposed architecture is depicted in Fig. 2. The log collector component is responsible for retrieving and storing the system execution data. The log transformer component transforms the available system execution data into event logs that can be used within ProMSecCo. The ProMSecCo component does the semantic process mining, as explained before. The ProMLet is a basic user interface for the web service component as it is integrated in the PoSecCo Integrated Environment. It provides a user interface to show the constraints that are checked automatically, and their results.

Figure 3 shows the results of the automated checking of the SoD constraint in this environment. In this case, the SoD constraint has been violated. By clicking on the link "Segregation of Duty on APP and DB", additional diagnostic information is provided to the end user (like who has violated this constraint, and when has it been violated). Using this diagnostic information, the end user can either inspect the corresponding event log and gain additional diagnostic information, or can inspect the raw execution data for this violation.

4   Conclusions

Auditing an entire service landscape, i.e., checking whether it complies to all regulations and agreements, is known to be a hard and time consuming task. Ensuring that the service landscape is configured correctly is an important task within auditing, but not sufficient to guarantee compliance, as configurations might have been temporarily changed in between two audits.

To overcome this risk, we present in this paper the ProMSecCo tool. ProMSecCo analyzes execution data generated by the service landscape in the form of event logs using semantic process mining techniques.

Structured log collection is essential for the use of ProMSecCo within auditing. Therefore, we propose in this paper a log-collecting architecture to integrate the tool within a service landscape. In this way, ProMSecCo allows to automate the compliance checking process, which is an essential next step towards continuous auditing.

References

1. van der Aalst, W.M.P.: Process Mining: Discovery Conformance and Enhancement of Business Processes. Springer, Berlin (2011)
2. van der Aalst, W.M.P., van Hee, K.M., van der Werf, J.M.E.M., Verdonk, M.: Auditing 2.0: Using Process Mining to Support Tomorrow's Auditor. IEEE Comput. **43**(3), 102–105 (2010)
3. van der Aalst, W.M.P., van Hee, K.M., van der Werf, J.M.E.M., Kumar, A., Verdonk, M.C.: Conceptual model for on line auditing. Decis. Support Syst. **50**(3), 636–647 (2011)
4. Arsac, W., Laube, A., Plate, H.: Policy chain for securing service oriented architectures. In: Di Pietro, R., Herranz, J., Damiani, E., State, R. (eds.) DPM 2012 and SETOP 2012. LNCS, vol. 7731, pp. 303–317. Springer, Heidelberg (2013)
5. Bezzi, M., Damiani, E., Paraboschi, S., Plate, H.: Integrating advanced security certification and policy management. In: Felici, M. (ed.) CSP EU FORUM 2013. CCIS, vol. 182, pp. 55–66. Springer, Heidelberg (2013)
6. Casalino, M.M., Mangili, M., Plate, H., Ponta, S.E.: Detection of configuration vulnerabilities in distributed (web) environments. In: Keromytis, A.D., Di Pietro, R. (eds.) SecureComm 2012. LNICST, vol. 106, pp. 131–148. Springer, Heidelberg (2013)
7. Haworth, D.A., Pietron, L.R.: Sarbanes-Oxley: Achieving compliance by starting with ISO 17799. Inf. Syst. Manage. **23**(1), 73–87 (2006)
8. Jans, M., Lybaert, N., Vanhoof, K., van der Werf, J.M.E.M.: Business process mining for internal fraud risk reduction: results of a case study. In: 9th International Research Symposium on Accounting Information Systems, Paris (2008)
9. Jans, M., van der Werf, J.M.E.M., Lybaert, N., Vanhoof, K.: A business process mining application for internal transaction fraud mitigation. Expert Syst. Appl. **38**(10), 13351–13359 (2011)

10. van Loon, J.H.W.: Design of a monitor for on-the-fly checking of business rules. Master's thesis, Technische Universiteit Eindhoven (2011)
11. Neri, M.A., Guarnieri, M., Magri, E., Mutti, S., Paraboschi, S.: A model-driven approach for securing software architectures. In: SECRYPT 2013, pp. 595–602. SciTePress (2013)
12. PoSecCo. D4.3 - Tailoring Semantic Process Mining Methods to Behavioral Landscape Models (2011)
13. Verbeek, H.M.W., Buijs, J.C.A.M., van Dongen, B.F., van der Aalst, W.M.P.: XES, XESame, and ProM 6. In: Soffer, P., Proper, E. (eds.) CAiSE Forum 2010. LNBIP, vol. 72, pp. 60–75. Springer, Heidelberg (2011)
14. van der Werf, J.M.E.M., Verbeek, H.M.W., van der Aalst, W.M.P.: Context-aware compliance checking. In: Barros, A., Gal, A., Kindler, E. (eds.) BPM 2012. LNCS, vol. 7481, pp. 98–113. Springer, Heidelberg (2012)

Privacy Preserving Business Process Fusion

Roberto Guanciale[✉] and Dilian Gurov

KTH Royal Institute of Technology, Stockholm, Sweden
{robertog,dilian}@csc.kth.se

Abstract. Virtual enterprises (VEs) are temporary and loosely coupled alliances of businesses that join their skills to catch new business opportunities. However, the dependencies among the activities of a prospective VE cross the boundaries of the VE constituents. It is therefore crucial to allow the VE constituents to discover their local views of the interorganizational workflow, enabling each company to re-shape, optimize and analyze the possible local flows that are consistent with the processes of the other VE constituents. We refer to this problem as *VE process fusion*. Even if it has been widely investigated, no previous work addresses VE process fusion in the presence of privacy constraints. In this paper we demonstrate how private intersection of regular languages can be used as the main building block to implement the privacy preserving fusion of business processes modeled by means of bounded Petri nets.

Keywords: Business process fusion · Petri nets · Privacy · SMC

1 Introduction

In the world of business, several potentially competitive enterprises can share their knowledge and skills to form a temporary alliance, usually called a virtual enterprise (VE), in order to catch new business opportunities. Virtual enterprises can be part of long-term strategic alliances or short-term collaborations. To effectively manage a virtual enterprise, receiving well-founded support from business process engineering techniques is critical. In particular, it is necessary to establish the cross-organizational business process, that is, to identify for each participant what can or is to be performed locally. In other words, one needs to compute the contributing subset of the existing local business process that is consistent with the processes of the other VE constituents. We refer to this problem as *VE process fusion*.

To illustrate VE process fusion, consider the following running example. Let a and b be two enterprises, with business processes as shown in Fig. 1a and 1b, respectively, modeled as labeled Petri nets. The two processes contain: (i) internal tasks and events of the enterprises (the boxes labelled E, D, G, H and P, standing for tasks such as the packaging of goods, the receipt of a payment and the like), (ii) shared events and interactions between the two enterprises (A, B and C, representing tasks such as the exchange of electronic documents or the departure of a carrier from the harbor), (iii) silent events (black boxes, usually

© Springer International Publishing Switzerland 2015
F. Fournier and J. Mendling (Eds.): BPM 2014 Workshops, LNBIP 202, pp. 96–101, 2015.
DOI: 10.1007/978-3-319-15895-2_9

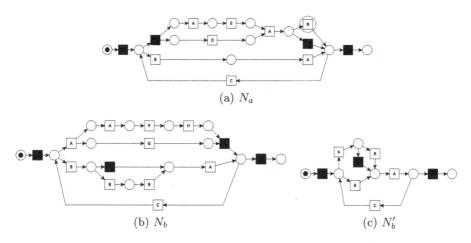

Fig. 1. Business processes modeled with Petri nets

used to simplify net structure). Intuitively, when the enterprise a is fused with enterprise b, its business process must be updated so as to satisfy the partner's constraints. For instance, an analysis of the fusion suggested above will reveal that the encircled activity B in Fig. 1a can not be executed any more after the fusion.

One of the main obstacles to VE process fusion is the perceived threat to the participants' autonomy. In particular, the participants can be reluctant to expose their internal processes, since this knowledge can be analyzed by the other participants to reveal sensitive information such as efficiency secrets or weaknesses in responding to a market demand. Moreover, the value of confidentiality of business processes is widely recognized, and many enterprises have started to use the patent mechanism to protect the investment required to optimize their workflows.

In this work we consider two mutually distrustful parties, each following a local business process, that wish to compute their local view of the VE process, assuming no trusted third party is available. The VE process is modeled as the synchronous composition of the participant work-flows, and each participant's local view is represented by a process that is trace equivalent to the VE process up to transitions that are not observable by the participant itself. The two parties are reluctant to reveal any information about their own business process that is not strictly deducible from the local view of the other party. For example, regardless whether enterprise b owns the business process N_b or N_b' from Fig. 1, the sub-process of N_a that is consistent with the observable partner's constraints is one and the same (Fig. 2); therefore, the mechanism used to implement process fusion should not allow party a to distinguish between N_b and N_b' or any other partner process that gives rise to the same local view of a.

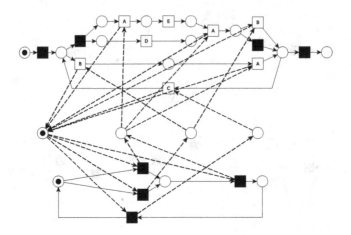

Fig. 2. The local view of a after its fusion with b

To satisfy these security constraints, our work is built on top of our previous results on private regular language intersection and process fusion in a secure multiparty computation setting (SMC) [4].

Here, we demonstrate how these results can be extended to deal with business processes that are formally modeled with bounded Petri nets. Furthermore, we provide a prototype implementation of our proposed technique, developed as a plug-in of PROM [8], a well known business process analysis platform.

2   Private Fusion of Virtual Enterprise Business Processes

We employ bounded labeled Petri nets to formally represent business processes. There is a general agreement (see e.g. [7]) that well-formed business processes correspond to bounded Petri nets (or more specifically, sound workflow nets), and several proposals (e.g. [3]) demonstrate techniques to convert high-level models (such as BPMN) to Petri nets.

Assume two enterprises a and b, with their own business processes, that cooperate to build a VE. For each of the two enterprises we are given a local alphabet, Σ_a respectively Σ_b. The symbols of the alphabets can represent various types of actions or events: (i) an internal task of the enterprise (e.g. packaging of goods), (ii) an interaction between the two enterprises (e.g. exchange of electronic documents), (iii) an event observed by one of the enterprises only (e.g. the receipt of a payment), or (iv) an event observed by both enterprises (e.g. that a carrier has left the harbor). Each enterprise also owns a local business process, representing all possible licit executions, that is given as a bounded labelled Petri net, N_a respectively N_b, defined over the corresponding local alphabet.

The problem of *VE process fusion* can be defined as computing the mapping:

$$N_i \mapsto N_i' \qquad (i \in \{a, b\})$$

Algorithm 1. $Protocol_i(N_a, N_b)$

1. $N_i^p := \mathbf{proj}_{\Sigma_a \cap \Sigma_b}(N_i)$ // project the private net on the common alphabet
2. $A_i^p := NFA(N_i^p)$ // obtain the equivalent nondeterministic automaton
          // by computing the reachability graph of the net
3. $A_i^d := SC(A_i^p)$ // determinize the automaton
4. send A_i^d to the secure multiparty protocol of [4]
5. receive $A := SMC_\times(A_a^d, A_b^d)$
6. $N := Reg(A)$ // synthesize the corresponding Petri net
7. return $N_i \times N$ // apply the external constraints to the initial net

where $N_i' \sim \mathbf{proj}_{\Sigma_i}(N_a \times N_b)$. and $\sim$ is trace equivalence. Here, the global VE business process is represented by the synchronous composition $\times$ and $\mathbf{proj}_{\Sigma_i}$ means making silent every transition that has label not in Σ_i.

Here we are interested in preserving the participants' privacy. In particular, we wish the two participants to obtain N_a' and N_b', respectively, without being able to learn about the other enterprise's processes more than what can be deduced from the own process (i.e., the *private input*) and the obtained result (i.e., the *private output*). Apart from the processes, we also consider private the alphabet differences; that is, we consider public just the common alphabet $\Sigma_a \cap \Sigma_b$ (i.e., the events of type (ii) and (iv)). Moreover, we assume that no trusted third party is available to serve as an intermediary.

To compute the VE process fusion without compromising the participants' privacy we take benefit from our previous result on private intersection of regular languages.

Algorithm 1 gives the protocol executed by the participant $i \in \{a, b\}$.

Our protocol is built on two main ideas. Since the input Petri nets are bound, their reachability graphs are finite and can be used to compute the DFAs representing the net languages (steps 1, 2 and 3). Moreover, as proved by Theorem 2, disclosing the intermediate language (step 5) does not leak any information that can not be directly deduced from the private output.

The following result establishes the *correctness* of the protocol, in the sense that the resulting network correctly represents the executions obtained by the synchronous product of the two business process after hiding all internal transitions of the other participant.

Theorem 1. $Protocol_i(N_a, N_b) \sim \mathbf{proj}_{\Sigma_i}(N_a \times N_b)$

The next result shows that the protocol preserves the participants' *privacy*, namely that the two participants are not able to learn about the other enterprise's processes more than what can be deduced from the own processes and the private output.

Theorem 2. Let N_a, N_b and N_b' be three labeled Petri nets defined over the alphabets Σ_a, Σ_b and Σ_b' respectively. If $\mathbf{proj}_{\Sigma_a}(N_a \times N_b) \sim \mathbf{proj}_{\Sigma_a}(N_a \times N_b')$ and $\Sigma_a \cap \Sigma_b = \Sigma_a \cap \Sigma_b'$ then $Protocol_a(N_a, N_b)$ is indistinguishable from $Protocol_a(N_a, N_b')$.

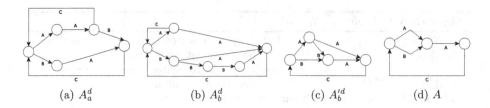

$$(a)\ A_a^d \qquad\qquad (b)\ A_b^d \qquad\qquad (c)\ A_b'^d \qquad\qquad (d)\ A$$

Fig. 3. DFAs

Example. We demonstrate the protocol using our running example. Starting from the input Petri nets N_a and N_b of Fig. 1, the two participants compute the DFAs A_a^d and A_b^d of Fig. 3 (steps 1, 2 and 3), hiding all transitions whose labels are not in $\Sigma_a \cap \Sigma_b$, computing the reachability graph, and then determinizing the result. Step 4 requires the execution of the secure multi-party protocol for regular language intersection of [4], which returns the automaton A to both participants. After the termination of the SMC protocol, the participants can proceed independently. Figure 2 depicts the final network obtained by the participant a, which is computed by synthesizing a Petri net from A, and by using the product operator $\times$.

Now, if the participant b owns the Petri net N_b', then the computed intermediate automaton is $A_b'^d$. Notice that the SMC protocol for regular language intersection still yields the automaton A. In fact, A is the minimal automaton of both $A_a^d \times A_b^d$ and $A_a^d \times A_b'^d$. This guarantees that the participant a learns nothing more than the expected result.

3   Prototype Implementation

We developed a prototype implementation by integrating the business process analysis platform PROM [8] with the secure multiparty computation platform SHAREMIND 2 [1]. Each enterprise hosts an instance of PROM. The enterprise business process can be imported either by using the native PROM support for standard Petri net file formats, or by using existing plug-ins (see e.g. [2,5]) that transform BPMN diagrams to Petri nets. Steps 1, 2, 3, 6 and 7 of the protocol are executed in PROM by using existing plug-ins (e.g. PNAnalisys and TSPetrinet) and a new plug-in encapsulates the functionality of the JAutomata Library.

The SMC protocol for regular language intersection has been implemented using SHAREMIND. To enable PROM (developed in Java) to interact with the SHAREMIND client (developed in C++) we encapsulated the latter in a REST web service and we used standard libraries to implement the HTTP protocol and data serialization.

The execution time of the algorithm is dominated by the SMC protocol for regular language intersection. In our experiments on a Linux virtual machine, the protocol requires 185 seconds to handle the Petri nets in Fig. 1.

4   Conclusion

In this paper we present the first privacy preserving protocol that allows the participants to discover their local views of the composition of their workflows, when the latter are modeled with Petri nets. Even if the composition of Petri nets has been widely studied in the contexts of business processes, concurrent systems and Web services, no previous work takes into account privacy from a workflow perspective.

Our ongoing research efforts includes the support for higher abstraction levels. The enterprises can use the existing techniques to transform high level models (e.g. BPMN diagrams) to Petri nets and to enable our protocol. We plan to identify suitable techniques to project back to the high level model the local view of the interorganizational workflow. Finally, the composition of workflows can yield unsound processes, such as interorganizational interactions that manifest deadlocks and livelocks. To support the creation of virtual enterprises, we plan to extend our results to enable suitable analysis techniques (e.g. [6]) without fully revealing the interorganizational workflow.

Acknowledgments. This work has been supported by the European Union Seventh Framework Programme (FP7/2007-2013) under grant agreement no. 284731 "Usable and Efficient Secure Multiparty Computation (UaESMC)".

References

1. Bogdanov, D., Laur, S., Willemson, J.: Sharemind: a framework for fast privacy-preserving computations. In: Jajodia, S., Lopez, J. (eds.) ESORICS 2008. LNCS, vol. 5283, pp. 192–206. Springer, Heidelberg (2008)
2. Bruni, R., Corradini, A., Ferrari, G., Flagella, T., Guanciale, R., Spagnolo, G.: Applying process analysis to the italian egovernment enterprise architecture. In: Carbone, M., Petit, J.-M. (eds.) WS-FM 2011. LNCS, vol. 7176, pp. 111–127. Springer, Heidelberg (2012)
3. Dijkman, R.M., Dumas, M., Ouyang, C.: Semantics and analysis of business process models in bpmn. Inf. Softw. Technol. **50**(12), 1281–1294 (2008)
4. Guanciale, R., Gurov, D., Laud, P.: Private intersection of regular languages. In: PST. IEEE (2014)
5. Kalenkova, A.: ProM BPMN conversions (2014). http://www.promtools.org/prom6/packages/BPMNConversions
6. Van der Aalst, W.: Loosely coupled interorganizational workflows: modeling and analyzing workflows crossing organizational boundaries. Inf. Manage. **37**(2), 67–75 (2000)
7. van der Aalst, W.M.: The application of petri nets to workflow management. J. Circuits, Syst. Comput. **8**(01), 21–66 (1998)
8. van Dongen, B.F., de Medeiros, A.K.A., Verbeek, H.M.W.E., Weijters, A.J.M.M.T., van der Aalst, W.M.P.: The ProM framework: a new era in process mining tool support. In: Ciardo, G., Darondeau, P. (eds.) ICATPN 2005. LNCS, vol. 3536, pp. 444–454. Springer, Heidelberg (2005)

PMC-MR 2014

Configuring Configurable Process Models Made Easier: An Automated Approach

D.M.M. Schunselaar[1]([✉]), Henrik Leopold[2], H.M.W. Verbeek[1],
Wil M.P. van der Aalst[1], and Hajo A. Reijers[1,3]

[1] Eindhoven University of Technology,
P.O. Box 513, 5600 MB Eindhoven, The Netherlands
{d.m.m.schunselaar,h.m.w.verbeek,w.m.p.v.d.aalst,h.a.reijers}@tue.nl
[2] WU Vienna, Welthandelsplatz 1, 1020 Vienna, Austria
henrik.leopold@wu.ac.at
[3] Perceptive Software, Piet Joubertstraat 4, 7315 AV Apeldoorn, The Netherlands

Abstract. Configurable process models have shown their usefulness for capturing the commonalities and variability within business processes. However, an end user will require an abstraction from the configurable process model, which is a highly technical artifact, to select a suitable configuration. Currently, the creation of such an abstraction requires considerable steps and technical knowledge. We provide an approach to construct such an abstraction automatically on the basis of an understanding of common concepts underlying process models on the one hand and automated analysis techniques on the other. Our approach also guarantees the consistency between the configuration choices of the end user. A positive yet preliminary evaluation with business users has been carried out to test the usability of our approach.

Keywords: Automatic · Configuring · Configurable process model · Concepts

1 Introduction

Configurable process models form a well-studied and highly evolved formalism for capturing the commonalities and variability between (similar) process models [1]. However, to obtain the exact configuration from a configurable process model that best suits a particular context is in many respects still a challenge.

Early approaches have mostly focused on the formalism to specify a configurable model and to keep configuration choices consistent, but did not guide an end user through the entire configuration process [2]. Later work incorporated so-called "auto-complete" features to automatically set configuration points which otherwise would lead to incorrect models [3]. More recent work has incorporated

D.M.M. Schunselaar, H.M.W. Verbeek, W.M.P. van der Aalst and H.A. Reijers—
This research has been carried out as part of the Configurable Services for Local Governments (CoSeLoG) project (http://www.win.tue.nl/coselog/).

© Springer International Publishing Switzerland 2015
F. Fournier and J. Mendling (Eds.): BPM 2014 Workshops, LNBIP 202, pp. 105–117, 2015.
DOI: 10.1007/978-3-319-15895-2_10

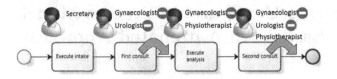

Fig. 1. Example configurable model consisting of 4 steps and 4 resources.

guidance by making end-users go through an electronic questionnaire: Its questions relate to the configuration options, while the answers to such questions can be mapped to configuration choices [4]. At this point, the creation and maintenance of such questionnaires to a large extent relies on manual work. For instance, in the questionnaire-based approach an expert has to define the questions to be posed to the end-user and must map the configuration settings to answer options. This is an intricate and laborious activity, particularly if the size of the configurable process model is large. Furthermore, changes to the configurable model may require elaborate inspection of the manual work that has already been conducted. Finally, questionnaire-based approaches rely on the help of experts to use the instrument and are thus not directly applicable off-the-shelf.

In this work, we provide support for the configuration process that is both automatically generated and universally applicable, i.e. independent of the model domain. To this end, we exploit the notion of general concepts that are at the core of many process modelling techniques. In this paper, we rely on the meta-model of APROMORE [5] to identify instances of these concepts, i.e. *resource* instances, *variable* instances, and *activity* instances. But our approach can be extended with other concepts. Our approach allows for an automatic identification of the concepts and their inter-relations in a configurable process model. The application-domain expert can then use these insights to make high-level decisions that tune the configurable model towards its intended use without the need to go through each and every element of the configurable model. For instance, if we take the model from Fig. 1 as our input, our approach would automatically deduce, amongst others, *gynaecologist* and *consult* as instances of the resource concept.

To optimally guide the user in setting their preferences, we developed a so-called *consistency graph*. This consistency graph is automatically constructed from the configurable model and signals users when they specify contradictory requirements. For instance, the user wants to include an activity but does not have the resources capable of executing it. Based on the requirements of the user, we infer the model(s) that best fit these. To show the business value of our approach, we have applied our approach on a real-life case study and evaluated its use with experts from a consultancy firm which is active in de healthcare ICT. In this evaluation, we used a configurable process model that captures the variety of process set-ups within Pelvic Floor Examination units in hospitals. From this configurable process model, we automatically distilled the concepts present. With the concepts, we automatically constructed the consistency graph without the need of any domain expert. Next, by presenting a view on the consistency graph and using this view to set their preferences, we demonstrated to the end-users how a model can be derived that best fits their needs. This paper discusses their feedback on this approach.

The structure of this paper is as follows: Sect. 2 lists the related work. In Sect. 3, we present the consistency graph, how we construct the consistency graph, and how we can deduce the configuration(s) using the consistency graph. Section 4 contains the implementation details of our approach. The evaluation of our approach is presented in Sect. 5. Finally, the conclusions and future work are presented in Sect. 6.

2   Related Work

Various approaches exist to provide an abstraction of the configurable process model as to simplify the configuration process [1]. In the approach that is described in [6], facts are set by posing questions to the user. For instance, "Shipping via DHL" is a question which is used to deduce the fact on the carrier for a package. Within the questionnaire-based approach, one can define constraints over the possible facts, e.g., at least one shipping company has to be selected. When the various facts have been set, these facts are used to set configuration options for the various configuration points. Within this approach, the questions about the facts have to be created by hand. Our approach can aid in this since the facts are related to instances of concepts, e.g., *Shipping* and *DHL* would both be concept instances.

In [7], the `Provop` approach is presented to use contextual information in the configuration of the configurable process model. Based on facts, various configuration options are selected, for instance, whether the "Quality Relevance" is high. Next to setting the facts directly, `Provop` also offer the possibility to reason over the facts, e.g., setting a particular value for a fact can have a cascading effect on another fact. Like the questionnaire-based approach, also `Provop` has been used in real-life case studies and its applicability and usability have been clearly demonstrated. Again, our approach can act as an intermediate approach to ease the manual work of distilling which facts to ask the user.

Various approaches exploit feature models to abstract from the configurable process model at hand. Feature models [8] are a way to capture aspects as well as the interdependencies between features. Feature models allow for a hierarchical decomposition of features making it possible to define one's preference at different levels of granularity. Various papers have brought the feature models to the area of configurable process models, e.g. [9–11]. As with other approaches, the construction of the feature model is a manual task. Our approach can indicate which features play a role in the process model.

Finally, in [12], the authors present an approach for querying a repository of models. In order to query this repository, the user has to design parts of a process model which are matched to process models in the repository and all process models containing these parts are returned. This approach is applicable to our setting, i.e., instead of querying a repository of models, the various models obtainable from the configurable process model are queried. However, this requires modelling skills from the end user, not necessarily present, and, the query being declarative in nature, requires the end user to inspect the returned process models to learn what is (not) possible in them.

In summary, the main limitation of existing approaches is the manual link between the configurable process model and the abstraction presented to the user, and requiring skills not necessarily present with the end user. In the next section, we present our way to improve on the state of the art by automatically deducing that abstraction without requiring particular skills of the end user.

3   Configuration Space Pruning

In this section, we introduce our configuration approach. We start by giving a general overview. Then, we discuss how we derive the concepts from the process model and how we use a consistency graph for the configuration.

3.1   Overview

As mentioned, we use the meta-model of APROMORE for the identification of instances of concepts. If we, for instance, consider the model in Fig. 1, we have 4 activities being executable by the resources as indicated, e.g., the activity *First consult* can be performed by the *Gynaecologist* and the *Urologist*. Taking a more detailed perspective, we can decompose activities into so-called business objects, actions, and business object modifiers. Hence, we associate the model in Fig. 1 with the resource instances *Secretary, Gynaecologist, Urologist*, and *Physiotherapist*, the business object instances *intake, consult*, and *analysis*, the object modifier instances *first* and *second*, and the action instance *execute*.

All these instances are combined into a single consistency graph such that the user can reason about these concept instances without going into each and every activity. We define the consistency graph on the entire configurable process model to present the user with a complete overview of the concept instances in the potential instantiation. By presenting a complete overview, the user can also indicate their preference on the non-configurable parts. If the non-configurable

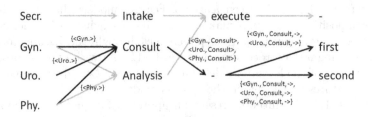

Fig. 2. The concept graph belonging to the model in Fig. 1. Some relations between the concepts have been grayed out to better indicate the contexts belonging to other relations.

part is incompatible with the user's organisation, this is notified at the earliest possible moment.

As not all the concepts have to be equally important, the user has the option to define a partial order on the concepts. In this way, we are able to present a view on the consistency graph starting from the most important concept. Let's assume the user has the following preferences with respect to the importance of concepts: (1) resource (the most important), (2) business object, (3) action, and (4) business object modifier (the least important). In that case, we would obtain the concept graph as depicted in Fig. 2. Note that we introduced a dummy "-" when a particular instance of the respective concept does not exist.

Apart from the concept instances, the consistency graph also contains relations (edges) between instances based on the ordering of concepts, e.g., the *consult* is performed by the *gynaecologist*. The relations are decorated with contexts. These contexts indicate when two concept instances are related, e.g., the relation between - and *first* only exists if the resource is either the *Gynaecologist* or the *Urologist*, the business object is a *consult*, and the action is -.

After having deduced the concept graph from the process model, the user can select which concepts, relations, and contexts are to be taken into account in the configuration process. For instance, the user might want to express that a gynaecologist and urologist are not present in their organisation and should therefore not play any part in the configuration. The concept graph from Fig. 2 is then annotated as depicted in Fig. 3. By storing this information in the concept graph, we do not return instantiations of the configurable process model which has a resource gynaecologist or urologist.

Next to indicating that certain concept instances are not present, the user also has the option to indicate an element (concept instance/relation/context) is highly relevant in a configuration context and should therefore be present in the configured model. This can be indicated in two ways; all and some. All indicates that an element is present and all elements related to it are all present. For instance, if the organisation would have indicated that the gynaecologist and urologist are present in all cases, then every cross in Fig. 3 would have

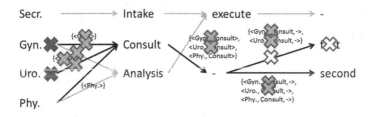

Fig. 3. The concept graph from Fig. 2 enriched with the information that the user does not have gynaecologists and urologists in their organisation. The completely filled crosses are the user's choice, the crosses filled with diagonal lines are directly deduced from the user's choice, and the crosses without a fill are deduced from the combination of the user's choices.

been substituted by a checkmark indicating they are present in All cases. Some
is in between all and none. For instance, taking Fig. 3 as an example, if the
user indicates that the physiotherapist is present in their organisation, then this
means *Consult* is set to some as it is present in some contexts but not in all.

In the concept graph in Fig. 3, we have crossed out *first* (set it to none)
although this was not explicitly encoded by the user. Rather, this is a result of
the user's action to eliminate the urologist and gynaecologist from the configuration process. By setting *first* to none, we make the user aware of this result.
The user could still opt to try and set *first* to some or even all. However, if
the user decides to do this, the graph becomes inconsistent. After all, there is
no qualified resource available anymore to execute a first consult. In order to
compute the transitive effect of choices in the configuration process, we defined
rules to transfer the selected answer to answers for other concepts, relations, and
contexts. Applying the consistency graph from Fig. 3 onto the model of Fig. 1
results in the model depicted in Fig. 4.

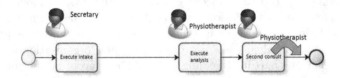

Fig. 4. The model obtained after applying the consistency graph of Fig. 3 to the model
in Fig. 1. All elements with a cross have been removed.

In the following, we elaborate how we obtain the concept instances from the
process model, we provide a formal definition of the consistency graph and rules
to transfer an answer, and how we use the consistency graph for configuration.

3.2   Obtaining the Concepts in the Consistency Graph

The consistency graph is obtained on basis of the process model. The resources
and data instances can be directly deduced from the process model. The decomposition of the activity labels is accomplished by using the language-based analysis technique from [13]. This technique builds on the insight that activity labels
follow regular structures, so-called labelling styles. By automatically recognising the varying labelling styles, it automatically decomposes every activity into
the underlying action, business object, and additional fragments. As an example, consider the activity "Notify customer via e-mail". As a result from the
label style recognition and the subsequent decomposition, the analysis technique
returns the action "notify", the business object "customer", and the additional
fragment "via e-mail". Note that this technique can be effectively adapted to
languages other than English [14].

3.3 The Consistency Graph

The consistency graph consists of two elements: a concept graph and a set of rules to ensure the consistency of that graph. In the concept graph, we have dontCare next to all, some, and none. DontCare is used as a default value and it can be used to indicate that the user is not interested in that particular element.

Definition 1 (Concept graph). *A concept graph G is a 5-tuple (V, E, C, QA, R) where:*

- *V is a set of vertices representing the different concept instances,*
- *$E \subseteq V \times V$ is a set of directed edges, denoting the relations*
- *$C : E \rightarrow 2^{V^*}$ are the contexts for each edge, denoting when a particular relation holds,*
- *$QA : V^* \cup E \cup V \rightarrow \{All, Some, None, DontCare\}$, the options selected for the contexts, vertices, and edges,*
- *(V, E) forms a DAG,*
- *$R \subseteq V$ are the roots (the most important concept instances).*

Prior to defining the rules for consistency, we first need a notion of subsumption on the contexts.

Definition 2 (Subsumption). *Let $lo, lo' \in V^*$ be two lists of concept instances, then we say lo' subsumes lo, denoted by $lo \sqsubseteq lo'$, if and only if: all concept instances in lo occur in lo' and they occur in the same order.*

In Table 1, the requirements to which the concept graph has to adhere to be a consistency graph are listed. The requirements reflect the intuitive meaning of each of the options a user has (all, some, none, dontCare).

The first three lines show the connection between the edges and the contexts on those edges. For instance, if an edge should be present in some cases, then there is at least one context which is either present for all or some but there should also be a context which is not all.

The next six lines connect the vertices with the incoming and outgoing edges. For instance, if a vertex is set to none, then all the incoming and outgoing edges are set to none. The last six lines are connecting the different contexts with each other, e.g., if a particular context is set to all, then all subsuming contexts are also set to all.

Definition 3 (Consistency graph). *Let $G = (V, E, C, QA, R)$ be a concept graph, we say G is a consistency graph if it adheres to the requirements in Table 1.*

To aid the user in creating the consistency graph, we apply the requirements from Table 1 after each choice of the user. In the application of the requirements, we take the user's choices done so far into account. For instance, if the requirements state that a concept instance has to be set to all but the user already set if to none, then the affected elements are denoted as inconsistent.

Table 1. The different requirements for transferring the selected answer.

$\forall_{e \in E}(QA(e) = \text{all} \Leftrightarrow \forall_{o \in C(e)} QA(o) = \text{all})$
$\forall_{e \in E}(QA(e) = \text{some} \Leftrightarrow \exists_{o \in C(e)} QA(o) \in \{\text{all, some}\} \wedge \exists_{o \in C(e)} QA(o) \neq \text{all})$
$\forall_{e \in E}(QA(e) = \text{none} \Leftrightarrow \forall_{o \in C(e)} QA(o) = \text{none})$
$\forall_{v \in V}(QA(v) = \text{all} \Leftrightarrow \forall_{(v,v') \in E} QA((v,v')) = \text{all})$
$\forall_{v \in V}(QA(v) = \text{all} \Leftrightarrow \forall_{(v',v) \in E} QA((v',v)) = \text{all})$
$\forall_{v \in V}(QA(v) = \text{some} \Leftrightarrow \exists_{(v,v') \in E} QA((v,v')) \in \{\text{all, some}\} \wedge \exists_{(v,v') \in E} QA((v,v')) \neq \text{all})$
$\forall_{v \in V}(QA(v) = \text{some} \Leftrightarrow \exists_{(v',v) \in E} QA((v',v)) \in \{\text{all, some}\} \wedge \exists_{(v',v) \in E} QA((v',v)) \neq \text{all})$
$\forall_{v \in V}(QA(v) = \text{none} \Leftrightarrow \forall_{(v,v') \in E} QA((v,v')) = \text{none})$
$\forall_{v \in V}(QA(v) = \text{none} \Leftrightarrow \forall_{(v',v) \in E} QA((v',v)) = \text{none})$
$\forall_{(v,v') \in E, lo \in C((v,v'))}(QA(lo) = \text{all} \Leftrightarrow \forall_{(v',v'') \in E, lo' \in C((v',v''))} lo \sqsubseteq lo' \Rightarrow QA(lo') = \text{all})$
$\forall_{(v',v) \in E, lo \in C((v',v))}(QA(lo) = \text{all} \Rightarrow \exists_{(v'',v') \in E, lo' \in C((v'',v'))} lo' \sqsubseteq lo \Rightarrow QA(lo') \in \{\text{all, some}\})$
$\forall_{(v,v') \in E, lo \in C((v,v'))}(QA(lo) = \text{some} \Leftrightarrow \exists_{(v',v'') \in E, lo' \in C((v',v''))} lo \sqsubseteq lo' \Rightarrow QA(lo') \in \{\text{all, some}\} \wedge$
$\exists_{(v',v'') \in E, lo' \in C((v',v''))} lo \sqsubseteq lo' \Rightarrow QA(lo') \neq \text{all})$
$\forall_{(v',v) \in E, lo \in C((v',v))}(QA(lo) = \text{some} \Rightarrow \exists_{(v'',v') \in E, lo' \in C((v'',v'))} lo' \sqsubseteq lo \Rightarrow QA(lo') = \text{some})$
$\forall_{(v,v') \in E, lo \in C((v,v'))}(QA(lo) = \text{none} \Leftrightarrow \forall_{(v',v'') \in E, lo' \in C((v',v''))} lo \sqsubseteq lo' \Rightarrow QA(lo') = \text{none})$
$\forall_{(v',v) \in E, lo \in C((v',v))}(QA(lo) = \text{none} \Rightarrow \exists_{(v'',v') \in E, lo' \in C((v'',v'))} lo' \sqsubseteq lo \Rightarrow QA(lo') \in \{\text{some, none}\})$

Next to verifying the consistency of the concept graph, we also verify that there is a possible instantiation from the configurable process model. This is a two-step approach, first based on the consistency graph, we can already configure certain parts, e.g., from the consistency graph, we can deduce which resources are allowed to execute which activities. In the second step, we iterate through possible instantiations of the configurable process model and verify if this instantiation adheres to the consistency graph.

In order to verify whether an instantiation adheres to the consistency graph based on the user's choices (G), we build the consistency graph of the instantiation (G_i). If an element in G is set to all or some, then we expect that this element is present in G_i. Note that, we know that by applying the requirements the user's choices have propagated and hence we can verify the presence locally. If an element in G is set to none, we expect that element is not present in G_i.

4   Implementation

The consistency graph has been implemented as part of *Petra* [15] (Process model based Extensible Toolset for Redesign and Analysis), a ProM plug-in and takes as input a configurable process model. It can be downloaded from www.processmining.org. *Petra* is a framework designed for the analysis of the configuration space of a configurable process model. Within *Petra*, different Key Performance Indicators (KPIs) and different tools for computing these KPIs can be used. The work presented here is used to prune the configuration space and thus reducing the computing power needed to analyse the configuration space. However, the ideas presented here transcend the use within *Petra* and can easily be made available to other formalisms, e.g., C-YAWL.

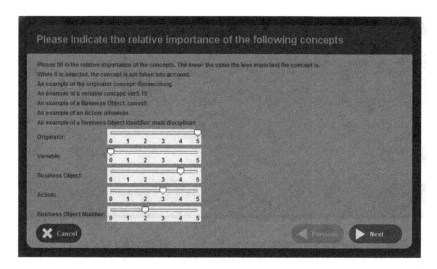

Fig. 5. The GUI presented to the user where they can indicate the relative importance of the various concepts.

We start with a configurable process model. Afterwards, prior to eliciting the requirements with the plug-in, the relative importance of the different concepts is to be elicited by the user (see Fig. 5). The screenshot shows the concepts present in a particular example. Next to the concepts, examples of instances of these concepts based on the configurable process model are provided to the domain expert. Using the sliders, the user can indicate their relative importance.

Based on the relative importance of the various concepts as indicated by the user, the concept instances are ordered. In the next screen (Fig. 6), the user can indicate which concept instances are to be preserved and whether there is a relationship between concept instances. The user has full freedom to explore the various concept instances and tailor these and their relationship to their preference. In Fig. 6, the user has indicated that *Bureau opname* (intake office) is related to **all**, which means that *Bureau opname* is related to *Afspraak* (appointment) and *Vragenlijst* (Questionnaire).

Next to this, the user can select, on a more fine-grained level, whether there is a relation between concept instances in a particular context (Fig. 7). In Fig. 7, the user has indicated that *multi disciplinair na* (*multi-disciplinary post*) is **all** in the context that the resource instance is a *Verpleegkundige* (*Nurse*) working on the Business Object *overleg* (*deliberation*), and the action *uitvoeren* (*execute*). By setting the use of *multi disciplinair na* to **all**, it can be automatically deduced on the basis of the consistency graph and the introduced rules that the other concept instances in this context have to be set to **some**. However, the user has set the *overleg* to **none**, resulting in an inconsistency as shown by the red parts. Note that, the inconsistency moves from context to edge to concept instances, resulting in signals of inconsistencies on a larger scale. By showing these inconsistencies, the user is notified of an impossibility. The impossibility can indicate for instance

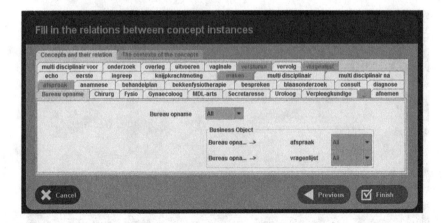

Fig. 6. The GUI presented to the user where they can indicate the relation between the concept instances, in this case the relations between *Bureau opname*, and *Afspraak* and *Vragenlijst*.

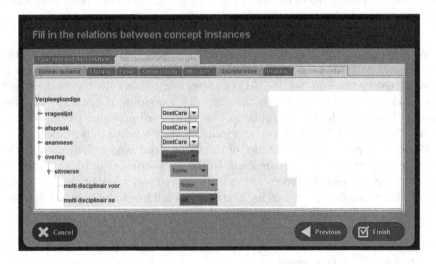

Fig. 7. The GUI presented to the user where they can indicate the relation between the concept instances, with a particular context. The context is build-up similar to the folder structure on a PC, e.g., *multi disciplinair na* is used in the context that the resource instance *Verpleegkundige* is working on Business Object *overleg*, and action *uitvoeren*. In this case, there is an inconsistency between *overleg* and *multi disciplinair na*.

that the user's requirements are not according to certain rules, but it can also indicate that the configurable model is not suitable for their organisation.

After pressing *Finish*, the tool automatically sets configuration points based on the settings by the user. This results in a (configurable) process model which is used in *Petra*. *Petra* checks for each instantiation if it adheres to the consistency graph.

5   Evaluation

For the evaluation of our approach, we cooperated with the consultancy agency iCON healthcare[1]. This agency advises hospitals, clinics, and other medical institutes on the improvement of their healthcare operations. We cooperated specifically with a consultant with deep knowledge on the way Pelvic Floor Examinations are carried out and a coach specialised in process modelling. Pelvic Floor Examinations are typically set up in an outpatient clinical setting, where various fields of medical expertise are brought together such as gynaecology, urology, physiotherapy, and surgery. Within the setting of Pelvic Floor examinations, there is considerable freedom to organise the diagnostic and treatment processes. Therefore, the consultants are seeking ways to guide their clients to a process set-up that best fits the local requirements but exploiting the options present in process set-ups within other hospitals. As a first step towards providing such services, the consultants held structured interviews with stakeholders within various hospitals to obtain an insight into these processes. This knowledge was codified in the form of process models. Using an extension to the techniques presented in [16], we were able to construct a configurable process model from these models.

In the evaluation of the approach we described in this paper, we went through 3 scenarios to expose the consultants to its characteristics. In the first scenario, we showed how the tool could be used to enable/disable a single concept, in casu a particular type of medical expert. In the second scenario, we went one step further by showing how the relations between concepts could be enabled/disabled. In particular, we showed the way to specify whether a surgeon would be allocatable to an activity involving a questionnaire. Finally, in the third scenario, we used a configurable process model obtained after merging a number of process models. Using this configurable process model, we were able to configure a specific process model which was applicable to one of the hospitals in their network. The presentation and discussion of the scenarios lasted approximately 80 min; the reflection on the approach 40 min.

The first outcome of our evaluation concerns the perceived usefulness of the tool. Both consultants looked highly favourable into this aspect. One of them stated that "the business case for this tool is that the information analysis phase can be strongly reduced", hinting at how the number of process set-ups to be evaluated could be highly reduced. As a precondition, it was noted that there should be an upfront investment in a database with configurable process models. The second point of reflection was the usability of the tool. According to one of the consultants "the interface is easy and intuitive". The notion of concepts in particular was well understood, as well as the meaning of the configuration choices. Finally, the third point of discussion related to potential improvements. The suggestions mostly involved the direct context of the toolkit: To improve the way to reach a sufficient amount of high-quality models from the hospital context and to provide support for bringing more detail to a model once it is

---

[1] www.iconhc.nl.

configured, e.g., the inclusion of work instructions and detailed resource constraints. One of the consultants even stated that: "The more we can fill in, the more valuable the tool becomes".

6 Conclusion

In this work, we showed an approach to automatically generate support to simplify and speed up the configuration of a configurable process model. We zoomed in on the use of general concepts, which can be recognised in most if not all process models, to specify those elements and relations that are relevant to the particular context of the model to be configured. We paid attention to safeguarding the consistency of the various choices an end user can make as well.

One of the main limitations of our approach at this moment is the lack of support for configuration constraints. Contrary to the configuration constraints present in related work, we intend configuration constraints from the end-user and between concept instances. For instance, for a hospital it does not matter which of two concept instances are present as long as at least one is present. In our current implementation, the user is not able to state conditional requirements between concept instances. We plan to add support for this using constraints in the spirit of a declarative modelling language. Next to supporting configuration constraints, we also plan to develop a *constructive* approach for deducing if there is an instantiation adhering to the consistency graph as defined by the user. When working with large amounts of variation points, the verification whether there is an instantiation adhering to the requirements of the end users can become a computational bottleneck.

In conclusion, we hope to contribute with this and future work to the further uptake and application of configurable process models.

Acknowledgements. The authors would like to thank Aukje Houben and Bram de Kort from iCON Healthcare for their cooperation in our case study.

References

1. La Rosa, M., van der Aalst, W.M.P., Dumas, M., Milani, F.P.: Business process variability modeling: a survey. ACM Comput. Surv. (2013). http://eprints.qut.edu.au/61842/
2. Rosemann, M., van der Aalst, W.M.P.: A configurable reference modelling language. Inf. Syst. **32**(1), 1–23 (2007)
3. van der Aalst, W.M.P., Lohmann, N., La Rosa, M.: Ensuring correctness during process configuration via partner synthesis. Inf. Syst. **37**(6), 574–592 (2012)
4. La Rosa, M., Lux, J., Seidel, S., Dumas, M., ter Hofstede, A.H.M.: Questionnaire-driven configuration of reference process models. In: Krogstie, J., Opdahl, A.L., Sindre, G. (eds.) CAiSE 2007. LNCS, vol. 4495, pp. 424–438. Springer, Heidelberg (2007)

5. La Rosa, M., Reijers, H.A., van der Aalst, W.M.P., Dijkman, R.M., Mendling, J., Dumas, M., García-Bañuelos, L.: APROMORE: an advanced process model repository. Expert Syst. Appl. **38**, 7029–7040 (2011)
6. La Rosa, M., van der Aalst, W.M.P., Dumas, M., ter Hofstede, A.H.M.: Questionnaire-based variability modeling for system configuration. Softw. Syst. Model. **8**(2), 251–274 (2009)
7. Hallerbach, A., Bauer, T., Reichert, M.: Capturing variability in business process models: the provop approach. J. Softw. Maint. Evol. Res. Pract. **22**(6–7), 519–546 (2010)
8. Kang, K.C., Cohen, S.G., Hess, J.A., Novak, W.E., Peterson, A.S.: Feature-oriented domain analysis (foda) feasibility study. Technical report cmu/sei-90-tr-21 esd-90-tr-222. Technical report, Software Engineering Institute, Carnegie Mellon University (1990)
9. Schnieders, A., Puhlmann, F.: Variability mechanisms in e-business process families. In: Abramowicz, W., Mayr, H.C. (eds.) BIS. LNI, vol. 85, pp. 583–601. GI (2006)
10. Acher, M., Collet, P., Lahire, P., France, R.: Managing variability in workflow with feature model composition operators. In: Baudry, B., Wohlstadter, E. (eds.) SC 2010. LNCS, vol. 6144, pp. 17–33. Springer, Heidelberg (2010)
11. Czarnecki, K., Antkiewicz, M.: Mapping features to models: a template approach based on superimposed variants. In: Glück, R., Lowry, M. (eds.) GPCE 2005. LNCS, vol. 3676, pp. 422–437. Springer, Heidelberg (2005)
12. Awad, A., Sakr, S., Kunze, M., Weske, M.: Design by selection: a reuse-based approach for business process modeling. In: Jeusfeld, M., Delcambre, L., Ling, T.-W. (eds.) ER 2011. LNCS, vol. 6998, pp. 332–345. Springer, Heidelberg (2011)
13. Leopold, H., Smirnov, S., Mendling, J.: On the refactoring of activity labels in business process models. Inf. Syst. **37**(5), 443–459 (2012)
14. Leopold, H., Eid-Sabbagh, R.H., Mendling, J., Azevedo, L.G., Baião, F.A.: Detection of naming convention violations in process models for different languages. Decis. Support Syst. **56**, 310–325 (2013)
15. Schunselaar, D.M.M., Verbeek, H.M.W., van der Aalst, W.M.P., Reijers, H.A.: Petra: A tool for analysing a process family. In Moldt, D., Rölke, H. (eds.) International Workshop on Petri Nets and Software Engineering (PNSE 2014). CEUR Workshop Proceedings, Aachen, vol. 1160, pp. 269–288. CEUR-WS.org (2014). http://ceur-ws.org/Vol-1160/
16. Schunselaar, D.M.M., Verbeek, E., van der Aalst, W.M.P., Raijers, H.A.: Creating sound and reversible configurable process models using CoSeNets. In: Abramowicz, W., Kriksciuniene, D., Sakalauskas, V. (eds.) BIS 2012. LNBIP, vol. 117, pp. 24–35. Springer, Heidelberg (2012)

When Language Meets Language: Anti Patterns Resulting from Mixing Natural and Modeling Language

Fabian Pittke$^{(\boxtimes)}$, Henrik Leopold, and Jan Mendling

WU Vienna, Welthandelsplatz 1, 1020 Vienna, Austria
{fabian.pittke,henrik.leopold,jan.mendling}@wu.ac.at

Abstract. Business process modeling has become an integral part of many organizations for documenting and redesigning complex organizational operations. However, the increasing size of process model repositories calls for automated quality assurance techniques. While many aspects such as formal and structural problems are well understood, there is only a limited understanding of semantic issues caused by natural language. One particularly severe problem arises when modelers employ natural language for expressing control-flow constructs such as gateways or loops. This may not only negatively affect the understandability of process models, but also the performance of analysis tools, which typically assume that process model elements do not encode control-flow related information in natural language. In this paper, we aim at increasing the current understanding of mixing natural and modeling language and therefore exploratively investigate three process model collections from practice. As a result, we identify a set of nine anti patterns for mixing natural and modeling language.

Keywords: Mixing of natural language and modeling language · Anti patterns · Business process models

1 Introduction

Nowadays, business process modeling is an essential part of organizational design. Many organizations document their operations in an extensive way that involves several modelers and may result in more than thousand separate process models [1]. The increasing number of process models gives raise to automated quality assurance techniques since the consistency in such large-scale modeling initiatives can be hardly assured in a manual way [2]. Indeed, process models from practice often suffer from inconsistencies with respect to layout, level of detail, terminology, and labeling [2–5].

Recognizing this, many techniques for automatically assuring the quality of process models have been introduced. There are techniques for checking structural properties such as deadlocks [6], techniques for checking the correctness of the data flow [7,8], and techniques for automatically refactoring the model structure [9,10]. Recently, also linguistic issues have been addressed. More specifically,

© Springer International Publishing Switzerland 2015
F. Fournier and J. Mendling (Eds.): BPM 2014 Workshops, LNBIP 202, pp. 118–129, 2015.
DOI: 10.1007/978-3-319-15895-2_11

available techniques recognize labeling styles [4,11] and rework them according to desired naming conventions [12]. However, in particular semantic issues caused by natural language have not been investigated in much detail. As an example, consider the activity label *Consult expert and prepare report*. Apparently, this label contains two separate activities, i.e., *consult expert* and *prepare report*, which are linked by the conjunction *and*. The problem is that the execution semantics between these separate activities is not clearly defined. In fact, the word *and* could imply a parallel as well as a sequential execution. The reason for this confusion is the usage of natural language for expressing control-flow related aspects. Since natural language is often ambiguous, the precise intention of the modeler is not fully transparent to the reader.

In this paper, we investigate the problem of mixing natural and modeling language in process models. As there is, to the best of our knowledge, no research that addressed this problem, we take an explorative approach and manually analyze three process model collections from practice. Our contribution is a classification of anti patterns, which summarizes and groups cases in which natural language is used for expressing semantics of modeling language constructs. For each anti pattern, we identify possible interpretations and describe the characteristics in detail. The overall goal is to provide the knowledge base for automatically detecting, resolving and preventing these cases in the future.

The rest of the paper is structured accordingly. Section 2 illustrates the problem and discusses related work. Section 3 explains our methodology of approaching the problem. Section 4 presents the anti patterns we identified as well as an overview of their occurrence in the investigated model collections. Finally, Sect. 5 concludes the paper.

2 Problem Statement

In prior research, different aspects of process model quality have been addressed. In particular, structural and behavioral problems are well-understood and can automatically be resolved using different techniques. Structural problems refer to the elements of a process model and their interconnection. Available techniques can automatically transform unstructured process models into structured ones [10] or automatically detect deadlocks [6,13]. Behavioral problems refer to control flow-related aspects of process models. Available techniques detect control-flow errors by using formal techniques [14] or check control-flow related properties of process models [15]. Additionally, the quality of natural language in process models has been addressed in current research. Existing techniques include, for instance, the refactoring of the activity label grammar [4] or the detection of ambiguous terminology [5]. In [16], the authors also investigate whether the natural language in activities violates the logic that is imposed by control flow splits. For example, an application cannot be rejected or accepted in the same process instance.

One aspect that has not been addressed in prior research are inconsistencies resulting from mixing natural language and modeling language in a single model

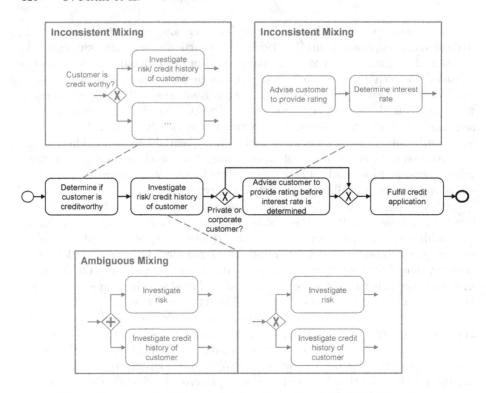

Fig. 1. Process with Elements Mixing Natural and Modeling Language

element. Figure 1 illustrates a number of typical problems which occur when the natural language is used to express semantics that are supposed to be communicated with constructs from the modeling language. The figure shows a short process model from a bank representing a credit application. The process starts by determining credit worthiness of the customer. Therefore, possible risks as well as the credit history are analyzed. In the next step, it is determined whether the customer is a private or a corporate customer. Depending on the status, he is advised to provide a rating. Finally, the credit application is fulfilled.

The figure illustrates different cases of mixing natural language and modeling language. The activity *Determine if customer is credit worthy* requires the model reader to evaluate the credit worthiness. However, since this activity implies a decision, it would be more consistent to model it as a gateway. The activity *Advise customer to provide rating before interest rate is determined* uses the word *before* for implementing a sequence of activities. Here, it would be more consistent to model two separate activities. Although both cases represent an inconsistent mix of natural and modeling language, it has to be noted that their are not ambiguous, i.e., the intention of the modeler is clear. Nevertheless, there are also less understandable cases. For example, the activity *Investigate risk/ credit history of customer* is highly ambiguous. Although we know that the activity involves an investigation of certain objects, it is unclear if the person is requested to investigate both the risk and the credit history or only one of these objects. The semantics of the slash symbol is simply not clearly defined and often used in different ways in practice.

The implications of mixing natural and modeling language are considerable. It may affect the ability of a reader to properly understand the model or to develop a solid understanding of the underlying process. Moreover, the performance of different analysis techniques might be affected. If the control flow semantics of a process are partially encoded using natural language, a structural check for deadlocks or other issues may erroneously evaluate the process as correct. Typically, such techniques simply assume that each activity contains a single piece of information that is not subject to additional conditions.

In order to address the problem of mixing natural and modeling language, techniques are needed that can detect and resolve affected process model elements. This, however, requires a precise understanding of these cases in the first place. So far, current research lacks a deeper understanding of such cases, their characteristics as well as their qualitative and quantitative extent. In order to close this gap, this paper investigates three model collections from practice. We use these collections to detect and classify linguistic anti patterns and to learn about their qualitative and quantitative extent. The overall goal is to provide the necessary knowledge for automatically detecting and resolving such cases in the future.

3   Research Design

The aim of this paper is to detect cases where natural language and modeling language are mixed. To achieve this goal, we adopt an explorative approach as conducted by Weber et al. for identifying refactoring opportunities in process models [9]. In particular, we perform an extensive manual analysis of industry process models to derive a list of generic anti patterns. Section 3.1 introduces our data set. Then, Sect. 3.2 gives an overview of our analysis methodology.

3.1   Selection Criteria and Data Collection

In order to maximize the external validity of our results, we select process model collections that vary with respect to different dimensions such as modeling language, domain, and the degree of standardization. The characteristics of the selected process model collections are summarized in Table 1. Our data set includes:

- **SAP Reference Model Collection:** The SAP Reference Model Collection (SRM) captures the business processes of the SAP R/3 system in its version from the year 2000 [17, pp. 145–164]. It includes 604 Event-driven Process Chains with in total 2433 activities. Since the SRM is a reference model collection, it has a relatively high degree of standardization.

Table 1. Demographics of the test collections

Characteristic	SRM	IMC	AI
No. of Models	604	349	1,091
No. of Labels	2,433	1,840	8,339
Modeling Language	EPC	EPC	BPMN
Domain	Independent	Insurance	Academic Training
Standardization	High	Medium	Low

- **Insurance Model Collection:** The Insurance Model Collection (IMC) contains 349 EPCs dealing with the claims handling activities of a large insurance company. It includes a total of 1840 activities and is less standardized than the SRM as the models were created for internal purposes only.
- **AI Collection:** The models from the BPM Academic Initiative (AI) stem from academic training (see http://bpmai.org). The selected English subset includes 1,091 process models with in total 8,339 activity labels. As the model have been mainly created by students, we expect the lowest degree of standardization in this collection.

3.2 Data Analysis

To analyze the model collections, we choose an incremental approach that consists of two separate steps: anti pattern extraction and anti pattern classification.

In the *anti pattern extraction phase*, we manually scanned the process model collections for linguistic constructs implying control flow semantics. By independently analyzing the collections, we made sure that we did not miss relevant anti patterns and reduced the probability of biased results.

In the *anti pattern classification phase*, we analyzed each anti pattern in detail and derived possible interpretations. As a result, we received a set of nine anti patterns. Based on the number of possible interpretations, we classified each anti pattern as *inconsistent* or *ambiguous*. Inconsistent anti patterns mix natural and modeling language in an inconsistent way, but still have only one possible interpretation. Ambiguous anti patterns, by contrast, mix natural and modeling language in such a way that two or more interpretations are possible.

4 Findings

This section presents the findings of our explorative study. Section 4.1 presents the anti patterns which inconsistently mix natural and modeling language, but still only have a single interpretation. Section 4.2 introduces the anti patterns which are ambiguous and, hence, allow for multiple interpretations. In Sect. 4.3, we give an overview of the quantitative extent of the identified anti patterns.

4.1   Anti Patterns with Inconsistent Mixing

In the following, we introduce the anti patterns having a single interpretation. In total, there are four anti patterns: *Logical Extra Information, Iteration, Skip*, and *If Evaluation*.

Anti Pattern 1 (Logical Extra Information). The *Logical Extra Information* anti pattern incorporates logical information into the label. This information imposes additional conditions on the task and, hence, has direct impact on the control flow. Typically, this anti pattern uses temporal prepositions such as *before* or *after* to clarify the order of activities. Figure 2 shows an example of this anti pattern and its corresponding consistent solution.

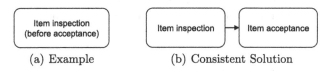

(a) Example   (b) Consistent Solution

Fig. 2. Anti Pattern 1 (Logical Extra Information)

Anti Pattern 2 (Iteration). The *Iteration* anti pattern is arranged in such a way that the natural language fragment asks for an iteration or a loop construct. In most of the cases, the iteration is expressed by the language pattern *repeat ... until* or a statement such as *per item*. In many cases, the label also contains the iteration condition. Figure 3 provides an example of this anti pattern and its corresponding consistent solution.

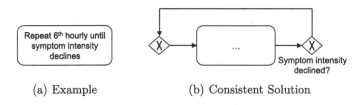

(a) Example   (b) Consistent Solution

Fig. 3. Anti Pattern 2 (Iteration)

Anti Pattern 3 (Skip). The activity of a *Skip* anti pattern generally implies a decision about an activity that must only be conducted under specific conditions. If the conditions are not met, the activity is skipped and the process continues without executing this activity. Our analysis showed that activity labels that follow this anti pattern combine prepositions with adjectives or the past participle of the verb *to require*. Thus, examples include *if necessary, if required*, or *as required*. Figure 4 shows an example and its corresponding consistent solution.

Anti Pattern 4 (If Evaluation). The *If Evaluation* anti pattern also implies a decision in the process flow. By contrast to the previously mentioned anti patterns, the If Evaluation anti pattern explicitly specifies the condition that has

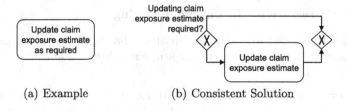

(a) Example   (b) Consistent Solution

Fig. 4. Anti Pattern 3 (Skip)

to be checked. In most cases, activities of this anti pattern contain a verb asking for the verification or investigation of certain conditions and the conditional word *if*. Examples of this anti pattern include *determine if, validate if, check if,* and *confirm if.* Figure 5 shows an example and its consistent solution.

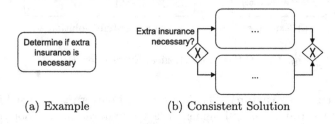

(a) Example   (b) Consistent Solution

Fig. 5. Anti Pattern 4 (If Evaluation)

4.2   Anti Patterns with Ambiguous Mixing

In the following, we introduce the anti patterns that allow for multiple interpretations. In total, they are 5 ambiguous anti patterns: *Wrong Label Class, Multiple Activities, Decision, Content-based Extra Information,* and *Temporal Extra Information.*

Anti Pattern 5 (Wrong Label Class). Process model elements suffering from the *Wrong Label Class* anti pattern erroneously combine labeling style and modeling construct, i.e., activity, event, or gateway. As an example, consider an activity that is labeled using an event label or vice versa. As a result, it remains unclear whether the natural language or the modeling language determines the meaning of the construct. As shown in Fig. 6, the activity *Tick box invoice entered* might refer to the event *Tick box invoice entered* or to the activity *Enter a tick box invoice.*

Anti Pattern 6 (Multiple Activities). Activities suffering from the *Multiple Activities* anti pattern combine several actions, business objects, or combinations of these in a single activity element. Hence, a single activity element instructs people to perform multiple streams of action. Typically, this anti pattern includes the conjunction *and,* or special characters such as *+,* or *&.*

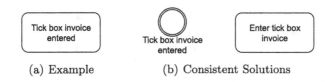

(a) Example   (b) Consistent Solutions

Fig. 6. Anti Pattern 5 (Wrong Label Class)

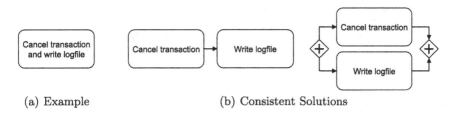

(a) Example   (b) Consistent Solutions

Fig. 7. Anti Pattern 6 (Multiple Activities)

The interpretation of this pattern is ambiguous. It may refer to a sequence of activities as well as to a parallel execution. Figure 7 illustrates this anti pattern using the activity *Cancel transaction and write logfile*.

Anti Pattern 7 (Decision). The *Decision* anti pattern implies a control flow split leading to several exclusive or inclusive streams of action. Similarly to the previous anti pattern, this anti pattern may use multiple actions, business objects, or combinations of these. Typically, this anti pattern occurs when two alternatives are linked with the conjunction *or*. Alternatively, the special character /may represent an indicator for this anti pattern. As shown by the activity *Negotiate liability or quantum* in Fig. 8, we cannot infer whether this anti pattern expresses an exclusive or an inclusive decision.

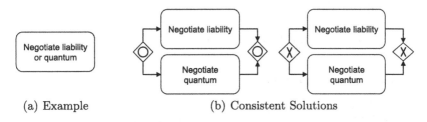

(a) Example   (b) Consistent Solutions

Fig. 8. Anti Pattern 7 (Decision)

Anti Pattern 8 (Content-based Extra Information). The *Content-based Extra Information* anti pattern refers to activities that ambiguously incorporate additional information into the label. This may include the specification of business objects or the refinement of entire activities. The most prominent examples are the use of brackets and the separation of information using a dash. As an example for this anti pattern, consider the activity *Capture Driver details* *(inc. licence, alcohol, questions etc.)* from Fig. 9. Here, the business object *driver details* is further specified in brackets. However, the interpretation of this label is unclear. This anti pattern may refer to a single activity as well as to multiple activities in form of a subprocess that are specified elsewhere. Figure 9 illustrates the possible interpretations of this activity.

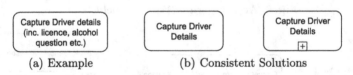

(a) Example   (b) Consistent Solutions

Fig. 9. Anti Pattern 8 (Content-based Extra Information)

Anti Pattern 9 (Temporal Extra Information). The *Temporal Extra Information* anti pattern is similar to the latter anti pattern. It, however, incorporates temporal instead of content-based information. This may include temporal prepositions that clarify the duration (e.g. in minutes, hours, or days) of an activity or other time-related constraints. Typically, the additional information is provided in brackets and, in many cases, unclear. The temporal information may represent waiting time, i.e., time that must pass before the process continues normally, or the temporal information could be interpreted in the sense of an attached intermediate event. The latter implies that the execution of the activity is canceled as soon as the time limit is reached (Fig. 10).

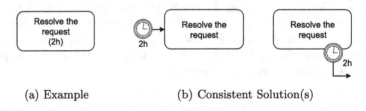

(a) Example   (b) Consistent Solution(s)

Fig. 10. Anti Pattern 9 (Temporal Extra Information)

4.3   Quantitative Findings

To get an impression of the quantitative extent of the previously introduced anti patterns, Table 2 gives an overview of the number of occurrences of the anti patterns for each investigated collection. The numbers reveal that all three collections particularly suffer from the anti patterns *Content-based Extra Information* and *Multiple Activities*. For the other patterns, we observe a more heterogeneous distribution. While the IMC and the AI collection also frequently suffer from the anti pattern *Wrong Label Class* and *If Evaluation*, the SRM collection is almost free from these issues. Reasons for such differences include a differing degree of standardization and a differing experience of the involved modelers. Especially, less experienced modelers may tend to use natural language for expressing more complex control-flow structures such as loops, skips, and decisions.

Table 2. Anti pattern frequencies

	Anti Pattern	SRM	IMC	AI
Inconsistent Anti Patterns	AP 1 - Logical Extra Information	0	10	7
	AP 2 - Iteration	0	0	15
	AP 3 - Skip	0	49	0
	AP 4 - If Evaluation	0	156	70
Ambiguous Anti Patterns	AP 5 - Wrong Label Class	0	18	104
	AP 6 - Multiple Activities	217	329	606
	AP 7 - Decision	2	125	52
	AP 8 - Content-based Extra Information	285	63	112
	AP 9 - Temporal Extra Information	0	1	68

In conclusion, we can state that the phenomenon of mixing natural and modeling language can be frequently encountered in practice. A detailed investigation also revealed that models containing one anti pattern tend to include further anti patterns. As pointed out earlier, this can significantly affect the understandability of the models as well as the performance of automated analysis techniques. Hence, the introduced classification represents an important step towards automatically cleaning process model repositories from this quality issue and preventing it in the future.

5   Conclusion

In this paper, we investigated the problem of using natural language for expressing modeling language constructs. We therefore manually analyzed three process model collections from practice in order to identify anti patterns. In total, we identified a set of nine different anti patterns, which we classified into *inconsistent* and *ambiguous* cases. While the latter category is particularly a problem for the understandability of humans, all these anti patterns may negatively affect the results of automated analysis techniques as they often assume that activities do not contain additional conditions encoded in natural language. A quantitative evaluation of the findings demonstrated that anti patterns for mixing natural and modeling language can be frequently found in process models from practice and that there is also a tendency for models to contain multiple anti patterns.

Altogether, this paper provides the foundations for automatically detecting and resolving issues related to mixing natural and modeling language. Furthermore, the identified anti patterns foster the creation of a canonical process model, i.e., a process model in which each activity refers to only one stream of action. Such a canonical process model would be highly beneficial for several process model analysis techniques as, for instance, the matching of activities [18], the matching of process models [19,20], and the calculation of process behavior [21]. Against this background, it is our goal to implement a technique for detecting and resolving the identified anti patterns in the future. In addition, we plan to validate our anti pattern classification against additional process model collections.

References

1. Rosemann, M.: Potential pitfalls of process modeling: part A. Bus. Process Manage. J. **12**(2), 249–254 (2006)
2. Becker, J., Rosemann, M., von Uthmann, C.: Guidelines of business process modeling. In: van der Aalst, W.M.P., Desel, J., Oberweis, A. (eds.) Business Process Management. LNCS, vol. 1806, pp. 30–49. Springer, Heidelberg (2000)
3. Davis, R.: Aris Design Platform: Advanced Process Modelling and Administration. Springer, Heidelberg (2008)
4. Leopold, H., Smirnov, S., Mendling, J.: On the refactoring of activity labels in business process models. Inf. Syst. **37**(5), 443–459 (2012)
5. Pittke, F., Leopold, H., Mendling, J.: Spotting terminology deficiencies in process model repositories. In: Nurcan, S., Proper, H.A., Soffer, P., Krogstie, J., Schmidt, R., Halpin, T., Bider, I. (eds.) BPMDS 2013 and EMMSAD 2013. LNBIP, vol. 147, pp. 292–307. Springer, Heidelberg (2013)
6. Fahland, D., Favre, C., Koehler, J., Lohmann, N., Völzer, H., Wolf, K.: Analysis on demand: instantaneous soundness checking of industrial business process models. Data Knowl. Eng. **70**(5), 448–466 (2011)
7. Sun, S., Zhao, J., Nunamaker, J., Liu Sheng, O.: Formulating the data-flow perspective for business process management. Inf. Syst. Res. **17**(4), 374–391 (2006)
8. Sidorova, N., Stahl, C., Trcka, N.: Soundness verification for conceptual workflow nets with data: early detection of errors with the most precision possible. Inf. Syst. **36**(7), 1026–1043 (2011)
9. Weber, B., Reichert, M., Mendling, J., Reijers, H.A.: Refactoring large process model repositories. Comput. Ind. **62**(5), 467–486 (2011)
10. Polyvyanyy, A., García-Bañuelos, L., Dumas, M.: Structuring acyclic process models. In: Hull, R., Mendling, J., Tai, S. (eds.) BPM 2010. LNCS, vol. 6336, pp. 276–293. Springer, Heidelberg (2010)
11. Leopold, H., Smirnov, S., Mendling, J.: Recognising activity labeling styles in business process models. Enterp. Model. Inf. Syst. Architect. **6**(1), 16–29 (2011)
12. Leopold, H., Eid-Sabbagh, R.H., Mendling, J., Azevedo, L.G., Baião, F.A.: Detection of naming convention violations in process models for different languages. Decis. Support Syst. **56**, 310–325 (2013)
13. Dehnert, J., Rittgen, P.: Relaxed soundness of business processes. In: Dittrich, K.R., Geppert, A., Norrie, M. (eds.) CAiSE 2001. LNCS, vol. 2068, pp. 157–170. Springer, Heidelberg (2001)
14. van der Aalst, W.M.P.: Workflow verification: finding control-flow errors using petri-net-based techniques. In: van der Aalst, W.M.P., Desel, J., Oberweis, A. (eds.) Business Process Management. LNCS, vol. 1806, pp. 161–183. Springer, Heidelberg (2000)
15. van der Aalst, W.M.P., de Beer, H.T., van Dongen, B.F.: Process mining and verification of properties: an approach based on temporal logic. In: Meersman, R., Tari, Z. (eds.) OTM 2005. LNCS, vol. 3760, pp. 130–147. Springer, Heidelberg (2005)

16. Gruhn, V., Laue, R.: Detecting common errors in event-driven process chains by label analysis. Enterp. Model. Inf. Syst. Architect. **6**(1), 3–15 (2011)
17. Keller, G., Teufel, T.: SAP(R) R/3 Process Oriented Implementation: Iterative Process Prototyping. Addison-Wesley, Boston (1998)
18. Dijkman, R.M., Dumas, M., van Dongen, B.F., Käärik, R., Mendling, J.: Similarity of business process models: metrics and evaluation. Inf. Syst. **36**(2), 498–516 (2011)
19. Dijkman, R., Dumas, M., García-Bañuelos, L.: Graph matching algorithms for business process model similarity search. In: Dayal, U., Eder, J., Koehler, J., Reijers, H.A. (eds.) BPM 2009. LNCS, vol. 5701, pp. 48–63. Springer, Heidelberg (2009)
20. Leopold, H., Niepert, M., Weidlich, M., Mendling, J., Dijkman, R., Stuckenschmidt, H.: Probabilistic optimization of semantic process model matching. In: Barros, A., Gal, A., Kindler, E. (eds.) BPM 2012. LNCS, vol. 7481, pp. 319–334. Springer, Heidelberg (2012)
21. Weidlich, M., Mendling, J., Weske, M.: Efficient consistency measurement based on behavioral profiles of process models. IEEE Trans. Softw. Eng. **37**(3), 410–429 (2011)

vrBPMN* and FM: An Approach to Model Business Process Line

Geraldo Landre[1]([✉]), Edilson Palma[1], Débora Maria Paiva[1],
Elisa Yumi Nakagawa[2], and Maria Istela Cagnin[1]

[1] Computing College, Federal University of Mato Grosso do Sul (UFMS),
Campo Grande, MS, Brazil
geraldo@facom.ufms.br
http://www.facom.ufms.br
[2] Department of Computer Systems, University of São Paulo (USP),
São Carlos, SP, Brazil
http://www.icmc.usp.br

Abstract. Recently, Business Process Management (BPM) has increasing demanded reuse of business process models. In order to represent these models, diverse techniques have been used, such as the variability management and business process configuration, arising the Business Process Line (BPL) area. In order to model BPL, the joint use of vrBPMN (varant-rich Business Process Model and Notation) and Feature Model (FM) has been considered as a relevant alternative. However, there is a kind of FM elements that does not have a properly correspondent in vrBPMN, that is, the IOR element. In addition to that, FM and vrBPMN have some redundant informations. The main contribution of this paper is to propose an extension to the vrBPMN notation, named vrBPMN*, and, together with FM, makes it possible to adequately model BPL. We conducted an empirical study to analyze the viability of using vrPBMN* and FM to model business process, as well as their building time and correctness. As main results, we have observed that the proposed notation favours business process modeling, reducing time and increasing correctness of produced models.

1 Introduction

Currently, the competition among companies has required a constant evolution in how business is conducted. In this scenario, Business Process Management (BPM) has as main goal to improve both understanding and optimization of existing business process, as well as design of new ones, making it possible to become companies more competitive and efficient [12]. In order to adequately represent these processes, the activity of business process modeling has been widely applied, representing such process from different perspectives [8].

In another perspective, reuse is a successful practice in several contexts, such as in Software Engineering area. Reuse of business process models is also interesting, as it can reduce time and, at the same time, increase productivity in

© Springer International Publishing Switzerland 2015
F. Fournier and J. Mendling (Eds.): BPM 2014 Workshops, LNBIP 202, pp. 130–141, 2015.
DOI: 10.1007/978-3-319-15895-2_12

business process modeling. Besides that, this reuse can increase the quality of the produced models, considering that such models have been already previously tested and used [11]. Intending to systematically reuse business process models, a new research area has been established: Business Process Line (BPL) [14,15]. Based on concepts and experiences from Software Product Line (SPL) [13], BPL also presents the challenge of being adequately represented. Several approaches can be found in the literature [2,7,10,14,15]. Among them, two techniques have been widely used: Feature Model (FM) [9], commonly used to represent commonalities and variabilities in BPL [7], and BPMN (Business Process Model and Notation), used to represent business process templates and considered one of the most adequate to describe business process [4]. Moreover, an extension of BPMN, the vrBPMN (variant-rich BPMN) [15], was proposed enabling to explicitly represent variability in business process models. Besides that, the joint use of vrBPMN and FM has been considered a relevant solution to represent such models. On this assumption, we conducted a study to observe capacity of vrBPMN and FM to support BPL modeling. From this study, we observed that it is not possible to represent Inclusive-OR (IOR) elements in vrBPMN, which is an important characteristic of variability elements.

In this context, the main contribution of this paper is to present an extension to the vrBPMN notation, named vrBPMN*, which together with FM, makes it possible to more completely model BPL. Additionally, the paper presents an empirical study conducted to analyze the viability of vrBPMN* and FM to support elaboration of business process models, as well as their building time and correctness. As main results, we have observed that the proposed notation favours business process modeling, increasing correctness of the produced models with a minimum impact in time spent in such activity.

The remainder of this paper is organized as follows. In Sect. 2 we present necessaries background concepts of this work as well as related work. In Sect. 3, we present key factors to BPL modeling, and also are presented the adherence of vrBPMN and FM for it. From observed limitations discussed in early sections, we present in Sect. 4 the vrBPMN extension, named vrBPMN*, proposed to model BPL properly. In Sect. 5, the empirical study conducted is presented. Finally, in Sect. 6, the conclusions and future work are presented.

2   Background and Related Work

BPM considers an organization as a system of interconnected process and involves a combination of efforts for mapping, improving, and adhering the organization's process [3]. Business processes are continuously improved through the continuous improvement cycle of business process. In this context, the business process modeling is an activity that has two main goals [4]: (i) to describe characteristics of business processes in order to support communication and get tacit knowledge about operations of an organization; and (ii) to map businesses process of a domain or organization to support business analysts to improve performance and reduce cost of the processes. However, despite the benefits offered by the business process modeling, this activity requires time and, consequently, cost to be performed.

A configurable process model describes a family of similar process models in a given domain, which can be configured to obtain a specific process model that is subsequently used to handle individual cases [1]. Such Business Process Family, or Business Process Line (BPL), is a concept originated from Software Product Line (SPL) [13] and aims at reusing business process models by using variability management.

A important key concept used in this paper follow the terminology of Pohl *et al.* [13]. Variability is composed by Variation Point and its Variants. Each variant is related to a variability mechanism, which represents "as" a variant is performed. In the BPL context, variants are performed through parts of a business process, for example, a slice of process, a subprocess, a specific task or even artifacts. It is also important to define the "Variability Dependence" and "Variability Restriction" terms. The first one refers to how a variation point is related with its variants and which the variants have relationships among themselves. A variant can be Mandatory, Optional, Alternative-XOR, or Inclusive-OR. There are also two types of variability restriction: include and exclude. In include type, a variant when selected for realization includes other variant (independent of the variation point) or includes a variation point, the variation point should be performed even though optional. In exclude type, when a variant is selected, other variant or variation point can not be selected.

According with Gröner et al. [7], a BPL consists of: a business process template, which represents the flow of business process; a variability model, which represents "what" e "how" the business process vary; and a mapping between both artifacts (business process template and variability model), representing the traceability between them. These authors propose the adoption of BPMN elements for modeling the business process template and the adoption of the FM model for modeling variabilities. However, the use of BPMN and FM does not make clear when decisions are made at runtime or at building time [5]. In this sense, vrBPMN notation [15] is an adaptation of the BPMN, adding possibility of representing both variation points and variability mechanisms directly in business process templates through UML 2 stereotypes [6]. Thus, elements that represent variability mechanisms in the template are explicit, facilitating their identification. This notation was designed for a software development process of a Process-Oriented Software Product Line called Process Family Engineering Process (PFEP) [15], in order to describe the variability mechanisms directly into a BPMN model. However, there is no evidence on how to represent IOR-Elements (i.e., when a variation point can be resolved for one or more variants) using vrBPMN. In next section, we analyzed in more details the possibility of using vrBPMN and FM.

3   BPL Modeling

In order to create and maintain a BPL, besides documenting and representing the whole business process that composes a covered domain (including variability mechanisms), it is also recommended to model [13]: (i) all variation points of each business process model; (ii) all variants of each variation point; (iii) all variability dependencies; and (iv) all variability constraints.

In order to meet such recommendations, Shcnieders and Puhlmann [15] proposed the combined use of two types of modeling. The first one enables the variability modeling and allows the construction of an artifact named Variability Model. The second one represents the business process modeling and allows creation of a Business Process Template, which consists an artifact composed by business process model together with related variability mechanisms. Each business process model that belongs to the set of organization business process, covered by BPL, must have a template that represents it.

In next subsections, the variability model and the business process template are presented and are represented using, respectively, the FM and vrBPMN. In addition, Sect. 3.2 presents limitations observed in vrBPMN. These limitations motivated the proposal of vrBPMN*, which is presented in Sect. 4.

3.1 Variability Model

The notation for modeling BPL's variability must contain elements to represent variation points, variants, and also variability dependency and variability constraints. The model shall not represent business behaviour, i.e., it shall not represent how each variant is realized (variability mechanisms).

Figure 1 illustrates variability represented in FM. It is possible to observe three variation points: (i) "Delivery", which is optional and has two alternative variants: "Car Delivery" and "Simple Delivery"; (ii) "Payment", which is mandatory and has three IOR variants: "Credit", "Debit", "Cash"; and (iii) "Receipt", which is mandatory and has two alternatives variants: "Manual Receipt" and "Electronic Receipt". Finally, it is possible to observe that there is a variability constraint of "Inclusion" type between "Credit" variant and "Electronic Receipt" variant.

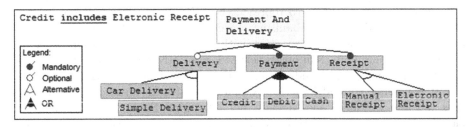

Fig. 1. FM example: Payment and Delivery features

3.2 Business Process Template

The notation used to represent business processes must have elements to represent business process, e.g., elements of BPMN or Activity Diagram [6]. This notation must also have elements to mark variation points in business process model, connecting them to variability model. Lastly, the notation must allow the variability mechanisms modeling in business process model [15], which could be done through the same elements used for business process modeling, e.g., BPMN elements.

In Fig. 2, we illustrated two vrBPMN diagrams associated to the FM of Fig. 1. "Delivery Process Template" ilustrates a business process template, in which an optional variation point, represented by ≪Null≫ stereotype, is marked on "Delivery" task, and also variability mechanisms (connected by ≪Extension≫ stereotype) corresponding to two variants (≪Variant≫): "Car Delivery" and "Simple Delivery". It is also possible to observe that "Receipt Process Template" has a mandatory variation point on "Receipt" task (represented with ≪Abstract≫ stereotype) and is connected with its variability mechanisms (≪Variant≫) through ≪Implementation≫ stereotype. With these examples, we presented the most important elements of vrBPMN. A complete list of vrBPMN elements is available in [15].

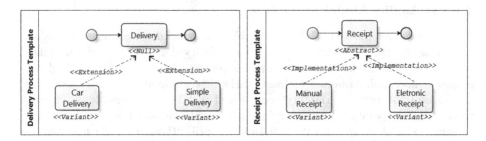

Fig. 2. vrBPMN examples: Delivery and Receipt Process Templates

Two of three variation points illustrated in Fig. 1 were modeled as business process templates by means of vrBPMN. However, when we try to model a business process template to represent the "Payment" variation point, and its respective variability mechanisms, we can notice that, because it is IOR, it is necessary to specify information with respect to the realization order of mechanisms when more than one is selected. vrBPMN does not provide stereotype for representing this kind of information. We observed also that with only FM, it is possible to model variability in a BPL with its variation points, variants and also variability dependency and constraint. But it is not possible to model neither the domain's business process nor the variability mechanisms. In the other hand, with vrBPMN, it is possible to model whole BPL's business process, including variability mechanisms. It also allows the modeling of variation points and different variability dependencies between a variation point and its variants. Nevertheless, it is recommended to document variability separately, that is, in a specific artifact [13]. In fact, variability constraints can not be modeled using vrBPMN, since there may exist variability in different abstraction levels of a business process, which may contain constraints between each other.

Therefore, the aforementioned models are complementary and, used together, can support complete modeling of a BPL.

Finally, we have observed that Inclusive-OR (IOR) elements of the FM model do not have an adequate correspondence in the vrBPMN notation and there is no evidences in the literature on how to resolve this issue.

4   Adaptations in FM and vrBPMN

As FM represents not only variabilities but also commonalities, and as commonalities in business process (e.g., the whole process, subprocess, tasks, flows, and data objects of the process) can be represented in vrBPMN models, commonalities are present in both of them. In face of this redundancy, we believe that excluding commonalities of FM is a way to simplify the models and provide a better support for process analysts.

On the other hand, due to limitations of vrBPMN presented in Sect. 3.2, we propose inclusion of new elements in this notation for suiting it to FM's elements, thereby creating a novel notation to model business process templates named vrBPMN*.

A new element, named "Combined Realization" that is represented by ≪Combined≫ stereotype, was then added to vrBPMN in order to represent an IOR variability dependency in the variation point of the BPL's business process template, as shown in Fig. 3. ≪Combined≫ stereotypes indicates that at least one variant must be realized. Representation of such variability dependency must considers that at least one and at most all variants shall be realized.

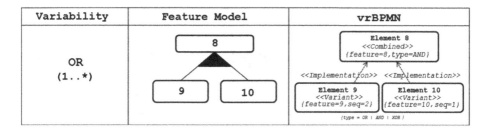

Fig. 3. vrBPMN extension - IOR variability representation (≪Combined≫ stereotype)

Additionally, we noticed the need to identify the temporal execution of business process when more than one variant is selected. For instance, as shown in Fig. 4 (left), a variation point in business process template "Make Payment", must be realized by one or more of the following variants: "Credit Card Payment", "Debit Card Payment" and "Payment with Cash". The right side of Fig. 4 shows a business process derived from presented template. It is possible to observe that the realization of these variants occurs in an *ad hoc* manner, i.e., no matter the sequence that these tasks are realized, as long as all the selected are realized.

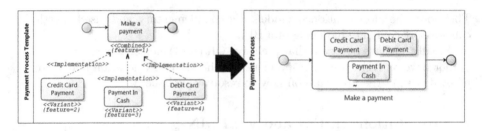

Fig. 4. Example of ≪*Combined*≫ stereotype usage: "Payment" Template and a derived model

However, it might be necessary to make explicit the execution order in case of more than one variant is selected. With this in mind, we added a parameter by means of UML's *tagged value* named *type*, which must contain one of the following values: "OR", "AND", "XOR" or empty (omitted).

The type of variability mechanism "OR" ({*type=OR*}) implies that selected mechanisms are connected by an inclusive gateway (Fig. 5). The variability mechanisms are connected through an exclusive gateway if the type is "XOR" (Fig. 6). In addition, if the type is "AND" ({*type=AND*}), the variability mechanisms is connected by a parallel gateway (Fig. 7) or, if mechanisms are realized in a sequential order, a parameter is added to the ≪*Implementation*≫ element, also as a *tagged value*, named *seq*, to define the realization order of the mechanisms (Fig. 8). These adaptations make the BPL modeling feasible through the joint use of vrBPMN* and FM.

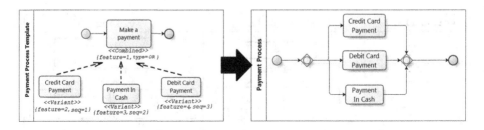

Fig. 5. BPMN model derived from "Payment", {*type=OR*} - with all variants selected.

5   Empirical Study

To evaluate the efficiency of modeling a business process from a BPL, modeled by the combined use of notation vrBPMN* and FM, we carried out an empirical study, planned according Wohlin *et al.* [16], comparing this approach with an approach for reusing business process models based on examples. For this, a domain was selected and three business processes in such domain were previously modeled. These three business process models were used to create a BPL, and

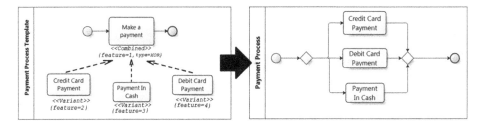

Fig. 6. BPMN model derived from "Payment", $\{type=XOR\}$ - with all variants selected.

were also used in the example-based approach. The four steps of our empirical study are presented below: Definition, Planning, Execution, and Presentation and Analysis of Data.

5.1   Definition, Planning, and Execution

The objective of the empirical study was to evaluate the impact of the adoption of a BPL model to support the reuse when creating a business process that is similar to the domain covered by such BPL, in relation to the creation of the same business process from example-based approach. The comparison was made in terms of "time" to perform the modeling and "correctness" of the business process model.

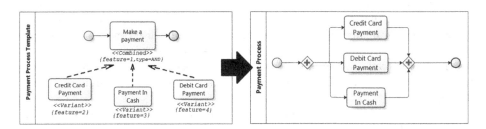

Fig. 7. BPMN model derived from "Payment", $\{type=AND\}$ - with all variants selected in parallel.

The dependent variables of the empirical study are the time employed in the business process modeling and the number of errors in the business process models.

This study included eight Master's students in Computer Science of Facom/UFMS, six of them representing participants with little or no experience in business process modeling and two of them representing participants with experience in business process modeling. In order to prevent that participants with different levels of expertise in business modeling favour some of the approaches, the profile of each participant was previously analyzed and participants were divided in two groups in order to balance the knowledge levels of each group. One group

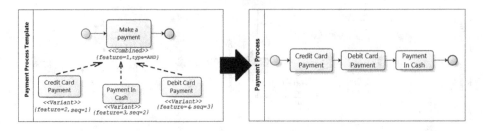

Fig. 8. BPMN model derived from "Payment", {*type=AND*} - with all variants selected.

used the BLP model and the other one used the example-based approach. They were named G-BPL and G-Examples, respectively.

We used a Rental BPL based on three models of business processes related to the loan of books, video rental, and vehicle rental. Participants of G-Examples group received the three models business processes, which could be consulted. Participants of G-BPL group did not have access to such models and received the BPL Rental, composed by: the business process template, the FM, and the configuration form of business process.

The execution plan for the empirical study consists of a single phase, in which participants of both groups had to individually model the process of Dresses Rental business. For this, both groups received a textual description of this business process and the aforementioned artifacts. This description was based on the description of a process in location domain, which has been studied in previous works [11].

Considering that time spent only for the modeling was selected to analyze efficiency, it can be argued that efficiency could be influenced by the time spent reading and understanding the description of the business process to be modeled by each participant. To eliminate this possibility, participants had 20 min to read the description and eliminate any doubts regarding the understanding of this description.

In Table 1, it is described the procedure of modeling business process used in the empirical study by each approach.

5.2   Presentation and Analysis of Data

Data collected during the empirical study, presented in Table 2, suggest that the G-BPL group was benefited by the use of BPL model both in terms of time and the correctness of the model produced.

(a) Time spent in the modeling of business process model: The time was recorded from start modeling, after 20 min used for reading of the description of the Dresses Rental business process, until the completion of the business process model. From results related to time spent by the participants during the modeling results, it is observed that the participants were influenced by the approach used. There was a decrease of 23.26 % in the average time spent by participants

Table 1. Procedure used in the study execution

	Adopted Procedure
Example-based	1.Read and understand the description of business process to be modeled (20 minutes) 2. Analyze existents business process models taken as example, from the perspective of the description of business process to be modeled 3.Model the business process using BPMN resorting to examples, when appropriate
BPL-based	1.Read and understand the description of business process to be modeled (20 minutes) 2. Analyze the vrBPMN* template of the BPL, paying attention to the variation points and variability mechanisms 3.Analyze the FM of the BPL 4. Identify in the process to be modeled the configurable elements at the BPL, based on the configuration form 5.Fill the configuration form with the pertinent values to each configurable element 6. Realize the variability of business process to be modeled, based on the vrBPMN* template and the FM, selecting the appropriated variability mechanisms to be adopted to business process modeling 7. Transcribe the workflow generated by realization, producing a business process model in BPMN

Table 2. Summary of Study Results.

Results: Group G-BPL				Results: Group G-Examples			
Reuse Support	Time Spent	Config. Mistakes	Semantic Mistakes	Reuse Support	Time Spent	Config. Mistakes	Semantic Mistakes
BPL	00:47	1	4	Example	00:38	8	6
BPL	00:28	0	2	Example	00:49	6	3
BPL	00:26	5	3	Example	00:42	3	4
BPL Avrg.	**00:33**	**2**	**3**	**Ex. Avrg.**	**00:43**	**6**	**4**

that used BPL model compare to those based on examples. This indicates the confirmation of the hypothesis *Ha0*.

(b) Correctness of the business process model obtained: To analyse the correctness of the models produced, we took into account the semantic analysis and the configuration analysis of the model elaborated by each participant. In the semantic analysis, we examined the compliance of the model elaborated with the description of the Dresses Rental business process. In the configuration analysis, we checked all occurrences of each configurable element and examined if the correct value in relation to the context of the model was used. The results related to the correctness of the elaborated business process model show that the approach influenced the participants. Group G-BPL had a higher performance compared to participants of group G-Examples. There was a decrease of 66.67 % of configuration errors and 25 % of semantic errors, indicating the confirmation of the *Ha1* hypothesis.

6   Conclusion

BPL has proved to be an important approach to create, manage, and mainly reuse models of business process. In this scenario, the main goal of this work was to provide a contribution to the area of BPL. In particular, we proposed a means to more adequately represent models of business process by extending the vrBPMN notation. For this, new elements were proposed and added to the original notation to suit the vrBPMN to the FM model. Despite the empirical study conducted be limited in relation to population, composed by only eight participants, it allowed the identification of important points about the use of BPL modeling with FM and vrBPMN* to support the business process reuse. For example, we observed that the BPL modeling has a tendency to accelerate the business process modeling, since even the inexperienced participants were able to complete the elaboration of the business process model in a shorter period of time. As future work, we intend to: (i) refine the documentation of the vrBPMN* syntax; (ii) conduct more experiments to observe the use of our approach in diverse scenarios; and (iii) develop a computational tool that supports the integrated use of vrBPMN* and FM.

References

1. van der Aalst, W., Lohmann, N., La Rosa, M., Xu, J.: Correctness ensuring process configuration: an approach based on partner synthesis. In: Hull, R., Mendling, J., Tai, S. (eds.) BPM 2010. LNCS, vol. 6336, pp. 95–111. Springer, Heidelberg (2010)
2. Boffoli, N., Caivano, D., Castelluccia, D., Visaggio, G.: Driving flexibility and consistency of business processes by means of product-line engineering and decision tables. In: 3rd International Workshop on Product Line Approaches in Software Engineering, Zurich, pp. 33–36 (2012)
3. Chang, J.F.: Business Process Management System - Strategy and Implementation, 1st edn. Auerbach Publications, Boca Raton (2006)
4. Chinosi, M., Trombetta, A.: Bpmn: an introduction to the standard. Comput. Stand. Interfaces **34**(1), 124–134 (2012)
5. Gottschalk, F., Aalst, W., Jansen-Vullers, M.: Configurable process models–a foundational approach. In: Becker, J., Delfmann, P. (eds.) Reference Modeling, pp. 59–77. Physica-Verlag, Heidelberg (2007)
6. OMG Object Management Group: Documents associated with uml version 2 (2005)
7. Grökovic, G., Parreiras, F., Gaevic, D.: Modeling and validation of business process families. Inf. Syst. **38**(5), 709–726 (2013)
8. Jablonski, S., Bussler, C.: Workflow Management: Modeling Concepts, Architecture and Implementation. International Thomson Computer Press, London (1996)
9. Kang, K.C., Cohen, S.G., Hess, J.A., Novak, W.E., Peterson, A.S.: Feature-oriented domain analysis (FODA): feasibility study. Technical report, SEI (1990)
10. La Rosa, M., Dumas, M., Hofstede, A., Mendling, J.: Configurable multi-perspective business process models. Inf. Syst. **36**(2), 313–340 (2011)
11. Ladeira, S., Penteado, R., Braga, R., Cagnin, M.I.: Business modelling reuse based on views: a case study. In: 22nd Brazilian Symposium on Software Engineering, Brazil, pp. 140–155 (2008). (In Portuguese)

12. Laudon, K., Laudon, J.: Essentials of Management Information Systems, 10th edn. Prentice Hall, Upper Saddle River (2012)
13. Pohl, K., Bockle, G., van der Linden, F.J.: Software Product Line Engineering: Foundations, Principles and Techniques, 1st edn. Springer, Heidelberg (2005)
14. Rolland, C., Nurcan, S.: Business process lines to deal with the variability. In: 43rd Hawaii International Conference on System Sciences, pp. 1–10 (2010)
15. Schnieders, A., Puhlmann, F.: Variability mechanisms in e-business process families. In: International Conference on Business Information Systems, Austria, pp. 583–601 (2006)
16. Wohlin, C., Runeson, P., Hst, M., Ohlsson, M., Regnell, B., Wessln, A.: Experimentation in Software Engineering. Springer, Heidelberg (2012)

BPCAS 2014

Context-Aware Programming for Hybrid and Diversity-Aware Collective Adaptive Systems

Hong-Linh Truong[(✉)] and Schahram Dustdar

Distributed Systems Group, Vienna University of Technology, Vienna, Austria
{truong,dustdar}@dsg.tuwien.ac.at

Abstract. Collective adaptive systems (CASs) have been researched intensively since many years. However, the recent emerging developments and advanced models in service-oriented computing, cloud computing and human computation have fostered several new forms of CASs. Among them, Hybrid and Diversity-aware CASs (HDA-CASs) characterize new types of CASs in which a collective is composed of hybrid machines and humans that collaborate together with different complementary roles. This emerging HDA-CAS poses several research challenges in terms of programming, management and provisioning. In this paper, we investigate the main issues in programming HDA-CASs. First, we analyze context characterizing HDA-CASs. Second, we propose to use the concept of hybrid compute units to implement HDA-CASs that can be elastic. We call this type of HDA-CASs h^2**CAS** (Hybrid Compute Unit-based HDA-CAS). We then discuss a meta-view of h^2**CAS** that describes a h^2**CAS** program. We analyze and present program features for h^2**CAS** in four main different contexts.

1 Introduction

Collective adaptive systems (CASs) have been researched intensively since many years [1–4]. For solving complex problems in business and society, new concepts of CASs have been emerging by utilizing human-based computing and software-based computing elements as basic building blocks of CASs. Among them, the Hybrid and Diversity-aware CAS (HDA-CAS) has emerged as a new type of CAS that consists of diverse machine- and human-based computing elements [5]. HDA-CASs promise a new way to solve complex problems that requires both human knowledge and machine capabilities, such as in simulation, urban planning, and city management.

While CASs can be built based on computing elements from different environments, in our research, we are particularly interested in HDA-CASs that are built from software-based services, thing-based services, and human-based services, following service-oriented and cloud computing models. In such models, machine-based and human-based elements provide fundamental computation, data, and network functions and these elements have well-defined service interfaces and are provisioned under cloud models. Atop diverse types of services

© Springer International Publishing Switzerland 2015
F. Fournier and J. Mendling (Eds.): BPM 2014 Workshops, LNBIP 202, pp. 145–157, 2015.
DOI: 10.1007/978-3-319-15895-2_13

in the cloud, new types of dynamic elasticity properties have emerged. First, a huge amount of diverse types of resources are available that can be taken into the construction of CASs on demand. Second, elasticity requirements from the consumer for whom a CAS is provided and problems being solved by the CAS force us to design CASs capable of handling cost and quality changes. Therefore, we believe that utilizing dynamic, on-demand service units from clouds to establish HDA-CASs is a promising direction.

Since HDA-CASs are designed to deal with complex problems in an adaptive way, examining elasticity mechanisms for building HDA-CASs using cloud resources, offering cloud computing models for HDA-CASs, and dynamically managing HDA-CASs at runtime is a very interesting but challenging problem. In our previous work, we have described cloud models for software and people, basic hybrid compute unit models for establishing computing systems including both software and people, and basic programming APIs for these units [6,7]. In this paper, we examine how such fundamental building blocks can be used to build HDA-CASs. We advocate the form of HDA-CASs being constructed from hybrid compute units (HCUs), which consist of software-, thing- and human-based service units. These units are provisioned under the service concept (with well-defined interfaces and utilization model), enabling dynamic programming features for utilizing them. To this end, this paper presents the following contributions:

– analysis and definition of context associated with HDA-CASs
– analysis of hybridity and elasticity properties of HDA-CASs,
– analysis of the utilization of hybrid compute units for implementing HDA-CASs, called h^2**CAS**,
– a meta-view of main building blocks for h^2**CAS**, and
– analysis of programming features for h^2**CAS** in four main high-level contexts.

Our contributions provide fundamental work for the development of program specification of h^2**CAS**, h^2**CAS** provisioning services, and h^2**CAS** elasticity techniques.

The rest of this paper is structured as follows: Sect. 2 defines the context of HDA-CAS and discusses the hybridity and elasticity of HDA-CASs. Section 3 defines HDA-CASs using hybrid compute units and a meta-view of our h^2**CAS** specification. Section 4 discusses issues in programming h^2**CAS**. Related work is presented in Sect. 5. We conclude the paper and outline our future work in Sect. 6.

2 Analyzing Contexts of HDA-CAS

2.1 Context of HDA-CAS

Our goals to support context-aware programming HDA-CASs are to provide (i) right constructs for specifying what constitutes a HDA-CAS, (ii) tools and middleware for deploying, provisioning and instantiating HDA-CASs based on their specifications, and (iii) means for programming the control and reconfiguration of HDA-CASs at runtime. Therefore, it is important to understand the context in which a HDA-CAS will be formed and operated as well as possible contexts inherent in the lifetime of HDA-CASs. We define a context of a HDA-CAS as follows:

Definition 1 (Context of HDA-CAS). *Context of a HDA-CAS describes situational information about tasks and quality of results (*What*), structures of the HDA-CAS and its constituting units for computation/data/network functions as well as for monitoring/control/management functions (*Who*), and the coordination and elasticity mechanisms that control the operation of the HDA-CAS (*How*) in a determined time frame (*When*).*

To support context-aware programming of HDA-CASs, we need to address several open questions of *When*, *What*, *Who/Which* and *How* characterizing contexts in which programming features for HDA-CASs play a crucial role:

- *When:* When a HDA-CAS is formed and instantiated? From when to when a HDA-CAS is in a particular context? When does a HDA-CAS switch its context?
- *What:* What are the tasks that a HDA-CAS has to solve in a particular context? What are the expected quality of results (QoRs) for these tasks?
- *Which/Who:* Which types of units are needed for performing computation/data/network functions and for monitoring/management/control functions in a HDA-CAS context? Which structures can be used to describe a HDA-CAS and its units?
- *How:* How does a HDA-CAS work? How does a HDA-CAS coordinate its units? How does a HDA-CAS support and control its elasticity?

Programming a HDA-CAS means that we need to be able to describe several types of information related to the above-mentioned questions in well-defined specifications. Based on that, via software-defined APIs, we can create, provision

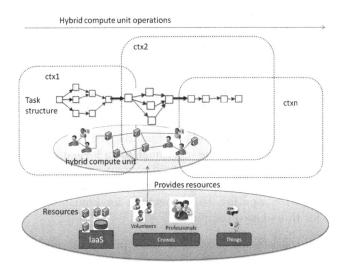

Fig. 1. High-level view of context (`ctx`), task structure and units associated with HDA-CAS

and control HDA-CASs to enable units within these HDA-CASs to interact and perform their tasks/roles.

Let us consider the case in which a HDA-CAS is built by using a hybrid compute unit (HCU) [6,7]. There are complex relationships among the *What* and *Who/Which* within a context and among contexts within the lifetime of a HDA-CAS, as shown in Fig. 1. A HCU is provisioned from different resources (via virtualization techniques). The HCU is the Who/Which of the HDA-CAS. The HCU is intended for solving problems which have complex, and possibly evolving, task structures, dependent on the context. Therefore, under a specific context in the lifetime of the HDA-CAS, HCU structures may be changed to assure the QoR associated with the tasks.

2.2 Hybridity in CASs

Hybridity is an intrinsic property of HDA-CASs. This property is due to the fact that HDA-CAS is formed to address complex problems, which require us to employ diverse and hybrid types of units and roles:

– Different types of resources, including machine-based, human-based and thing-based resources that offer computation, data, and network functions as well as monitoring, control and management functions.
– Different roles performed in the same collective: including performing computation/data/network functions and supporting management, monitoring and control functions. Different types of resources or a single resource might perform different roles or the same role at different time based on different capabilities.

Therefore, techniques for programming HDA-CASs must support fundamental programming constructs and algorithms to deal with the hybridity of computing models in HDA-CASs. In terms of hybridity, the following aspects are important:

– We must be able to execute, coordinate, and manage computation/data/network functions using hybrid processing units (e.g., CPU/core for machine-based computing, human brain for human-based computing, and sensor for thing-based computing),
– We must be able to program hybrid architectures (e.g., the cluster of machines for machine-based computing, the individual/team for human-based computing, and the web of things for thing-based computing), and
– We must be able to program hybrid communication protocols (e.g., TCP/IP for machine-based computing, social network for human-based computing, and MQTT for thing-based computing).

A HDA-CAS will consists of a mixture of these processing units, architectures and communications.

2.3   Elasticity in HDA-CASs

One of the main issues in programming and provisioning HDA-CAS is to support the elasticity principles, covering resource, quality, and cost/benefit elasticity. These principles should be the core mechanisms for, e.g., managing and controlling the operations of HDA-CASs (thus, addressing the *How* aspect of HDA-CAS contexts). The main reason is that HDA-CAS is a dynamic entity whose structures, tasks, and QoRs are dynamically changed. The type of resource elasticity can be seen through the change, reduction and expansion of units for computation/data/network functions. Other types of elasticity can be observed through the following aspects:

- Mixture of different QoRs from a single collective, given a specific goal: a collective is dynamic w.r.t. structures, interactions, and performance, thus, it can produce different QoRs, depending on different settings (e.g., time, availability, incentives, to name just a few).
- Mixture of cost/benefit models: a collective might perform a goal (offering a capability) with different cost/benefit models with different or the same quality.

Such elasticity capabilities must be captured, modeled and associated with HDA-CASs, enabling the management and control of HDA-CASs via programming features. For example, we must be able to program the selection and utilization of suitable units for different types of tasks and QoRs (e.g., specifying expected performance, cost, and quality of data). Overall, we foresee the following levels of elasticity:

- *Processing Units:* The basic mechanisms are (i) to add/remove new processing units based on the load and (ii) to replace existing processing units with new processing units. If units are humans, then we can search clouds of human-based services to find relevant units. If it is software then we can find new software based on service selection techniques.
- *Architecture:* the architecture reflects how different units performing computation/data/network functions and monitoring/control/management functions can be glued. The basic mechanisms are (i) to provision different static and runtime topologies for different types of units, and (ii) to change different protocols/algorithms within monitoring/control/management units.
- *Communications:* There will be multiple communication protocols among different types of units, e.g., communications among units performing computation/data/network functions and among monitoring/control/management units. The basic mechanisms are (i) adding/removing communication protocols, (ii) reconfiguring existing protocols, and (iii) replacing existing protocols with new protocols.

3 h^2CAS– HDA-CAS Using Hybrid Compute Units

3.1   Hybrid Compute Units and HDA-CAS

Based on the two main properties of hybridity and elasticity of HDA-CASs, to specify and program HDA-CAS's structures, we rely on the hybrid compute unit (HCU) concept – a unified model that is able to capture different types of service units and their relationships. Using service units and relationships modeled in the HCU, the HDA-CAS programmer can define HDA-CAS structures, including topologies and communications, and configure other elements, such as algorithms for selecting units for performing computation/data/network functions, for evaluating quality of results, and for controlling the elasticity of units by considering costs and benefits. The HCU model is described in detail in [7]. Service units are associated with elasticity capabilities; each capability can be programmed via software-defined APIs. A general concept is that the consumer of HDA-CASs acquires a HCU representing the HDA-CAS structure. Then consumer can control the elasticity of the HDA-CAS via APIs, triggering suitable set of actions, each mapped to some primitives of units. We define a model of HDA-CAS based on the HCU as follows:

Definition 2 (HCU-based HDA-CAS). *A HCU-based HDA-CAS (h^2CAS) includes a set of service units which can be software-based services, human-based services and thing-based services that can be provisioned, deployed and utilized as a collective on-demand based on different quality, pricing and incentive models.*

In our work, programming h^2CAS means that: (i) we are able to specify relevant information of h^2CAS, (ii) h^2CAS specification will be compiled and executed by some middleware, and (iii) h^2CAS operations will be controlled at runtime by the h^2CAS itself or by external controllers via software-defined APIs. Main programming features that a h^2CAS programming framework should support:

- *Initialization:* we must be able to describe the structure of h^2CAS including units, architectures and communications. The *Who/Which* must be structured based on types of the tasks and the QoRs (the *What*). We must be able to initiate the h^2CAS based on the structure, deployment, and configuration.
- *Elasticity Management:* we must be able to understand elasticity contexts of h^2CAS, which must be monitored. The elasticity of h^2CAS will be used to control dynamic changes of h^2CAS structures to meet the expected QoR. During runtime, depending on specific contexts, we can measure/monitor/predict QoRs and perform elasticity actions by calling elasticity APIs of h^2CAS.

3.2   Meta-Program for h^2CAS

To specify h^2CAS, we need to determine the types of units needed for performing computation/data/network functions and for performing management/control/ monitoring functions, possible coordination and communication protocols/models among different types of units and elasticity capabilities of these units to control the elasticity of h^2CAS. They can be determined before the initialization of a h^2CAS or during the lifetime of a h^2CAS, based on specific contexts of h^2CAS. In this section, we discuss h^2CAS meta-view and leave the detailed design and implementation of the meta-view specification for the future work.

Figure 2 presents a meta-view of h^2CAS programs describing possible service units and interactions. h^2CAS includes four main building block specifications:

- *Task Management:* three main types of units should be specified for task management. `InputTaskStorageUnit` is used to manage input tasks (e.g., from the consumer of h^2**CAS**) that need to be solved by h^2**CAS**. `TaskMatchingUnit` and `TaskControlUnit` are used to match tasks to units performing computation/data/network functions and to manage tasks performed by such units, respectively.
- *Result Management:* at least three main types of units should be specified. `OutputResultStorageUnit` is used to manage results of h^2**CAS** that will be sent to the consumer. `QoREvaluationMatchingUnit` and `QoREvaluation ControlUnit` are used to find units for performing the QoR evaluation and manage QoR evaluation tasks.
- *Computation/Data/Network Task Execution and Control:* types of possible units used for performing computation/data/networks should be specified. Three main units for managing computation/data/network units (`CDNElas ticityControlUnit`), for supporting communications (`CDNCommunication Unit` and for interacting with clouds of services (`CloudConnectorUnit`) should be specified.
- *Elasticity Monitoring and Control:* two main units should be specified. First, `MonitoringUnit` is used for performing different monitoring activities, including monitoring task management, result management, computation/data/

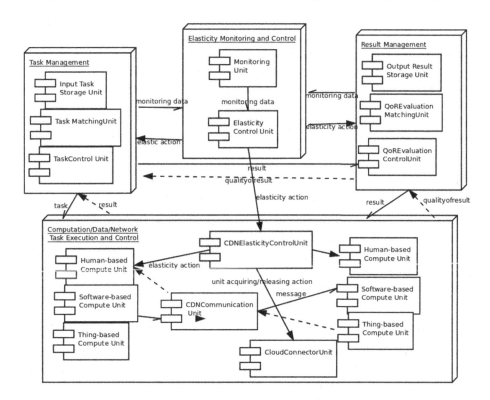

Fig. 2. h^2**CAS** meta-view

network functions, etc. Second, `ElasticityControlUnit` is specified for performing elasticity controls, such controlling units for performing computation/ data/network functions, communication units, task management units, etc.

In terms of programming, these types of units are "class" and when initialized, we can have different instances of these units based on different implementations and configurations. Each building block will require different ways to specify and program units, architectures and protocols. Among different building blocks, there will be protocols for their interactions. Similar to the types of units, these protocols can also have different instances. It is important to note that these units can be software-based, thing-based, or human-based. For example, `TaskControlUnit` or `CDNElasticityControl` can be human-based services. Therefore, h^2**CAS** operations are not fully automatically managed and controlled. Instead, these operations are carried out through a combination of human and machine activities.

4 Context-Aware Programming Features for h^2CAS

In the following, we discuss programming features for h^2**CAS** that are centered around four main specific contexts:

- *consumer-generated independent continuous task context:* in this context, a h^2**CAS** is established and used for solving independent tasks sent continuously by the consumer of the h^2**CAS**.
- *consumer-generated dependent task context:* in this context, a h^2**CAS** is established and used for solving a task graph sent by the consumer of the h^2**CAS**.
- *evolving independent task context:* in this context, a h^2**CAS** is established and used for solving a set of independent tasks but during the problem solving time, several new independent tasks are created by the h^2**CAS**.
- *evolving dependent task context:* in this context, a h^2**CAS** is established and used for solving a set of dependent tasks and during the problem solving several dependent tasks are created newly by the h^2**CAS**.

They are high-level contexts which can be subdivided into different types of sub-contexts based on the *What* aspect (e.g., a sub-context in which only the same type of tasks is solved), the *Who/Which* aspect (e.g., a context in which all tasks are solved by human-based compute units), and/or the *How* aspect (e.g., a context in which only cost elasticity is needed).

4.1 Consumer-Generated Independent Continuous Task Context

Context Description. In this context, a h^2**CAS** is provisioned for solving a flow of independent tasks from its consumers. All the tasks are atomic and the tasks are created by the consumer of the h^2**CAS**. QoR is associated with individual tasks. It is possible to have different types of tasks, which require different types of units performing computation/data/network functions. Tasks are continuously given to h^2**CAS**. This kind of task delivery is highly related to works in crowdsourcing tasks [8]. However, the main difference is that the task flow is continuous.

Initialization. For independent tasks, h^2**CAS** will receive a flow of independent tasks which are put into `InputTaskStorageUnit` by the consumer of the h^2**CAS**. We can safely assume that there is only one service unit working on a specific task at a given time. If the QoR of a task does not match the requirement (e.g., the task cannot be finished by a unit), the task should be reassigned and performed by another unit. For this reason, we can also decide not to include `CDNCommunicationUnit` for units performing computation/data/network functions. Thus, h^2**CAS** could be programmed by forming h^2**CAS** based on general task descriptions without `CDNCommunicationUnit`.

A minimum set of units for performing tasks can be established by programming/configuring suitable (pre-)runtime/static unit formation algorithms within `CDNElasticityControlUnit`. The h^2**CAS** can coordinate task execution based on different coordination models programmed in `TaskControlUnit`.

Elasticity. Depending on the task types, h^2**CAS** could be deployed to use only clouds of human-based services or clouds of hybrid services. At runtime, based on monitoring information, especially QoR (e.g., higher or lower QoR than expected), `ElasticityControl` and `CDNElasticityControlUnit` can apply elasticity controls to individual units performing computation/data/network functions, to change coordination protocols within task management and output management units, or to interact with other clouds to negotiate pricing models and acquire/release resources. Elasticity controls can be performed via different control algorithms and can be also programmed via elasticity APIs.

4.2   Consumer-Generated Dependent Task Context

Context Description. This context is quite similar to the previous context in Sect. 4.1, except a complete task graph is given to the h^2**CAS**. The task graph includes dependent tasks, e.g., in terms of data or control dependencies.

Initialization. Similarly to the previous context, a h^2**CAS** can be established with a minimum cost and a limited number of units performing computation/data/network functions. Thus, initially the h^2**CAS** can be just enough for solving a sub-graph and then eventually be extended to solve other tasks, e.g. followed the strategies in [6]. Although tasks are dependent, communications among h^2**CAS** units performing tasks may or may not be established. When `CDNCommunicationUnit` is not needed, the dependencies among tasks can be managed by `TaskManagementUnit`. All task results have to be routed back to the *TaskControlUnit*. Otherwise, the dependencies can also be managed by units performing tasks and using `CDNCommunicationUnit` to send/receive messages about task results to other units. Another benefit of using `CDNCommunicationUnit` is to facilitate the discussion among units performing tasks, when these units are human-based.

Elasticity. The elasticity in this context is similar to the previous context in Sect. 4.1. However, the elasticity of units performing computation/data/network functions could be relied on different strategies, such as expanding and reducing units by considering Business-as-Usual and corrective action cases [6].

4.3   Evolving Independent Task Context

Context Description. In this context, a set of independent tasks needs to be solved by a h^2**CAS**; each task has its own expected QoR. However, solving an independent task might lead to the creation of sub-tasks. This requires two ways of interactions among a unit performing a task in h^2**CAS**, `TaskControlUnit` and `QoREvaluationControlUnit` to decide how sub-tasks should be assigned, executed and evaluated.

Initialization. We could start with a common strategy of initializing a h^2**CAS** with a minimum capability (e.g., based on costs) and later on we can use elasticity mechanisms to expand or reduce the h^2**CAS**. Since a unit performing a task needs to interact with `TaskControlUnit` to decide how to assign, execute and evaluate sub-tasks, two different possibilities can be configured: (i) the unit performing a task returns the outcome – either sub-tasks or the result of the task – to management units in `TaskManagement` and let them to manage the outcome and (ii) the unit performing a task coordinates the execution of sub-tasks it creates. In the latter, the initialization requires `CDNCommunicationUnit` and another protocol to allow the unit to call `TaskMatchingUnit` and `CDNElasticityUnit` to assign and manage its sub-tasks.

Elasticity. When a unit performing computation/data/network functions or QoR evaluation is not responsible for its newly-created tasks, the typical elasticity mechanisms in previous contexts (Sects. 4.1 and 4.2) could be utilized. Otherwise, different elasticity mechanisms can be performed by the unit by calling `CDNElasticityControlUnit`. When the unit is a human-based compute unit, the elasticity actions are manually done by the human. In case, the unit is a software-based compute unit, we need to program suitable algorithms for executing, managing and evaluating sub-tasks. Note that when a unit utilizes elasticity controls to acquire other units to perform its sub-tasks, it is possible that the newly acquired units are the core elements for a new h^2**CAS**. In other words, a unit can create a new h^2**CAS** to solve its sub-tasks.

4.4   Evolving Dependent Task Context

Context Description. In this context, a set of dependent tasks is given to h^2**CAS**. Usually the number of tasks is small but the complexity of the task is high. Furthermore, QoR is associated with the whole set of tasks. While solving tasks, new tasks, also dependent on other tasks, could be created. Overall, the task graph will be expanded and reduced until the h^2**CAS** completes all the tasks in the graph.

Initialization. A h^2**CAS** could be formed based on the task graph using strategies similar to thos in Sect. 4.3.

Elasticity. The elasticity can be carried out in a similar way to the context in Sect. 4.3. Since the QoR is associated with the whole task and tasks are strongly dependent by each other, elasticity control mechanisms need to be programmed in such a way that takes into account these strong dependencies.

5   Related Work

In [1], a formal model for socio-technical CAS is discussed. It discusses how to specify CAS using different formal models. Generally, there is no software framework for programming h^2**CAS** as we describe in this paper. In the state-of-the art, typically a specific CAS is built with several components and it is used for different purposes by varying inputs into the CAS. Another way to solve complex problems by using human-based services and software-based services is to design a specific middleware/platform to manage and distribute tasks to different resources, which can be software or humans. An example of such platforms is Jabberwocky [9] which allows specifying types of people based on personal properties and expertise and route tasks and combing humans with machines. These platforms are not systems for HDA-CAS. Our work actually aims at generalizing these platforms by providing techniques for programming and provisioning such specific CASs or middleware using service units.

Software architectures describing the interactions between humans and other software service units have been discussed, e.g. in [10]. They aim at supporting design techno-social software systems that allow people to work with machines. Our work is different as, in the programming perspective, we support the developer to write h^2**CAS** program of which, in addition to other types of information, some architectures of software-based and human-based units are specified by the developer.

Several task management models, coordination and communication protocols for collaborative complex problem solving have been developed. For example, two approaches in designing task processes for humans are studied in [8] but managing task processes is just one feature that influences the design and operation of a collective in our work. In fact a major related work in human computation focus on designing task processes and distributing tasks to different human compute units [11,12]. Our work differs from them as we focus on programming systems that enable the execution of different task processes and on the elasticity of these systems to deal with elasticity requirements of tasks. In [13] several researchers have discussed several issues for supporting collaborative, dynamic and complex tasks performed by crowds. In general, they analyze several research challenges and we believe that certain types of collectives built atop human units should address these challenges. Our $h^2\mathbf{CAS}$ model built for elasticity and based on hybrid compute units could be used to program platforms to support some of these mentioned challenges.

In our previous work, we focus on HCU and service unit models [6,7]. We have presented the hybridity and elasticity of different types of units in HCU in general. In this paper, we examine how to implement $h^2\mathbf{CAS}$ using HCUs, therefore, our hybridity and diversity analysis of $h^2\mathbf{CAS}$ is bound to the context from/in which $h^2\mathbf{CAS}$ is formed and operates.

6   Conclusions and Future Work

HDA-CAS is a new form of collective adaptive systems (CASs) built for solving complex problems by utilizing diverse and hybrid service units offering well-defined cloud provisioning models. However, we need to support the right programming features to simplify the creation, provisioning and execution of HDA-CAS. In this paper we analyze possible contexts associated with HDA-CAS and propose the utilization of hybrid compute units to program HDA-CAS. In doing so, we focused on context aspects – such as *When, What, Who/Which* and *How* – in programming HDA-CASs. We presented $h^2\mathbf{CAS}$ as one way of implementing HDA-CASs as well as outlined a meta-view for specifying $h^2\mathbf{CAS}$ and programming features for $h^2\mathbf{CAS}$ in some general contexts.

Currently, we are working on a specification of programming constructs and models that can be used to specify $h^2\mathbf{CAS}$ in detail. Furthermore, we are working on tools and middleware for compiling $h^2\mathbf{CAS}$ specification and deploying, controlling and provisioning techniques for $h^2\mathbf{CAS}$.

Acknowledgments. We thank Muhammad Z. C. Candra, Mirela Riveni, Ognjen Scekic and Vincenzo (Enzo) Maltese for fruitful discussions on hybrid compute units, elasticity, and collective adaptive systems. The work mentioned in this paper is partially supported by the EU FP7 SmartSociety project under grant $N°$ 600854.

References

1. Coronato, A., Florio, V.D., Bakhouya, M., Serugendo, G.D.M.: Formal modeling of socio-technical collective adaptive systems. In: Proceedings of the 2012 IEEE Sixth International Conference on Self-Adaptive and Self-Organizing Systems Workshops. SASOW 2012, pp. 187–192. IEEE Computer Society, Washington, DC, USA (2012)
2. Fundamentals of collective adaptive systems. http://focas.eu/
3. Andrikopoulos, V., Saez, S.G., Karastoyanova, D., Weiss, A.: Towards collaborative, dynamic and complex systems (short paper). In: SOCA, pp. 241–245. IEEE (2013)
4. Bruni, R., Corradini, A., Gadducci, F., Lafuente, A.L., Vandin, A.: Modelling and analyzing adaptive self-assembly strategies with Maude. Sci. Comput. Program. **99**, 75–94 (2015)

5. Hybrid and diversity-aware collective adaptive systems. http://www.smart-society-project.eu/
6. Truong, H.L., Dustdar, S., Bhattacharya, K.: Conceptualizing and programming hybrid services in the cloud. Int. J. Coop. Info. Syst. **22**, 1341003 (2013)
7. Truong, H.-L., Dam, H.K., Ghose, A., Dustdar, S.: Augmenting complex problem solving with hybrid compute units. In: Lomuscio, A.R., Nepal, S., Patrizi, F., Benatallah, B., Brandić, I. (eds.) ICSOC 2013. LNCS, vol. 8377, pp. 95–110. Springer, Heidelberg (2014)
8. Little, G., Chilton, L.B., Goldman, M., Miller, R.C.: Exploring iterative and parallel human computation processes. In: Proceedings of the ACM SIGKDD Workshop on Human Computation. HCOMP 2010, pp. 68–76. ACM, New York, USA (2010)
9. Ahmad, S., Battle, A., Malkani, Z., Kamvar, S.: The jabberwocky programming environment for structured social computing. In: Proceedings of the 24th Annual ACM Symposium on User Interface Software and Technology. UIST 2011, pp. 53–64. ACM, New York, USA (2011)
10. Dorn, C., Taylor, R.N.: Coupling software architecture and human architecture for collaboration-aware system adaptation. In: Notkin, D., Cheng, B.H.C., Pohl, K. (eds.) ICSE, pp. 53–62. IEEE / ACM, San Francisco (2013)
11. Quinn, A.J., Bederson, B.B.: Human computation: a survey and taxonomy of a growing field. In: Tan, D.S., Amershi, S., Begole, B., Kellogg, W.A., Tungare, M. (eds.) CHI, pp. 1403–1412. ACM, New York (2011)
12. Kulkarni, A.P., Can, M., Hartmann, B.: Turkomatic: automatic recursive task and workflow design for mechanical turk. In: Proceedings of the 2011 Annual Conference Extended Abstracts on Human Factors in Computing Systems. CHI EA 2011, pp. 2053–2058. ACM, New York, USA (2011)
13. Kittur, A., Nickerson, J.V., Bernstein, M., Gerber, E., Shaw, A., Zimmerman, J., Lease, M., Horton, J.: The future of crowd work. In: Proceedings of the 2013 Conference on Computer Supported Cooperative Work. CSCW 2013, pp. 1301–1318. ACM, New York, USA (2013)

Towards Cognitive BPM as the Next Generation BPM Platform for Analytics-Driven Business Processes

Hamid R. Motahari Nezhad[(⊠)] and Rama Akkiraju

IBM Almaden Research Center, San Jose, CA, USA
{motahari,akkiraju}@us.ibm.com

Abstract. Human-centric business processes in the enterprise are knowledge-intensive, and rely on human judgment for decision making. This reliance impacts the integrity, uniformity, efficiency and consistency of the process enactment over time. We describe our experience and challenges in driving the adoption of business process management tools in the sales process at a large IT services provider. We argue that in knowledge-driven and human-centric activities such as IT services sales, current technologies do not meet the needs. They do not support data capture and analytics around process and using it to reason about and take action on the process. Process definition and enactment, both, needs to be dynamic, flexible and adaptive based on the understanding of the state of affairs. We present a vision and a framework for a *cognitive BPM system* where the knowledge management, user interaction and analytics are employed to dynamically assess and proactively adapt the process based on the results of data analytics and continuous learning from the actions taken.

Keywords: Human-centric BPM · Management issues and empirical studies · Non-traditional BPM scenarios · Analytics-driven BPM · Cognitive Computing

1 Introduction

The field of business process management (BPM) has gone through many waves of insight and innovation in its journey. From work simplification concepts originated in early 1900s through quality control and quality management awareness in the late 1980s and early 2000s to management theory frameworks such as Balanced Score Card, and process and IT frameworks (SCOR, CIBIT, eTom) to the recent social, mobile, smart (sensor-based) and adaptive BPM themes - all have emerged to adapt to the business and technological innovations in the industry. The latest insight in BPM field, driven by today's market dynamics and the need to be agile and adaptive, is analytics-driven BPM.

Driven by market momentum around social, mobile and cloud based technological innovations, companies are under constant pressure to be agile, and to proactively respond to changes in the marketplace by adapting their business processes in near real-time. For example, client relationship management (CRM) products these days can no longer rely on structured enterprise data and pre-defined processes alone. They have to monitor, mine and analyze the continuous feedback being received through various social channels such as Facebook posts, Twitter tweets, and other public and private

F. Fournier and J. Mendling (Eds.): BPM 2014 Workshops, LNBIP 202, pp. 158–164, 2015.
DOI: 10.1007/978-3-319-15895-2_14

discussion forum postings. By continuously collecting and analyzing real-time data from social, mobile and other platforms together with the more traditional enterprise data, companies can observe trends, take corrective actions and improve business outcomes. Analytics of various kinds including predictive, prescriptive, discovery, descriptive and diagnostic [2] play a critical role in business processes.

In this position paper, we report on observations from our efforts and experiences in developing and deploying BPM tools at a large IT services provider. We argue that in knowledge-driven and human-centric activities such as IT services sales where data-driven understanding leads to decisions in the process, rigid, pre-defined process definitions do not meet the needs. Process definition and enactment, both, have to be dynamic, flexible and adaptive based on the understanding of the state of affairs. We present a framework and approach for a *cognitive BPM system* where the process dynamically adapts to the situation at hand based on the results of data analytics and continuously learns from the actions taken (as articulated in newly emerged cognitive computing paradigm [1]).

The rest of the paper is structured as follows. In Sect. 2, we provide a brief overview of advances in BPM space is support of human-centric processes. In Sect. 3, we describe our observation of the challenges for supporting analytics-driven human processes. Section 4 presents a framework and our vision of cognitive BPM for supporting analytics-driven BPM, and discusses current progress and the steps toward defining and developing cognitive BPM. Finally, we conclude in Sect. 5.

2   BPM Advances in Support of Human-Centric Processes

Traditional business process management [5], workflow management systems [4] and process-aware information systems [6] excel at supporting the automation of well-specified, repetitive and highly automatable business processes. There has been a considerable effort in supporting flexibility in business processes [7] and supporting human-centered work in the context of case management applications [8], artifact-centric processes [9], and process analytics and predictive monitoring [10]. These efforts have been focused on using information of the process execution in order to adapt or change its course of execution. Another category of existing work focuses on analyzing the past execution data of the process in order to recommend future course of actions for new execution cases [7, 8]. However, information from the bigger context that is a container for the execution of process, and analytics using this data has less been explored for supporting the automation of human-centric processes, and not only to adapt the execution but to adapt the process model by creating different variations of the process model for different contexts, where each perform well.

The challenges of supporting human-centric processes in the enterprise is also studied in [11]. The major shift that we witness today is that the decisions on how to define, refine, enact and adapt the process is made as the result of data analytics, with data that comes from the context of the process, and all external channels such as social media, devices, Internet, enterprise repositories, etc. These are the basis for defining a cognitive business process management system in which analytics results enable process management systems to sense, analyze, learn and as a result constantly and automatically adapt the system to reflect the context and situation that it is running in, and achieve situational awareness, self-learning and adaptiveness.

3   Analytics-Driven Enactment of Human-Centric Processes

We are into a new era of computing, where an enormous volume of data is generated and gathered around us, and used to make business decisions. In the following, we discuss how people in today's data-rich environment work in the context of human-centric sales processes in an IT service provider environment.

The main characteristic of human-centric processes is that they are described at a high level of abstraction (reference level), and the detailed activities are decided upon, performed and orchestrated by humans. One of the main reasons that such processes have still remained as "human-centric" is the need for capturing, interpreting and reasoning on the data that drives process decisions, and the need for continuous evaluation of the situation to adapt the actions, create variations of the process for different purposes, and re-execute some process steps with new knowledge. That is, partly, why traditional process automation solutions and their flexible and adaptive variations have not yet got wide-spread adoption in the industry. It is important to study how people work today in the absence of process automation tools for human-centric processes. How humans take their understanding of work context into account, and what are the desired features for such tools. We take as an example the IT service sales process, in which people form multiple departments inside an enterprise services organization get involved and collaborate.

The need for a business-aware automation solution for human-centric processes: A survey of sales professional in the studied IT service provider company asking about priority areas for sales process improvements ranks automation and tool support right after few important changes to the reference process itself, which can be considered as cognitive feedback on the process. While the need for process automation tools has a productivity-gain motivation, as a secondary criteria, as the sales executives and teams expect to eliminate the need for manual tracking of activities, they stress that the tool should capture and understand the business context, and use this information to make dynamic suggestions based on gained insights on what works better, and when to achieve better business outcome. This is a key factor in making the business case for deployment of BPM tools.

Multiple data sources feeding process decisions: there are multiple information systems, data repositories and data sources (social media, news, financial information) and information from interactions with internal and external people (email, social networking, chat, client interactions, etc.) that are used as feeds by sales people to make decisions proactively and reactively. These decisions may have major impact on process activities, and therefore require flexibility of process automation systems in adapting the process definition and execution in a continuous manner.

Inbox used a work management system: The lack of automation support for sales process has driven sales people to use their email, an unstructured knowledge and interaction management tool, into a work and process management system through a combination of defining folders, rules, tagging and taking various feeds into their inbox and categorization. Nonetheless, this approach is still manual, error-prone and requires a high level of discipline and organization.

Changes to process guidelines and templates are commonplace and communicated through email: As more data has become available, and therefore agile decisions made in various parts of the business, the description of the overall sales process and guidelines on process steps and also document templates are updated more frequently, and in a faster pace. While these changes are posted to corresponding websites, the main method for communicating process changes is through emails, which highlights the need for processing unstructured information in order to understand the need for changing process definitions and process execution instances.

4 Future BPM Platforms for Supporting Analytics-Driven BPM

Two key shortcoming of current BPM suite of technologies for supporting human-centric are: lack of data-driven understanding of the context to drive process decisions, and using the result of analytics to adapt the process execution and process model (including annotating it, and creating multiple variations of it for different contexts) to accommodate continuous data and process decision updates.

Analytics-driving process model definition and adaptation: the first observation is that often process cannot be modeled in details in advance. Based on the reference process model, and a library of available actions, defined or learned, the concrete activities and decision on the dynamic composition of process activities is driven by analytics results. A research question in this context is how to learn process activities, and compose the process automatically based on results of an analytics? For example, reacting to a customer churn prediction, how to adapt/compose a process that reduces the chances of customer leaving (finds what customers like and puts together the best set of actions to attract or retain the customers).

Analytics supporting the adaptation of process enactment: As new information become available, new analytics results become available in different classes of predictive, descriptive, prescriptive and discovery analytics. Each class of analytics, may impact what process activities and how they are executed. In particular, predictive analytics need to be extended in the context of the processes to identify what process steps and resources may be needed as the result of certain business-focused predictions. For instance, based on such predictions, to suggest to create alternative paths (or variations of the process) in the process for different set of customers to maximize business outcome. Other types of analytics should be also reconsidered in the context of process enactment on how they would impact the process and business outcome.

The need for flexibility may comprise addressing the following requirements, though in a new analytic-driven approach: (i) ability to start from reference process and activities, and compose the process in a data-driven approach, (ii) ability to adapt the reference process, and create additional annotations to show e.g., the business performance of actions, in an automated approach. (ii) typical to other human-centric activities, ability to adapt the process step, e.g., re-execute a step (or a fragment of the process) in a context-aware manner, (iii) ability to make reasoning, and answer questions about the what-if-scenarios about the process based on analytics (predictive, discoveries, descriptive, etc.), and support proactive vs. reactive paradigm for decision makings. (iv) ability to process unstructured information available in personal communication, interaction and news feeds (social) and across multiple channels and devices in order to support process automation, (v) integrated artifact (structured data) and process management: today the artifacts and processes are managed separately by different systems. Analytics-driven BPM needs a holistic view on how data is relevant to process execution, (vi) revisiting main process notions and definitions, for example revisiting the notion of task completion. Current workflow systems consider a task instance closed once it is marked as completed. However, in practice, the task may not be completed and be subject to several (unplanned) revisions before the process ends.

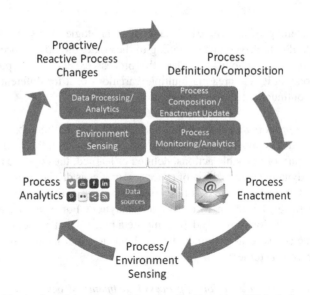

Fig 1. Our vision for the lifecycle of a Cognitive BPM platform

We believe that BPM field is about to undergo profound transformations in the coming few years into what we call a cognitive BPM. Our vision for such a cognitive BPM platform is shown in Fig. 1. The advancement of Big Data tools and platforms, and the success of cognitive computing [1] platforms such as IBM Watson make it possible to analyze massive amounts of data in real-time to provide insights at a scale and magnitude that was not possible before. As noted from our experiences with IT services sales domain, those domains that have to deal with large amounts of (unstructured) data to understand the process updates over different channels to dynamically adapt business processes. We have taken the first step in this direction by processing sales people interactions over email and chat to automatically identify process tasks, and any update to them, reported in [12]. We envision a self-learning, cognitive sales process that is fully instrumented with probes and data collected from both internal and external sources. As the world becomes more instrumented and more data gets generated, and as enterprises' capabilities improve to mine their own internal data, the need to combine all this to make sense and to take actions that lead to desired outcomes becomes even more prominent. BPM vendors must make plans for enabling their BPM platforms with these cognitive capabilities to support analytics-driven business processes.

5 Conclusions

In this position paper, we have presented our observations and challenges noted in deploying business process management (BPM) tools in IT services sales process at a large IT services provider organization. We argue that in knowledge-driven and human-centric activities such as IT services sales where data-driven understanding leads to decisions in the process, rigid, pre-defined process definitions do not quite work. Process definition and enactment, both, have to be dynamic, flexible and adaptive to the results of analytics. We presented a framework for cognitive BPM as a next generation platform for analytics-driven business processes.

References

1. Cognitive Computing: http://www.research.ibm.com/cognitive-computing
2. Corocoron, M. The five types of analytics. http://www.informationbuilders.es/intl/co.uk/presentations/four_types_of_analytics.pdf
3. Mukherjee, D., Blomberg, J., Akkiraju, R., Raghu, D., Gupta, M., Ghosal, S., Qiao, M., Nakamura, T.: A case based approach to serve information needs in knowledge intensive processes. In: Basu, S., Pautasso, C., Zhang, L., Fu, X. (eds.) ICSOC 2013. LNCS, vol. 8274, pp. 541–549. Springer, Heidelberg (2013)
4. van der Aalst, W., van Hee, K.: Workflow Management: Models, Methods, and Systems. MIT Press, Cambridge (2002)
5. Dumas, M., La Rosa, M., Mendling, J., Reijers, H.A.: Fundamentals of Business Process Management. Springer, Heidelberg (2013)
6. Dumas, M., van der Aalst, W.M., ter Hofstede, A.H.: Process-Aware Information Systems: Bridging People and Software Through Process Technology. Wiley, New York (2005)
7. Reichert, M., Weber, B.: Enabling Flexibility in Process-Aware Information Systems: Challenges, Methods, Technologies. Springer, New York (2012)
8. Motahari Nezhad, H.R., Keith, D.: Swenson: adaptive case management: overview and research challenges. In: CBI, pp. 264–269 (2013)
9. Hull, R.: Artifact-centric business process models: brief survey of research results and challenges. In: Meersman, R., Tari, Z. (eds.) OTM 2008, Part II. LNCS, vol. 5332, pp. 1152–1163. Springer, Heidelberg (2008)
10. zur Muehlen, M., Shapiro, R.: Business process analytics. In: Rosemann, M., vom Brocke, J. (eds.) Handbook on Business Process Management, vol. 2, pp. 137–157. Springer, Berlin (2009)

11. Kabicher-Fuchs, S., et al.: Human-Centric Process-Aware Information Systems (HC-PAIS), CoRR abs/1211.4986 (2012)
12. Kalia, A.K., Motahari Nezhad, H.R., Bartolini, C., Singh, M.P.: Monitoring commitments in people-driven service engagements. In: IEEE SCC, pp. 160–167 (2013)

Towards Ensuring High Availability in Collective Adaptive Systems

David Richard Schäfer[1](✉), Santiago Gómez Sáez[2], Thomas Bach[1],
Vasilios Andrikopoulos[2], and Muhammad Adnan Tariq[1]

[1] Institute of Distributed and Parallel Systems (IPVS),
University of Stuttgart, Stuttgart, Germany
{david.schaefer,thomas.bach,adnan.tariq}@ipvs.uni-stuttgart.de
[2] Institute of Architecture of Application Systems (IAAS),
University of Stuttgart, Stuttgart, Germany
{gomez-saez,andrikopoulos}@iaas.uni-stuttgart.de

Abstract. Collective Adaptive Systems support the interaction and adaptation of virtual and physical entities towards achieving common objectives. For these systems, several challenges at the modeling, provisioning, and execution phases arise. In this position paper, we define the necessary underpinning concepts and identify requirements towards ensuring high availability in such systems. More specifically, based on a scenario from the EU Project ALLOW Ensembles, we identify the necessary requirements and derive an architectural approach that aims at ensuring high availability by combining active workflow replication, service selection, and dynamic compensation techniques.

Keywords: Workflows · High availability · Service discovery · Process fragment injection

1 Introduction

Collective Adaptive Systems (CAS) comprise heterogeneous entities collaborating towards the achievement of their own objectives, and the overall objective of the collective [1]. Such large-scale systems are usually constituted by physical and virtual entities that interact with each other towards achieving individual and collective goals. In the EU ALLOW Ensembles[1] Project we aim to provide support for modeling, executing, and adapting such interactions among entities. We propose to model and manage entities as collections of *cells* encapsulating their functionalities. Entities collaborate with each other to achieve their objectives in the context of *ensembles* describing the interactions among them.

In [1] we proposed the usage of service orchestrations and choreographies to specify the behavior of cells and to define the interactions within ensembles, respectively. However, the achievement of individual and collective goals through interactions among entities raises further challenges for such a system.

---

[1] EU ALLOW Ensembles: http://www.allow-ensembles.eu/.

© Springer International Publishing Switzerland 2015
F. Fournier and J. Mendling (Eds.): BPM 2014 Workshops, LNBIP 202, pp. 165–171, 2015.
DOI: 10.1007/978-3-319-15895-2_15

More specifically, we focus our work on ensuring high availability of cells by means of ensuring the continuation of their execution. Moreover, in case of system failures, errors of any type must be handled effectively and efficiently. For this purpose, we present our vision and ongoing work to target such challenges by analyzing and proposing an approach based on workflow replication, service selection and execution, and dynamic service compensation. Existing work ensures high availability in different ways. Parallel service execution focuses on ensuring activity deadlines [2]. However, such approaches increase the overall cost due to the number of accessed services. Logging and checkpointing mask computing node failures but introduce delays during the recovery phase of the system [3]. Another approach is the primary-backup strategy, where a primary node executes the workflow and transfers its state to all backups [4]. Failures of the primary first have to be detected and a new primary has to be selected, which again introduces delays and, thus, unavailability. In previous work, we targeted declarative workflow replication and restructuring to increase availability [5]. In this work, we build on the service-oriented architecture and imperative workflow description for our proposal.

The contributions of this work can be summarized as follows: (1) the identification of requirements based on the EU ALLOW Ensembles motivation scenario and (2) the design of a reference architecture synthesizing workflow replication, service selection, and dynamic compensation techniques to support high availability. The remainder of the paper is structured as follows: starting from a motivation scenario in Sect. 2, we introduce our architectural approach in Sect. 3, and conclude with a summary and future research challenges in Sect. 4.

2   Motivation

To motivate our work, we use the example illustrated in Fig. 1a based on the FlexiBus scenario [1]. Consider employee Adam gets a call from his boss that he needs to attend a meeting on the other end of the city in half an hour. To reach his destination, the workflow depicted in Fig. 1a needs to be executed on a device capable of executing workflows. In the following, we call such devices *nodes*. Consider that the workflow is executed on Adam's mobile device. Mobile environments in specific but any environment in general might endure node, service, and communication link failures. In the best case, these failures lead to temporal unavailability. In the worst case, the execution fails. We address this by executing multiple workflow instances on different nodes (*replicated workflow execution*) and invoking several services for the execution of one activity (*service selection and execution*). In general, replication is highly desirable for increasing availability as mentioned by Schaefer et al. [5] and depicted by the replicated execution of Adam's workflow in Fig. 1b. The service needed by the first activity is only available on the internet. When the mobile phone loses connectivity, it does not receive the reply from the service and cannot proceed. However, the replica on the server in the internet continues execution. If the replicas reconnect and synchronize before the execution reaches the last activity, which has to be executed locally on the phone, the availability is then never affected.

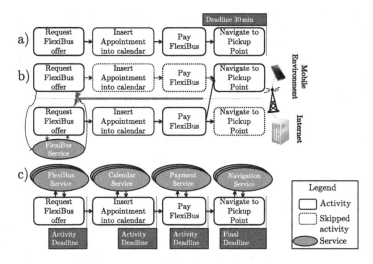

Fig. 1. (a) The workflow of Adam to get to the appointment in time. (b) Example of a replicated execution. (c) Workflow with activity level deadlines and multiple services.

As shown in Fig. 1c, we assume that every activity of the workflow can be satisfied by a number of different services. To guarantee that the workflow deadline is met, we invoke several services for one activity staggered over time. This means we give services time to reply before calling additional services. Both, the workflow replication and the service execution strategy, can lead to the invocation of multiple services which might change the outcome of the workflow execution. In order to compensate for the additional service executions, we propose the dynamic and automated discovery and injection of compensation handlers into the workflow instance during run-time.

3   Approach

In this section, we explain how to use *replicated workflow execution*, and *service selection and execution* to increase availability. Furthermore, our strategies dynamically discover services at run-time making it hard to specify the respective compensation operations at design time. To solve this, we present a dynamic compensation mechanism. Our proposed architecture (cf. Fig. 2) consists of a cluster of *Execution Engines* (EE) (where the replicated workflow instances are executed) each placed on a different node and an *Enterprise Service Bus* (ESB). We add a *Replication Layer* to the EE and the ESB to handle workflow replication. To enable service selection and execution, we add a *Service Selection and Execution Layer* (SEL) to multiple components of the ESB. The components of these layers will be discussed in detail in the remainder of this section.

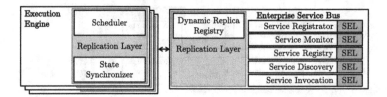

Fig. 2. Our architecture extends the EE and the ESB by a Replication Layer and adds a Service Selection and Execution Layer (SEL) to multiple components of the ESB.

3.1   Workflow Replication

We use replicated workflow executions to increase availability (cf. Sect. 2). Executing a workflow multiple times on different EEs, placed on different computing nodes, can lead to inconsistencies. Thus, we appropriately schedule the activities and synchronize the processes, e.g., the payment activity, confirming the offer and transferring the money, is executed only by one EE. Otherwise, Adam pays multiple times. In principle, when executing an activity multiple times, it either can cause inconsistencies (*non-replicable*) or never causes inconsistencies (*replicable*). If the activity is non-replicable, the *Scheduler* (cf. Fig. 2) coordinates to ensure exactly one execution of the activity avoiding any inconsistency in advance. After the activity's execution, the *State Synchronizer* transfers the changed state to all other EEs. To enable seamless communication, all EEs executing workflow replicas are registered in the *Dynamic Replica Registry* (cf. Fig. 2).

To increase availability further, we also allow temporal inconsistencies. Therefore, we further divide the non-replicable activities into compensable and non-compensable. In the case that the EEs cannot synchronize (e.g., because of network partitioning), each EE can proceed executing compensable and replicable activities. When the EEs reconnect, all but one EE have to compensate all non-replicable activities to regain consistency. The Scheduler will coordinate and trigger the necessary compensations. This strategy, however, leads to a new problem. We cannot define the compensation handlers at design time because the compensation logic depends on the used service, which is dynamically discovered during run-time. Thus, our idea is to inject the compensation logic into the workflow instance at run-time (cf. Sect. 3.3).

3.2   Selection and Execution of Services

To guarantee the workflow level deadline, we derive optimal sub-deadlines for all activities (cf. Fig. 1c). To make sure these activity deadlines are met, we investigate the response time characteristics and costs of all services registered in the Service Registrator of the ESB (cf. Fig. 2). For each activity, we invoke a number of services, staggered over time, such that the deadline is met with high probability (i.e., 99.99 %) and the expected execution cost (e.g. monetary or energy) is minimized. If an activity is non-replicable but several services are invoked for execution, we need to compensate the additionally executed services dynamically during run-time (cf. Sect. 3.3). This is reflected in additional compensation cost. Currently we investigate approaches of assigning activity level deadlines and invoking services respectively. Preliminary results of a staggered execution, calculated with simulated annealing, promise to decrease the expected execution cost by $\sim 30\%$, compared to invoking all services at the same time.

We plan to extend the existing components of the ESB by a SEL (cf. Fig. 2). For example, the Service Monitor records the response times of the different services and stores that data in the extended Service Registry.

3.3 Dynamic Compensation Handling

The workflow technology natively supports compensation capabilities and proposes the usage of compensation spheres as a mechanism to group transactional and non-transactional activities into a new unit of work [6]. When a compensation sphere is executed unsuccessfully, the workflow system executes the compensation logic defined in the process model for the grouped unit of work. However, two main disadvantages arise when specifying the compensation logic at design time: (1) the process modeler must completely know the external services rollback operations and (2) there exists limited flexibility to dynamically cope with services' compensation logic modifications (e.g., due to service versioning).

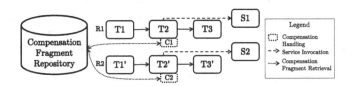

Fig. 3. Retrieval and Injection of Process Compensation Fragments

The replication and service discovery mechanisms previously presented require dynamic and adaptable compensation capabilities to rollback operations from different services (or service replicas) which are dynamically discovered during run-time. Figure 3 depicts the proposed approach for enabling an adaptive orchestration of compensation operations based on enabling run-time process refinement and the usage of process fragments presented in [7]. Process fragments partially or completely specify a concrete functionality and are typically persisted and discovered from fragment repositories during the process design time. Process fragments can be used during run-time to refine a process model partially specified during modeling time.

In Fig. 3, two process replicas R1 and R2 discover two services S1 and S2, respectively, which provide similar functionalities. As described in Sect. 3.1, all replicas might execute their discovered services. However, if the activity is non-replicable and compensable, only one execution is selected eventually. This selection leads to the need for compensating state modifications that activities, e.g., T2', perform on the external services. For instance, the compensation logic for a credit card payment varies depending on the payment gateway and credit card issuer. The proposed approach considers the usage of the *Abstract Activity* proposed in [8] to specify compensation fragments placeholders which are refined during run-time. The *Compensation Fragment Repository* enables the storage and retrieval of compensation fragments for different services and their corresponding versions. Therefore, the Replication Layer in both the EE and ESB (cf. Fig. 2) must be aware of such constructs and interact with the compensation fragment repository.

4   Conclusions and Future Work

Collective Adaptive Systems are characterized by the interactions among multiple heterogeneous entities towards achieving individual and collective goals. A system capable of supporting such interactions at the different phases, i.e., modeling, provisioning, and execution, must guarantee high availability and robustness of the functionalities consumed and exposed by such entities. In this work we present our vision towards ensuring such characteristics based on the FlexiBus motivation scenario from the EU ALLOW Ensembles Project.

Based on the requirements identified in the motivating scenario, we present an architectural approach which relies on the usage of workflows and SOA-based approaches and technologies. Moreover, we propose the usage of workflow replication, and service selection and execution strategies towards fulfilling the deadlines which may be imposed by the individual entities. However, such techniques infer the necessity of ensuring an adaptable compensation functionality for the multiple workflow replicas and consumed services, which can be addressed by enabling the dynamic retrieval and injection of compensation fragments. In future work, we plan to identify concrete solutions that can be used for realizing the presented concepts.

Acknowledgement. This work has been partially funded by the EU Project ALLOW Ensembles (600792).

References

1. Andrikopoulos, V., Bucchiarone, A., Sáez, S.G., Karastoyanova, D., Mezzina, C.A.: Towards modeling and execution of collective adaptive systems. In: Lomuscio, A.R., Nepal, S., Patrizi, F., Benatallah, B., Brandić, I. (eds.) ICSOC 2013 Workshops. LNCS, vol. 8377, pp. 69–81. Springer, Heidelberg (2014)
2. Stein, S., Payne, T.R., Jennings, N.R.: Robust execution of service workflows using redundancy and advance reservations. IEEE Trans. Serv. Comput. 4(2), 125–139 (2011)
3. Elnozahy, E.N.M., Alvisi, L., Wang, Y.M., Johnson, D.B.: A survey of rollback-recovery protocols in message-passing systems. ACM Comput. Surv. 34(3), 375–408 (2002)

4. Lau, J., Lung, L.C., da Fraga, J., Santos Veronese, G.: Designing fault tolerant web services using bpel. In: Seventh IEEE/ACIS International Conference on Computer and Information Science, ICIS 2008, pp. 618–623, May 2008
5. Schäfer, D.R., Bach, T., Tariq, M.A., Rothermel, K.: Increasing availability of workflows executing in a pervasive environment. In: Proceedings of IEEE SCC 2014. IEEE Computer Society, June 2014
6. Leymann, F., Roller, D.: Production Workflow: Concepts and Techniques. Prentice Hall, Upper Saddle River (2000)
7. Eberle, H., Unger, T., Leymann, F.: Process fragments. In: Meersman, R., Dillon, T., Herrero, P. (eds.) OTM 2009, Part I. LNCS, vol. 5870, pp. 398–405. Springer, Heidelberg (2009)
8. Bialy, L.: Dynamic Process Fragment Injection in a Service Orchestration Engine. Diploma thesis No. 3564, University of Stuttgart, Germany (2014)

DAB 2014

Analytics Process Management: A New Challenge for the BPM Community

Fenno F. (Terry) Heath III and Richard Hull[(✉)]

IBM T.J. Watson Research Center, Yorktown Heights, NY, USA
{theath,hull}@us.ibm.com

Abstract. Today, essentially all industry sectors are developing and applying "big data analytics" to gain new business insights and new operational efficiencies. Essentially two forms of analytics processing support these business-targeted applications: (i) "analytics explorations" that search for business-relevant insights in support of description, prediction, and prescription; and (ii) "analytics flows" that are deployed and executed repeatedly to apply such insights to support reporting and enhance existing business processes. The human environment that surrounds business-targeted analytics involves a multitude of stake-holder roles, and a number of distinct processes are required for the development, deployment, maintanence, and governance of these analytics. This short paper presents preliminary work on a framework for Analytics Process Management (APM), a new branch of Business Process Management (BPM) that is intended to address the central challenges managing analytics flows at scale. APM is focused on the processes that manage the overall lifecycle of analytics flows and their executions, and their integration into "operational" business processes that have been the traditional domain of BPM. The paper identifies key meta-data that should be maintained for analytics flows and their executions, and identifies the core business processes that are needed to create, apply, compare, and maintain such flows. The paper also raises key research questions that need to be addressed in the emerging area of APM.

1 Introduction

Today, essentially all industry sectors are developing and applying "big data analytics" to gain new business insights and new operational efficiencies. Essentially two forms of analytics processing support these business-targeted applications: (i) "analytics explorations" that search for business-relevant insights in support of description, prediction and prescription; and (ii) "analytics flows" that are deployed and executed repeatedly to apply such insights to support reporting and enhance existing business processes. The human environment that surrounds business-targeted and related analytics involves a multitude of stake-holders, ranging from executives focused on return on investment, to data scientists focused on extracting relevant information and insights; and from Subject Matter Experts (SMEs) who deeply understand an application area, to user experience

© Springer International Publishing Switzerland 2015
F. Fournier and J. Mendling (Eds.): BPM 2014 Workshops, LNBIP 202, pp. 175–185, 2015.
DOI: 10.1007/978-3-319-15895-2_16

experts, to the user community that consumes the analytics outputs as a part of their own business processes. A fundamental challenge is: How can businesses effectively create, apply, measure, compare, configure, adapt, and govern these analytic activities at a large scale and as an on-going part of their activities? It is essential that the solution developed provide rich, flexible, and intuitive mechanisms for managing the full lifecycle of analytics flows and their executions, including (a) incorporating the results of analytics explorations into analytics flows, (b) measuring, (re-)configuring, improving, and expanding the scope of the analytics flows over time, and (c) incorporating the outputs of the analytics flows into the business operations and processes in meaningful and measurable ways. We use the term *Analytics Process Management* (*APM*) to refer to the processes these processes. APM focuses on the analytics activities that are often performed to enhance *operational* business processes, that is, processes that are focused on the core operations of an enterprise.

The focus of this paper is quite timely, because the need for data scientists who actually perform deep statistical analytics is much smaller than the need for people who can manage the creation, application, and improvement of the analytics. For example, according to a McKinsey report from 2011 [8], in the United States the demand for "deep analytical positions in the big data world could exceed the supply being produced by current trends by 140,000 to 190,000 positions." But, the report goes on to say that "we project a need for 1.5 million additional managers and analysts in the United States who can ask the right questions and consume the results of the analysis of big data effectively." Further, there is "a need for ongoing innovation in technologies and techniques that will help individuals and organizations to integrate, analyze, visualize, and consume the growing torrent of big data." A prime motivation for developing the field of APM is to streamline those activities, so that the creativity in finding new ways to apply, validate, compare, and refine analytics is not hampered by the more mundane activities needed to support on-going execution, maintenance, and evolution of the analytics flows.

Up until now, the academic research community has focused largely on the challenges of statistical analysis, information extraction, and data "extract, transform, load" (ETL), and not on the challenge of managing analytics processes within the business context. For example, [3] provides an in-depth survey of techniques and challenges for applying analytics on the data produced by businesses. The focus is on using the analytics to produce reports and visualizations for human consumption. But the challenge of embedding the analytics outputs into operational business processes, and refining the analytics through experiences gained, is largely overlooked. Similarly, a recent survey on technical challenges in Big Data [5] focuses on analytics outputs for human consumption. This contrasts sharply with trends for applying analytics in industry sectors such as e-commerce and marketing, where online customer interactions are guided in realtime by analytics derived from huge volumes of data. Also, [14] points out that "[r]esearch on how to manage analysis algorithms ... is quite open."

Popular analytics processing suites such as IBM's SPSS or RapidMiner [10] (which is also available open source [11]) provide capabilities that are central to APM. In particular, they provide visual tools for specifying rich varieties of analytics flows, for storing and sharing them, and for version management. However, they do not emphasize a number of capabilities that are relevant to managing the overall lifecycle of these flows in the context of long-term production-level usage. For example, there is little built-in support for recording and accessing the provenance of how data outputs have been produced by different versions of a flow. Also, there is little emphasis on seamlessly integrating measurement and continuous improvement into flow creation and maintenance. As a result, it is challenging for typical non-IT users to work with keep track of how measurements, comparative testing (e.g., A/B testing), and re-configurations of aspects of analytics flows fit together.

This short paper presents preliminary work on a framework intended to provide the foundation for Analytics Process Management. The framework builds upon and extends several established disciplines, including data integration/federation; knowledge representation and semantic web; scientific workflow and data provenance; the CRoss-Industry Standard Process for Data Mining (CRISP-DM); BPM including business artifacts and Case Management; and Information Technology governance. The framework involves two main layers: (i) analytics flows, which provide the core data structure that provides an anchor for APM, and (ii) a family of processes that manage different aspects of the full lifecycles of flows and their executions. Analytics flows are described in terms of three fundamental dimensions: functionality, variation, and provenance. A key application of this framework is to suggest guidelines around what meta-data should be stored about analytics flows and their executions, to enable better governance, auditability, comparisons, maintenance, and explanation of analytics as applied in business contexts.

This paper introduces two illustrative examples based on analytics projects being developed at IBM Research (Sect. 2), and uses them to illustrate the primary aspects of managing analytics flows from a process management perspective (Sect. 3). The paper then describes the key building blocks of analytics flows and introduces the three dimensional framework for managing them (Sect. 4). The paper concludes by mentioning some of the key open challenges in this area (Sect. 5).

2   Two Representative Analytics Applications

This section briefly introduces two examples of analytics processes that can be used in conjunction with operational business processes to improve their performance. Prototype systems for both applications are under development at IBM Research.

The LARIAT [2] system is focused on using web-accessible media, along with conventional business data, to identify and prioritize business-to-business (B2B) sales leads. The system crawls the web for publically available information about businesses and performs several steps of processing, which are illustrated in the box in Fig. 1 (see also Fig. 3). The LARIAT flow begins by filtering a stream of documents (news articles, government filings, analyst reports, etc.) both syntactically (using keywords) and then semantically (using AQL [6], to find occurrences of business patterns that suggest that a company may have interest in purchasing a given product. Entity resolution is used to match company names against standard names (namely, from Dunn and Bradstreet), to create "signals". For example, an article that describes a company with many knowledge workers that shows intention to expand might generate a "signal" that matches the company with potential to buy social business communications platform. Next, all of the signals found about a single company are aggregated (or "fused") to form "company descriptions". These are augmented with data from Dunn and Bradstreet and from another analytics flow that yields "propensity-to-buy" information. The company descriptions are then prioritized by a configurable family of rules. Optionally, workers may validate (and possibly delete) the signals, due to the possibility of false hits by the semantic filtering and the entity resolution, after which prioritization is again performed. The output can be delivered to sales teams on an on-going basis, and incorporated into banner-ad placement and other online marketing activity.

The second application is focused on providing a detailed understanding of the "customer satisfaction" (which is sometimes equated to the "Net Promoter Score") of business customers of a large telecommunications company.[1] The approach taken draws from [15] and elsewhere, and involves the identification of a handful of key "drivers" (see Fig. 4) that are combined to help infer the overall satisfaction score for each customer. Representative drivers include provisioning experience, trouble ticket experience, and contract renewal experience; statistical models for these are derived based on available data and can be refreshed periodically (e.g., monthly or quarterly). Yet another statistical model can be created to infer the overall customer satisfaction scores, based on the driver scores and training data about customer satisfaction. Importantly, knowledge of the individual driver scores can be used to identify mitigating actions that have a good probability of improving customer satisfaction.

3   Analytics from the BPM Perspective

We now consider how the processes needed to support the overall lifecycle of the analytics applications described in the preceding section are created and maintained, and used to augment operational business processes.

Figure 1 shows a broad range of stakeholders that may be involved with a B2B leads identification system such as LARIAT; we provide some highlights about these stakeholders here. "Data scientists", that is, experts in analytics, are

---

[1] The authors thank Dashun Wang and Jeff Robinson, who are collaborators in this prototyping effort, for numerous discussions and insights about the approach to analytics taken.

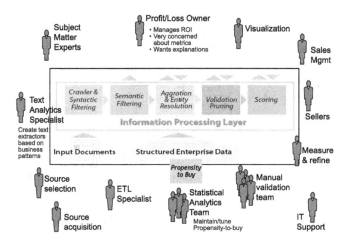

Fig. 1. Representative stakeholders surrounding B2B leads identification analytics

definitely present, both to help with statistical analysis around propensity-to-buy, and with text analytics to create AQL extractors based on relevant business patterns. Extract-Transform-Load (ETL) specialists and other IT support staff are also needed.

But numerous roles are needed in addition. A key role is Subject Matter Expert (SME); people in this role identify key business patterns that can reveal potential causality between observable events and likelihood of a company to need a given kind of product. Different kinds of users, including Sellers, Sales Management, and the executive(s) with profit and loss responsbility, will all have valuable suggestions with regards to the patterns, policies and prioritizations that are being incorporated. On-going manual validation is needed because of imprecise algorithms for text extraction and the entity resolution. This will impact both the outputted results, and feed back to the text extractors, the entity resolution algorithm, and elsewhere. Finally, the quality and effectiveness of the leads generated by the analytics flow need to be measured, to enable improvement over time.

The customer satisfaction analytics application will also involve a large number of stakeholders having analogous roles.

How can the activity of the people in these many roles be organized and managed? A key first step is to realize that all of the activity is centered around one or more analytics flows and executions of them. The next question is: what kinds of process are needed to manage the full lifecycle of such flows and executions? Figure 2 shows the eight main kinds of process needed to manage these lifecycles. These are the core of "Analytics Process Management".

The eight kinds of APM processes are largely complimentary to the CRISP-DM Reference Model [12] That model is focused on the creation, refinement, and deployment of a data mining project, whereas the listing here incorporates the application and management of the lifecycle of analytics flows and their

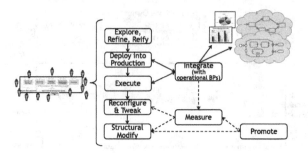

Fig. 2. The eight kinds of process at the core of Analytics Process Management

executions over long periods of time. The eight kinds of business process are as follows:

Explore, Refine, and Reify: This focuses on the initial creation of an analytics flow (or family of related flows). The several steps of the CRISP-DM method are typically performed here. The typical outcome of this process is a prototype system that embodies an analytics flow.

Deploy into Production: Deployment into production involves additional steps, mainly around hardening the various procedures and activities that go into the analytics flow. Some of these activities are IT-intensive, but others may involve establishing procedures whereby SMEs and users can provide feedback and/or refinements over time. This phase may include the design and deployment of targeted business processes, e.g., to incorporate on-going manual validation activities.

Integrate (with operational business processes): The outputs of the analytics flow may be used to create reports, and to directly impact operational business processes (including both process- and data-centric ones).

Execute: Execution of the analytics flow includes both the continuous or periodic creation of the key flow outputs, but also the periodic maintenance of different flow components, such as the statistical models for the drivers in the customer satisfaction application, or the lead prioritization rules in the B2B leads identification application. (Execution is discussed further in Sect. 4.)

Measure: On-going measurement of analytics flows and their application is crucial to justifying the investment into analytics, and to continuous improvement. Activities here include setting up measurement regimes, on-going performance monitoring, comparisons between flow versions, and reporting.

Reconfigure & Tweak: Analytics flows typically have numerous areas that can be adjusted without disrupting the overall structure of the flow. For example, in the LARIAT flow the prioritization rules and the entity resolution algorithm are configurable. Reconfiguring and tweaking these areas will fall to SMEs, analytics experts, and IT specialists, and needs to be performed in a systematic and recorded manner.

Structural Modify: Analytics flows may also be modified at a more structural level, to provide new features or to address changes in the underlying business context. Issues reminiscent of software engineering, such as version control and backwards compatibility, must be addressed.

Promote: A crucial element in the success of analytics projects is their adoption and expanded usage within a business environment. This typically requires active promotion and salesmanship by the analytics team. Further, the needs and interests of potential users may impact how the flow outputs are measured, and the overall nature of the flows.

All of the APM processes are knowledge-worker driven. They potentially involve SMEs, data scientists, BPM modeling experts, and/or the users of the analytics flows. Further, the tasks that may be relevant will vary depending on the kind of analytics flow involved, how well the flow is performing in terms of the measurements, and the new kinds of applications and users that the flow has. As a result, it appears that a declarative, data-centric approach to BPM, as found in the modern Case Management and business artifacts approaches [9,13] will be most suitable for supporting these processes. These approaches focus on key business-relevant entities (also called "cases" or "artifacts") that progress through a process, including both data that is accumulated by the entity, and the possible lifecycle that the entity might follow. In the case of managing analytics, the analytics flow itself serves as a kind of "meta-entity", an anchor that supports all of the processes. Individual processes will typically focus on additional entities; for example the Measure process might focus on "measurement plan" entities (that include information about the goal of the measurement activity, the instrumentation of the analytics flow needed, the data collected, etc.), whereas the Deploy Into Production process might focus on a "deployment plan" entities (that include information about all the tasks that need to be performed, the physical systems used, the software components that are deployed, the responsible parties, etc.)

4   Analytics Flows: A Data-Centric Perspective

This section provides a data-centric basis for supporting the kinds of business processes described in the preceding section for managing analytics flows. This includes a more detailed look at the analytics flows themselves and their execution. The section also introduces a high-level three-dimensional framework for structuring the data relavent to analytics flows and their execution.

Figures 3 and 4 provide (simplified) sketches of analytics flows underlying the LARIAT and customer satisfaction prototype applications described in Sect. 2. These flows are essentially directed graphs that include three primary kinds of node: Processing Steps, Repositories, and Policies.

Processing Steps (depicted as squares): These computation steps (automated or manual) may be fast or slow, and correspond to the application of some algoirthm to previously computed data. A processing step may be guided by one or more Policies. A processing step may produce data that is placed into a Repository and/or it may produce information relevant to a Policy (e.g., a new statistical model, or a new set of rules).

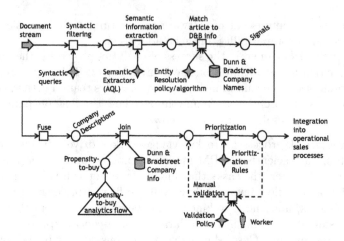

Fig. 3. Sketch of analytics flow for LARIAT B2B leads identification

Repositories (depicted as circles): These data stores will hold raw or derived objects. In some cases a processing step may augment existing objects by adding attributes or aggregating in additional information; in other cases the processing step may create essentially new objects (e.g., creating an object to hold information about a company not previously recognized, based on one or more newly discovered documents about that company).

Policies (depicted as 4-pointed stars): Here the term 'policy' is to be understood very broadly, to include, e.g., an algorithm (e.g., for entity resolution, or for automatic clustering), a statistical model (e.g., for one of the drivers relating to customer satisfaction), a set of manually created rules (e.g., for prioritizing sales leads), a family of syntatic queries or semantic (e.g., AQL) text extractors, or a procedure to be followed in a manual process.

Other nodes may also be included, e.g., corresponding to input data streams, structured data used by the flow, or workers used by the flow.

Unlike traditional flowcharts and workflows, the execution of an analytics flow may be *segmented over time*. For example, in the LARIAT flow, the Propensity-to-Buy repository might be refreshed on a monthly basis, whereas new documents are processed as they become available. Also, the manual validation step may be performed on a daily or weekly basis, but only for a fraction of the overall set of companies and documents processed by the flow. In the Customer Satisfaction application, the Policies for different drivers might be refreshed occasionally, on a monthly or quarterly basis, whereas other parts of the flow are executed daily.

We use the term *inquiry* to refer to an execution of part or all of a flow, based on particular input data (typically held in selected repositories of the flow) and based on particular versions of the relevant policies. An inquiry typically produces derived analytics *products*, which are placed into appropriate repositories, or become new versions of selected policies. (The term 'inquiry' is used, because

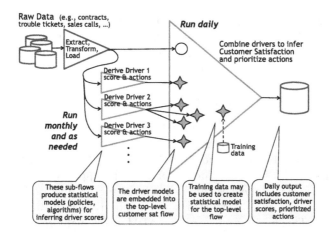

Fig. 4. Sketch of analytics flow for Customer Satisfaction application

it suggests an activity that uses established techniques in a focused attempt to obtain new information or conclusions based on existing information.)

We propose a three-dimensional framework for keeping track of analytics flows, the inquiries performed against them, and the evolution of the flows over time. This is based on "functionality", "variation", and "provenance". The *functionality* dimension is focused primarily on the different kinds of functions that Processing Steps might perform. These include incorporating different kinds of input data (e.g., structured data, document streams, event streams), ETL, entity resolution and other data fusion, automated statistical analytics (e.g., clustering, correlations), aggregations, visualizations, and monitoring and measurement. Each kind of Processing Step will involve different types of meta-data that should be maintained, to support normal execution, modifications over time, and maintenance of provenance information.

The *variation* dimension is focused on version control at the level of analytics flows. A given flow will be re-configured over time, as dictated by measurement outcomes and requests from users. Eventually, structural changes to the flow will be implemented, even though it is supporting many of the same operational business processes. It is important that all of the variations are tracked, can be examined, and can be compared.

Finally, the *provenance* dimension is focused on tracking exactly how any given (intermediate or final) output from an analytics flow was produced. The area of provenance is well-studied in the context of scientific workflow [4], and much of that work can be re-used for analytics flows. However, analytics flows emphasize measurement of flow outputs vis-a-vis their performance in operational business processes (e.g., efficiency gains in a supply chain or uplift in sales), and the impact of refinements. As a result, some extensions to existing support for provenance may be needed. Also, in the case of analytics flows it is sometimes useful to build in the rationale behind certain steps, so that explanations about analytics outputs can be explained to users more easily. For example, in the LARIAT system, each prioritization rule includes a manually created "explanation"; these are combined to create an overall explanation for the prioritization score computed for each company.

5   Open Research Challenges

This paper describes the key challenges that businesses will face as they bring "big data analytics" more fully into their day-to-day activities, and proposes a new research area centered around *Analytics Process Management (APM)*. The paper presents two illustrative examples of analytics applications, highlights key process management challenges raised by managing production-level analytics flows, and proposes core data structures and perspectives that can be used as the basis for APM. This initial framework for APM raises many research questions, a few of which are highlighted here.

The biggest question is how to manage the lifecycle of analytics flows and their executions in the context of large scale production, and in particular in the context of measurements, comparative testing, and evolution. This paper proposes some very high-level constructs to support that management, but a much more refined model and understanding will need to be developed, through experiential learning, targeted human factors and performance experiments, and conceptual and theoretical investigation.

There are two challenges relating to the creation of new flows. First, as pointed out in [7], somewhere between 50 % to 80 % of analytics work is characterized as "data wrangling" or "data janitor work". More specifically, this refers to an ad hoc form of "extract-transform-load (ETL)" work that is needed to find, understand, clean, and transform the data, so that it is suitable for analytics exploration. Second, when data scientists explore data using analytics tools (e.g., MatLab or R) it is rare for them to track, reproduce and/or re-use the steps they have taken. However, the algorithms developed in analytics explorations will increasingly be used as the starting point for production analytics flows. It is thus important to provide more systematic ways for ETL and analytics exploration to be recorded and made accessible for re-use. Tools such as VisTrails [1] may provide a useful starting point, but the ultimate solution will need to be very light-weight and non-intrusive.

A final challenge, also mentioned in [14], is to collaboratively develop expressive mechanisms and tools for multiple parties to develop, search, and share analytics flows and subflows. This will be increasingly important as the size of analytics flows continues to grow, and numerous teams will be contributing components into them. This is an especially rich challenge because of the depth and intricacy of the semantics implicit in these flows, and the need to continually demonstrate how the flows enable measurable performance gains in support of diverse business objectives.

Acknowledgements. The perspective described here developed through discussions and projects with many people, including: Matt Callery, Richard Goodwin,

Elham Kabhiri, Mark Linehan, Pietro Mazzoleni, Danny Oppenheim, Krishna Ratakondra, Jeff Robinson, Anshul Sheopuri, Piwadee (Noi) Sukaviriya, Roman Vaculín, Chitra Venkatramani, and Dashun Wang.

References

1. Callahan, S.P., Freire, J., Santos, E., Scheidegger, C.E., Silva, C.T., Vo, H.T.: Vistrails: visualization meets data management. In: Proceedings of the ACM SIGMOD International Conference on Management of Data, Chicago, Illinois, USA, 27–29 June 2006, pp. 745–747 (2006)

2. Callery, M., et al.: Towards a plug-and-play B2B marketing tool based on time-sensitive information extraction. In: IEEE International Conference on Services Computing, SCC 2014, Anchorage, AK, USA, June 27–July 2 2014, pp. 821–828 (2014)

3. Chaudhuri, S., Dayal, U., Narasayya, V.R.: An overview of business intelligence technology. Commun. ACM **54**(8), 88–98 (2011)

4. Davidson, S.B., Freire, J.: Provenance and scientific workflows: challenges and opportunities. In: Proceedings of the ACM SIGMOD International Conference on Management of Data, pp. 1345–1350 (2008)

5. Jagadish, H.V., Gehrke, J., Labrinidis, A., Papakonstantinou, Y., Patel, J.M., Ramakrishnan, R., Shahabi, C.: Big data and its technical challenges. Commun. ACM **57**(7), 86–94 (2014)

6. Krishnamurthy, R., et al.: Systemt: a system for declarative information extraction. SIGMOD Rec. **37**(4), 7–13 (2008)

7. Lohr, S.: For Big-Data Scientists, 'Janitor Work' is Key Hurdle to Insights, 17 August 2014. http://www.nytimes.com/2014/08/18/technology/for-big-data-scientists-hurdle-to-insights-is-janitor-work.html?_r=0

8. Manyika, J., et al.: Big data: the next frontier for innovation, competition, and productivity, May 2011. McKinsey Global Institute report. http://www.mckinsey.com/insights/business_technology/big_data_the_next_frontier_for_innovation

9. Marin, M., Hull, R., Vaculín, R.: Data centric BPM and the emerging case management standard: a short survey. In: La Rosa, M., Soffer, P. (eds.) BPM Workshops 2012. LNBIP, vol. 132, pp. 24–30. Springer, Heidelberg (2013)

10. RapidMiner. RapidMiner Studio Manual. www.rapidminer.com/documentation/

11. RapidMiner Opensource Development Team. RapidMiner - Data Mining, ETL, OLAP, BI. http://sourceforge.net/projects/rapidminer/

12. Shearer, C.: The CRISP-DM model: the new blueprint for data mining. J. Data Warehous. **5**(4), 13–22 (2000)

13. Swenson, K.D.: Mastering the Unpredictable: How Adaptive Case Management will Revolutionize the Way that Knowledge Workers Get Things Done. Meghan-Kiffer Press, Tampa (2010)

14. Truong, H.L., Dustdar, S.: A survey on cloud-based sustainability governance systems. IJWIS **8**(3), 278–295 (2012)

15. Wang, T., Wang, D., Wang, F.: Quantifying herding effects in crowd wisdom. In: The 20th ACM SIGKDD International Conference on Knowledge Discovery and Data Mining, KDD 2014, New York, NY, USA - 24–27 August 2014, pp. 1087–1096 (2014)

Towards Location-Aware Process Modeling and Execution

Xinwei Zhu[1]([✉]), Guobin Zhu[1], Seppe K.L.M. vanden Broucke[2],
Jan Vanthienen[2], and Bart Baesens[2]

[1] International School of Software, Wuhan University,
Luoyu Road 37, Hongshan, Wuhan, Hubei, China
xinwei.zhu@whu.edu.cn
[2] Department of Decision Sciences and Information Management, KU Leuven,
Naamsestraat 69, 3000 Leuven, Belgium

Abstract. Business Process Management (BPM) has emerged as one of the abiding systematic management approaches in order to design, execute and govern organizational business processes. Traditionally, most attention within the BPM community has been given to studying control-flow aspects, without taking other contextual aspects into account. This paper contributes to the existing body of work by focusing on the particular context of geospatial information. We argue that explicitly taking this context into consideration in the modeling and execution of business processes can contribute to improve their effectiveness and efficiency. As such, the goal of this paper is to make the modeling and execution aspects of BPM location-aware. We do so by proposing a Petri net modeling extension which is formalized by means of a mapping to coloured Petri nets. Our approach has been implemented using CPN Tools and a simulation extension was developed to support the execution and validation of location-aware process models. We also illustrate the feasibility of coupling business process support systems with geographical information systems by means of an experimental case setup.

Keywords: Business process management · Geographical information systems · Location-aware processes · Process modeling · Process execution · Coloured petri nets

1 Introduction

Throughout the past two decades, Business Process Management (BPM) has emerged as one of the abiding systematic management approaches in order to align organizational business processes and workflows to the needs of clients [1]. Traditionally, most attention within the BPM community has been focused on studying control-flow aspects of business processes, i.e. the aspects governing the flow of business activities (i.e. the sequence in which activities can be performed). In recent years, however, integrating other perspectives and "contexts" within this view has received increased attention, as support systems which adopt a

© Springer International Publishing Switzerland 2015
F. Fournier and J. Mendling (Eds.): BPM 2014 Workshops, LNBIP 202, pp. 186–197, 2015.
DOI: 10.1007/978-3-319-15895-2_17

control-flow view only are unable to adequately capture human behavior due to lack of descriptions of possible constraints against activity modeling. As such, many scholars have shifted towards studying various approaches that integrate control-flow with other contexts. In this paradigm, processes can be rapidly changed and adapted to a new external data-governed context (e.g., location, weather, etc.).

This paper contributes to the existing body of work by focusing on the particular *context of geospatial information*. We argue that taking this context into account in the various life cycle steps of BPM can contribute to improve the effectiveness and efficiency of process management. Especially in environments were a need arises to apply both process-aware and Geographical Information Systems (GIS), it makes sense to combine and integrate these two perspectives instead of keeping them isolated. Such an approach would help to increase understandability and objectiveness of designed process models, govern and constrain control-flow and process behavior based on location driven constraints, and allow for better location based monitoring and feedback support during execution of such processes. The goal of this paper is thus to make the modeling and execution aspects of BPM "location-aware". We do so by proposing a Petri net modeling extension which incorporates location aspects and ways to constrain the execution of activities based on location-based constraints. Next, we formalize the execution semantics of our extension by describing a mapping to coloured Petri nets. Finally, we have implemented our approach using CPN Tools [2]; a simulation extension was developed to support the execution and validation of models created using our approach and to illustrate the feasibility of coupling business process support systems with geographical information systems.

The remainder of this paper is structured as follows. Section 2 provides an overview of related work and preliminaries. Section 3 outlines a running example which will be used to illustrate the developed artifacts. Next, Sect. 4 introduces the Petri net modeling extension to model location-aware processes, after which Sect. 5 discusses the execution semantics of such models by means of a mapping to coloured Petri nets. Section 6 discusses the developed implementation. Section 7 concludes the paper.

2 Preliminaries

2.1 Related Work

We regard location as one of the key variables in the wider context of a business process. In the layered process context model proposed by Rosemann et al. [3], location describes an important variable situated in the environmental context layer, which describes process-related variables that reside beyond the business network in which an organization is embedded, but still pose a contingency effect on the business processes. Scholars have argued that the inclusion of location contextual variables in business process management practices help to improve dependency aspects (constraining activity executions based on location aspects, for instance) [4], increase the adaptability and flexibility of running processes (by reconfiguring and modifying models and tasks based on location aspects) [5], and improve the efficiency (performance and cost-effectiveness) of organizational processes [6].

However, works around the connection of location services with principles of business process management are scarce in the literature. Many researchers focus on connecting spatial-based information with scientific workflows [7–11] (i.e. describing a series of scientific-oriented computational or data manipulation steps), but not with business workflows. As a notable exception, [12] discusses map metaphors that are used to visualize work items and resources in process-aware information systems (using the YAWL workflow language). This technique specifies that users could check geographical positions and distances based on a geographical map, but does not indicate how geographical aspects can influence the behavioral aspects of the process. Decker et al. [4,13] have defined location constraints for individual workflow activities when modeling a workflow schema to restrict the location where an activity can be performed, but the location constraints lack comprehension and expressiveness.

Some existing BPM tool suites allow for the definition and capture of additional variables in the modeling of business processes [14,15]. Such attribute fields could be used to capture location-based information, but only in the form of secondary constructs or text-based annotations for readers to understand the graphical diagram, which do not impact the semantics or execution of the modeled process in a direct way. Our approach aims to make location-based constructs first-class citizens in the modeling and execution of process models.

2.2   Definitions and Notations

This section outlines some preliminary concepts and definitions which will be utilized in the remainder of the paper. We assume readers to be familiar with the concept of Petri nets [16,17] and their execution semantics. A particular subclass of Petri nets which we utilize hereafter are called WorkFlow nets (or WF-nets) [18]. A WF-net specifies the behavior of a single process instance in isolation and is defined as follows.

Definition 1. WF-net *[18]. A Petri net* (P, T, F) *is a WF-net iff:*

- *There is a single source place* $i \in P$ *such that* $\bullet i = \emptyset$;
- *There is a single sink place* $o \in P$ *such that* $o\bullet = \emptyset$;
- *The net* $(P, T \cup \{t'\}, F \cup \{(o, t'), (t', i)\})$ *is strongly connected, i.e. every* $x \in P \cup T$ *lies on a path from* i *to* o.

To define the execution semantics of our Petri net modeling extension, we will provide a formalized mapping to coloured Petri nets (CPN) [2]. CPNs are an extension of Petri net which allow for tokens of multiple types ("colors"), add guard transitions to constrain the execution of transitions and add arc expression to govern the input and output flow of tokens.

Definition 2. Coloured Petri net *(see [2]). A CPN is a tuple* $(P, T, A, \Sigma, C, V, N, G, E, M, I)$ *with* P *the set of places,* $P = \{p_1, p_2, ..., p_{|P|}\}$; T *the* set of transitions, $T = \{t_1, t_2, ..., t_{|T|}\}$ with $P \cap T = \emptyset$; A the set of arcs, $A = \{a_1, a_2, ..., a_{|A|}\}$; Σ the set of color sets defined within the model; V the set of variables used in the model, $V = \{v_1, v_2, ..., v_{|V|}\}$; $C : P \cup V \rightarrow \Sigma$ returning the color set associated to a place or a variable; $N : A \rightarrow P \times T \cup T \times P$ mapping arcs to a place-transition or transition-place flow. $G : T \rightarrow \{GExpr\}$ is the guard expression function mapping a transition $t \in T$ to a boolean expression $GExpr$, denoting whether the transition is permitted to fire. Evaluating this expression yields a boolean result $GExpr^* \in \{true, false\}$. $E : A \rightarrow \{AExpr\}$ is the arc expression function mapping an arc $a \in A$ to an expression $AExpr$. Evaluating an arc expression yields a multiset of tokens, $AExpr^*_{MS}$ to be produced (transition to place arcs) or consumed (place to transition arcs). $M : p \in P \mapsto C(p)_{MS}$ is the marking function, returning the multi set of tokens contained in a place with $\forall p \in P : [\forall \sigma \in M(p) : [\sigma \in C(p)]]$ and $I : P \rightarrow \{IExpr\}$ is the initialization function, initializing places in the model with a state, expressed as colored tokens. The evaluation of an $IExpr$ yields a token multi set: $IExpr^*_{MS}$ with $\forall p \in P : [\forall \sigma \in IExpr^*_{MS} : [\sigma \in C(p)]]$.

The execution semantics of a CPN differ from those of a regular Petri net. For a transition $t \in T$ to be enabled, all expressions of the incoming arcs should be satisfied and the guard condition of the transition must evaluate to true, $G(t)^* = true$. When firing an enabled transition, output and input places are updated accordingly given the input and output arc expressions.

Next, we shift our attention to the formalization of locations. The definition of our concept of location corresponds with a so called "feature" as applied by most geographical information systems [19]. A feature is describes something that can be drawn on a map, i.e. something in the real world—a monument, a landmark or even moving objects such as cars or trains. Additionally, it is reasonable to group certain features together if they share a number of properties. For example, China, Belgium and Germany can all be regarded as features of the type "Country". In addition, apart from a semantic description (a name and other properties), features can also be represented in physical terms, i.e. as a mathematical expression of an object's location in terms of points, lines, paths (multiple line segments) or polygons, associated with a well-defined coordinate reference system.

Definition 3. *Feature, feature type.* *Our definition of location corresponds with a so called feature. Features are defined in terms of a geometry, a feature type, and an arbitrary number of additional attributes (such as a human-readable name). Let FT_L be a set of feature types, $FT_L = \{ft_1, ft_2, ..., ft_{|FT|}\}$; let F_L be a set of features, $F_L = \{f_1, f_2, ..., f_{|L|}\}$; let $Type : F_L \rightarrow FT_L$ be a function mapping features to a type. We will also denote this using the shorthand $f : ft$ with $f \in F_L$ and $ft \in FT_L$. Let $Geometry : f \in F_L \mapsto g$ be a function which returns the geometry (g) for a given location with g a point, line, path or polygon and let f^a indicate some attribute a associated with a feature $f \in F_L$. This can be data of any type, e.g. a name or even other features.*

In our definition, a feature is only represented by one geometry type only, although this can be easily extended (and is already supported in an indirect

manner by construction of additional features which serve as attributes for the
feature at hand).

Finally, we introduce the concept of a "geospatial relationship". By defining
the concept of a geometry and establishing relationships over them, we are able
to answer queries such as "Is one feature contained in another?" Many definitions
for such relationships exist, but many of the most widely used GIS toolkits, e.g.
GeoTools, PostGIS, ArcGIS, SQL Server etc., define geospatial relationships
based on the "Topic 8" standard proposed by the OpenGIS Consortium (OGC)
[19]. We will also utilize these relationships towards the construction of location
constraints, as will be illustrated later. Note that, in some cases, geospatial
relationships are categorized in separate sets, such as topological, measurement,
sequential or complex relationships [6,20], but for the sake of simplicity, we use
one global moniker (a "geospatial relationship") in this work.

3   Running Example

To illustrate our location-aware Petri net modeling extension and its execution
semantics, we will utilize a running example throughout this paper, inspired on
the case examples provided in [13]. The basic WF-net is depicted in Fig. 1. The
example process describes a technical maintenance service, which is executed as
follows. The process is started once a customer call is received in a particular
call center (Receive Customer Call, RCC and Accept Customer Call, ACC). The
call center evaluates the complaint, based on which the user is remotely assisted
(Remote Assist, RAS) or an inspector is dispatched from the call center to the
customer's location to investigate the problem on-site (Dispatch, DIS). Based on
the results of the investigation (On-site Inspection, OSI), the inspector can solve
the problem whilst investigating, or calls-in a mobile repair team to perform on-
site repair work (Call Repair Team, CRT and On-site Work, OSW). If the repair
cannot be performed on-site, the repair team heads to a repair shop to perform
repairs there (Shop-floor Repair, SFR), before returning to the customer and
continuing the on-site work (this can occur multiple times). After the repair is
finished, the repair team is called back (Release Repair Team, RTT). Finally,
independent of the nature of the solution offered, some administrative follow-up
work (Follow-up Administration, FUA) needs to be performed to close the case.

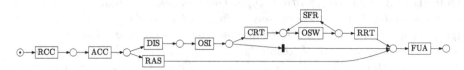

Fig. 1. WF-net model of "repair" process used as a running example throughout the
paper.

The description of this process highlights some locational aspects which can
not be captured by control-flow alone. In particular, we list the following locational concerns which need to be adhered to:

- Call centers may only handle customer calls when the customer is located within the region a call center is responsible for;
- The call center performing the follow-up work should be situated in a different region then call center handling the customer call;
- Requests can only be made to repair teams which are located in the customer's region or 50 Km around it. Naturally, a repair team which is already working for another customer cannot be requested;
- Shop-floor repairs should be made in the repair station closest to the customer's location; this should be based on navigational routing information, not on beeline distance.

4   Location-Aware Workflow Modeling

This section discusses our proposed Petri net modeling extension to model location-aware processes. Our methodology includes two main extensions, namely *location dependent transitions* and *location constraints*.

Figure 2 shows the running example modeled using our location-aware extension. Location dependent transitions are indicated with a flag (⚑), together with the feature name and type for the location which will be bound to the transition after executing. The shaded boxes represent location-aware constraints, used to constrain the locations which can be bound to a location dependent transition. Visually, the constraints are connected with all the transitions which bound location will be used as an input in the constraint, and with one transition which is bounded by the constraint (using dashed arcs).

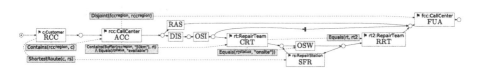

Fig. 2. The running example of Fig. 1 modeled using our location-aware extension.

Definition 4. *Location-aware WF-net (LAWF-net). Formally, a location-aware WF-net (LAWF-net) is represented as a tuple $(P, T, F, F_L, FT_L, T_L, C_L, CF_L)$ with P, T and F unchanged with regards to the definition of a WF-net (places, transitions and flows); F_L and FT_L the sets of features and their type (see before); $T_L \subseteq T$ the set of location dependent transitions C_L the set of location constraints (a set of expressions); $CF_L \subseteq (T_L \times C_L) \cup (C_L \times T)$ a finite set of directed arcs linking location dependent transitions to a constraint.*

We also define the function $LM : T_L \to F$ to get the feature bound to a particular location dependent transition (the location marking). Initially, i.e. before execution of a transition, $\forall t \in T_L : [LM(t) = \emptyset]$. Most location constraints are formulated directly in the form of a geospatial relationship (when the relationship returns a boolean result), but generally there are no strict criteria for the definition of a location constraint $c \in C_L$ except for the following.

Definition 5. *Location constraint.* *A location constraint is an expression $c \in C_L$ which evaluates to a boolean result $c^* \in \{true, false\}$. The expression involves exactly one output transition, i.e. $\exists!(x, y) \in CF_L : [x = c \wedge y \in T]$. $C_L^t = \{c \in C_L | \exists!(x, y) \in CF_L : [x = c \wedge y = t]\}$ is used as a shorthand to return all constraints defined on $t \in T$. The expression can involve zero or more location dependent input transitions. The feature bound to such input transitions, given by LM will be used as an input for the expression at the time of evaluation.*

As stated in the preliminaries section, we mainly apply the geospatial relationships as defined by the "Topic 8" standard proposed by the OpenGIS Consortium (OGC) [19] towards formulating location constraints. As an example, in Fig. 2, the constraint "$Contains(rcc^{region}, c)$" contains one output transition (ACC) and one input transition (RCC)". Instead of using the transition labels in the expression, we use a short name ("rcc" or "c") as a way to indicate bound features for location dependent transitions directly. "rcc^{region}" should thus be read as "the region attribute (another feature) of rcc (the feature bound to the ACC transition). We also define a feature type for each location dependent transition indicating the type of the features which can be bound to the transition. This means that, even when no constraints are modeled, an intrinsic "$Type(LM(t)) = x$" constraint is present for any $t \in T_L$ with $x \in FT_L$ the defined feature type. We can thus also define $Type : T_L \rightarrow FT_L$ as a shorthand function returning the feature type for a location dependent transition. Note also that constraints can also be defined over a non-location dependent transition, as is the case with "$Equals(rt^{status}, "onsite")$". Such constraints govern the execution of non-location dependent transitions without binding a location to them.

The execution semantics of LAWF-nets are similar to those of a normal Petri net.

Definition 6. *LAWF-net execution semantics.* *A transition $t \in T$ is enabled in a LAWF-net iff: the control-flow properties for being enabled are satisfied (i.e. a token in all input places) and all constraints $c \in C_L^t$ are satisfied, i.e. $\forall c \in C_L^t : [c^* = true]$ if $t \in T \backslash T_L$. If $t \in T_L$ (i.e. t is a location-dependent transition), evaluating the satisfyability of the constraints involves checking whether there exists a feature which can be bound to the transition, i.e. $\exists f \in F_L : [\forall c \in C_L^t : [c^* = true]]$[1].*

---

[1] Naturally, when evaluating the conditions for a transition to be enabled, the currently bound feature to that transition reflects the previous (or unset) feature, whereas the evaluation of the constraint satisfyability requires a location marking where the feature under consideration is bound to the location dependent transition. To resolve this, every $f \in F_L$ is evaluated under a location marking $LM_{t,f}$ such that $LM_{t,f}(t) = f$ and $LM_2(x) = LM_1(x)$ for all $x \in T_L \wedge x \neq t$. In case that all constraints hold under this candidate location marking and this feature is chosen to be bound, $LM_{t,f}$ will be finalized as the new marking after firing the transition.

Firing a location dependent transition causes a normal token movement and additionally brings the location marking in a new state $LM_1 \xrightarrow{t} LM_2$ such that $LM_2(t) = f$ and $LM_2(x) = LM_1(x)$ for all $x \in T_L \wedge x \neq t$. That is, a satisfiable feature is bound to the location dependent transition.

5   Execution of Location-Aware Process Models

Our LAWF-net modeling extension provides a straightforward and understandable means to merge location aspects with control-flow concerns. Although we have provided execution semantics in the section above, we also provide a mapping from LAWF-nets to CPN models, due to the following reasons. First, as we will see later, mapping LAWF-nets to CPN models enables to use existing tools to drive the execution of location-aware processes. Second, it also allows for easier integration with existing GIS platforms. Third, by providing an approach which is fully compatible with CPN, we can build open a large existing body of work concerning validation of such models (i.e. ensuring the correctness of the designed model). Finally, formulating location-aware process models in terms of CPN models also allows for integration with other contexts, i.e. timing or social (organizational) aspects.

Figure 3 shows the result of the conversion of a LAWF-net to a CPN model. The following definitions provides the formalization of this mapping.

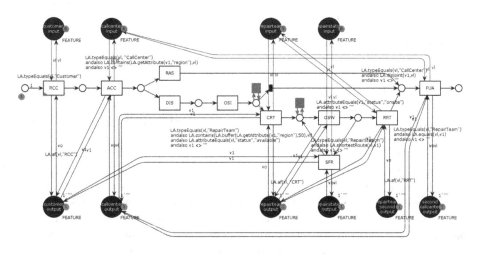

Fig. 3. LAWF-net of Fig. 2 converted to a CPN model.

Definition 7. *LAWF-net to CPN mapping.* A LAWF-net $(P^L, T^L, F^L, F^L_L, FT^L_L, T^L_L, C^L_L, CF^L_L)$ is mapped to a CPN model $(P, T, A, \Sigma, C, V, N, G, E, M, I)$ as follows:

- $\Sigma = \{U, F_L^L\}$ with $U = \{unit\}$ (color sets);
- $\forall p \in P^L : [p \in P]$ with $C(p) = U$. $I(p) = \{unit\}$ iff $\bullet p = \emptyset$, $I(p) = \emptyset$ otherwise and $\forall t \in T^L : [t \in T]$ (control-flow places and transitions);
- $\forall t \in T_L^L : [p_L^t \in P]$ with $C(p_L^t) = F_L^L$ and $I(p_L^t) = \emptyset$ (the places in the bottom row labeled "output" in Fig. 3) (location output places);
- $\forall ft \in FT_L^L : [p_L^{ft} \in P]$ with $C(p_L^{ft}) = F_L^L$ and $I(p_L^{ft}) = \{f \in F_L^L | Type(f) = ft\}$ (the places in the bottom row labeled "input" in Fig. 3) (location input places);
- $\forall (x,y) \in F^L : [a_{(x,y)} \in A]$ with $N(a_{(x,y)}) = (x,y)$ and $E(a_{(x,y)}) = unit$ (control-flow);
- $v_L \in V$ with $C(v_L) = F_L^L$ and $v_O \in V$ with $C(v_O) = F_L^L$ (binding and overriding variable);
- $\forall t \in T^L : [a_t^{input}, a_t^{return}, a_t^{output}, a_t^{override} \in A]$ with $N(a_t^{input}) = (p_L^{Type(t)}, t)$, $N(a_t^{return}) = (t, p_L^{Type(t)})$, $N(a_t^{output}) = (t, p_L^t)$ and $N(a_t^{overrid}) = (p_L^t, t)$. $E(a_t^{input}) = E(a_t^{return}) = E(a_t^{output}) = v_L$ and $E(a_t^{override}) = if |M(p_L^t)| = 0$ then empty else $M(p_L^t)$ (this arc consumes the feature token from the output place if it is present) (input, output, return and override arcs);
- $\forall t \in T^L : G(t) = \bigwedge_{c \in C_L^{L^t}}(c)$ (a conjunction of all the constraints with this transition as the output) (guards);
- $\forall t \in T^L : [\forall c \in C_L^{L^t} : [\forall (x,y) \in \{(x,y) \in CF_L^L | x \in T_L^L \wedge y = c\} : [v_L^{(x,y)} \in V, a_i^{(x,y)}, a_o^{(x,y)} \in A]]]$ with $C(v_L^{(x,y)}) = F_L^L$ and with $N(a_i^{(x,y)}) = (p_L^x, t)$ and $N(a_o^{(x,y)}) = (t, p_L^x)$. $E(a_i^{(x,y)}) = E(a_o^{(x,y)}) = v_L^{(x,y)}$ (constraint input arcs).

6   Implementation and System Integration

The converted running example shown in Fig. 3 was implemented as a CPN model using CPN Tools [2]. Note that, due to the limitations of this tool, the CPN model in contains some additional constructs which are not part of the formalization. First, the addition of "dummy" invisible transitions before CRT and OSW. This is due to the fact that CPN Tools only performs a check for enabling tasks immediately after a marking change, and does not repeat this check when the user requests to execute a particular transition. Therefore, the invisible transitions are used as a workaround to force CPN Tools to perform the check again. Second, we can modify the arc expression of output arcs a_t^{out} for any $t \in T^L$ which still returns a multiset of tokens equal to v_L, but also triggers external events. This might be useful for logging purposes, or—as we do here— fire an event to an underlying GIS system which sends a repair team on their way. Third, as it is impossible to formulate the expression for the $a_t^{override}$ arcs using CPN Tools, we instead initialize each location output place with a dummy (empty) placeholder, and add constraints to prevent this dummy feature to be used as an input (we also explicitly perform a feature type check in the guard of each location dependent transition, but this is just for the sake of clarity).

Modelers are free to extend a converted CPN model. If so desired, for instance, modelers might opt to use one global location input pool place instead of creating an input place per feature type. Such system would make it possible for instance to allow more than one feature type to become bound to location dependent transitions. Secondly, end users might opt to remove overriding $a_t^{override}$ arcs for some location dependent transition, for example to keep track of multiple bound transitions in the case of recurrent transitions. Finally, modelers might also desire for location dependent (or any) transitions to output other features apart from the one being bound to the location dependent transition. This can also easily be achieved by adding more output places and formulating appropriate arc expressions.

The question remains how the various location constraints were implemented in the CPN model. To do so, a simulation extension was developed using CPN Tools RPC (remote procedure call) functionality. The reason this approach was chosen instead of using CPN Tools' built-in SML language is twofold. First, both practitioners and academics are more familiar with Java (the language of the simulation extension) than SML, allowing for easier understanding and extension. Second, this approach allows to easily integrate location-aware business process models with existing GIS systems, both for evaluating the geospation relationships (constraining and driving the process) and to react to activities as they are being executed (within the GIS system). To illustrate this, we have created an experimental set-up using the GeoTools Java package[2]. Figure 4 shows the running CPN model running with a GIS system. A map is shown based on real-life shapefiles which were imported in the set-up. As illustrated, the GIS system is able to impose geospatial constraints restricting the control-flow of the

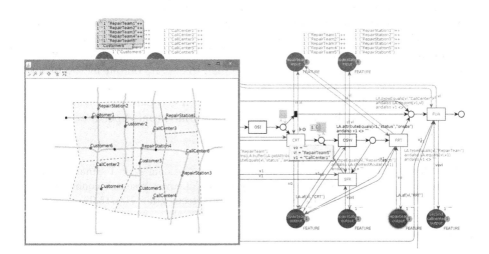

Fig. 4. CPN model running in tandem with a GIS system. The GIS system is able to impose geospatial constraints restricting the control-flow of the process. Vice versa, execution of activities can impose effects on features in the GIS system.

---

[2] See: http://geotools.org. This toolkit offers support for all geospatial relationships defined by the "Topic 8" standard proposed by the OpenGIS Consortium (OGC) [19].

process (some activities can only be started once the repair team is on-site, for instance). Vice versa, execution of transitions in the process also drives changes in the GIS system, e.g. sending out a request to a repair team causes this repair team to head to the customer's location using the shortest route available (as is shown in Fig. 4). This illustrates the feasibility and validity of our proposed methodology[3].

7   Conclusion

For the most part, the modeling and execution of business process models has been studied and performed in practice in a rather limiting environment, dealing mainly with control-flow aspects only, without taking other contextual aspects into account. In this paper, we have focused our attention towards making the modeling and execution of business processes location-aware, i.e. on the particular context of geospatial information. A Petri net modeling extension was proposed which incorporates location aspects and ways to constrain the execution of activities based on location constraints. This approach was formalized by means of a formalized mapping to coloured Petri nets and implemented in combination with an experimental GIS setup to illustrate the feasibility of coupling business process support systems with geographical information systems.

We believe our contribution to be a first valuable step towards incorporating location aspects in business processes, hence allowing stake holders to execute such processes in a more effective and efficient manner, with application areas in logistics, transportation and others. Indeed, the ability to make processes flexible and adaptive in terms of their ability to react to road, traffic or weather conditions is put forward as a promising area of study. Therefore, in future work, we plan to set up a number of case studies to elaborate on the feasibility and robustness of our approach. In addition, we plan to expand on our methodology, both by investigating more location-based patterns which play a role in business process environments (the focus here was mainly on geospatial constraints) and how these aspects can be combined with other contextual aspects other than geographical information as well.

Acknowledgment. This work is supported by the National Key Technology R&D Program, China (grant 2012BAH01F02), by the KU Leuven research council (grant OT/10/010) and the Flemish Research Council (Odysseus grant B.0915.09).

References

1. Vom Brocke, J., Rosemann, M.: Handbook on Business Process Management: Strategic Alignment, Governance, People and Culture. Springer, New York (2010)

---

[3] Full source code of the developed implementation can be found at: http://processmining.be/locationaware.

2. Jensen, K., Kristensen, L.M., Wells, L.: Coloured Petri nets and CPN tools for modelling and validation of concurrent systems. Int. J. Softw. Tools Technol. Transf. **9**(3–4), 213–254 (2007)
3. Rosemann, M., Recker, J.C., Flender, C.: Contextualisation of business processes. Int. J. Bus. Process. Integr. Manage. **3**(1), 47–60 (2008)
4. Decker, M.: Modelling location-aware access control constraints for mobile workflows with UML activity diagrams. In: UBICOMM 2009, pp. 263–268, October 2009
5. Georgoulias, K., Papakostas, N., Chryssolouris, G., Stanev, S., Krappe, H., Ovtcharova, J.: Evaluation of flexibility for the effective change management of manufacturing organizations. Robot. Comp.-Integr. Manuf. **25**(6), 888–893 (2009)
6. Zhu, X., Recker, J., Zhu, G., Santoro, F.: Exploring location-dependency in process modeling. Bus. Process. Manage. J. **20**(6), 794–815 (2014)
7. Medeiros, C., Vossen, G., Weske, M.: Geo-wasa-combining GIS technology with workflow management. In: Proceedings of the Seventh Israeli Conference on Computer Systems and Software Engineering, pp. 129–139, June 1996
8. Alonso, G., Hagen, C.: Geo-opera: workflow concepts for spatial processes. In: Scholl, M.O., Voisard, A. (eds.) SSD 1997. LNCS, vol. 1262, pp. 238–258. Springer, Heidelberg (1997)
9. Seffino, L.A., Medeiros, C.B., Rocha, J.V., Yi, B.: Woodss—a spatial decision support system based on workflows. DSS **27**(1), 105–123 (1999)
10. Ludäscher, B., Altintas, I., Berkley, C., Higgins, D., Jaeger, E., Jones, M., Lee, E.A., Tao, J., Zhao, Y.: Scientific workflow management and the Kepler system. Concurrency Comput. Pract. Exp. **18**(10), 1039–1065 (2006)
11. Jäger, E., Altintas, I., Zhang, J., Ludäscher, B., Pennington, D., Michener, W.: A scientific workflow approach to distributed geospatial data processing using web services. In: SSDBM 2005, SSDBM, pp. 87–90 (2005)
12. de Leoni, M., van der Aalst, W.M.P., ter Hofstede, A.H.M.: Visual support for work assignment in process-aware information systems. In: Dumas, M., Reichert, M., Shan, M.-C. (eds.) BPM 2008. LNCS, vol. 5240, pp. 67–83. Springer, Heidelberg (2008)
13. Decker, M., Che, H., Oberweis, A., Sturzel, P., Vogel, M.: Modeling mobile workflows with bpmn. In: 2010 Ninth International Conference on Mobile Business and 2010 Ninth Global Mobility Roundtable (ICMB-GMR), pp. 272–279, June 2010
14. Recker, J.C.: "Modeling with tools is easier, believe me": the effects of tool functionality on modeling grammar usage beliefs. Inf. Syst. **37**(3), 213–226 (2012)
15. Recker, J.C., Rosemann, M., Indulska, M., Green, P.: Business process modeling: a comparative analysis. J. Assoc. Inf. Syst. **10**(4), 333–363 (2009)
16. Murata, T.: Petri nets: properties, analysis and applications. Proc. IEEE **77**, 541–580 (1989)
17. Peterson, J.L.: Petri Net Theory and the Modeling of Systems. Prentice-Hall, Inc., New Jersey (1981)
18. van der Aalst, W.M.P.: The application of Petri nets to workflow management. J. Circuits Syst. Comput. **8**(01), 21–66 (1998)
19. OGC: The opengis abstract specification-topic 8: Relationships between features (1999)
20. Zhu, X., Zhu, G., Guan, P.: Exploring location-aware process management. In: Bian, F., Xie, Y., Cui, X., Zeng, Y. (eds.) GRMSE 2013 Part II. CCIS, vol. 399, pp. 249–256. Springer, Heidelberg (2013)

Extending CPN Tools with Ontologies to Support the Management of Context-Adaptive Business Processes

Estefanía Serral, Johannes De Smedt, and Jan Vanthienen[✉]

Department of Decision Sciences and Information Management,
KU Leuven Faculty of Economics and Business, Naamsestraat 69,
3000 Leuven, Belgium
{Estefania.SerralAsensio,Johannes.Smedt,Jan.Vanthienen}@kuleuven.be

Abstract. Colored Petri Nets (CPN) are a widely used graphical modeling language to manage business processes. Business processes often appear in dynamic environments; therefore, context adaptation has recently emerged as a new challenge to explicitly address fitness between business process modeling and its execution environment. Although CPN can introduce data by defining internal data records, this is not enough to capture the complexity and dynamics of the execution context data. This paper extends CPN tools to support the management of context-adaptive business processes. To achieve this challenge, CPN tools are integrated with ontology-based context models that properly represent and manage the business process context. This allows context to be appropriately modeled at design time, and queried and updated at runtime. The combination of ontologies with CPN tools presents a way to bridge business processes management with context data management while treating data and behavior as separate concerns. In this way, system design, reuse, and maintenance are also improved.

Keywords: Colored Petri Nets · Context adaptivity · Ontologies · CPN tools

1 Introduction

Colored Petri Nets (CPN) [1] are a mathematical modeling language that has a graphical notation and very powerful analysis techniques. For these reasons, the importance of this language is undeniable in Business Process Management (BPM) [2].

Since users and organizations as well as their software systems operate more and more in dynamic environments, context adaptation has recently emerged as a new perspective in BPM to explicitly address fitness between business process modeling and its execution context. Thus, the behavior in the information system could automatically adapt in order to effectively operate in environments where context changes frequently. In BPM, context is usually defined as data

© Springer International Publishing Switzerland 2015
F. Fournier and J. Mendling (Eds.): BPM 2014 Workshops, LNBIP 202, pp. 198–209, 2015.
DOI: 10.1007/978-3-319-15895-2_18

that can influence and change business process execution, data that is normally highly dynamic, such as: equipment state and location, time, season, temperature, stakeholders' location and preferences, etc. [3].

To represent data, CPN allows the declaration of internal data structures and the assignation of values as tokens embedded inside the net. For instance, Fig. 1 shows a workflow example of a product sale in a shop using CPN. Sellers (SEL), customers (CUST), and products (PROD) are color sets represented by an id. The tokens of these colour sets are indicated as input in the corresponding net transitions. In the process, a seller approaches a customer and explains a product. The customer can either buy it or leave the shop. The seller will be redirected to the seller pool after a successful sale or when the customer leaves. If a products gets sold, its registry is updated; otherwise, it returns to the product pool.

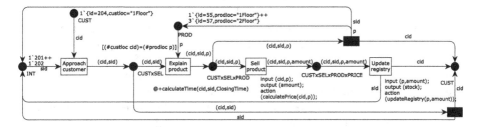

Fig. 1. Example workflow of a shop.

As shown in the example, CPN allows the use of data in processes; however, the data records are focused on defining the types of data that need to be passed across the net, and the token values need to be manually specified in the corresponding transitions. This does not offer a proper support and expressiveness for representing dynamic context information: the execution environment is continuously changing and the data should reflect the current values to allow the Petri net adaptation. Also, reuse of data is not possible since it is internally defined for each workflow.

Therefore, CPN needs to be extended with suitable context modeling techniques that properly define and manage context as a separate concern to: (a) allow context data to be dynamically updated; (b) facilitate system design, reuse, and maintenance; (c) allow better and more informed decisions, e.g., the current location of the customers, sellers and products, can be combined to make a better match and increase the chances of selling products; (d) provide reasoning to infer knowledge relevant for the process execution, e.g.: sellers are available if they are currently working and not assisting any customer, or heating devices are promoted in unexpected cold periods; etc.

In this paper, we extend CPN tools [4] and integrate them with ontology-based context models to properly support context adaptation in CPN. By using ontologies, it becomes possible to: represent context data with a high degree of expressiveness, update it at runtime, automatically infer new knowledge, and incorporate context data in multiple workflows throughout the system. While previously all tokens and variables needed to be specified using basic data structures and needed to be process model specific, this approach lifts the workflow data management to a higher level.

The remainder of this paper is organized as follows. Section 2 presents the related work. Section 3 explains the extended CPN to describe context-adaptive business processes. Section 4 describes the developed tool to support the extension. Finally, Sect. 5 discusses the presented contributions and further work, and Sect. 6 presents the conclusions.

2   Related Work

In [3,5,6], the different kinds of business process context properties are analyzed. These works acknowledge the need of analyzing business process context to make BPM more effective. However, they only focus on identifying which context properties are relevant, and they do not provide support for context adaptation. Also, works such as [7,8] emphasize the need for process flexibility through the support of adaptations during process execution; however, none of them focus on providing context adaptation in Petri nets.

Several approaches have been proposed to extend Petri nets in order to support context adaptation in business processes. Lu et al. [9] present a scenario-based method to design context-aware service models in which Petri nets are used as the formalism for building a logic model of context-aware services. Petri nets are extended with context functions that can be linked to states or transitions. This work focuses on system design, not paying attention to how context should be represented and managed to be used in order to adapt the Petri nets execution.

Feilong Tang et al. [10] present a context model and a context-aware workflow management algorithm for ubiquitous campus navigation. They extend Petri nets with the context concept; however, the proposed context model and execution algorithm are tied to the campus navigation application and the integration of the context concept in Petri nets is rather abstract.

Ardissono et al. [11,12] present a framework for the context-aware management of applications based on the composition of Web Services in complex workflows. The context-aware workflow execution is based on the introduction of abstract activities. Each abstract activity has an associated set of context-dependent implementations representing the alternative courses of action that the workflow engine should select depending on the context. Thus, instead of representing context adaptation in Petri nets, each alternative is represented using a different Petri net. In addition, no detail is given about how context is specified and managed.

Although these works advance the state of the art towards supporting context-adaptive business processes with Petri nets, none of them provides either a proper support for context management or any tool support for managing context-adaptive business processes using Petri nets.

3 Modeling Context-Adaptive Business Processes

We integrate two models to represent context-adaptive business processes: (a) an ontology-based context model, where the business context is semantically described; and (b) an extended CPN where the business process can refer to the context described in the context model.

3.1 Context Modeling

In order to describe the business context, we use ontologies since several studies [13–15] state that the use of ontologies to model context is one of the best approaches for this purpose. Ontologies guarantee a high degree of expressiveness, formality and semantic richness, and exhibit prominent advantages for reasoning and reusing context as well as facilitating the interoperability of different systems.

An ontology is a formal representation of a set of concepts within a domain and the relationships between those concepts. An ontology mainly contains the following elements:

- **Classes:** all kinds of entities or concepts. A class usually refers to a collection or a category of objects sharing some common character and well accepted under common sense; e.g., the classes product and location.
- **Data properties:** properties that identify a class itself from other classes and has a basic type, such as int, string, time, etc.; e.g., name and age.
- **Object properties:** properties that identify a relation between two ontology classes, i.e., identifies how an object is connected to other object in an ontology, e.g., product_location, which relates the product class and the location class.
- **Constraints:** rules that must be satisfied for the elements for which are defined; e.g., the cardinality of a certain property must be 1; the class A is subclass of the class B; the object property is_in (which relates one location object to other location object) is transitive (i.e., if a location X is in the Y location and the Y location is in the Z location, then, X is inside Z too); etc.
- **Individuals:** instances or objects of the defined classes; e.g., the individual Dell_latitud_e6410_16 of the class product, with name Dell_laptop, and which product_location is office236, which is an individual of the location class.

In order to specify the context of the application, first the context classes, properties, and constraints for the domain should be identified (this should be reusable for each application within the domain). Afterwards, the specific context application should be specified as individuals of the defined classes.

To represent the ontology-based context model, we use the Web Ontology Language (OWL)[1]. OWL is a machine-interpretable semantic markup language for publishing and sharing ontologies and is an open World Wide Web Consortium (W3C) standard. OWL is designed to provide a vocabulary along with a

---

[1] http://www.w3.org/TR/owl-ref/.

formal semantics in order to facilitate the management and processing of knowledge at runtime. Thus, it provides a great support to represent context and deal with its dynamicity.

Figure 2 shows a simplified OWL implementation of the context model for the running business process example. From letf to right the figure shows some classes (such as *Product*, *ProductType*, *Customer* and *Seller*); some data properties (such as *name*, *price* and *inPromotion*); some instances of the *ProductType* and *Product* classes; and the property values of the product instance *AirConditionrLex125_6*.

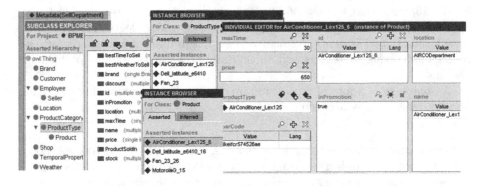

Fig. 2. Snapshot of the context model created for the running example.

3.2   CPN Extension

CPN is defined is as follows [1]:

- P the places.
- T the transitions.
- $F \subseteq (P \times T) \cup (T \times P)$ the arcs in the model.
- $\sum$ the color sets of the tokens.
- V the set of typed variables, such that $Type[v] \in \sum, \forall v \in V$.
- $C : P \rightarrow \sum$ the color set functions.
- $G : T \rightarrow EXPR_V$ a guard function, such that for each transition t $Type[G(t)] =$ $Bool$.
- $E : F \rightarrow EXPR_V$ an arc expression function such that for each arc a $Type$ $[E(a)] = C(p)_{MS}$ where p is the place connected to a.
- $I : P \rightarrow EXPR_\emptyset$ an initialization function that assigns an initializations expression to each p such that $Type[I(p)] = C(p)_{MS}$.

As such, CPN is a tuple $(\sum, P, T, F, C, V, G, E, I)$ with $EXPR$ the set of expressions provided by the inscription language, e.g., CPN ML. $Type[e]$ resembles the *type* of an expression $e \in EXPR$. Timing is considered as one of the color sets and is not explicitly introduced.

After analysing this definition, we determine that context can be introcuced in the following constructs in CPN:

- **Transition guards:** can contain context data to enforce dynamic conditions on tokens.
- **Transition timing:** context can express time constraints and conditions, which can be incorporated into the transitions.
- **Transition actions:** can contain functions whose parameters are context data
- **Arc expressions:** arcs determine the flow relationships between places and transitions and may have expressions that contain context data, for instance, for indicating a delay in the flow, for indicating the number of tokens, etc.
- **Place inicial marking:** can contain context data to enforce dynamic values on tokens.

By taking into account the extensions of these constructs to enable the use of context, our extension can be defined as follows:

- $\sum_A$ the context-aware color sets, which are defined in the context model.
- V_A the variables of the color sets for which $Type[v_a] \in \sum_A, \forall v_a \in V_A$. In this definition, all the variables are defined in the context model to obtain maximal flexibility.
- P_A the context-aware places for which $C_A : P_A \to \sum_A$ are the context-aware color set functions.
- T_A the context-aware transitions with $G_A : T_A \to EXPR_{V_A}$ their guards.
- F_A the context-aware arcs with $E_A : F_A \to EXPR_{V_A}$ their expressions.

By this definition, context is introduced as a special case of data-awareness in the CPN. It can cover all of the behavior which is represented by colors in the model. With $EXPR_{V_A}$, the context has its own way of incorporating data operations outside of the CP-net. This separates the workflow logic from the data logic, but connects them in a call-and-response approach. It is also possible to apply extra reasoning in the context model. For example, OWL provides great facilities for inferring new information by using, e.g., SWRL rules[2]. This extends the inscription language $EXPR_{V_A}$ to a more powerful subject in the workflow.

The context-awareness does not change the marking of transitions in a particular way, as we do not interfere with the occurrence rules. However, the extension is now able to retrieve the data from an instantiation of the context model, which allows the workflow to be aware of the current execution context and properly deal with the context dynamicity. Also, by using ontologies, it becomes possible to define data that can be used throughout different workflows of a system. Moreover, ontologies provide a very high expressiveness for defining data, which makes the data-awareness of the workflow much stronger; for instance, the locatedIn relationship can be specified as a transitive property in order to indicate, e.g., that when a seller is in a specific department in the shop, her/his location is not only the deparmet but also the shop where the department is.

---

[2] http://www.w3.org/Submission/SWRL/.

4   Tool Support

In order to support the modeling and execution of context-adaptive business processes, we have extended CPN Tools [4]. Although there are other software packages such as, ExSpect [16] and GreatSPN [17], we chose CPN Tools because it has been widely used and supported, which results in timely updates and the introduction of new features such as the incorporation of declarative constraints and extensions. CPN Tools is a free of charge tool that provides state-space analysis, simulation, and the generation of event logs that can be used for further process analysis (e.g., process mining). The tool relies on the functional programming language *Meta Language* (ML) to incorporate simulation and analysis, and enables the user to implement custom functions and probability distributions that can be used throughout the model. The modeling tool that we have developed to manage context-adaptive business processes is composed by a Context Management Plug-in and an extension of CPN Tools.

4.1   Context Management Plugin

Context is managed as a separate concern in order to facilitate system design, reuse, and maintenance. We have developed a plug-in that allows the OWL model to be interpreted, updated, and saved. Specifically, the API allows opening and saving an OWL context model as well as managing its context instances (i.e., individuals) independently of their classes, such as methods for retrieving and updating data and object properties of a certain instance.

To implement this class, we have used Jena 2.4[3], and the Pellet reasoner 1.5.2[4]. Jena is a Java framework for building Semantic Web applications that provides a programmatic environment for creating, examining, and modifying an OWL ontology. Pellet is an open-source tool that provides reasoning services for OWL ontologies. Pellet facilitates accessing to the information stored in the ontology. For example, the *getDataPropertyBool()* method, which retrieves the value of a boolean data property, is implemented as follows:

```
public static boolean getDataPropertyBool(String
    individualID, String attributeID) {
  boolean attributeValue=false;
    try {
        dataset.begin( ReadWrite.READ);
        Individual ind=
            ontModel.getIndividual(prefixURI +
            individualID);
        Property prop=
            ontModel.getProperty(prefixURI +
            attributeID);
```

---

[3] https://jena.apache.org/.
[4] http://clarkparsia.com/pellet/.

```
    try{
    attributeValue= ind.getPropertyValue(prop).
        asLiteral().getBoolean();
    } catch(Exception e){
        System.out.println("The context property
            identifiers are not correct");
    }
  dataset.close();
  } finally {dataset.end();}

  return attributeValue;
}
```

4.2 CPN Tools Extension

We have developed a Java extension in CPN Tools 4.0 which recently added a framework for this purpose [4]. By implementing an extension, it is now possible to use Java methods in the modeled Petri nets by means of remote procedure calls (RPC). These calls reach the ML engine which executes them and inputs the returned values into the model. Thus, context represented in the OWL context model can be injected into the Petri net model as data by means of these RPCs. Using this functionality, we have implemented a CPN Tool extension, called CM, that provides methods to interpret and update the context model. These methods use the Context Management plug-in explained above, which contains the proper logic to manage the context model. This tool, ready for supporting the modeling and execution of context-adaptive business processes can be downloaded at https://perswww.kuleuven.be/~u0095631/.

Using the presented extension, Fig. 3 shows the context-aware enriched solution of the running example in Fig. 3. Various ML functions are referring to the CM name space, which communicates with the Java code that calls OWL data. The specific ML functions that are shown in the figure are:

- *retrieveInstances(contextClassID):* this function retrieves all instances of a particular context class. They are transformed by the ML function *deserialize* and inputted as tokens into the system as can be seen for customers, sellers and products.
- *contextProp{Int/Bool/String}(IndividualID,PropertyID):* this function retrieves the value (integer, boolean or string) of the property for the entered context instance.
- *setContextProp{Int/Bool/String}(IndividualID,PropertyID,New value):* this function sets the value (integer, boolean or string) of the property for the entered context instance.
- *ContextObjProp(IndividualID,PropertyID):* this method retrieves the identifier of the object that is related with the *IndividualID* by the *PropertyID*.

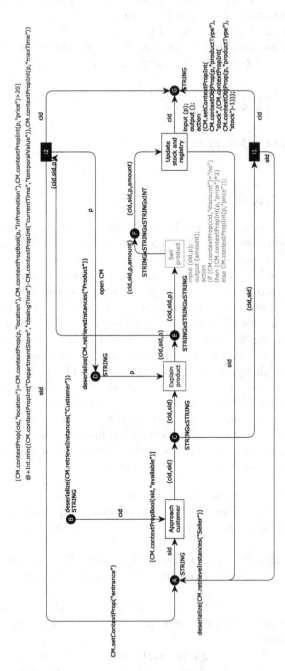

Fig. 3. Implementation example which extends the workflow of the shop with context data.

They are aligned with the Java methods, which implement the functionality of calling the OWL database. For example *contextPropBool()* is implemented as follows:

```
public boolean contextPropBool(String instanceID,
   String contextPropertyID){
    return
        contextModel.getDataPropertyBool(instanceID,
        contextPropertyID);
};
```

Thus, the running example is now expressed in a context-adaptive way. The id of the seller *sid* is now linked with the shifts of the individuals, which are retrieved in the guard of *Approach Customer*. The transition *Explain product* is bound heavily with various context constraints and are indicated in blue: the seller will offer guidance to customers when the product is in promotion, the price is higher than a certain amount (which can also be defined in the context), and the customer that is visiting the store is currently at the right location. Otherwise, this transition will be skipped and the customer leaves the system through the invisible transition. The seller and the product become available again. Also, the duration of the transition is dependent on the time that is left until closing time. The price of the product is calculated in *Sell product* and depends on the information that resides within the context of the customer. For instance, if the customer has already bought numerous products, s/he might benefit from a discount. Finally, the stock levels are changed in the net by updating the data of the corresponding product in the context model. This is an example of how the context gets changed by the model and offers two-way synchronization of the data. Overall, all the data contributions in the colored Petri net are made dynamic and semantically defined in the OWL ontology, which is superior to the static approach of CPN Tools for enactment. Previously, all the data had to be stored in the separate records within CPN Tools or a file where they could be retrieved from. In our approach, the data is inputted at runtime from the OWL model, where the context is stored in a semantic and highly expressive way.

5   Discussion

While CPN Tools offers great support for modeling and enacting CPN, not all the benefits of context adaptation can be leveraged by its implementation. The calculation of the current context state is done upon a change in the places surrounding a transition. As such, other transitions can manipulate the context and render it unfit for the enabling of the transition, while the context was already verified and enabled it. This also avoids inputting tokens into the CPN after its initialization.

In addition, the syntactics to incorporate context properties into the CPN are rather complex and perhaps not immediately user-friendly. This can be solved by explicitly declaring the context in color sets. However, this creates the need of syncronizing the context model and the color set every time the net is executed.

Furthermore, the extensions framework of CPN tools is still constrained by the usage of the boolean, integer, and string (BIS) types, which limits the incorporation of high-level or generic data types. This implies that only simple context can be incorporated, and a separation between ontology variables and CPN variables exist. This boils down to a change in the definition to $A \subseteq \sum$ the color sets in the context with V_A the variables for the color sets consisting of $Type[v_a] \in Bool, String, Integer, \forall v_a \in V_a$. The two data typologies need to be merged and made compatible, which limits the implementation to manage the context by using the identifiers of each ontology element instead of the elements themselves; e.g., instead of getting an object of a product class and retrieving the information directly from the object, only its identifier is retrieved. Therefore, it is necessary that the context functions make a search to find the intance that matches the identifier in order to retrieve or modify the corresponding data.

Finally, CPN Tools allow for state-space analysis, which enables modelers and users to search for unwanted behavior such as dead locks and infrequent or overly-frequent execution paths. However, context-aware workflows may bring new requirements and challenges for performing this analysis that will be investigated as further work.

6   Conclusions

In this paper, we have presented a tool that supports the management of context-adaptive business processes enabling their use in dynamic environments. The tool extends CPN Tools with ontologies in order to support the modeling and execution of context-adaptive CPN. Using the extended tool, the data that is already available in the information system context can be used in the Petri nets of the system with minimal effort; while using ontologies, the context of the system can be semantically represented and properly managed at runtime. Ontology-based context models also make it easy to navigate the data structure that is present in the information system and add it to the Petri nets.

As such, workflows can be enriched with the context defined in the context ontology models, and in the other way around, the process can also reach the context and update data that is encountered within the workflow.

Acknowledgments. This work has been funded by the KU Leuven Research Fund (F+ Fellowship J:BOF/MS/F+/13/032) and the FWO (Fonds voor Wetenschappelijk Onderzoek) Project G0804 13N.

References

1. Jensen, K.: Coloured petri nets. In: Brauer, W., Reisig, W., Rozenberg, G. (eds.) Petri Nets: Central Models and Their Properties. LNCS, vol. 254, pp. 248–299. Springer, Heidelberg (1987)
2. van der Aalst, W.M.P.: Making work flow: on the application of petri nets to business process management. In: Esparza, J., Lakos, C.A. (eds.) ICATPN 2002. LNCS, vol. 2360, p. 1. Springer, Heidelberg (2002)
3. Rosemann, M., Recker, J.C., Flender, C.: Contextualisation of business processes. Int. J. Bus. Process Integr. Manag. 3(1), 47–60 (2008)
4. Westergaard, M.: CPN tools 4: multi-formalism and extensibility. In: Colom, J.-M., Desel, J. (eds.) PETRI NETS 2013. LNCS, vol. 7927, pp. 400–409. Springer, Heidelberg (2013)
5. Saidani, O., Nurcan, S.: Context-awareness for adequate business process modelling. In: RCIS, pp. 177–186 (2009)
6. de la Vara, J.L., Ali, R., Dalpiaz, F., Sánchez, J., Giorgini, P.: Business processes contextualisation via context analysis. In: Parsons, J., Saeki, M., Shoval, P., Woo, C., Wand, Y. (eds.) ER 2010. LNCS, vol. 6412, pp. 471–476. Springer, Heidelberg (2010)
7. Goedertier, S., Vanthienen, J.: Compliant and flexible business processes with business rules. In: 7th Workshop on Business Process Modeling, Development and Support (BPMDS 2006) at CAiSE 2006, pp. 94–104 (2006)
8. Dadam, P., Reichert, M.: The adept project: a decade of research and development for robust and exible process support–challenges and achievements. Comput. Sci. Dev. 23(2), 81–97 (2009)
9. Lu, T., Bao, J.: A systematic approach to context aware service design. J. Comput. 7(1), 207–217 (2012)
10. Tang, F., Guo, M., Dong, M., Li, M., Guan, H.: Towards context-aware workflow management for ubiquitous computing. In: 2008 International Conference on Embedded Software and Systems, ICESS 2008, IEEE, pp. 221–228 (2008)
11. Ardissono, L., Furnari, R., Goy, A., Petrone, G., Segnan, M.: A framework for the management of context-aware workflow systems. In: WEBIST (1). (2007) 80–87
12. Ardissono, L., Furnari, R., Goy, A., Petrone, G., Segnan, M.: Context-aware workflow management. In: Baresi, L., Fraternali, P., Houben, G.-J. (eds.) ICWE 2007. LNCS, vol. 4607, pp. 47–52. Springer, Heidelberg (2007)
13. Chen, H., Finin, T., Joshi, A.: An ontology for context-aware pervasive computing environments. Spec. Issue Ontol. Distrib. Syst. Knowl. Eng. Rev. 18, 197–207 (2004)
14. Baldauf, M., Dustdar, S., Rosenberg, F.: A survey on context-aware systems. Int. J. Ad Hoc Ubiqui. Comput. 2(4), 263–277 (2007)
15. Ye, J., Coyle, L., Dobson, S., Nixon, P.: Ontology-based models in pervasive computing systems. Knowl. Eng. Rev. 22(4), 315–347 (2007)
16. van der Aalst, W.M.P., de Crom, P.J.N., Goverde, R.R.H.M.J., van Hee, K.M., Hofman, W.J., Reijers, H.A., van der Toorn, R.A.: Ex*Spect* 6.4 an executable specification tool for hierarchical colored petri nets. In: Nielsen, M., Simpson, D. (eds.) ICATPN 2000. LNCS, vol. 1825, pp. 455–464. Springer, Heidelberg (2000)
17. Baarir, S., Beccuti, M., Cerotti, D., De Pierro, M., Donatelli, S., Franceschinis, G.: The greatspn tool: recent enhancements. ACM SIGMETRICS Perform. Eval. Rev. 36(4), 4–9 (2009)

Using Data-Object Flow Relations to Derive Control Flow Variants in Configurable Business Processes

Riccardo Cognini$^{(\boxtimes)}$, Flavio Corradini, Andrea Polini, and Barbara Re

University of Camerino, Camerino, Italy
{riccardo.cognini,flavio.corradini,andrea.polini,barbara.re}@unicam.it

Abstract. Focusing on the relationship between behavioural and information perspectives in this paper we present an approach to support flexibility of Business Processes. The approach extends Feature Model descriptions with data-objects in order to derive process fragments and process variants. The approach has been applied to a data-intensive scenario such as the reporting activity of EU projects with encouraging results.

Keywords: Business process · Variability · Data object management

1 Introduction

Flexibility of Business Processes (BP) is a hot topic that has received increasing interest in the last years [13]. Motivations that drive flexibility can be classified as endogenous, when they relate to aspects that are internal to the organization itself, or exogenous, when they relate to external aspects. Flexibility issues can also be categorized according to the phases of the BP life cycle to which they relate. Each type of flexibility needs specific instruments, both in terms of modelling notations, and run-time supporting mechanisms. In particular, variability is the general term used to identify the ability of providing different BP model variants from the same process structure and/or behavior.

Focusing on BPs describing the control flow, flexibility is an issue influencing data objects and data flows between activities [13]. In term of flexibility this two perspectives cannot be managed in isolation and they have to be integrated. In this context an approach supporting the modelling of BP and data objects in a flexible way is a need. Too often data objects are not considered in a changing scenario, so we propose a novel approach extending the concept of Feature Model (FM) with reference to BP activities and data objects.

In this paper we propose business process Feature Model (bpFM) to deal with data objects in flexible BPs. In bpFM features are activities that can differentiate a BP from another in term of BP structure and execution paths. In bpFM data

---

This research has been partially founded by EU project LearnPAd GA: 619583 and by the Project MIUR PRIN CINA - 2010LHT4KM.

F. Fournier and J. Mendling (Eds.): BPM 2014 Workshops, LNBIP 202, pp. 210–221, 2015.
DOI: 10.1007/978-3-319-15895-2_19

objects can be modeled as input/output of activities, then the life cycle of data objects can be deduced from a bpFM model. Starting from the bpFM model a designer can choose the activities she needs in her BP in order to generate BP fragments in BPMN 2.0, and according to predefined mapping rules. To derive a complete BP variant, the designer will need then to provide the execution order of fragments. To do that data objects play a fundamental role because from the data object life cycle the execution order of the activities can be deduced.

The paper is organized as follows. Section 2 presents some background material, whereas Sect. 3 describes a case study that can help in the comprehension of the approach. Section 4 describes the proposed approach. Section 5 describes the modelling activities and Sect. 6 introduces the mapping solution we adopted. Finally, Sect. 7 presents relevant related works, while Sect. 8 draws some conclusion and opportunities for future work.

2   Background - Feature Modeling

Feature modelling is an approach emerged in the context of Software Product Lines to support the development of a variety of products from a common platform. The approach aims at lowering both production costs and time in the development of individual products sharing an overall reference model, while allowing them to differ with respect to specific features to serve, e.g. different markets [12]. FMs are suitable to represent a family of software products, nevertheless in the last years feature modelling has been used also to represent commonality and variability in Business Information Systems, introducing the concept of a BP family, that is a set of BPs sharing the same goal.

A FM is a graphical model used to express different relationships among features using a tree representation. In particular, in the first feature modeling approach, named Feature-oriented Domain Analysis (FODA), *mandatory*, *optional* or *alternative* features can be introduced [6]. *Mandatory* features represent characteristics that each product must have (i.e. each mobile device has a screen) (Fig. 1-A). *Optional* features represent characteristics that a product can have but a fully functional product can also be derived without including such a feature (i.e. a mobile device can have a 3G connection or not) (Fig. 1-B). *Alternative* features represent characteristics that cannot be present together in a product (i.e. a mobile device can have a standard screen or a touch screen, not both) (Fig. 1-C). Researchers have proven that basic FM models are too restrictive to represent all the relationships between features which are useful to characterize a family of products [3]. As a result the FM notation has been extended to permit the definition of feature cardinality, defining how many features in a set are needed to have a working product. For instance it is possible to express relationships such as *"at least one feature in a set of features is needed in each product"*. This is done via *OR features* (Fig. 1-D). Additionally, *include relationship* is used to express that a feature selection implies the selection of another feature that is on a different part of the tree (Fig. 1-E), and *exclude relationship* is used to express that a feature selection requires to discard another one that is on a different part of the tree (Fig. 1-F).

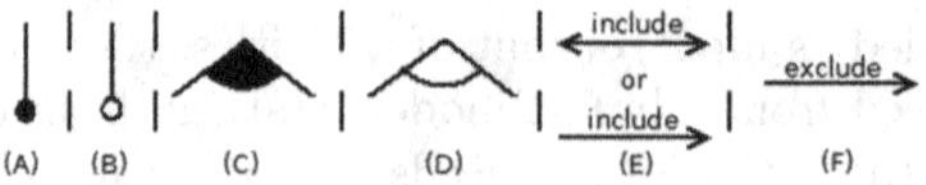

Fig. 1. Feature models constraints.

3   Case Study - EU Project Reporting

Over the last years the Seventh Framework Program (FP7), and now Horizon 2020, are funding opportunities for many organizations in Europe in order to support innovation, and collaboration. The participation to a EU financed project oblige the beneficiary in budget reporting activities as an evidence of the tasks performed within the project. Introducing simplification in Horizon 2020, the European Commission itself recognized the complexity of the reporting procedures for FP7. Nevertheless such complexity is still high for running projects.

Submitting a EU project the organizations have to be aware of the dynamic environment in which they are working. They have to be able to manage variability considering the different programs, funding and reporting schemes, etc. The ability to deal with this variability is critical for the success of the project where the organization is involved.

Moreover, it is worth noting that it is often the case that the participation to successful proposal requires to involve a unit of administrative personnel to support administrative reporting activities. There is typically high mobility in this administrative role. Mobility means being able to support organizations with different profiles and different constraints according to EU guideline. For instance, enterprises and universities fit with different procedures in order to reach the same goal. The availability of a flexible learning platform considering such complexity is therefore highly desired.

According to such scenario grant management has been chosen as the running examples of our work since it is quite simple, and at the same time sufficiently complex to validate the proposed approach. BPs involved in the grant management need to react at the different scenarios in order to set up the most suitable configuration. Just to give some examples we can refer to different implementation of the BPs such as reporting, both periodic and final, payment, and amendment.

Among the several BPs, we consider the *periodic budget reporting*. This refers to the activities that an organization (in reference to its administrative offices) has to put in place in order to manage the administrative procedures related to the participation to a European Research Project. Regarding such BP we considered the following basic architectural requirements.

Req1 all participants must fill the Form C with their direct costs.
Req2 all participants must fill the Form C with their indirect costs. They may
be calculated using four possible criteria that are *actual indirect costs, actual*

indirect costs - but using a simplified method, flat rate of 20% and flat rate of 60% of the total direct eligible costs.

Req3 The Form C is related to the funding scheme and project type. For instance, they are Network of Excellence (NoE), Collaborative Project (CP) and Coordination and Support Action (CSA).

Req4 If the financial contribution requested exceeds 375.000 euros, the participant must provide a Certificates of Financial Statement (CFS).

Req5 Each participant must sign their own Form C.

Req6 Each participant must submit to the project coordinator the signed Form C and, in case the financial contribution requested exceeds 375.000 euros, also the CFS.

Focusing on the information perspective we consider the following data objects.

Form C contains all the information related to financial cost claim. The form is adapted to take into account information such as the beneficiary, the funding schemes, etc. The general structure is extended by two main parts, the first one contains all the direct cost of a participant, whereas a second one contains all the indirect cost of a participant. Form C can be signed by the participant or not, as soon as it is signed it can be submitted to the project coordinator.

CFS is a form completed by an external auditor. It contains a number of questions which the auditor must answer to verify the beneficiary accounting, and control system or document, in relation to the execution of the project.

CFS Copy is a scanned version of the original CFS.

4   Modeling Business Process Variability

In order to model variability of BPs and data objects we propose an extended version of FM, named bpFM. In bpFM features are BP activities, whereas feature constraints express if an activity must, or can be, inserted in a BP variant, and if it must or can be included within an execution path. Data objects included in bpFM express information to be used to support designer in the modelling of control flow relations in a BP variant.

To model variability using the proposed approach the modeler will follow a three stage process. The first step foresees the identification of the features and data objects to be included in the bpFM (configuration). At this stage the designer chooses the features representing the activities she considers necessary to reach the objectives pursued by a family of BPs. Implicitly this leads to data objects identification needed for a specific variant. Selected activities and data objects are included in a configuration that is the input for the second step where BP fragments are automatically generated thanks to a set of mapping rules. In particular, for each configuration different BP fragments can be generated. The final step concerns the modelling of BP variants. At this stage the designer will add control flow relationships among the generated BP fragments, data objects relations contribute to the BP variant design defining a partial order relation among generated activities in order to derive a BP with a meaningful data flow. Nevertheless, in teh current version of the approach, it is possible that the selection done by the designer leads to an inconsistent data-flow. The derived variant should be then verified to discover possible data-flow errors. Possible extensions of the approach could investigate the derivation of variants correct-by-construction.

5   Modeling Activities and Data Object via bpFM

Modeling Activities via bpFM. bpFM provides support to express constraints and relationships among the activities that can be included in a BP variant. Feature constraints can be single or multiple depending on how many activities they refer to. In bpFM we include the following constraints.

- A *Mandatory Activity* constraint requires that the activity must be inserted in each BP variant, and it has also to be included in each execution path (Fig. 2-A).
- An *Optional Activity* constraint requires that the activity can be inserted (or not) in each BP variant and it could be included (or not) in each execution path (Fig. 2-B).
- A *Domain Activity* constraint requires that the activity must be inserted in each BP variant but it could be included (or not) in each execution path (Fig. 2-C).
- A *Special Case Activity* constraint requires that the activity can be inserted (or not) in each BP variant. When it is inserted it has to be included in each execution path (Fig. 2-D).
- An *Inclusive Multi Activities* constraints requires that at least one of the activities must be inserted in each BP variant, and at least one of them have to be included in each execution path (Fig. 2-E).
- An *One Optional Activity* constraint requires that exactly one of the activities has to be inserted in each BP variant, and it could be included (or not) in each execution path (Fig. 2-F).
- A *One Selection Activity* constraint requires that exactly one of the activities has to be inserted in each BP variant, and it has to be included in each execution path (Fig. 2-G).
- A *XOR Activities* constraint requires that all the activities must be inserted in each BP variant, and exactly one of them has to be included in each execution path (Fig. 2-H).
- A *XOR Selection Activities* constraint requires that at least one of the activities has to be inserted in each BP variant, and exactly one of them has to be included in each execution path (Fig. 2-I).

Finally, *Include* and *Exclude* relationships between features are also considered according to the base definition of FM (Fig. 2-J and Fig. 2-K).

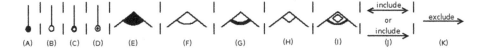

Fig. 2. bpFM Constraints.

Modelling Data Object via bpFM. Focusing on BP variability, modelling data objects plays a fundamental role since variability has to be expressed also at the data level. This means that each BP variant could include completely different sets of data objects.

bpFM manages all types of BPMN 2.0 data objects and uses the same notation. In particular:

- The *Data Object* element models data in a general way;
- The *Data Object Collection* element refers to multi-instance data objects; using this a designer can express the involvement of more than one data object;
- The *Data Input* element is used to express (external) input data, and it can be read by an activity;
- The *Data Output* element is used to express output data, and it can be generated by an activity;
- The *Data Store* element represents data that will persist after the process instance finishes.

A data object looks like a document icon whereas a Data Store looks like a database icon. Connectors are represented using arrows from data object to the activity or vice-versa. Data Input and data output are marked in order to make clear that they are input and output for the whole BP with white or black arrow respectively. Finally, data object collection is data object with the multi instances marker.

As well as in BPMN 2.0 data object elements can be connected as inputs and outputs to activity, that in our case are features. To represent inputs and outputs of each activity in bpFM we introduce a particular semantic for data objects. This is inspired by the semantics presented in [1]. According to such semantics to execute an activity it is needed that all the data objects in input are available, and as soon as all the data objects in output are generated the activity can be completed. Child features also inherit data objects, in the sense that if a data object is linked as input to a feature, all the child activities need such data object to be executed. This is also valid for the output.

In modelling data we also include state representation. An activity can require or can generate a data object in a specific state. If the state is not explicitly reported the activity is state independent. A data object cannot be in two different states at the same time (Fig. 3-B). If the same object is linked to the same activity specifying two different states, this means that states are exclusive with respect to each other and they have to be resolved during the modelling of a variant. A state of a data-object is represented with square brackets under the data-object name.

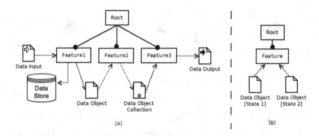

Fig. 3. Data object in bpFM.

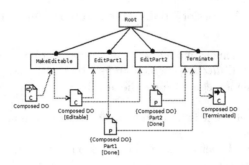

Fig. 4. Composed data object in bpFM.

Even though BPMN 2.0 deals with data, it does not provide a way to represent composed data object. In bpFM we introduce the notion of composite and *part − of* data object that can be extended for each type of BPMN 2.0 data object.

- A composed data object indicates that the data object is composed by a set of specific block of data, and it is marked with the letter *C*.
- *Part − of* data object indicates that the data object is contained in a specific block of data, and it is marked with the letter *P*. It also explicitly refers to the data-object of which it is part reporting the name of it inside curly brackets.

For example, in Fig. 4 we show a data object named *Composed DO* composed by two parts (*Part1* and *Part2*). Considering the editing of the two parts an independent activities, even if it refers to the same document, the notion of *part − of* give the possibility to explicitly make them independent also from the data point of view.

The *part − of* notion can also be extended to data-object state and it makes possible that a data object that is *part − of* a composed data object can change its own state without impacting on the global state of the composed data object. This means that in bpFM we make possible that the state of a composed data object is not directly deduced from the state of the single data objects composing it.

Modelling bpFM into Practice. For the sake of comprehension we report here the application of the approach to the EU projects periodic report BP (Fig. 5) according to the requirements described in Sect. 3.

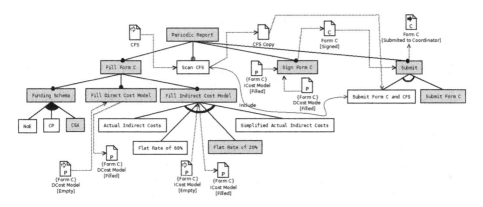

Fig. 5. EU participant periodic report bpFM model.

The data object that drives the execution of the BP is the *Form C* that is composed by the *DCost Model* (Direct Cost Model) and the *ICost Model* (Indirect Cost Model). *Form C* can fit one or more of the three available funding schema, they are *NoE*, *CP* and *CSA*, then we model it using an *Inclusive Multi Activities*. Each participant needs to fill both the cost models (*Fill Direct Cost Model* and *Fill Indirect Cost Model*). The data objects *DCost Model* and *ICost Model* are initially empty (state *Empty*), but after the filled activities they become filled (state *Filled*). More in details the Indirect Cost Model can be based in four different policies depending by the project, the type of participants, etc. They can be based on *Actual Indirect Cost*, *Simplified Actual Indirect Cost*, at a *Flat Rate of 20 %* or at a *Flat Rate of 60 %* of the total direct eligible costs. So, they are represented using *One Selection Activity*. When both the *DCost Model* and the *ICost Model* are filled the *Form C* can be signed by the participant (state *Signed* on data object *Form C*). When it is signed it can be submitted to the coordinator of the project. In case, the financial contribution requested exceeds 375,000 euros, the participant needs also to scan his/her *CFS*. *Scan CFS* activity is modelled using a *Special Case Activity*. In the case the CFS is needed it must be sent to the coordinator jointly with *Form C*. For this reason there are two alternatives to submit the document (*Submit Form C and CFS* or *Submit Form C*).

6   Deriving BP Fragments and BP Variants

Mapping Rules Definition. The automatic generation of BP fragments from a bpFM model is based on the application of specific mapping rules according to activity constraints. The generation step takes in input a bpFM including activities and data objects and the configuration defined by the designer on the bpFM model (in gray in the Figures). As a result a set of BP fragments in BPMN 2.0 are returned.

The transformation we have defined permits to derive the fragment according to the possible selection or not of a feature and according to the semantic of the various constraints. In particular:

- A *Mandatory Activity* rule impose the selection of the feature (activity) and results in the inclusion of the activity (possibly including a related data object) in the execution path of any variant.
- An *Optional Activity* rule asks for a combination of an activity (possibly with data object) and gateway conditions when the activity is selected, so that two execution paths of the fragment are possible, one including the activity and the other one not. When the activity is not selected it results with no mapping.
- A *Domain Activity* rule asks for a combination of the selected activity (possibly with data object) and gateway conditions, so that two execution paths of the fragment are possible, one including the activity and the other one not.
- A *Special Case Activity* rule asks for including the activity (possibly with data object) in the execution path of the fragment if selected. When the activity is not selected it results with no mapping.
- A *Inclusive Multi Activities* rule asks for a combination of the selected activities (possibly with data object) and inclusive gateway conditions, so that multiple paths in the fragment are supported considering selection. In case only one activity is selected it is mapped as an activity (possibly with data object) in the execution path of the fragment.
- A *One Optional Activity* rule asks for the activity that is selected (possibly with data object) and exclusive gateway conditions, so that two paths are supported by the fragment, one including the activity and the other one not.
- A *One Selection Activity* rule asks for including the selected activity (possibly with data object) in the execution path of the fragment.
- An *XOR Activities* rule ask for a combination of the selected activities (possibly with data object) and exclusive gateway conditions, so that alternative paths are supported in the execution path of the fragment.
- An *XOR Selection Activities* rule ask for a combination of the selected activities (possibly with data object) and exclusive gateway conditions, so that alternative paths are supported; in case only one activity is selected rule ask for an activity (possibly with data object) in the execution path of the fragment.

Considering bpFM notion of inheritance, when a data object is connected as an input/output to a feature, child features inherit it. In this case the child feature is connected to the activity that is introduced in the fragment according to the bpFM constraint and related mapping rule. For instance, in Fig. 6 the data object *Data Object 4* is associated as input to the feature named *Root*. It means that *Data Object 4* must be mapped as input of the selected child features *Feature1* and *Feature2*. The mapping rule are not affected by composed data definition. We manage component and part-of data-object as well as the other data objects since BPMN does no provide composed data (Fig. 7).

Deriving BP Fragments and BP Variants into Practice. For the sake of comprehension we report here the application of the approach to the European Budget Report.

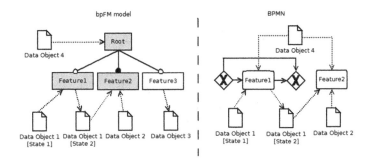

Fig. 6. Mapping data object (selected activities are in gray).

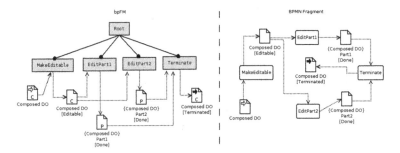

Fig. 7. Mapping composed data object (selected activities are ingray).

Starting from the given bpFM, and applying the modeling approach we propose, the designer can concentrate at a first stage on the definition of a configuration selecting the activities, and the data-objects that are needed to reach specific objectives that is EU reporting. To support the fragment definition, the configuration results in the selection of the features as represented in the bpFM model (Fig. 5). Using the mapping rules BP fragments are generated (Fig. 8). Finally, the designer manually models the final BP integrating and connecting the generated BP fragments (Fig. 9). Designer can define control flow relationships among the various fragments in order to derive a fully defined BP variant. The derived BP has three main phases the first one manage the founding schema, the second phase refers to the filling form C, whereas the last phase refers to the signing and submitting of the form C.

7 Related Works

BP variability is a hot topic that has been broadly considered during the last years [2,4,8,15]. Here we report the papers that are closer to our approach.

Configurable integrated EPC (C-iEPC) considers variability in term of behavioral, information, and organization perspectives [7]. From this work we took inspiration for the management of data-object in bpFM. Moreover every

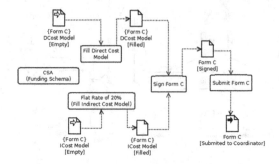

Fig. 8. BP fragments resulting from the configuration and the mapping.

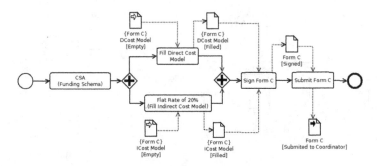

Fig. 9. A possible BP variant.

approach that includes BPMN 2.0 can manage data. Therefore they typically consider the notion of variability in relation to the information perspective (i.e. the PESOA approach [14]).

Some papers emphasize the combination between FM and BP to represent variability. In [5] FM are used for customizing process models combining FM with process model template. In this case the FODA basic notation is used. According to the domain knowledge (and its feature selections), in [5] a BP variant is derived combining FM and process model template, but differently from us no specific rules are given. The Corepro framework provides an interesting approach for modelling data structure and states changes [9,10]. It introduces a part-of relationship in order to allow the representation of composed data object. From the application of this approach we recognized that composed data objects should be management in each BP modelling approach.

To introduce mechanisms for variability with reference to the information perspective we took inspiration also from the work presented in [11].

8 Conclusions and Future Work

In this paper we illustrated a novel approach to model BP variability focusing on control flow and data. To do this we introduce an extended version of FM supporting input-output data representation. Starting from bpFM the designer can select different features, and thanks to the definition of specific mapping rules, it is possible to obtain BP variants for which the precise definition of the final control flow structures can also be driven by data object flow relations. The approach has been applied to a data intensive scenario, such as EU project budget reporting, with encouraging results.

In the future we plan to explore the possibility of enlarging domain analysis with the evaluation of additional real case studies. Moreover we intend to explore consistency verification for derived variants in particular with reference to data-object consistency. Finally, we aim at developing a tool-chain to have an integrated development environment.

References

1. Awad, A., Decker, G., Lohmann, N.: Diagnosing and repairing data anomalies in process models. In: Rinderle-Ma, S., Sadiq, S., Leymann, F. (eds.) BPM 2009. LNBIP, vol. 43, pp. 5–16. Springer, Heidelberg (2010)
2. Ayora, C., Torres, V., Weber, B., Reichert, M., Pelechano, V.: VIVACE: a framework for the systematic evaluation of variability support in process-aware information systems (in press)
3. Capilla, R., Bosch, J., Kang, K.C.: Systems and Software Variability Management. Springer, Heidelberg (2013)
4. Cognini, R., Corradini, F., Gnesi, S., Polini, A., Re, B.: Research challenges in Business Process Adaptability. In: SATTA@SAC, pp. 1049–1054 (2014)
5. Gröner, G., Bošković, M., Silva Parreiras, F., Gašević, D.: Modeling and validation of business process families. Inf. Syst. **38**(5), 709–726 (2013)
6. Kang, K., Cohen, S.G., Hess, J.A., Novak, W.E., Peterson, A.S.: Feature-oriented domain analysis feasibility study. Technical report, DTIC Doc (1990)
7. La Rosa, M., Dumas, M., ter Hofstede, A.H.M., Mendling, J., Gottschalk, F.: Beyond control-flow: extending business process configuration to roles and objects. In: Li, Q., Spaccapietra, S., Yu, E., Olivé, A. (eds.) ER 2008. LNCS, vol. 5231, pp. 199–215. Springer, Heidelberg (2008)
8. La Rosa, M., van der Aalst, W.M., Dumas, M., Milani, F.P.: Business process variability modeling: a survey (2013)
9. Müller, D., Reichert, M., Herbst, J.: Flexibility of data-driven process structures. In: Eder, J., Dustdar, S. (eds.) BPM Workshops 2006. LNCS, vol. 4103, pp. 181–192. Springer, Heidelberg (2006)
10. Müller, D., Reichert, M., Herbst, J.: Data-driven modeling and coordination of large process structures. In: Meersman, R., Tari, Z. (eds.) OTM 2007, Part I. LNCS, vol. 4803, pp. 131–149. Springer, Heidelberg (2007)
11. Nigam, A., Caswell, N.S.: Business artifacts: an approach to operational specification. IBM Syst. J. **42**(3), 428–445 (2003)
12. Pohl, K., Böckle, G., Van Der Linden, F.: Software Product Line Engineering, vol. 10. Springer, Heidelberg (2005)
13. Reichert, M., Weber, B.: Enabling Flexibility in Process-Aware Information Systems: Challenges, Methods, Technologies. Springer, Berlin (2012)
14. Schnieders, A., Puhlmann, F.: Variability mechanisms in e-business process families. BIS **85**, 583–601 (2006)
15. Valença, G., Alves, C., Alves, V., Niu, N.: A systematic mapping study on BP variability. Int. J. Comput. Sci. Inf. Tech. **5**(1) (2013)

The BE^2 model: When Business Events meet Business Entities

Fabiana Fournier and Lior Limonad$^{(\boxtimes)}$

IBM Research - Haifa, Carmel Mountain, 31905 Haifa, Israel
{fabiana,liorli}@il.ibm.com

Abstract. This work presents a unified modelling approach based on two declarative models which integrates event- and entity-driven paradigms while preserving a clear separation of concerns between their executions. The proposed approach provides business users with a unified model that is both sufficiently equipped to capture the inherent complexity of realistic business operations, and still enables gaining a complete overview of the entire business arena. This was attained building upon the business-entity-model and the-event-model as two complementary modeling paradigms yielding the BE^2 model. In this paper we describe how these two models have been systematically unified using an ontological formalism as a common conceptual baseline. The approach also derives a set of modeling guidelines to preserve the consistency across the two specifications. We demonstrate the actual instantiation of the proposed BE^2 model in the Transport and Logistics domain.

Keywords: Event processing · The event model · Business entity · Business artifact · Ontology

1 Introduction and Motivation[1]

In today's competitive and dynamic landscape, business managers are continuously forced to effectively react to any event that has the potential to affect the expected course of their business processes. To cope with this requirement, companies are increasingly adopting business process engines alongside with event processing engines, to manage their business process and get real-time alerts once a situation requiring a course of action occurs. In this work, we propose a unified modelling approach, based on two declarative models, that integrates event- and entity-driven paradigms while preserving a clear separation of concerns between their executions. Our approach is demonstrated in the Transport and Logistics (T&L) domain using a classic example of an area which is event driven by nature.

We selected the *Business Entity Model* (BEM) [5, 10, 13] for the design and implementation of all ordinary business operations and *The Event Model* (TEM) [7] for the design and implementation of all irregularities and any additional event-driven situations that require careful attention. Both models are declarative, were developed as

---

[1] The research leading to these results has received funding from the FIspace FP7-FI-PPP project (Number 604123).

F. Fournier and J. Mendling (Eds.): BPM 2014 Workshops, LNBIP 202, pp. 222–234, 2015.
DOI: 10.1007/978-3-319-15895-2_20

computation independent models [2], and have formal semantics [1, 10] to enable their automatic transformation to specific platform specifications.

While BEM is instrumented to cope with event-driven business processes, it lacks the capability to express the business logic of complex events. On the other hand, TEM is dedicated to cope with all the complexity in defining an event-driven application, while lacking support to express high-level and cross-cutting business process orchestrations [6]. Our experience from several conducted use cases using both models [9] has shown that the two are complementary to one another such that their unified expressiveness can substantially promote the construction of a more effective and consumable enterprise modeling means.

2   Two Paradigms: Business Entities and Business Events

2.1   The Business Entity Model (BEM)

The Business-Entity Model (BEM) (*a.k.a.* Business Artifacts) conceptualizes the organizational domain as being composed of key conceptual entities. The fundamental concept in the BEM is a *BE type*, specified as a key conceptual dynamic entity that arises in and flows through a portion of the operations of a business. The internal form of a BE type is a marriage of process and data, such that its execution (namely, a *BE instance*) has access to all relevant information that has been created by the business as the instance moves through the business operations. Correspondingly, a BE type specification comprises an *Information model* and a *Lifecycle model*.

A *BE's Information model* is further classified into two subsets of attributes—*data attributes*, which hold all business-relevant data about the instance as it moves through the business, and *status attributes*, which hold information indicating the current 'phase' in the lifecycle the instance is at. A *BE's Lifecycle model* describes the possible ways an entity of that type might progress through a business by responding to events and invoking services, including human activities. Various modeling grammars may be used to describe the lifecycle part. The most recently developed formalism, also used here, is the Guard-Stage-Milestone (GSM) model [10]. The GSM model comprises a forest of hierarchical *stages*, each designating possible changes between a set of preconditions ('*guards*') and a set of goals ('*milestones*'). More precisely, the enactment of a specific GSM instance is governed by the notion of a *sentry* as a unique type of an Event-Condition-Action (ECA) rule. Specifically, the GSM model constitutes four concrete types of sentries: *achiever, invalidator, guard,* and *terminator.* The former two conditionally toggle the status of milestones (i.e., achieved or invalidated), while the latter two conditionally toggle the status of stages (i.e., open or closed). Events may include either external occurrences such as user activities or incoming service calls, or internal events such as stage termination or milestone achievement. Each tree branch in the hierarchy has an *atomic stage* in its end (namely, a *task*). Tasks may include service calls, value updates to attributes in the information model, and activities to be performed by external human actors. A summary of all key model constructs in the BEM is detailed in Table 1.

Table 1. BEM main constructs

Model construct	Definition
Business Entity Type	A key conceptual dynamic entity (or object) that arises in and flows through a portion of the operations of a business [1].
Business Entity Instance	A particular execution of an entity type.
Data Attribute	Some business-relevant information.
Status Attribute	Some information indicating the lifecycle 'phase' the BE instance is at.
(sub)Stage	One or more activities, including calls to external services and possibly sub-stages, intended to achieve some milestone [11].
Milestone	A business-relevant operational objective expressed using a condition over the information model and possibly a triggering event [11].
Sentry (abstract construct)	An ECA rule, where: Event – might be from the external world (e.g., from a human performer or an incoming service call), might be from another BE instance, or might be the result of some milestone or stages changing their status [11]. Condition – an (OCL) expression ranging over the information model of the BE instance [11]. Action – depending on the type of sentry (see rows below).
Guard Sentry	A *sentry* whose action triggers the opening of a stage.
Terminator Sentry	A *sentry* whose action triggers the closing of a stage.
Achiever Sentry	A *sentry* whose action attains a milestone.
Invalidator Sentry	A *sentry* whose action revokes the attainment of a milestone.

2.2   The Event Model (TEM)

The Event Model (TEM) is a novel way to model, develop, validate, maintain, and implement event-driven applications. TEM is based on a set of well-defined principles and building blocks, and it is targeted at business users, thus does not require substantial programming skills. For a deep description of TEM refer to [7].

TEM is composed of the following five building blocks:

1. *TEM Concepts*: Everything in TEM is a concept, which can be either a glossary concept or a logic concept. A glossary concept is a term in the specific domain which has a meaning. Some of the concepts denote computational entities, and a logic concept is a description of how such a computational entity is computed.
2. *TEM Glossary*: The knowledge model that stores all application glossary concepts.
3. *TEM Diagrams*: The set of diagrams that describes the event causality dependencies (and hence the event flow) in the event-driven application.
4. *TEM Logic*: The knowledge model that describes all logic concepts of a specific event-driven application.
5. *TEM Principles*: The set of assertions and integrity constraints that determine the semantics of the model's interpretation and sets restrictions on the various models.

Table 2. TEM main logic constructs

Model construct	Definition
Actor	Anyone or anything that plays a role in an event processing application.
Producer actor	An actor that emits events having some relevance to a certain *situation* in the context of a specific event processing application.
Consumer actor	An actor that subscribes to *situations*.
Event type [8]	A collection of *event instances* in the domain that have some common meaning and structure. Specified as a container of fact types.
Event instance [8]	The computerized entity that denotes a specific occurrence of an *event type*.
Raw event type [8]	An event originating from an *event producer*.
Derived event type [8]	An event whose instances are created by applying a function on event (s) instances over time.
Situation event type	A derived event of interest that may require a course of action. A Situation is consumed by an *event consumer*.
Fact type	A named atomic piece of data. This is analogous to the attribute of an entity or of an event in most data models. Further classification of fact types can be found in [8].
Context [8]	A specification of processing relevance conditions to partition the event instances so these partitions can be processed separately.
Condition	Expressions executed against input event instances.
Partition-by context (a.k.a Segmentation Context, [8])	Context partition criterion based on the values of one or more *Fact Types* contained in event(s) instances.
When context (a.k.a Temporal Context, [8])	Context partition criterion based on the instance time of events, also known as temporal context.
Filter-on event	An expression evaluated against the content of a single event instance, to determine whether an event instance should participate in the event derivation.
Pattern	An expression on related event types' instances such as Detected, Absent, Thresholds over Aggregations, or Fact Type value changes. A pattern is used to detect the specified relationships among event instances.
Filter-on pattern	An expression on multiple event instances, including comparisons, memberships, and time-relationships. A filter on pattern is used to filter the pattern result based on conditions among the different events that issued the specific pattern.

In this paper, we focus only on TEM logic. A summary of all key model logic constructs is detailed in Table 2. The event business logic is expressed in Excel-like tables that, in turn, can be transformed into code. The other constructs are required to build a consistent and complete model but not relevant for this paper.

TEM Logic is represented by two tables as follows:

Event Derivation Table (EDT) is a two-dimensional representation of logic leading to a *derived event*, based on *events* and *facts*. Thus, an EDT designates the circumstances under which a derived event of interest is reached. There exists a single logic table for each derived event. The table specifies the conditions for generations of new instances of this event type.

Computation Table is a two-dimensional representation of the logic leading to a *computed fact type*. A computation table is a logic artifact that specifies the computation of assignments of the values of fact types (attributes) associated with a derived event. The derived fact type mentioned in the name of the computation table is associated with the table in the sense that it describes the value assignment for its fact types. If the value of a derived fact type equals the fact type value of the input event, then the computation table for this derived fact type can be omitted.

3 Illustrative Example – The Import and Export Scenario

We use a scenario taken from the transport and logistics domain to illustrate our contribution. Specifically, we use an adaptation of one of the trial scenarios observed in the FIspace FP7 EU project [9] related to the import and export of consumer goods from China to the UK. The scenario and the exception handling are typical to any logistics scenario therefore are representative enough to generalize on our ideas. End-to-end collaborative supply chain execution, along with enhanced visibility, and pro-active deviation management, are necessary to ensure on-time delivery and customer satisfaction. This may sometimes require compensations to customers in cases of deviations from the anticipated schedule.

In the BEM, the *Shipment* entity was identified as centric to the business operation modeled. Correspondingly, its lifecycle model in GSM is illustrated in Fig. 1. The scenario is broken down into three sub-stages which depict warehousing at port of origin, overseas transit, and warehousing again at port of destination.

Complementary to this specification, shipment exceptions handling is modeled by TEM. Specifically, TEM alerts upon a delay situation if the actual arrival time has gone beyond a certain tolerance time. The Event Derivation Table for the delay situation is given in Table 3 along with the corresponding computation in Table 4.

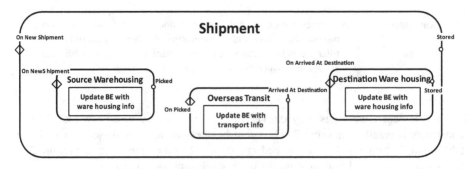

Fig. 1. GSM model for the import and export scenario

The temporal context extends between the time the shipment is picked (OnPicked event) and the Expected Time of Arrival (ETA) at destination plus a delay tolerance. The segmentation context partitions the events by Shipment ID (i.e., Shipment ID is a *Fact Type* according to which event instances are grouped). The event pattern the EDT is specified for is Absence [8]. Consequently, the EDT row yields a *Shipment-delay* event upon the situation of failing to observe shipment arrival before the (ETA + tolerance time) for a specific shipment. In our illustrative example, let's assume that the *Shipment delay* derived event type is associated with a *Delay message* fact type. The alert message is computed as shown in Table 4.

Table 3. Shipment delay derivation table

	Shipment delay Logic						
Row #	When Expression	When Start	When End	Partition by	Filter on event	Pattern	Filter on pattern
				Shipment ID		Shipment actual	
1		OnPicked	ETA at destination + delay tolerance	same		is Absent	

Table 4. Delay message computation table

	delay message Computation	
Row #		Row in Event Derivation Table
1	"Shipment " + Shipment ID+ " is delayed in " +tolerance time+ "hours "	1

4 Our Integration Approach

To guide the integration of the two models, we employed an ontology based approach, following the principles of ontological expressiveness from [19]. We used Bunge's ontology [3, 4] as the common conceptual ground according to which both models can complement one another to accommodate richer grammatical expressiveness. Although there are several other ontological frameworks in the literature (e.g., [14, 15, 17]), the one of Bunge is equipped to handle the realistic and materialized view of the world of which all business domains are a part. That is, this view fits well with the business domain as the target of the two models composed. In addition, the Bunge ontology was already employed to direct the development and evaluation of modeling languages in the Information Systems field [18, 19].

The Bunge's ontology postulates both about the structural and dynamic views of the world. In the context of the structural view, the world is considered to be made of *things* which possess *properties*. According to the dynamic view, the set of properties possessed by each thing is perceived at any point in time through *state variables* for which their collective set is termed the *state* of that thing. When a thing changes one or more of its state variable values, humans perceive this change as a change of state, termed an *event*. For additional core ontological concepts refer to [4]. In this work, we further extend the fundamental conceptualizations given in Bunge's ontology with additional terms developed in the *Generic Process Model* (GPM) [16] and in the *WaaSaBE* model [12]. Both conceptualizations rely on Bunge's ontology as the core conceptualization, and provide additional terminology which can be used to provide meanings to the constructs in the two models we integrate in this work.

Ontology based approach can be used as a means to systematically assess the quality of a modeling grammar [19]. Particularly, analyzing the mappings between a grammar's constructs and ontological concepts could lead to the identification of two key deficiencies that may undermine the clarity of the language: *construct overload* and *construct redundancy*. The former deficiency exists when one modeling constructs has two (or more) corresponding ontological interpretations. The latter deficiency exists when two (or more) modeling constructs have the same ontological interpretation. Such deficiencies are probable when combining modeling grammars in an aim to accommodate richer expressiveness. Hence, aiming to integrate BEM and TEM, we used ontological expressiveness to determine the quality of the unified grammar. First, we iterated over the constituent constructs in the two models, populating an ontological interpretation which matches the original definition given for each. Next, we carefully reviewed the correspondences between construct interpretations in the two models, looking for the above deficiencies. This analysis has identified a particular case of construct overload, which was resolved by augmenting the grammar of the BEM with a more specific construct.

5 Integrating Events and Entities: Formal Semantics

We used the ontological concepts described in the previous section as a common conceptual reference from which semantic similarities among the constructs in the two models can be drawn. For each of the key constructs in the BEM and TEM, we used its original definition to devise its corresponding ontological meaning as summarized in Tables 5 and 6, respectively.

Several possible semantic correspondences were observed after using the ontological terminology as a baseline. Our analysis has looked for constructs that have some ontological concepts shared in their definition as a signal to having some potential grammatical deficiency.

– Status attribute ↔ Fact type: Both modeling constructs refer to the representation of *state variables*. As such, the information model in BEM can also be considered a means to record context related TEM facts. For each fact type in TEM related to context, there may exist a status attribute corresponding to it in the BEM information model.

– Status attribute ↔ When context: the temporal context in TEM is determined by some (temporal) logic expression which relies on state variables. Ontologically, a state variable corresponds to the status attribute construct in BEM. Hence, the expression of each 'When context' in TEM is constructed as some logical combination consisting of status attributes in the BEM. However, it is also possible to include some temporal indicators in the When context which are not explicitly modeled as status attributes in BEM.

Table 5. Ontological semantics for BEM constructs

Model construct	Ontological meaning
Business Entity instance	A concrete realization of a business *commitment*.
Business Entity type	A set of possible realizations corresponding to a *commitment type*.
Data Attribute	A *property* of a thing.
Status Attribute	A *state variable*.
(sub)Stage	A *work-type* is a set of *transitions* from a certain *initial state* to a certain *goal state* (ontologically, may also be considered a *complex event*).
Milestone	A *hard goal* of a stage.
Sentry (abstract construct)	Sentry is a *transition-law*, as in Bunge's ontology, specified in the form of an ECA rule <*event, condition, action*>, where *event* corresponds to Bunge's ontological notion of event (i.e., a pair of states), *condition* is some logical combination of *state-* and *event-laws*, and *action* is a state-transition that depends on the specific type of the sentry.
Guard	A *sentry* whose action specifies a change to one or more state variables of a corresponding *stage*, transforming its current stable goal state to an *unstable state*.
Terminator	A *sentry* whose action specifies a change to one or more state variables of a corresponding *stage*, transforming its current unstable state to one of its *stable goal states*.
Achiever	A *sentry* whose action specifies change to one or more state variables of a corresponding *milestone*, transforming its current unstable state to one of its *stable goal states*.
Invalidator	A *sentry* whose action specifies a change to one or more state variables of a corresponding *milestone*, transforming its current goal state back to an *unstable state*.

– (sub)Stage ↔ Situation event type: This is probably the most significant correspondence identified. According to our analysis, both constructs correspond to the ontological notion of a *complex event* [4]. Each situation event in TEM is equivalent to the construct of a stage in BEM, such that each complex event can also be modeled as a stage in BEM that is triggered by some raw event that conforms to one of that stage's guarding sentries, and is concluded by a derived event which also signifies the attainment of one of that stage's milestones. Having this correspondence in the meaning of the two modeling constructs may lead to a deficiency referred to as *construct overload* [19] in BEM if the two modeling grammars of BEM and TEM are to be integrated. That is, the general notion of a *stage* in BEM may become ambiguous as it may be interpreted either as some *work type* or as some *situation event type*. In order to eliminate this potential ambiguity, an explicit modeling construct was derived as a specialization to the general notion of a stage in the BEM's GSM model (see Section 6.1).

Table 6. Ontological semantics for TEM constructs

Model construct	Ontological meaning
Actor	Any *thing* in the *environment* of the event processing system's *domain* which can interact with it. *Interaction* means that a thing's own state can cause changes in another thing's state (e.g., turning it from being *stable* to *unstable*).
Producer actor	An actor whose own change in state can cause a state change (namely, an *external event*) in the domain of the event processing system.
Consumer actor	An actor whose own state may become unstable as a result of some state change (namely, a *situation event*) taking place within the domain of the event processing system.
Event type	An *event space* (i.e., a set of *events*).
Event instance	An *event* (i.e., a pair of *states*).
Raw event type	A specific *event space* consisting of a set of possible *external events* created as a result of *interaction* between the event processing system and some *producer actor*.
Derived event type	A specific *event space* consisting of a set of possible *internal events* arising in the event processing system.
Situation event type	A specific *event space* consisting of a set of possible *complex events* which trigger some *interaction* with a *consumer actor*. Each such complex event is some conceivable composition of *external* (i.e., raw event type) and *internal* (i.e., derived) events.
Fact type	A *state variable* (e.g., age of a person in a certain point in time), represented by a function whose domain includes a set of substantial individuals.
Context	Some functional specification of an *event space*, whose domain includes some conceivable event space.
Condition	Some logical combination of *state-* and *event-laws*.
Partition By context [8] (a.k.a Segmentation Context)	A partitioning function over a set of *events* (i.e., an input *event space*) and selection properties, partitioning that domain into *lawful* and *unlawful event spaces*.
When context [8] (a.k.a Temporal Context)	Some partitioning function over a set of *events* and times (i.e., *state variables*), fragmenting that domain into *lawful* and *unlawful events spaces*.
Filter on event	A propositional function for an event space.
Pattern	A partially ordered set of events in a given event space. This ordering defines a set of equivalent processes (namely, a *process type*). The ordering may be specified as a combination of event transformation laws.
Filter on pattern	A propositional function whose input domain constitutes the context (i.e., an event space) and pattern.

- Milestone ↔ Situation event type: In line with the previous correspondence, the after state in a situation event type corresponds to a milestone in BEM.
- Sentry ↔ Condition: Conditions are used in both models to filter out irrelevant events. The realization is also equivalent, using some linguistic formalism which reflects some logical combination of *state-* and *event-laws*. However, in the case of BEM, condition expressions are always a part of some sentry, so the risk of having some grammatical deficiency is not existent.
- Guard ↔ Raw event type: Similar to the previous correspondence, the internal triggering event in each BEM guard is semantically equivalent to the notion of a raw event in TEM.

6 Augmenting the BEM Lifecycle Model with Situation Stages

Based on the semantic equivalences identified in the previous section, we introduce the construct of a *Situation Stage* as a new GSM construct in the BEM.

Definition 1: A *Situation Stage* is a specific type of a stage in GSM which corresponds to a single *situation event type* in TEM.

Unlike simple stages in the GSM lifecycle model in the BEM for which their realization is described either by some further decomposition into sub-stages or by some atomic stages (a.k.a., tasks), situation stages are 'opaque'. This means that each situation stage in BEM is simply a syntactic sugar, for which the details about its internal computation are illustrated in a corresponding TEM. Pragmatically this also means that the internal execution of a situation stage is governed by the execution of an event processing engine and not by the engine running the BEM.

The modeling of a situation stage in BEM abstracts away the business event driven logic of a specific situation. This logic is then modeled in a corresponding TEM. Consequently, there are several modeling principles implied from introducing the situation stage construct that need to be adhered to in order to maintain consistency across the two models. This includes the following:

- For each *Situation Stage* modeled in BEM:
    - All triggering events in the *guards* of that stage should match the relevant *raw events* which can trigger the derivation of the corresponding situation event type in TEM.
    - The situation stage should include a *milestone* whose triggering event type should match the situation event type in TEM.
- For each *Situation Event Type* modeled in TEM:
    - The *Partition by* field in the TEM Derivation table should be modeled as the BE type which consist of the corresponding situation stage in its lifecycle model.
    - The *Temporal context* in the TEM Derivation table is determined by the guarding events in the corresponding BEM situation stage. Specifically, the event component in each ECA rule of a guard sentry should be modeled a corresponding "When context" expression in TEM.

In order to meet the principles presented above as derived from our own experience with the modeling of the illustrative example, we propose the following high-level modeling steps to be carried out in the context of any organizational unit being analyzed (the first two steps may be followed in a non- deterministic fashion, being succeeded by the third step):

1. "Sunny day scenario": The first modeling step should conform to capturing the core of the business operation while staying ignorant of any situation exception handling. This mainly includes the identification and modeling of key business commitments as BEs.
2. Modeling of exceptional situations with TEM: For each business event which calls for exception handling or for any additional event-driven situation that requires an action, model a corresponding TEM.
3. Modeling the integration:

   - For each situation in TEM add a corresponding *situation stage* in BEM conforming to the aforementioned principles, such that the stage's level coincides with the temporal context in TEM, and the BE instance corresponds to the segmentation context in TEM. If there is no such BE type modelled in BEM, then create one or seek for one with identical business meaning. Note that it is assumed that the original design doesn't contain any overlapping in the business logic.
   - As implied for the insertion of the Situation Stage in BEM, add a new Stage which will handle the action to be carried out as a result of the situation detected.

We now return to the illustrative example to demonstrate the implications of the above guidelines. The BEM illustrated in Fig. 1 was designed in adherence to step one above, showing only the default 'sunny day operation', while being mute with respect to the handling of delays. The latter concern was modeled separately in TEM as illustrated in Table 3, adhering to step two above. Hence, prior to the application of the third integration step as proposed, there is zero visibility of the delay handling procedure in the BEM. This situation may eventually either lead to ambiguity in the modeling of the logic for the identification of shipping delays (e.g., adding an additional stage for it which coincides with the specification in TEM). More importantly, there is also the risk of failing to include an explicit business procedure for the handling of shipping delay (e.g., customer compensation). Adherence to the third modeling step results in the BEM illustrated in Fig. 2. This accounts for the aforementioned risks, leading to the inclusion of:

- A *Shipment Delay Derivation* situation stage – indicating explicitly that the derivation of the *OnShipmentDelay* event is specified in TEM, whose execution is the responsibility of the event processing engine. We also denote each situation stage with a designated 'flag' symbol to make its visual appearance different than the one of a regular stage in the BEM. The flag is the visual icon used in TEM diagrams to denote a situation.
- A *Shipment Delay Handling* stage – indicating explicitly how delays are handled by the organization as part of its operational processes.
- A *Customer Compensated* milestone – indicating a possible termination of the lifecycle due to a delay.

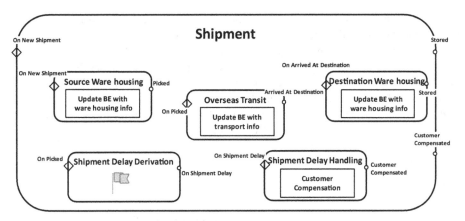

Fig. 2. The BE^2 model – visibility of the entire import and export scenario

Adherence to the proposed modeling guidelines forms a holistic view of the business operation being captured in the BEM (e.g., process termination after the customer has been compensated for a delay), while consistently also accommodating for the conceptual correspondences between the BEM and TEM.

7 Conclusions and Future Work

We introduced the BE^2 model which unifies the views of two declarative models: BEM for entity-centric processes and TEM for event-driven applications. Both models are intended for business users to alleviate the complexity in business operations. However, the BEM was originally aimed at illustrating high-level, event-driven business processes that span across different organizational units, while TEM was developed to express the logic of complex events typically associated with the handling of irregularities and deviations from the ordinary course of actions. Correspondingly, the grammar of each model was developed to account for these concerns; however, leading to a burden in the need to maintain consistency across independent specifications. Furthermore, there was also a risk of incompleteness in the specification of operational decision making, potentially missing to include in BEM decision making upon significant situations that require reaction in real-time.

The developed BE^2 model provides a kind of a 'semantic bridge' to ensure consistency and to eliminate redundancy across the specifications. We have systematically adjusted the grammar and devised guidelines to facilitate integration of the two grammars in a way which exploits the original expressive power in each model, while aligning the conceptual correspondences between the two. Furthermore, by augmenting the BEM, we adhere to the intention to use it as a means to express the pivotal view of the business, while TEM is used to provide deeper dive into the intrinsic complexity associated with some operations. We believe that the visibility gained in the unified model enables the business user to have a "better picture" of all its operations, while maintaining a separation of concerns and avoiding redundancy or omission of important steps in the process.

Our contribution in this work was guided by the ontological approach to accommodate for the internal validity of the unified grammar. We acknowledge that our unified modeling language has not yet been empirically validated. Our hope is that peer discourse and review of our contribution will constitute a preliminary form of validation both for the correctness and effectiveness of the developed model. Next, we plan to expose the BE^2 model to some of the business users in the domain of T&L and agrifood who take part in the FIspace EU project to obtain their feedback as a further mechanism for empirical validation of our work.

References

1. ACSI: The ACSI FP7 EU Project, http://www.acsi-project.eu/deliverables/
2. Brambilla, M. et al.: Model-Driven Software Engineering in Practice. (2012)
3. Bunge, M.: A World of Systems, Treatise on Basic Philosophy, Vol. 4. Reidel (1979)
4. Bunge, M.: The Furniture of the World, Treatise on Basic Philosophy, Vol. 3. Springer (1977)
5. Cohn, D., Hull, R.: Business artifacts: A data-centric approach to modeling business operations and processes. IEEE Data Eng. Bull. 32(3), 3–9 (2009)
6. Etzion, O., Adkins, J.M.: Tutorial: why is event-driven thinking different from traditional thinking about computing? DEBS. pp. 269–270 (2013)
7. Etzion, O., von Halle, B.: The Event Model, http://www.slideshare.net/opher.etzion/er-2013-tutorial-modeling-the-event-driven-world
8. Etzion, O., Niblett, P.: Event Processing in Action. (2010)
9. FIspace: The FIspace FP7 EU Project, http://www.fispace.eu/deliverable.html
10. Hull, R. et al.: Business Artifacts with Guard-Stage-Milestone Lifecycles: Managing Artifact Interactions with Conditions and Events. ACM Intl. Conf. on Distributed Event-based Systems (DEBS). (2011)
11. Hull, R. et al.: Introducing the Guard-Stage-Milestone Approach for Specifying Business Entity Lifecycles. Proc. of 7th Intl. Workshop on Web Services and Formal Methods (WS-FM 2010). Springer, LNCS (2010)
12. Limonad, L. et al.: The WaaSaBE Model: Marrying WaaS and Business-Entities to Support Cross-Organization Collaboration. SRII. pp. 303–312 (2012)
13. Nigam, A., Caswell, N.S.: Business artifacts: An approach to operational specification. IBM Syst. J. 42(3), 428–445 (2003)
14. Searle, J.R.: Social ontology. Anthropol. Theory. 6(1), 12–29 (2006)
15. Smith, B., Welty, C.: Ontology: Towards a new synthesis. Form. Ontol. Inf, Syst (2001)
16. Soffer, Pnina, Wand, Yair: Goal-Driven Analysis of Process Model Validity. In: Persson, Anne, Stirna, Janis (eds.) CAiSE 2004. LNCS, vol. 3084, pp. 521–535. Springer, Heidelberg (2004)
17. Sowa, J.F.: Knowledge representation: logical, philosophical, and computational foundations. Brooks Cole Publishing Co. (1999)
18. Wand, Y., Weber, R.: On the Deep Structure of Information Systems. Inf. Syst. J. 5(3), 203–223 (1995)
19. Wand, Y., Weber, R.: On the Ontological Expressiveness of Information Systems Analysis and Design Grammars. Inf. Syst. J. 3(4), 217–237 (1993)

Extending Process Logs with Events from Supplementary Sources

Felix Mannhardt[1,2]([⊠]), Massimiliano de Leoni[1,3], and Hajo A. Reijers[1,2]

[1] Eindhoven University of Technology, Eindhoven, The Netherlands
{f.mannhardt,m.d.leoni,h.a.reijers}@tue.nl
[2] Perceptive Software, Apeldoorn, The Netherlands
[3] University of Padua, Padua, Italy

Abstract. Since organizations typically use more than a single IT system, information about the execution of a process is rarely available in a single event log. More commonly, data is scattered across different locations and unlinked by common case identifiers. We present a method to extend an incomplete main event log with events from supplementary data sources, even though the latter lack references to the cases recorded in the main event log. We establish this correlation by using the control-flow, time, resource, and data perspectives of a process model, as well as alignment diagnostics. We evaluate our approach on a real-life event log and discuss the reliability of the correlation under different circumstances. Our evaluation shows that it is possible to correlate a large portion of the events by using our method.

Keywords: Process mining · Event correlation · Data Petri nets · Process logs

1 Introduction

Information about the execution of processes is stored in event logs of information systems that support, monitor or enact business processes in organizations. Such event logs contain recorded sequences of events (i.e., traces). Each trace typically records the execution of a process instance (i.e., case). As organizations typically use multiple information systems, the information about a single case may be recorded across several event logs that are stored in different locations. We consider one of those logs as the main event log (e.g., the event log written by a central process management system (PMS)) whereas the other event logs are seen as supplementary sources. In such a set-up, insufficient information may be available to link the events from the supplementary sources to cases in the main event log. Most existing process mining techniques require a single event log with the events grouped by cases as input [1], and, as a result, cannot make

The work of Dr. de Leoni is supported by the Eurostars - Eureka project PROMPT (E!6696).

F. Fournier and J. Mendling (Eds.): BPM 2014 Workshops, LNBIP 202, pp. 235–247, 2015.
DOI: 10.1007/978-3-319-15895-2_21

use of such unlinked data. Clearly, it would be beneficial to include supplementary events in an analysis as theses events or the corresponding data may help to get a better understanding of the overall business process.

The goal of this research is to correlate unlinked events from supplementary data sources, i.e., events that have been recorded by additional systems, to the traces of the main event log. The setting for our approach is that of large organizations, e.g., hospitals, banks, car manufacturers, where various semi-autonomous units need to cooperate while using a heterogeneous set of information systems. We assume that supplementary events do not contain data that allows them to be trivially associated to a single trace in the main event log. Hence, simple relational methods that exploit direct dependencies between data cannot be used to solve the problem. Furthermore, we assume that an expert provides domain knowledge about the entire process in the form of a process model, as to identify opportunities to link the various events.

We propose an approach that uses an alignment of the process model and the main event log to correlate supplementary events to the correct traces of the main event log (cf. [2]). Figure 1 gives an overview of the proposed technique. We use existing techniques to compute alignments for the

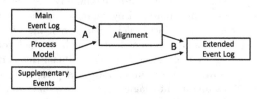

Fig. 1. Overview of the proposed approach

first step, (A). The alignments indicate which traces of the main event log have missing events according to the process model. We assume that those missing events may be found in a set of supplementary events by leveraging information about the control-flow, time, resource, and data perspective of the process model as captured in the alignment. We use this information in the second step, (B), to correlate supplementary events to traces in the main event log. For example, a PMS handling credit requests may require the execution of a *financial check* activity if the *amount* of the credit exceeds €10,000. The *financial check* activity is handled by a financial system and its execution is recorded yet disconnected from the event log of the PMS. Our approach uses the constraint regarding the credit *amount* to correlate the correct events e.g., the supplementary *financial check* events will only be correlated to traces referring to credit requests of more than €10,000.

In the literature, a few techniques have already been proposed to solve similar problems. In [3] a genetic approach, based on an artificial immune system, is used to merge multiple traces that most likely belong to the same case. While this work displays similarities to ours, it does not use an existing process model as input. As such, it cannot exploit available expert knowledge. Moreover, being a genetic approach, it is likely to be slow when applied to a large data set. In fact, [3] reports an execution time of up to 10 min on a small data set of 8,500 traces. The approach in [4] tries to group events that belong to a case from a relational database of an ERP system by using the foreign-key relations in such databases. The work [5] describes a method to correlate events based an common attributes in the setting of web service interactions. The common assumption in [4,5] is that there is a conceptual diagram (e.g. an ER model) that can be used to link events from different sources. These approaches would not be applicable in our setting, as we explicitly assume that no such relation is defined. In [6], the input is a stream of events without case identifiers that are clustered into traces by using sequence partitioning. This technique builds only on the event name, does not make use of other data associated to the event and, therefore, only returns traces of events without data attributes. The approach presented in [7] can be used to build an event log with uniform event names out of two event logs recording executions of the same process, where events referring to the same activity have different names. This work differs from ours as traces in the first event log are not extended with events from the second event log.

This paper contributes a new technique that addresses the problem of disconnected data sources for event data. The technique employs both an alignment of observed event data with a process model and constraints defined by the control-flow, time, resource, and data perspectives of the process model to correlate events.

The remainder of the paper is organized as follows. Section 2 introduces preliminaries such as process models and event logs. In Sect. 3 the technique is presented. A short evaluation using a real-life event log is discussed in Sect. 4. Finally, Sect. 5 concludes with a summary and sketches future work.

2   Preliminaries

We introduce preliminaries such as *Petri net with data* (DPN-net), *Event-Log* and *Alignment* that are needed to describe our approach.

A DPN-net extends a Petri net [8] with transitions that can write variables [2]. Transitions perform *write operations* on a set of given variables and may define a data-dependent guard. Transitions can fire only if all their input places are marked and their guard is satisfied. A guard can be formulated as an expression over the process variables. We denote with *Formulas(X)* the universe of such expressions defined over a set X of variables.

Definition 1 (DPN-net). *A DPN-net $N = (P, T, F, V, U, Val, W, G)$ is defined as:*

- *a Petri net (P, T, F);*
- *a set V of variables;*
- *a set U of variable values;*
- *a function $Val : V \rightarrow 2^U$ that defines the values admissible for each variable $v \in V$, i.e. $Val(v)$ is the domain of variable v;*
- *a write function $W : T \rightarrow 2^V$ that labels each transition with a set of write operations, i.e. with the set of variables whose value needs to be written/ updated;*
- *a guard function $G : T \rightarrow Formulas(V \cup \{v' \mid v \in V\})$ that associates each transition with a different guard.[1]*

---

[1] If a transition t should be associated with no guard, we set $G(t) = $ true.

When a variable $v \in V$ appears in a guard $G(t)$, it refers to the value just before the occurrence of t. If $v \in W(t)$, it can also appear as v' and refer to the value after the occurrence of t. Constraints on the resource and time perspective of a process can be encoded by using variables, write operations and guards of a DPN-net as shown in [2].

In the following we give an example of a DPN-net adapted from [2], which models the handling of road traffic fines by the local police in Italy.

Example 1. The DPN-net of this example is shown in Fig. 2, whereas Table 1 shows the guards associated with the DPN-net transitions. The process starts with recording the *Amount* that needs to be paid and possibly any *Points* to be deducted from the driver's license. Throughout the process the offender can pay the full fine or parts of it; the actual payment is recorded in the *Payment* variable. Whenever the fine is sent to the offender, additional postal *Expenses* need to be paid. Moreover, if the offender does not pay the fine timely, a penalty amount can be added to the fine. The offender can appeal against the fine, both

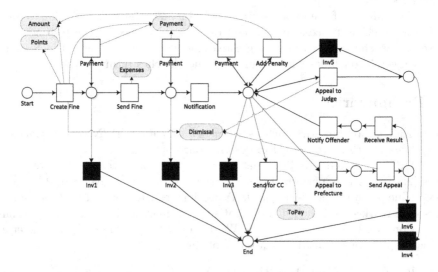

Fig. 2. DPN-net of the road traffic fine management process [2]

Table 1. Guards of the road traffic fine management DPN-net.

Transition(s)	Guard
Send for CC	ToPay' = Amount + Expenses − Payment ∧ ToPay' > 0
Inv2, Inv3	Payment = Amount + Expenses
Inv1	(Dismissal != NIL) ∨ (Payment = Amount ∧ Points = 0)
Receive Result, Inv5	Dismissal = NIL
Inv4	Dismissal = #
Inv6	Dismissal = G

through a judge or the prefecture. The result is recorded in the variable *Dismissal* and used to decide whether the process may stop. Finally, if the fine is not paid in full, the amount *ToPay* is send for credit collection (transition *Send for CC*).

Given a set X, $\mathbb{B}(X)$ denotes the set of all multi-sets over a set X. The set of possible *states* of N is formed by all pairs (M, A) where $M \in \mathbb{B}(P)$ is a marking of Petri net (P, T, F), i.e. a multi-set of the places in P, and A is a function that associates a value with each variable, i.e. $A : V \rightarrow U \cup \{\bot\}$, with $A(v) \in Val(v) \cup \{\bot\}$ for each $v \in V$. A special value $\bot$ is assigned to variables that have not been initialized.

A *transition firing* s is a pair $(t, w) \in T \times (V \nrightarrow U)$.[2] We introduce the following functions to easily access the components of a transition firing $s = (t, w)$: $\#_{vars}(s) = w$ and $\#_{act}(s) = t$. Function $\#_{vars}$ is also overloaded such that $\#_{vars}(s, v) = w(v)$ if $v \in \mathsf{dom}(\#_{vars}(s))$, or $\#_{vars}(s, v) = \bot$ if $v \notin \mathsf{dom}(\#_{vars}(s))$. We denote the set of possible transition firings, both valid and invalid, for a DPN-net N as S_N, i.e. $S_N = T \times (V \nrightarrow U)$. A sequence $\sigma \in S_N^*$ is called a **process trace**. Each DPN-net defines two special markings M_I, M_F: the initial and final marking. The initial state of a DPN-net is (M_I, A_I) with $A_I(v) = \bot$ for each $v \in V$. A non-empty set of *final states* exists and includes every state (M, A) with $M = M_F$. In any state, zero or more transitions of a DPN-net may be able to fire (i.e., occur). In the remainder, $\mathcal{P}_{N,M_I,M_F}$ denotes the **set of valid process traces** of a DPN-net N, i.e. the sequence of transition firings that, from the initial marking M_I, lead to final marking M_F. Readers are referred to [2] for more details.

Definition 2 (Event & Event Log). *Let $N = (P, T, F, V, U, Val, W, G)$ be a DPN-net and let S_N be the set of possible transition firings of N. An event $s_L \in S_N$ is the recording of a transition firing. A log trace $\sigma_L \in S_N^*$ is a sequence of events. An* event log *over N is a multi-set of traces: $L \in \mathbb{B}(S_N^*)$.*

Each event writes a value for a special variable *time* $\in V$ that indicates the timestamp of its occurrence; we use $\#_{time}(s_L) = \#_{vars}(s_L, time)$ to easily access the timestamp of any event s_L. We assume that L only contains events that are part of the DPN-net N. Any event referring to a transition that is not part of the process model is filtered out.

We can relate a trace σ_L of an event log L to a process model N by computing an alignment that shows where the trace deviates from the allowed behavior according to the process model. Such an alignment relates "moves" in the firing sequences of the trace to "moves" in firing sequences of the model. In case a "move" cannot be related, we explicitly denote such "no moves" by $\gg$. Table 2 shows such an alignment between a log trace and the DPN-net from Example 1.

Definition 3 (Alignment). *Let $N = (P, T, F, V, U, Val, W, G)$ be a DPN-net with initial marking M_I and final marking M_F. Let $S_N^{\gg} = S_N \cup \{\gg\}$. A legal move in an alignment is represented by a pair $(s_L, s_M) \in (S_N^{\gg} \times S_N^{\gg}) \setminus \{(\gg, \gg)\}$ such that*

---

[2] We use $\nrightarrow$ to denote a partial function.

Table 2. Alignment of a log trace the road fines management DPN-net

Event-log trace	Process
Create Fine {**Amount** = 36.0, **Payment** = 0.0, **Points** = 0}	Create Fine {**Amount** = 36.0, **Payment** = 0.0, **Points** = 0}
≫	Send Fine {**Expenses** = 10.0}
Notification	Notification
Payment {**Payment** = 46.0}	Payment {**Payment** = 46.0}
≫	Inv3

- (s_L, s_M) *is a* move in log *if* $s_L \in S_N$ *and* $s_M = \gg$,
- (s_L, s_M) *is a* move in model *if* $s_L = \gg$ *and* $s_M \in S_N$,
- (s_L, s_M) *is a* move in both with correct write operations *if* $s_L \in S_N$, $s_M \in S_N$ *and* $\#_{act}(s_L) = \#_{act}(s_M)$ *and* $\forall v \in V$ $\#_{vars}(s_L, v) = \#_{vars}(s_M, v)$,
- (s_L, s_M) *is a* move in both with incorrect write operations *if* $s_L \in S_N$, $s_M \in S_N$ *and* $\#_{act}(s_L) = \#_{act}(s_M)$ *and* $\exists v \in V$ $\#_{vars}(s_L, v) \neq \#_{vars}(s_M, v)$,

All other moves are considered as illegal. $\mathcal{A}_N = \{(s_L, s_M) \in (S_N^{\gg} \times S_N^{\gg}) \setminus \{(\gg, \gg)\} \mid s_L = \gg \vee s_M = \gg \vee \#_{act}(s_L) = \#_{act}(s_M)\}$ *is the set of all legal moves. The alignment of two execution traces* $\sigma', \sigma'' \in S_N^*$ *is a sequence* $\gamma \in \mathcal{A}_N^*$ *such that, ignoring all occurrences of* $\gg$, *the projection on the first element yields* σ' *and the projection on the second yields* σ''. *An alignment is a complete alignment of a log trace* σ_L *and a DPN-net N, if* $\sigma' = \sigma_L$ *and* $\sigma'' \in \mathcal{P}_{N, M_I, M_F}$.

Given an alignment γ of a log trace σ_L and a process trace σ_P, $\gamma|_L = \sigma_L$ and $\gamma|_P = \sigma_P$ are referred to as the log and the process projection of γ. Each alignment is associated with a cost that accounts for deviations; the cost of an alignment is the sum of the cost of its constituent moves. The cost of moves is defined by a process analyst since it depends on the specific domain. It can be abstracted as a cost-function $\kappa : \mathcal{A}_N \to \mathbb{R}_0^+$, which associates a non-negative cost to each potential move.

Work [2] reports on a technique to compute a so-called **optimal alignment**, i.e. one of the alignments with the lowest cost. Given a log trace and a DPN-net, this technique returns a complete alignment such that any other possible complete alignment has the same or higher cost.

3   Extending Process Logs Based on Alignments

This section describes our technique to extend process logs with events that are extracted from additional sources. The main input of the algorithm is *(1.)* a DPN-net $N = (P, T, F, V, U, Val, W, G)$ with a given initial and final marking; *(2.)* an event log $L \in \mathbb{B}(S_N^*)$ that records the firings of transitions belonging to some set $T' \subset T$; and *(3.)* a multiset of events $C \in \mathbb{B}(S_N)$, called *event candidates*, which records the firings of transitions belonging to some set $T \setminus T'$.

Our technique aims to extend log traces in $\sigma_L \in L$ by adding events in C to σ_L in the most likely position, while guaranteeing that the alignment is still a complete one. The event candidates are assumed to not contain data that allows us to trivially associate them with a trace of L (such as a trace identifier compatible with those in L).

The alignment of any log trace $\sigma_L \in L$ with N may contain a number of moves in model, each of which indicates a transition firing that was not recorded in σ_L but *should* have been observed. This missing transition firing can have two causes. The first is that it did not happen in reality at all (e.g., a process participant did not execute the expected activity deliberately or by mistake); the second reason is that it did happen but was not recorded in σ_L. Our technique elaborates a basic idea according to which a missing event (i.e. a recording of a transition firing) can possibly be found among the event candidates if it occurred. Often, this is not as easy as it may seem. On the one hand, many event candidates may be found suitable; therefore, additional criteria need to be considered to restrict them further. On the other hand, for some missing events no candidate may be found because, for example, the transition did not fire in reality.

To give the reader an idea on how we restrict the number of suitable event candidates, we restrict the suitable event candidates in the three following steps:

1. compute the event set $C_1 \subseteq C$ of the events that relate to the correct missing activity;
2. compute the event set $C_2 \subseteq C_1$ that contains events that have compatible timestamps with the missing event;
3. compute the event set $C_3 \subseteq C_2$ with events that conform to all data requirements of the DPN-net and, thus, are allowed to be performed in that position in the trace.

In the following, we describe our technique stepwise as shown in Algorithm 1. First, we compute an optimal alignment of each trace $\sigma_L \in L$ and N and add them to a set $\mathcal{I}$, using, e.g., the technique discussed in [2]. Variable k denotes the maximum number of event candidates that can be associated with a model move in order for a candidate to be chosen in that set. Initially, k is set to 1, which indicates that no event candidate is selected if there are potentially more than 1. The idea is that, if there are more suitable candidates, each has a lower probability to be the right one. Therefore, we only allow a candidate to be associated with a move in model if it is the only candidate. At each step of the iteration, we double this number (see line 18). This relaxation of the constraint continues until the user-defined matching limit l_M is reached, or all event candidates have been matched.

As described before, the set of *matching events* for each *move in model* $(\gg, s_m^i)$ of every alignment $\gamma \in \mathcal{I}$ is refined stepwise. From line 6 to line 10, we compute the set C_1, C_2, C_3 introduced above. As mentioned after Definition 2, each event e is associated with the timestamp $\#_{time}(e)$ of its occurrence. To determine whether an event candidate should be retained for a model

---

Algorithm 1. extendLogTraces

Input: DPN-net (N), Initial and Final Marking (M_I, M_F), Event Log (L), Event
       Candidates (C), Matching Limit (l_M)
Result: Extended Event Log (L_C)

1   $\mathcal{I} \leftarrow \bigcup_{\sigma_L \in L}$ align(N, M_I, M_F, σ_L)
2   $k \leftarrow 1$
3   **while** $k \leq l_M$ and $C \neq \varnothing$ **do**
4   **foreach** $\gamma \leftarrow \langle (s_L^1, s_M^1), \ldots, (s_L^n, s_M^n) \rangle \in \mathcal{I}$ **do**
5   **foreach** $(s_L^i, s_M^i) \in \gamma$, s.t. $s_L^i = \gg$ **do**
6              $C_1 \leftarrow \{s_C \in C \mid \#_{act}(s_C) = \#_{act}(s_M^i)\}$
7              $t_E \leftarrow$ earliestTime$_N (\gamma, s_M^i)$
8              $t_L \leftarrow$ latestTime$_N (\gamma, s_M^i)$
9              $C_2 \leftarrow \{s_C \in C_1 \mid t_E < \#_{time}(s_C) < t_L\}$
10            $C_3 \leftarrow \{s_C \in C_2 \mid$ replaceMove$(\gamma, i, (s_C, s_C))|_P \in \mathcal{P}_{N, M_I, M_F}\}$
11   **if** $1 \leq |C_3| \leq k$ **then**
12                $s_L \leftarrow$ selectEvent$(\frac{t_E + t_L}{2}, C_3)$
13                $C \leftarrow C \setminus \{s_L\}$
14                $\mathcal{I} \leftarrow (\mathcal{I} \setminus \gamma) \cup$ replaceMove$(\gamma, i, (s_L, s_L))$
15   **end**
16   **end**
17   **end**
18      $k \leftarrow 2k$
19 **end**
20 **return** $\bigcup_{\gamma \in \mathcal{I}} \gamma|_L$

---

move $(\gg, s_m^i)$, we determine the earliest time and latest time in which transition firing s_m^i can occur (lines 7–8). The earliest time is the largest timestamp in the process projection of γ that refers to transitions that in DPN-net $N = (P, T, F, V, U, Val, W, G)$ comes before $\#_{act}(s_M^i)$. We call such a set[3]:

$$\mathbf{preS}_N(\gamma, s) = \{s' \in \gamma|_P \mid \#_{time}(s') < \#_{time}(s)$$
$$\wedge \exists p \in {}^\bullet \#_{act}(s), \ \#_{act}(s') \in {}^\bullet p\}.$$

Given a user-defined time interval b_E, the earliest time function is defined as follows:[4]

$$\mathbf{earliestTime}_N(\gamma, s_M^i) = \begin{cases} \#_{time}(\mathbf{first}(\gamma|_L)) - b_E & \text{if } \mathbf{preS}_N(\gamma, s_M^i) = \varnothing \\ max_{s_M^j \in \mathbf{preS}_N(\gamma, s_M^i)}(\#_{time}(s_M^j)) & \text{else.} \end{cases}$$

The latest time is the earliest timestamp in the process project of γ. Space limitation prevents us from discussing the latest time in detail. However, the latest timestamp refers to the smallest timestamp in the process projection of γ that refers to transitions that in DPN-net $N = (P, T, F, V, U, Val, W, G)$ comes after $\#_{act}(s_M^i)$.

In sum, the subset C_1 of C has been computed by considering the control-flow perspective, whereas subset C_2 of C_1 (and of C) has been determined by considering the time perspective. To reduce the set of possible candidate of C further, the data perspective is also taken into account. A candidate s_C in C_2

---

[3] The preset of a transition t is the set of its input places: ${}^\bullet t = \{p \in P \mid (p, t) \in F\}$.
  The preset of a place p is the set of its input transitions: ${}^\bullet p = \{t \in T \mid (t, p) \in F\}$.
[4] We use $\mathbf{first}(\sigma)$ to indicate the first element of the sequence σ.

is also part of C_3 if we can replace the i-th move (in model) in alignment γ with $(s_C, s_C)^5$, and the resulting alignment is such that the process projection is still a valid process trace. This guarantees that event s_C at the i-th position conforms to the data, time and resource-perspective constraints as defined by the DPN-net N. Therefore, C_3 is the final set of event candidates.

As mentioned before, if the number of candidates is fewer than k, one is chosen. Otherwise, no candidate is chosen; possibly, one will be chosen at one of the subsequent iterations with increased k. The reason why we decide to use an incrementing k is related to fact that, first, we want to associate event candidates with traces that have higher certainty to represent the correct matching. In this way, the event candidate set becomes smaller, which also decreases the level of uncertainty for those matchings that were not sufficiently certain beforehand.

If one candidate needs to be chosen, we select the one s_L closer to the middle point between the earliest and latest time (line 12).[6] We use the middle point assuming that the waiting time between events is similar for each event. Event s_L is removed from the event candidates (line 13) and alignment is substituted by one in which the i-th move is replaced with (s_L, s_L) (line 14).

We conclude by sketching an informal discussion about the computational complexity of Algorithm 1. In the worst case, the *while* loop is repeated $\log(l_M)$ times; internally, the double *for-each* loop is repeated as many times as the overall number of model moves, which are of the same order of magnitude as the number of events in the event log. Each iteration of the double for-each loop is composed by steps that are either linear in the length of the alignments (e.g., line 7) or in the size of the event-candidate set (e.g., line 6, 9 or 10). In light of this, computing the set $\mathcal{I}$ of alignments dominates the worst-case complexity: as discussed in [2], computing optimal alignments is, in the worst case, double exponential in the size of the log trace and number of variables and guards.

4   Evaluation

We implemented the approach as a plug-in for the open-source process mining framework ProM[7]. This section reports on the evaluation on a real-life case study about the process to manage road-traffic fines by an Italian local police. The process follows the process model discussed in Example 1. The event log contained 543,583 events grouped into 145,800 traces, out of which 76,600 are recorded process executions that are compliant with the process model[8].

The process is managed through a single information system and, hence, a single event log has been extracted from the transactional database underneath. To validate our technique, we assumed four scenarios:

---

[5] The replacement operation is represented in the algorithm as function `replaceMove`$(\gamma, i, move)$ that return a variation of the alignment γ where the i-th move is replaced by *move*.

[6] `selectEvent`(C, t) denotes the operation of returning the event in a set C with the closest timestamp to t.

[7] http://www.promtools.org.

[8] Available at http://dx.doi.org/10.4121/uuid:270fd440-1057-4fb9-89a9-b699b47990f5.

A: Send Fine (Compliant). An independent system records the execution of transition *Send Fine*. The execution of the other process transitions is supported by a process management system. The latter generates an event log, whereas the former system only logs events without any reference to the trace to which they would belong in the event log. All events from non-compliant traces have been removed.

B: Send Fine. As above, but without removing non-compliant executions.

C: Send for CC (Compliant). The same as in A, but assuming that transition *Send for CC* was logged in a different system, instead of *Send Fine*.

D: Send for CC. As above, but without removing non-compliant executions.

We applied our technique to the four scenarios. For each scenario, we split the original event log L into an event set C and a new event log L' with the remaining events. We defined the cost function for the alignment such that a *move in model* step with events in C is cheaper than any other deviation. Then, we applied our algorithm in this way obtaining a new event log L''. Our goal is to correlate the events in C to the correct traces in L'. In the optimal case the returned event log L'' is equal to L. We evaluate the performance of our approach by using the following four types of correlations:

Perfectly correlated. Events are *perfectly correlated*, if every variable (including time) takes on the same value as in the respective event in the original trace.

Approximately correlated. Events are *approximately correlated*, if the original event refers to the same transition, and the position in the extended trace is the same as in the original trace, but at least one variable has a different value from the one assigned in the original trace.

Wrongly correlated. Events are *wrongly correlated* in case the event was not recorded at the same position in the original trace.

Ignored. All events that remain in the candidate set C and, thus, are not correlated to any trace are *ignored*.

For the evaluation, we express those criteria relative to the number of events in the *candidate set* C. If all events were *perfectly correlated*, the returned event log L'' would be indistinguishable from the original event log L. In reality, the correlation cannot always be perfect. However, for some analysis types, *approximately correlated* events are still valuable, as they are indistinguishable from the original events according to the process model. For example, the exact time that *Send for CC* was executed does not matter for some purposes. It is also possible that an event is correlated to a trace that originally did not contain such an event. We do aim to minimize the number of such *wrongly correlated* events.

The results of the experiments are shown in Table 3 for three different matching limits l_M: 512, 1024 and 2048. Looking at the *% Perfectly* column, the percentage of *perfectly correlated* events, we can see that our approach performs better on perfectly fitting event logs, but still is able to extend up to 40 % of the traces in scenario D. Moreover, in scenario C, with a perfectly fitting log there are no *wrongly correlated* events in contrast to up to 7.3 % wrongly correlated

Table 3. Extending an event log in different scenarios

Scenario	|C|	l_M	% Perfectly	% Approx.	% Wrongly	% Ignored
A: Send Fine (Compliant)	33178	512	22.0	13.9	1.5	62.6
		1024	34.0	30.3	3.1	32.2
		2048	38.6	44.8	5.2	11.3
B: Send Fine	101950	512	5.1	5.1	0.4	89.5
		1024	11.6	15.5	0.8	72.1
		2048	14.1	31.5	1.7	52.8
C: Send for CC (Compliant)	28049	512	29.1	4.3	0	66.6
		1024	51.8	6.1	0	42.1
		2048	69.6	12.4	0	18.1
D: Send for CC	54232	512	20.8	3.6	3.8	71.7
		1024	29.9	4.7	5.6	59.8
		2048	40.3	6.9	7.3	45.5

events in scenario D with a non-perfect log. This could be expected: the problem of having *wrongly correlated* events tends to occur more often if deviations exists between the observed behavior and what the process model allows for, e.g., an event has not occurred. For example, if an original trace in scenario D does not contain the event *Send for CC* even though the fine is unpaid, then the alignment will contain a *move in model* step for *Send for CC*, and an event may get *wrongly correlated*.

It is noteworthy that the *match limit* l_M can be used to steer the reliability of the result. For lower values of l_M, fewer events are *approximately* and *wrongly correlated* at the price of an increase in *ignored* events that are not correlated. Comparing scenario A and scenario B, we noticed the fact that both the percentage of approximately and wrongly correlated events is higher in scenario A, even though only compliant traces have been considered. Moreover, in scenario B, more events are ignored, i.e. 55.8 % in comparison to 11.3 % in scenario A, both for $l_M = 2048$. This observation can be explained by the larger candidate set in scenario B and the choice of the matching limit. For lower values of l_M, fewer events are *approximately* and *wrongly correlated* at the price of an increase in *ignored* events that are not correlated. Using the same matching limit, it is likely that more events are ignored for a larger candidate set, and, conversely, fewer events are approximately or wrongly correlated.

Overall, the approach seems of value. If the process executions are always conformant to the model, log traces are extended with the events referring to the right transition firings (i.e. events) 80 % of the time, although the variable assignments are not always perfect (i.e. approximate correlations). If the process executions are not always conformant, the accuracy of the matching degrades, yet roughly 50 % of the event candidates are perfectly or approximately correlated.

Please note that matching the right events is not straightforward for this event log. For instance, if a trace is extended with an event at the time 9/9/2014 instead of the correct time 8/9/2014, or with an amount of €81 instead of €80, we would already consider it as approximate matching. This difference could be negligible from a domain viewpoint. Especially small time deviations happen often for this particular event log, as there are hundreds of traces concerning the same type of infringement, thus, requiring the same amount to be paid by the offender. There is not enough information in the event log to distinguish between any two of these traces if they are being executed within the same time frame.

Regarding the execution time to extend the event logs with the set of event candidates, each scenario did not take more than 10 min, which we believe to be reasonable given the large sizes of the candidate sets, the number of traces, and the complexity of the approach.

5   Conclusion

In this paper we proposed a novel technique to extend process logs with events from supplementary sources that cannot be trivially linked to specific traces in a main event log. The problem of disconnected event sources is relevant in practice, as organizations typically use multiple information systems, which record events in separate event logs. We use an alignment of a process model and a main event log so that we can leverage on the control-flow, data, and time perspective of the process model to correlate events to a specific case. Our approach ensures that the supplementary events are correlated to traces of the main event log without violating the constraints on the different perspectives. We assume that supplementary events do not contain data that allows to easily associated them to a trace of the main event log.

A few approaches have been proposed in the literature to solve similar problems, but to the best of our knowledge no other research work makes use of the diverse perspectives of a user-supplied process model. A prototype of the technique has been realized in the ProM framework as *LogEnhancement* package. The evaluation shows promising results for a challenging real-life event log.

We acknowledge that our current evaluation is far from complete. For instance, we have only limited ourselves to remove events referring to one single transition type, such as *Send Fine* or *Send for CC*. It would be interesting to evaluate the correlation accuracy when an increasing number of transition types is removed. Similarly, we also aim to verify the approach in more real-life cases to reduce the subjectivity of the results. We aim to have a more thorough evaluation in the near future. For example, we would like to directly compare our technique with the approach proposed in [3]. However, our preliminary evaluation shows that the approach seems to be relevant in real business cases, such as the road-traffic process, which we used for our evaluation. Finally, we want to build on estimations of activity durations and use it to further restrict the possible event candidates based on timestamps.

References

1. van der Aalst, W.M.P.: Process Mining - Discovery, Conformance and Enhancement of Business Processes. Springer, Heidelberg (2011)

2. Mannhardt, F., de Leoni, M., Reijers, H.A., van der Aalst, W.M.P.: Balanced multi-perspective checking of process conformance. Technical report, BPM Center Report BPM-14-07 (2014). BPMcenter.org
3. Claes, J., Poels, G.: Merging computer log files for process mining: an artificial immune system technique. In: Daniel, F., Barkaoui, K., Dustdar, S. (eds.) BPM Workshops 2011, Part I. LNBIP, vol. 99, pp. 99–110. Springer, Heidelberg (2012)
4. Nooijen, E.H.J., van Dongen, B.F., Fahland, D.: Automatic discovery of data-centric and artifact-centric processes. In: La Rosa, M., Soffer, P. (eds.) BPM Workshops 2012. LNBIP, vol. 132, pp. 316–327. Springer, Heidelberg (2013)
5. Motahari-Nezhad, H., Saint-Paul, R., Casati, F., Benatallah, B.: Event correlation for process discovery from web service interaction logs. VLDB J. **20**(3), 417–444 (2011)
6. Walicki, M., Ferreira, D.R.: Sequence partitioning for process mining with unlabeled event logs. Data Knowl. Eng. **70**(10), 821–841 (2011)
7. Zhu, X., Song, S., Wang, J., Yu, P.S., Sun, J.: Matching heterogeneous events with patterns. In: Proceedings of the 2014 30th IEEE International Conference on Data Engineering, ICDE 2014, IEEE, pp. 376–387 (2014)
8. Desel, J., Esparza, J.: Free Choice Petri Nets. Cambridge University Press, Cambridge (1995)

BPI 2014

A Case Study in Workflow Scheduling Driven by Log Data

Mirela Botezatu[1]([✉]), Hagen Völzer[1], and Remco Dijkman[2]

[1] IBM Research – Zurich, Zurich, Switzerland
bot@zurich.ibm.com
[2] Eindhoven University of Technology, Eindhoven, The Netherlands

Abstract. This paper shows through a case study the potential for optimizing resource allocation in business process execution. While most resource allocation mechanisms focus on assigning resources to the tasks that they are authorized to perform, we assign resources to the tasks that they can provably perform most efficiently, by mining the execution logs. This gives rise to the minimization of the cost of the process execution. We present various cost measures and how hybrid algorithms can balance their conflicting goals. Our case study indicates significant potential for further research into optimal resource allocation mechanisms.

Keywords: Mathematical optimization of business processes · Static and dynamic optimization · Performance measurement of business processes · Resource allocation in business processes

1 Introduction

A workflow management system assigns work items to human resources, based on rules that are defined in the resource perspective of a process model [8,22]. This can also be called *scheduling* or *dispatching*. Various forms of scheduling have been studied from a theoretical perspective, by providing patterns of work item assignment that can be supported by workflow management systems [14]. In current workflow management systems, scheduling is primarily based on the availability of resources that match a role that is authorized to execute a work item. In addition, there exist other algorithms that take qualitative properties into account, such as the suitability of a resource for a particular work item [12], or the appropriateness of a resource, given other resources that worked on the same case [7]. All these approaches could be labeled as *qualitative scheduling*.

Because human resources are one of the most significant factors in the operational cost of workflow, it is also interesting to study *quantitative* approaches to scheduling. Scheduling can be quantitative in at least two different ways. First, it can be seen not only as a constraint satisfaction problem but as an optimization problem to minimize certain measures of cost or maximize certain measures of service quality. Second, the suitability of a resource is not a qualitative relation anymore but becomes a measure.

© Springer International Publishing Switzerland 2015
F. Fournier and J. Mendling (Eds.): BPM 2014 Workshops, LNBIP 202, pp. 251–263, 2015.
DOI: 10.1007/978-3-319-15895-2_22

In this paper, we consider the time a person needs to complete a certain type of work item as such a measure of resource suitability. It is clear that such a measure can be obtained and adapted over time from information in execution logs. There are very few prior studies for BPM systems that take work item scheduling as an optimization problem and use a measure of resource suitability. We are not aware of any approaches where work item scheduling is based on execution log data, cf. also Sect. 5.

This approach raises the question to what extent scheduling could be improved if suitability measures and log data is taken into account. In this paper, we show that this approach has substantial potential for saving costs. To do so, we conduct a case study on real data that shows such potential cost savings. The case study also illustrates a typical trade-off between different cost measures and shows how they can be reconciled.

The remainder of the paper is structured as follows. In Sect. 2 we present the concrete scheduling problem, the cost measures and the solution approach. In Sect. 3, we present the case study, how the data was processed and the experiments were conducted. We evaluate our solution by discussing the results in Sect. 4. The related work and the conclusions are presented in Sects. 5 and 6 respectively.

2   A Concrete Scheduling Setting

In this section, we present the setting of the scheduling problem - a high level view of the architecture, and our approach for solving it (i.e. the cost measures considered, the scheduling policies, the event log mining approach, etc.).

2.1   A Scheduling Problem

Scheduling problems can vary considerably as there are many potential parameters that can be considered.

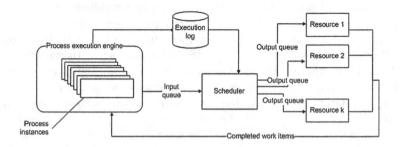

Fig. 1. Setting

Figure 1 illustrates our setting. A process engine executes a set of process instances, which can be multiple instances of multiple process models. The execution produces a stream of instances of user tasks. An instance of a user task is also called a *work item* henceforth. The stream of work items produced complies with the ordering specified by the process models. The stream of work items flows in a queue to a separate component, which we call the *scheduler*. The mentioned queue is the *input queue* of the scheduler.

The scheduler has also n *output queues*, one for each resource. The scheduler successively takes a work item from its input queue and puts it, based on all information available to it, into exactly one of its output queues. Each resource successively takes out a work item from its queue, works on it and completes it before the worker can take a new work item. We assume that every work item needs exactly one worker and the worker completes the item atomically without interruption. We assume that the following information is available to the scheduler:

(a) Out of a finite pool R of resources, the set $A_d \subseteq R$ of those that are *available* on a particular day d.
(b) The next item in its input queue. The scheduler does not know any further items in its input queue, i.e., it cannot buffer work items or look ahead in the queue, i.e., it is an *online scheduler*.
(c) The entire state of each of the output queues as well as their histories.
(d) A static binary relation between workers and work items specifying who can execute which work items. This may specify skill and/or authorization restrictions.
(e) A static mapping that maps each pair of a worker and a work item to an estimated duration of how long this worker needs to complete an work item.

Items (d) and (e) are denoted with the following matrix:

$$
\delta_{r,w} = \begin{pmatrix} \delta_{1,1} & \delta_{1,2} & \cdots & \delta_{1,k} \\ \delta_{2,1} & \delta_{2,2} & \cdots & \delta_{2,k} \\ \vdots & \vdots & \ddots & \vdots \\ \delta_{n,1} & \delta_{n,2} & \cdots & \delta_{n,k} \end{pmatrix} \qquad \delta_{r,w} = \begin{cases} x \in \mathbb{N}, & \text{resource } r \text{ is authorized to work on} \\ & \text{work item type } w \\ \text{Null}, & \text{otherwise.} \end{cases}
$$

When $\delta_{r,w}$ has an integer number as a value, it represents the median duration for the resource r to complete the work item type w.

We assume that we observe this system for a finite number of days. Let σ_r for $r \in R$ denote the history of the r-th output queue, and $\sigma_r[i], i = 1, \ldots, |\sigma_r|$ denote its i-th work item. By σ_d we denote the history of the output queue on a particular day d. By $\sigma_{r,d}$ we denote the history of the output queue of resource r restricted to day d. A *schedule* can be seen as the collection $\sigma = \{\sigma_r \mid r \in R\}$ of the history of the output queues. A schedule gives rise to various definitions of *cost* of a schedule $C(\sigma)$ such as the service time, makespan and load balance, which will be defined in the following. The goal of the scheduler is to minimize the cost of the schedule.

2.2   The Cost Measures

We evaluate various scheduling policies based on the following cost metrics. To this end, we assume that the durations of work item executions are recorded. We denote the execution duration of work item $\sigma_r[i]$ as $\delta(\sigma_r[i])$.

1. *Service time* - the total number of human working hours needed for executing all the work items of a given period. This cost measure is relevant for settings where the resources are paid per hour and one wants to minimize the labor costs.

$$S(\sigma) = \sum_{r \in R} \sum_{i=1}^{|\sigma_r|} \delta(\sigma_r[i])$$

2. *Makespan* - the time difference between the start and end of the execution of all work items in the system measured on a daily basis. This cost measure is important for when it is desirable to minimize the maximum total processing time of any resource, and thus have the set of work items finished as soon as possible. If we denote by t_e the time when the last work item is completed and by t_0 the time when the first work item is started, then for every day d, the makespan is defined as:

$$M_d(\sigma) = t_e(\sigma_d) - t_0(\sigma_d)$$

3. *Variance in the resource load, on a daily basis* - the difference between the most and the least loaded resources in one day. This cost measure is important for when it is wanted to minimize the discrepancies of different resources load.

$$V_d(\sigma) = max|C_{r,d} - C_{p,d}|r, p \in A_d \text{ where } C_{r,d} = \sum_{i=1}^{|\sigma_{r,d}|} \delta(\sigma_{r,d}[i])$$

2.3 Mining Resource Performance

Our approach is based on mining an estimation of the time a resource needs to complete a work item from an execution log. In this paper, we take one of the simplest approaches to this. A work item is an instance of a task, its approximate duration under resource r is the median duration of all instances of the same task in the execution log that were executed by resource r. As usual, we assume that the log identifies for each task instance, who executed it as well as its actual duration. In more refined approaches, one could take into account finer classes of work items that not only take into account which task was instantiated but also task properties such as data values. More sophisticated data mining approaches are required in that case to define suitable work item classes.

2.4 Scheduling Policies

We selected a set of scheduling policies that are relevant for the cost measures we considered and that are simple and fast for being a good fit in an online setting.

Random dispatching - benchmark. This policy dispatches the work items to the available resources randomly. This policy is used as a baseline to assess the benefits of having a data-driven scheduling policy in place.

Greedy exploit best resource. This policy, also named greedy-EBR henceforth, dispatches a newly arrived work item w to the resource that is the most efficient (time wise) in executing it from all the resources that are available that day, i.e. $r \in A_d$, such that $\delta_{r,w}$ is minimal.

Workload balancing. This policy dispatches a newly arrived work item to the resource that has the least accumulated load (within the day) at the moment of the arrival of the new work item from all the resources that are available that day. This policy is also known as list scheduling [6] (work items dispatched upon arrival and the resource is selected to have the minimum load) but on non identical machines. This greedy policy has an important theoretical property - it is a 2-approximation for *makespan scheduling* on identical machines. If resources had identical performance in executing work items, this policy would be at most two times worse than the optimal solution. Note that finding the optimal solution for makespan minimization in job shop scheduling is an NP-hard problem.

A hybrid policy. This policy dispatches work items to the resources taking into account both the performance of one resource in executing a particular work item, and the distribution of load across resources. Thus, we introduce the notion of *suitability* which is defined as follows: For each resource r, the suitability s_r, at time i, has the following value:

$$s_{r,i} = \delta_{r,w_i} * l_{r,i}$$

$s_{r,i}$ represents the suitability of resource r, for working on the work item w_i that has to be executed at time i. On the right side of the equality, δ_{r,w_i} represents the time needed for resource r to execute work item w_i, retrieved from the matrix of estimated durations, and $l_{r,i}$ represents the daily accumulated load of resource r at moment i.

As selecting the best formula based on which we implement the hybrid policy is not straight forward, one could try to find an optimal rule by weighting the factors involved in the product, i.e. $s_{r,i} = f(\delta_{r,w_i}) * g(l_{r,i})$ with suitable functions f and g. Therefore, we also looked at four variants of this formula, where the f and g we involve are $\sqrt{\cdot}$ and log. These functions are representatives of different decaying methods, the *polynomial decay* and the *exponential decay* respectively. These transformations will have also as consequence making the variance more uniform across resources with respect to their performance or load (depending on which metric we apply the function).

We will use the acronyms "Hyb" for the unaltered hybrid policy, and "Hyb_x_y" for the others.

1. Down-weighting the influence of the resource load "Hyb_sq_l":

$$s_{r,i} = \delta_{r,w_i} * \sqrt{l_{r,i}}$$

2. Down-weighting the influence of the resource performance "Hyb_sq_p":

$$s_{r,i} = \sqrt{\delta_{r,w_i}} * l_{r,i}$$

3. Aggressively down-weighting the influence of the resource load "Hyb_lg_l":

$$s_{r,i} = \delta_{r,w_i} * log(l_{r,i})$$

4. Aggressively down-weighting the influence of the resource performance "Hyb_lg_p":

$$s_{r,i} = log(\delta_{r,w_i}) * l_{r,i}$$

3   Case Study

In the following, we present a case study where we show how the resource performance was mined for this particular log, and further compare the policies which are run using as input also the mined resource performance information.

3.1   Data and Data Pre-processing

The data [18] originates from a Dutch Financial Institution, and it consists of events generated along a loan approval process. The logs consist of 262200 events in 13087 cases collected along 6 months. Among the events, we keep the *work item* events which are events that capture the substantial, manual work of the resources (58 in total) of the institution. The work item events are labeled with the state in their life-cycle, namely: "schedule", "start", and "complete". We further keep only "start" and "complete" events. The data contained in each event is the event id, the step in the approval process, whether it is a start/complete or schedule event, the resource id, the time-stamp and the case identifier.

By analyzing [1] the data one can notice that there are more "complete" events than "start" events. As we are interested in the duration of execution of an work item, this discrepancy is misleading. We kept only the first "complete" event associated to the start "event" for the execution of one work item. This choice is motivated by the fact that the second "complete" event was generated at the first hour, the second day, and we assumed it was a system generated event. Having equal number of "start" and "complete" events we compute a vector of durations. Using the pre-processed data we can populate the items (d) and (e) from Sect. 2. We build the matrix $\delta_{r,w}$ which stores the median execution time for each resource for each work item. We use the median as the measure of the center of the distribution because as shown in Fig. 2, the data has a skewed

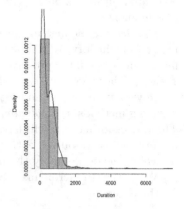

Fig. 2. Distribution of the duration of execution of work item "W_Completeren aanvraag" by resource 11189

distribution and the median is a better measure for the center of the distribution as it is not sensitive to outliers. When populating the matrix, certain entries are

Null. When $\delta_{r,w}$ is Null, it means that there are no records in the data of resource r working on item w, thus we assume that resource r is not authorized to work on work items of type w.

3.2 Running the Experiments

In order to evaluate our scheduling policies, we use the same historical data, both as a training set - to use as input for the scheduling policies - and as a test set - to compare the performance of the policies that we enumerated in Sect. 2.4 on the data. The implementations of the scheduling policies all align to our following assumptions:

1. The maximum working hours of a resource is less than 8 h. When a resource reaches the 8 h of work in one day, the resource is removed from the pool of available resources to which work items can be dispatched on that day.
2. No work items are passed from one day to another. This assumption is enforced by the original data, where the work items are started and completed the same day.
3. When summing up for the total duration of execution (service time) we did not add any waiting time in any of the four policies.

Point 3 is a limitation of our data set and evaluation approach, in which we did not have a process model for the process represented by the log data and hence no information about work item dependencies, which could change the arrival times of the work items in case of our re-assignment. This means that our evaluation assumes that any dependencies between any work items within one particular day are negligible, i.e., do not exist or can be canceled out by finding a suitable re-ordering for the work items of a single resource such that no waiting times arise. This is one (but not the only) aspect where we abstract from the reality of the data set, which points out a direction of refinement in a subsequent future study.

Please note however that all scheduling policies considered here, inclusively the random assignment, work under the same assumption and are in that sense comparable. Note that we do not compare with the actual schedule that the log itself represents.

For the implementation of the policies, we split the data in chunks that cover one working day. For each such chunk, we store a list with all the resources available that day by mining the log for resources that have work items associated to their id in that particular day. We also maintain a queue with the work items that need to be completed that day by extracting from the logs the list of work items that were recorded as started and completed that day.

We run the scheduling policies (Sect. 2.4) on the data. We record the values after running the policies for the service time and makespan, and we analyze the variation of resource load under each policy.

4   Results and Discussion

In the following we will compare the random policy, the greedy-EBR, the work-load balancing and the *baseline version* of the hybrid policy against the performance metrics proposed in Sect. 2.2. We analyze the computational complexity of the policies and finally we discuss the variations of the hybrid policy.

4.1   Comparative Analysis of the Four Different Scheduling Policies

(1) **Service time.** As we can see from Fig. 3, the greedy-EBR policy minimizes the total number of human working hours, being two times better than the hybrid policy, four times better than the workload balancing policy and nine times better than the random dispatching policy.

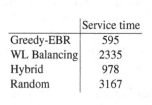

	Service time
Greedy-EBR	595
WL Balancing	2335
Hybrid	978
Random	3167

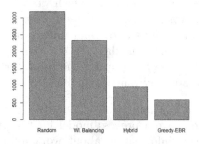

Fig. 3. Service time for the different scheduling policies

(2) **Makespan.** We computed the median makespan as an aggregate measure. We used the median because from Fig. 4 we see again outliers in the daily makespan for the greedy-EBR and random policies.

Table 1. Median makespan

	Makespan
Greedy-EBR	2.64
WL Balancing	1.09
Hybrid	1.10
Random	2.8

As we may see in Table 1, the best makespan is achieved implementing the workload balancing policy. The hybrid policy performs almost equally well. As it tries to load the resources considering both the performance and the occupancy of each resource, it exploits well the parallelism that the existence of multiple resources offers. We notice that the workload balancing policy and the hybrid

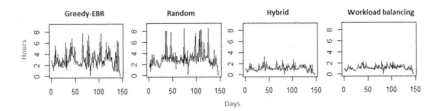

Fig. 4. Plot of the daily makespan for the 4 policies

policy are approximately two times better than both the greedy-EBR and the random policy in terms of daily makespan. The same reality is reflected in the plots in Fig. 4. Also, in Fig. 4, we may see that the makespan is not smooth for the greedy-EBR or in the random policy and this may be also explained by the variance in the workload in the institution.

(3) **Variance in the resource load.** The plots in Fig. 5 represent the smoothed daily difference between the most and the least loaded resource (left) and the standard deviation in the resource load (right), for the four dispatching policies. We smoothed the graph, as we want to depict the important trend in the data, while minimizing the noise generated when representing the "signal" at a very fine granularity. For smoothing, we used the simple moving average filter with time window of five days.

The discrepancy is more stable on a daily basis when the hybrid policy or the workload balancing policy are in place, as for these policies, we can see a rather smooth plot, with very few spikes. The random policy causes the largest discrepancies, as it randomly samples resources disregarding both load balancing and the resources performance. The greedy-EBR policy also causes high discrepancies as it greedily loads the best resource in executing a certain work item.

Computational complexity of the policies: In the following we analyze the complexity of each policy. This is relevant as in an online setting the policies should provide the decision of who works on which work item fast.

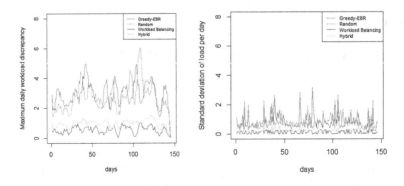

Fig. 5. Maximum difference (left), Standard deviation (right)

We assume the matrix with median duration for the execution of the work items by resources was computed offline and we don't take the complexity of computing it into account. We will note as n the total number of resources.

Greedy-EBR: The matrix with the median durations for resources executing work items can be modified once offline, so that each column vector is sorted by duration. In order to implement the greedy-EBR policy, whenever a new work item needs to be dispatched to a resource, one needs to select the column in the durations matrix that corresponds to the type of the work item that has arrived and select among the available resources that day, the one with the minimum duration. Having the columns sorted, retrieving the minimum can be achieved in constant time.

Workload balancing: For the workload balancing policy, one needs to dispatch the work item to the least loaded resource at that moment. Therefore again, the minimum has to be selected from the values of occupancies per resource. With an appropriate data structure for updating/retrieving the min of the occupancies of the resources (such as a balanced binary search tree), this operation can be performed in logarithmic time, therefore $O(log(n))$.

Hybrid: For the hybrid policy, one needs to update the resources vector of suitability for each work item and extract the minimum from it. As mentioned in the workload balancing policy complexity analysis, with appropriate data structure, the operations can be executed in logarithmic time in the size of the vector. Therefore two $O(log(n))$ operations need to be executed thus the complexity is $O(log(n))$.

The random dispatching policy is not considered for its time complexity because it is only used as a comparison and not intended to be used in a real scheduler.

4.2   Comparative Analysis of the Variations of the Hybrid Policy

After analyzing the policies based on the measures proposed in Sect. 2, we look further into the performance of the variations of the hybrid policy, based on two metrics: service time and makespan. The computational complexity is roughly the same for the variations (the run-time difference would be given by the additional cycles incurred by the weighting functions log and $\sqrt{\cdot}$).

Table 2. Results for the variants of the hybrid policy

	Hyb	Hyb_sq_l	Hyb_sq_p	Hyb_lg_l	Hyb_lg_p
Service time	978	798	1140	712	1280
Makespan	1.1	1.58	0.81	2.2	0.67

As shown in Table 2, none of the variants improves both metrics simultaneously but improves one at the cost of a degradation in the other. Thus "Hyb_sq_l" out-performs "Hyb" in terms of human working hours, achieving 18 % improvement while increasing the median of the daily makespan by 43 %. Also "Hyb_sq_p" outperforms "Hyb" in terms of the median of the daily makespan, decreasing it by 16 %, at the cost of 26 % increase in the number of human working hours. "Hyb_lg_l" improves the number of human working hours achieved using "Hyb" by 27 %, but it doubles the makespan. Implementing "Hyb_lg_p" results in 30 % increase in the number of human working hours, but achieves the best makespan - 40 % lower than the one obtained implementing "Hyb".

5   Related Work

Scheduling in workflows for performance gains has received attention along the years and it has been tackled mostly through analytical methods such as queuing theory, linear programming [2,4,15] or through algorithmic approaches which devise a formula as a function of suitability, urgency, conformance, availability, load [5,8,18]. We identified that not too much attention was paid to leveraging logged data for optimal scheduling.

Data mining can be used in the context of scheduling either for mining existing rules either for proposing scheduling solutions. We have seen that this combination of data mining and scheduling was exploited in the field of manufacturing or production planning in works such as [3,11] where the authors use it to decide the most appropriate dispatching rule at a certain moment, or at a certain state of the system. Authors in [16,17] use data mining to identify patterns for optimal dispatching rules engaging supervised machine learning algorithms.

Recently, data mining for work dispatching has been investigated also on workflow event logs either by mining existing dispatching rules produced by mathematical optimization techniques such as tabu search [10,13] or by proposing the suitable resources [9,20,21]. Through our work we also aim at proposing suitable resources to effectuate a certain work item, but our approach is different in the sense that while in [9,20] the focus falls on a more accurate prediction of resource performance our focus is on optimizing cost investigating online dispatching rules, with a satisfactory approximation matrix of resource performance. The authors in [21] dispatch a set of resources for the whole business process at a time, while we work on a different granularity, dispatching a resource for each ready work item, as it is mandated in an online setting.

6   Conclusion

While this is only a first case study for a novel approach where we take some but not all aspects of a realistic data set into account, our experimental results confirm the relevance of considering execution log data in a dispatching policy. The greedy-EBR policy achieves a 5 times improvement in the service time compared to the random policy and the workload balancing policy achieves a 2.7 times reduction of the makespan compared to the random policy. The trade-offs are also apparent in the results, as the benefit in service time achieved by the greedy-EBR policy is paid with the large makespan and the large discrepancies in the resources load. We showed to what extent a hybrid policy can trade off these conflicting goals by devising a weighted formula that can be adjusted to fit the business needs.

A scheduling component could be easily embedded into the architecture of a business process execution engine. In order for the scheduler to make use of the new data generated by the engine, we would propose an incremental schema to feed the scheduler by sending the new data to it in batches, one at a time, so that the scheduler can update itself appropriately.

Our study does not consider the preference of a particular resource in executing a certain work item. This could be considered in future work. We would further look into modeling of the resource performance as a time series and investigate whether patterns could be extracted (trend, seasonal variation) that could give additional insight. We would also analyze the effect the dependencies have on the metrics we proposed.

References

1. Code for the analysis. https://www.dropbox.com/s/kzl847rk0f48lbt/code.zip.pgp - pwd: P$P3119-515-FF$ $sdcB8-1
2. Baggio, G., Wainer, J., Ellis, C.: Applying scheduling techniques to minimize the number of late jobs in workflow systems. In: Proceedings of the 2004 ACM Symposium on Applied Computing, SAC 2004, pp. 1396–1403. ACM, New York (2004)
3. Baykasoğlu, A., Göçken, M., Özbakir, L.: Genetic programming based data mining approach to dispatching rule selection in a simulated job shop. Simulation **86**(12), 715–728 (2010)
4. Buzacott, J.A., Yao, D.D.: On queueing network models of flexible manufacturing systems. Queueing Syst. **1**(1), 5–27 (1986)
5. Combi, C., Pozzi, G.: Task scheduling for a temporalworkflow management system. In: 2006 Thirteenth International Symposium on Temporal Representation and Reasoning, TIME 2006, pp. 61–68, June 2006
6. Graham, R.L.: Bounds for certain multi-processing anomalies. Bell Syst. Tech. J. **45**(9), 1563–1581 (1966)
7. Kumar, A., Dijkman, R., Song, M.: Optimal resource assignment in workflows for maximizing cooperation. In: Daniel, F., Wang, J., Weber, B. (eds.) BPM 2013. LNCS, vol. 8094, pp. 235–250. Springer, Heidelberg (2013)
8. Kumar, A., Van Der Aalst, W.M.P., Verbeek, E.M.W.: Dynamic work distribution in workflow management systems: How to balance quality and performance. J. Manage. Inf. Syst. **18**(3), 157–193 (2002)
9. Liu, Y., Wang, J., Yang, Y., Sun, J.: A semi-automatic approach for workflow staff assignment. Comput. Indus. **59**(5), 463–476 (2008)
10. Ly, L.T., Rinderle, S., Dadam, P., Reichert, M.: Mining staff assignment rules from event-based data. In: Bussler, C.J., Haller, A. (eds.) BPM 2005. LNCS, vol. 3812, pp. 177–190. Springer, Heidelberg (2006)
11. Priore, P., De La Fuente, D., Gomez, A., Puente, J.: A review of machine learning in dynamic scheduling of flexible manufacturing systems. AI EDAM **15**(3), 251–263 (2001)

12. Reijers, H.A., Jansen-Vullers, M.H., zur Muehlen, M., Appl, W.: Workflow management systems + swarm intelligence = dynamic task assignment for emergency management applications. In: Alonso, G., Dadam, P., Rosemann, M. (eds.) BPM 2007. LNCS, vol. 4714, pp. 125–140. Springer, Heidelberg (2007)
13. Rinderle-Ma, S., van der Aalst, W.M.P.: Life-cycle support for staff assignment rules in process-aware information systems. Technical report, TU Eindhoven (2007)
14. Russell, N., van der Aalst, W.M.P., ter Hofstede, A.H.M., Edmond, D.: Workflow resource patterns: identification, representation and tool support. In: Pastor, Ó., Falcão e Cunha, J. (eds.) CAiSE 2005. LNCS, vol. 3520, pp. 216–232. Springer, Heidelberg (2005)
15. Jin, H.S., Myoung, H.K.: Improving the performance of time-constrained workflow processing. J. Syst. Softw. 58(3), 211–219 (2001)
16. Baskar, N., Premalatha, S.: Implementation of supervised statistical data mining algorithm for single machine scheduling. J. Adv. Manage. Res. 9(2), 170–177 (2012)
17. Shahzad, A., Mebarki, N.: Data mining based job dispatching using hybrid simulation-optimization approach for shop scheduling problem. Eng. Appl. Artif. Intell. 25(6), 1173–1181 (2012)
18. van Dongen, B.F.: Event log for the bpi challenge (2012). http://dx.doi.org/10.4121/uuid:3926db30-f712-4394-aebc-75976070e91f
19. Xu, J., Liu, C., Zhao, X., Yongchareon, S.: Business process scheduling with resource availability constraints. In: Meersman, R., Dillon, T.S., Herrero, P. (eds.) OTM 2010. LNCS, vol. 6426, pp. 419–427. Springer, Heidelberg (2010)
20. Xu, Z., Song, B.: A machine learning application for human resource data mining problem. In: Ng, W.-K., Kitsuregawa, M., Li, J., Chang, K. (eds.) PAKDD 2006. LNCS (LNAI), vol. 3918, pp. 847–856. Springer, Heidelberg (2006)
21. Yang, H., Wang, C., Liu, Y., Wang, J.: An optimal approach for workflow staff assignment based on hidden markov models. In: Meersman, R., Tari, Z., Herrero, P. (eds.) OTM-WS 2008. LNCS, vol. 5333, pp. 24–26. Springer, Heidelberg (2008)
22. Muehlen, Z.: M.: Organizational management in workflow applications - issues and perspectives. Inf. Technol. Manage. 5(3–4), 271–291 (2004)

Decomposed Process Mining: The ILP Case

H.M.W. Verbeek[✉] and Wil M.P. van der Aalst

Department of Mathematics and Computer Science,
Eindhoven University of Technology, Eindhoven, The Netherlands
{h.m.w.verbeek,w.m.p.v.d.aaalst}@tue.nl

Abstract. Over the last decade process mining techniques have matured and more and more organizations started to use process mining to analyze their operational processes. The current hype around "big data" illustrates the desire to analyze ever-growing data sets. Process mining starts from event logs—multisets of traces (sequences of events)—and for the widespread application of process mining it is vital to be able to handle "big event logs". Some event logs are "big" because they contain many traces. Others are big in terms of different activities. Most of the more advanced process mining algorithms (both for process discovery and conformance checking) scale very badly in the number of activities. For these algorithms, it could help if we could split the big event log (containing many activities) into a collection of smaller event logs (which each contain fewer activities), run the algorithm on each of these smaller logs, and merge the results into a single result. This paper introduces a *generic framework* for doing exactly that, and makes this concrete by implementing algorithms for decomposed process discovery and decomposed conformance checking using Integer Linear Programming (ILP) based algorithms. ILP-based process mining techniques provide precise results and formal guarantees (e.g., perfect fitness), but are known to scale badly in the number of activities. A small case study shows that we can gain orders of magnitude in run-time. However, in some cases there is tradeoff between run-time and quality.

Keywords: Process discovery · Conformance analysis · Big data · Decomposition

1 Introduction

The current attention for "big data" illustrates the spectacular growth of data and the potential economic value of such data in different industry sectors [1,2]. Most of the data that are generated refer to *events*, e.g., transactions in financial systems, interactions in a social network, events in high-tech systems or sensor networks. The incredible growth of event data provides new opportunities for process analysis. As more and more actions of people, organizations, and devices are recorded, there are ample opportunities to analyze processes based on the footprints they leave on event logs. In fact, we believe that the analysis of purely *handmade* process models will become less important given the omnipresence of event data [3].

© Springer International Publishing Switzerland 2015
F. Fournier and J. Mendling (Eds.): BPM 2014 Workshops, LNBIP 202, pp. 264–276, 2015.
DOI: 10.1007/978-3-319-15895-2_23

Process mining aims to *discover*, *monitor*, and *improve* real processes by *extracting knowledge* from *event logs* readily available. Starting point for any process mining task is an event log. Each event in such an event log refers to an *activity* (i.e., a well-defined step in some process) and is related to a particular *case* (i.e., a *process instance*). The events belonging to a case are *ordered* and can be seen as one "run" of the process. It is important to note that an event log contains only *example behavior*, i.e., we cannot assume that all possible runs have been observed. In fact, an event log often contains only a fraction of possible behavior [3].

Petri nets are often used in the context of process mining. Various algorithms employ Petri nets as the internal representation used for process mining. Examples are the region-based process discovery techniques [4–8], the α-algorithm [9], and various conformance checking techniques [10–13]. Other techniques use alternative internal representations (C-nets, heuristics nets, etc.) that can easily be converted to (labeled) Petri nets [3].

In this paper, we present a generic framework for *decomposing* the following two main process mining problems:

Process discovery: Given an event log consisting of a collection of traces, construct a Petri net that "adequately" describes the observed behavior.

Conformance checking (or replay): Given an event log and a Petri net, diagnose the differences between the observed behavior (the event log) and the modeled behavior (the Petri net) by replaying the observed behavior on the model.

To exemplify the use of this framework, we have implemented a decomposed discovery algorithm and a decomposed replay algorithm on top of it that both use ILP-based techniques [8,10]. We have chosen these ILP-based techniques as they provide formal guarantees and precise results. Since ILP-based techniques scale badly in the number of activities, there is the desire to speed-up analysis through smart problem decompositions.

The remainder of this paper is organized as follows. Section 2 briefly introduces basic concepts like event logs and Petri nets. Section 3 presents the generic framework, which consists of a collection of objects (like event logs and Petri nets) and a collection of algorithms (to import, export, visualize these objects, and to be able to create new objects from existing objects). Section 4 introduces the specific ILP-based discovery and replay algorithms implemented using our generic framework. Section 5 introduces a small case study, which shows that we can achieve better run-times, but that there are also tradeoffs between speed and quality. Section 6 concludes the paper.

2   Preliminaries

This section introduces basic concepts such as event logs, accepting Petri nets, discovery algorithms, log alignments, and replay algorithms.

2.1 Event Logs

Event logs are bags (or multisets) of event sequences (or traces). Events in an event log may have many attributes (like the activity, the resource who executed the activity, the timestamp the execution was completed, etc.). In the context of this paper, we are only interested in the activity an event refers to and abstract from other information. For this, we introduce the notion of a *classifier*, which maps every event onto its corresponding activity. As a result, we can map an entire trace onto an activity sequence, and an event log onto an activity log, where activity logs are bags of activity sequences.

Table 1. Activity log L_1^A in tabular form.

Name	Trace	Frequency
c_1	$\langle a_1, a_2, a_4, a_5, a_6, a_2, a_4, a_5, a_6, a_4, a_2, a_5, a_7 \rangle$	1
c_2	$\langle a_1, a_2, a_4, a_5, a_6, a_3, a_4, a_5, a_6, a_4, a_3, a_5, a_6, a_2, a_4, a_5, a_7 \rangle$	1
c_3	$\langle a_1, a_2, a_4, a_5, a_6, a_3, a_4, a_5, a_7 \rangle$	1
c_4	$\langle a_1, a_2, a_4, a_5, a_6, a_3, a_4, a_5, a_8 \rangle$	2
c_5	$\langle a_1, a_2, a_4, a_5, a_6, a_4, a_3, a_5, a_7 \rangle$	1
c_6	$\langle a_1, a_2, a_4, a_5, a_8 \rangle$	4
c_7	$\langle a_1, a_3, a_4, a_5, a_6, a_4, a_3, a_5, a_7 \rangle$	1
c_8	$\langle a_1, a_3, a_4, a_5, a_6, a_4, a_3, a_5, a_8 \rangle$	1
c_9	$\langle a_1, a_3, a_4, a_5, a_8 \rangle$	1
c_{10}	$\langle a_1, a_4, a_3, a_5, a_8 \rangle$	1
c_{11}	$\langle a_1, a_4, a_2, a_5, a_6, a_4, a_2, a_5, a_6, a_3, a_4, a_5, a_6, a_2, a_4, a_5, a_8 \rangle$	1
c_{12}	$\langle a_1, a_4, a_2, a_5, a_7 \rangle$	3
c_{13}	$\langle a_1, a_4, a_2, a_5, a_8 \rangle$	1
c_{14}	$\langle a_1, a_4, a_3, a_5, a_7 \rangle$	1

Table 1 describes the activity log $L_1^A = [c_1, c_2, c_3, c_4{}^2, c_5, c_6{}^4, c_7, c_8, c_9, c_{10}, c_{11}, c_{12}{}^3, c_{13}, c_{14}]$ defined over $A_1 = \{a_1, \ldots, a_8\}$. Activity sequence $c_6 = \langle a_1, a_2, a_4, a_5, a_8 \rangle$ occurs 4 times in L_1^A.

In the remainder of this paper, we will still often use the term event log, but we will use it often in conjunction with a classifier, which induces an activity log that will be used by the discovery and replay algorithms.

2.2 Accepting Petri Nets

For discovery algorithms, labeled Petri nets would suffice. However, for replay algorithms, we also need information on the initial marking of the net and of its possible final (or accepting) markings. For this reason, we introduce the concept of accepting Petri nets, which correspond to labeled Petri nets with an initial marking and a collection of final markings.

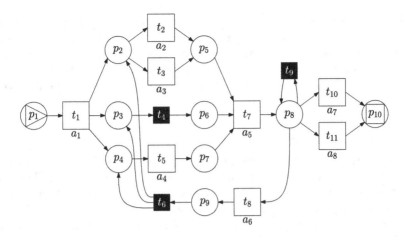

Fig. 1. An example accepting Petri net $N_1 = (P_1, T_1, F_1, l_1, \triangleright, \square)$.

For example, Fig. 1 shows an accepting Petri net $N_1 = (P_1, T_1, F_1, l_1, \triangleright_1, \square_1)$ over A_1, where $\triangleright_1 = [p_1]$ and $\square_1 = \{[p_{10}]\}$. As a result of the labeling, the transitions t_4, t_6, and t_9 are invisible. The firing sequence $\langle t_1, t_2, t_4, t_5, t_7, t_{10} \rangle$ runs from the initial marking to the only final marking and generates the trace $\langle a_1, a_2, a_4, a_5, a_7 \rangle$.

2.3 Discovery Algorithms

A discovery algorithm [4–9] is an algorithm that takes an event log (with classifier) as input, and generates an accepting Petri net as output. It is typically assumed that the behavior of the resulting accepting Petri net *fits* the behavior as captured by the event log in some way. However, also other quality dimensions like precision, generalization and simplicity need to be considered [3].

2.4 Log Alignments

Log and trace alignments are used by the replay algorithms to match the trace at hand with a valid firing sequence from the accepting Petri net. For this reason, a *trace alignment* contains a series of *moves*, which can be divided into three types:

Synchronous move: The trace and the net agree on the next action, as the next event (activity) in the trace matches an enabled transition in the net.
Log move: The next action is the next activity in the trace, which cannot be mimicked by the net.
Model move: The next action is an enabled transition in the net, which is not reflected by an event in the log.

A trace alignment is *valid* if the sequence of activities in synchronous and log moves equals the trace, if all transitions in synchronous moves have the corresponding activity as label, and if the sequence of transitions in synchronous and model moves equals some valid firing sequence in the net (which starts in the initial marking and ends in some final marking). We cannot always guarantee this latter requirement (valid firing sequence) when merging trace alignments. A trace alignment for which only the first two requirements hold is called a *weak* trace alignment. A *log alignment* maps every trace of the log onto a trace alignment.

2.5 Replay Algorithms

A replay algorithm is an algorithm that takes an event log (with classifier) and an accepting Petri net as input, and generates a log alignment as output. Typically, a replay algorithm assigns costs to the different moves. These costs are configurable. However, in this paper we use the following default costs. Synchronous moves have cost 0 as these correspond to a perfect match. A log move costs 5 and a visible model move costs 2. Model moves corresponding to invisible transitions have cost 0 (as these are not captured by the log) [10].

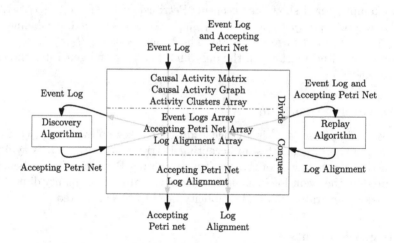

Fig. 2. Framework overview.

3 Generic Divide and Conquer Framework

This section introduces the generic framework for decomposed discovery and replay. Key ingredients for the framework are: *objects* (matrices, graphs, cluster arrays, etc.) and *algorithms* to process these objects (importing, exporting, visualizing, and creating a new object from existing objects) [14].

Figure 2 shows an overview of the framework, which contains many of the objects supported by the framework. The algorithms in the framework allow the user to create new objects from existing objects. The Discovery and Replay Algorithms on the sides symbolize existing discovery and replay techniques that can be connected to the framework.

3.1   Objects

To decompose an event log or an accepting Petri nets into sublogs or subnets, we need to divide the set of activities into so-called *clusters*. Then, we can create a sublog and a subnet for every cluster. There are different approaches that can be used to create an array of clusters. In this paper, we take a three-step approach:

1. Discover from the event log (or create from the accepting Petri net) a *causal activity matrix*. This matrix M maps every combination of two activities onto a real number in $[-1.0, 1.0]$, where $M[a, a'] \approx 1.0$ means that we are quite sure that there is a causal dependency from a to a', $M[a, a'] \approx -1.0$ means that we are sure that there is no causal dependency from a to a', and $M[a, a'] \approx 0.0$ means that we do not really know whether or not there is a causal dependency from a to a'.
2. Create a causal dependency graph from this matrix by taking the causal dependencies of which we are most certain.
3. Create an array of clusters from this graph using the technique as described in [14].

After having obtained the clusters, we can decompose the event log and accepting Petri net in an *event log array* and an *accepting Petri net array*, where the i-th sublog and subnet correspond to the i-th cluster in the array.

For the discovery case, we can then run the target discovery algorithm on every sublog, and merge the resulting subnets into a single accepting Petri net.

For the replay case, we can then replay every sublog on the corresponding subnet, and merge the resulting log alignments into a single log alignment. Although this approach provides various formal guarantees (e.g., the fraction of fitting cases computed in this manner is exact [14]), there may be some complications:

- Experiments have shown [15] that replaying a sublog on a subnet *which is obtained by removing all transitions that do not correspond to an activity in the cluster* can take more time than replaying the original log on the original net. For this reason, the framework also supports subnets that are obtained by making all transitions that do not correspond to an activity in the cluster *invisible*. This also reduces the number of activities in the subnets, but keeps the structure of the net intact.
- The current implementation of the replay algorithms uses integer costs. This is a problem, as we need to divide the costs of an activity evenly over the clusters where the activity appears (see [14]). If the activity appears in three clusters, how can we divide the costs of its log move (5) evenly over the clusters? For this reason, we introduce a *cost factor* in the framework. Every cost in the replay problem will first be multiplied by this factor, and the replay algorithms will run using these multiplied costs.

3.2   Algorithms

All objects in the framework can be exported, imported, and visualized. Furthermore, it is possible to create new objects from existing objects. Some of the algorithms supported in our framework:

Create Accepting Petri Net: Create an accepting Petri net from a Petri net.

Create Activity Clusters: Create a (valid maximally decomposed [14]) activity cluster array from an accepting Petri net.

Create Clusters: Create an activity cluster array from a causal activity graph.

Create Matrix: Create a causal activity matrix from an accepting Petri net.

Determine Activity Costs: Determine the cost factor for an activity cluster array.

Discover Accepting Petri Nets: Discover an accepting Petri net array from an event log array using a (wrapped) existing discovery algorithm.

Discover Clusters: Discover an activity cluster array from an event log.

Discover Matrix: Discover a causal activity matrix from an event log.

Filter Graph: Filter a causal activity graph from a causal activity matrix.

Filter Log Alignments: Filter a log alignment array using an accepting Petri net array. All uncovered transition are filtered out.

Merge Accepting Petri Nets: Merge an accepting Petri net array into an accepting Petri net. One supported way to merge nets (the one used in this paper) is by copying all objects (transitions, places, arcs) into a new net, and then fuse all visible transitions with the same label. However, other ways to merge nets are also supported.

Merge Log Alignments: Merge a log alignment array into a log alignment. The result will be a weak alignment. The supported way to merge alignments is to (1) accumulate costs and (2) 'zip' both alignments in such a way that in case of a conflict always the cheapest option is 'zipped in'.

Replay Event Logs: replay an event log array on an accepting Petri net array.

Split Accepting Petri Net: Create an accepting Petri net array from an activity cluster array and an accepting Petri net. The most straightforward supported way to split a net into subnets is by copying the net and removing all parts that do not correspond to the cluster at hand. However, as mentioned, this may result in excessive replay times. An alternative supported way is by copying the net and making all visible transitions that do not correspond to the cluster at hand invisible. This alternative way is used in this paper.

Split Event Log: Create an event log array from an activity cluster array and an event log. The most straightforward supported way to split a log is by starting with an empty log and adding all events that correspond to the cluster at hand. However, this may introduce additional causal dependencies between exit and entry activities of loops. An alternative supported way is by copying the log and renaming all events that do not correspond to the cluster at hand with a special activity, say γ. This paper uses the first way.

Please note that every one of these plug-ins may have its own set of parameters. Some parameters will be mentioned (and given actual values) later on.

3.3   Implementation

The entire framework and all algorithms have been implemented in the Divide-AndConquer package[1] of ProM 6[2]. For every framework object (like a causal

---

[1] The DivideAndConquer package is available through https://svn.win.tue.nl/trac/prom/browser/Packages/DivideAndConquer.

[2] ProM 6 is available through http://www.promtools.org/prom6.

activity matrix), this package does not only implement the object itself, but it also implements an import plug-in, an export plug-in, and at least one visualizer plug-in. Every algorithm is implemented as a regular plug-in, and comes with variants for both the UITopia context (that is, the ProM 6 GUI) and the headless context (which allows the plug-ins to be used from scripts and the like).

4   Decomposed Discovery and Replay Using ILP

Figure 3 shows how the "Discover with ILP using Decomposition" plug-in has been implemented on top of the framework, using a Petri net. In this Petri net, the places correspond to the framework objects, whereas the transitions correspond to framework plug-ins. The numbers in the plug-ins indicates the order in which the "Discover with ILP using Decomposition" plug-in invokes the framework plug-ins, where "Merge Clusters" (step 4) is an optional step that is only needed to merge all clusters into a single cluster. This optional step is only used to run the discovery algorithm on the entire event log, as filtering the event log on a single cluster containing all activities would result in the same event log. This way, it is certain that the discovery plug-in used is similar in both the decomposed and the non-decomposed setting.

However, there is one exception, one situation where the decomposed discovery uses a different setting than the regular discovery. The regular ILP-based discovery algorithm depends on the causal dependencies that are detected in an event log. For every casual dependency, it will search for a corresponding place [16]. As a result, if no causal dependency is detected from one activity to another, then the algorithm will not search for a place from the corresponding first transition to the second. In the presence of loops, this may be problematic in the decomposed setting, especially if small clusters are involved. Because of the loop, a transition a' that exits the cluster will typically be followed by a transition a that enters it. If in the cluster a can directly be followed by a', no causal dependency between a and a' will be detected as a can be directly followed by a' and vice versa. For this reason, the decomposed discovery algorithm does not use these causal dependencies to search for places. Instead, it uses a way of searching which is described as *basic* in [16].

Figure 4 shows the same for the "Replay with ILP using Decomposition" plug-in. Note that this plug-in is more complex than the "Discover with ILP using Decomposition", which is mainly caused by the two catches on the replay mentioned earlier:

1. It is better to obtain subnets by hiding external (to the cluster at hand) transitions. Steps 6, 7 and 11 are the result of this. Step 6 filters the subnets by hiding external transitions, whereas step 7 filters the subnets by removing external transitions. Step 11 uses the result of step 7 to filter the subalignments, which is required by step 12, as merging the log alignments assumes that all external transitions have been removed from the subalignments.

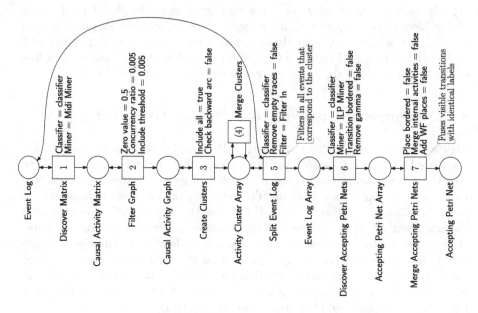

Fig. 3. Discover with ILP using Decomposition.

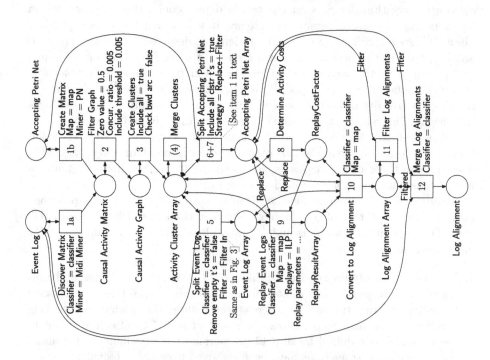

Fig. 4. Replay with ILP using Decomposition.

Table 2. Case study results.

Description	Event log	Place search	Nr. of clusters	Time (in seconds) average	95 % interval		Replay costs
regular discovery	aligned	causal	1	2245.72	2223.46	2267.99	N/A
decomposed discovery	aligned	basic	34	97.33	95.92	98.74	N/A
regular replay	aligned	N/A	1	12.04	11.86	12.22	0.00
decomposed replay	aligned	N/A	11	12.83	12.68	12.97	0.00
regular replay	original	N/A	1	92.75	91.57	93.94	14.49
decomposed replay	original	N/A	11	68.37	67.84	68.90	9.39

2. We need to scale up costs before the replay, and scale them down afterwards. Step 8 determines the cost factor, that is, the amount by which so scale up an down, step 9 scales the costs up before replay, and step 10 scales them down again.

Except for the underlying ILP-based discovery algorithm (step 6 in Fig. 3) and the underlying ILP-based replay algorithm (step 9 in Fig. 4), all plug-ins have been implemented in the framework, that is, in the `DivideAndConquer` package. This includes the "Discover with ILP using Decomposition" and "Replay with ILP using Decomposition" plug-ins.

5 Case Study

For the case study, we use an event log[3] based on the BPI Challenge 2012 [17]. As the ILP discovery algorithm requires an event log that is free of noise, we have aligned the event log to the model that was used in [15]. This may sound artificial, but we feel that for testing the discovery this is justified, as one of the requirements of the original ILP discovery algorithm is that the log is free of noise. For testing the discovery, we will only use the aligned event log, for testing the replay, we will use both event logs. For sake of completeness, we mention that the aligned log contains $13,807$ traces, $383,836$ events, and 58 activities.

The case study was performed on a Dell Optiplex 9020 desktop computer with Inter(R) Core(TM) i7-4770 CPU @ 3.40 GHz processor, 16 GB of RAM, running Windows 7 Enterprise 64-bit, Service Pack 1, and using revision 13851 of the `DivideAndConquer` package.

Table 2 shows the results of the case study. For the decomposed plug-ins in this table, the times reported are the times it takes the entire plug-in (all steps in Fig. 3 or Fig. 4) to finish after the user has provided the required additional information, like the classifier. For the regular plug-ins, the times reported are the times it takes only the discovery (only step 6 in Fig. 3) or only the replay (only step 9 in Fig. 4) to finish.

---

[3] The event logs used for this case study can be downloaded from
https://svn.win.tue.nl/trac/prom/browser/Documentation/DivideAndConquer.

5.1 Discovery

Regular discovery (without decomposition) using the ILP miner takes about 37.5 min, whereas decomposed discovery takes only 1.5 min (using 34 clusters). Both result in the same accepting Petri net, which shows that the decomposed discovery clearly outperforms the regular discovery for this case.

As a side note, we mention that we have also ran the regular discovery on the aligned log using the basic place search (cf. Section 4). This run took just under 3 hrs (178 min), and resulted in a so-called *flower* model [3]. This indicates that this way of searching for places in the ILP discovery algorithm is not suitable for regular discovery, as it takes a long time and yields bad results.

5.2 Replay

Regular replay takes about 12 s for the aligned event log, resulting in no costs, and takes 1.5 min for the original event log, resulting in 14.49 costs.[4] In contrast, the decomposed replay takes about 12 s for the aligned event log, using 11 clusters and resulting in no costs, and takes about 68 s for the original event log, using also 11 clusters but resulting in 9.39 costs. Note that decomposed replay by definition provides a lower bound for the alignment costs (due to local optimizations) [14]. How good the lower bound is depends on the decomposition.

So, the decomposed replay is faster on the regular event logs, but may result in only a lower bound of the actual answer (9.39 instead of 14.49 for the original event log).

6   Conclusions

This paper introduced a generic framework for decomposed discovery and replay. The framework is based on objects (matrices, graphs, arrays, etc.) required for the decomposed discovery and replay, and a collection of algorithms to create these objects, either from file or from existing objects. The framework can be used for any decomposed discovery and replay technique.

To illustrate the applicability of the generic framework, we showed how the ILP-based discovery and replay algorithms can be supported by it. The resulting ILP-based discovery is straightforward, but the resulting ILP-based replay algorithm is more complex because of efficiency and implementation issues. Both ILP-based process discovery and conformance checking are supported by our framework.

For the BPI2012 Challenge log, the ILP-based decomposed discovery algorithm has shown to be much faster than the regular discovery algorithm, while resulting in the same model. For the same log, the ILP-based replay algorithm

---

[4] Please note that, by changing the cost structure as suggested in [14], we can accumulate costs when merging subalignments into a single alignment. However, we do not have a way yet to accumulate fitness when merging subalignments. For this reason, we restrict ourselves to costs here.

has shown to be faster, but resulting in a less accurate answer. Clearly, there is often a tradeoff between running times and quality.

At the moment, the framework only supports a limited set of discovery and replay algorithms. As an example, only the α-algorithm and the ILP-based algorithm are supported as discovery algorithms. In the near future, we plan to extend this set to include other complex algorithms, like, for example, the evolutionary tree miner and the inductive miner.

Furthermore, the current framework is currently restricted to using a maximal decomposition of a net (or an event log). A coarser decomposition may be faster, as the algorithm may run faster on a single slightly larger cluster instead of on a collection of small clusters. The approach supports any valid decomposition; therefore, we are looking for better techniques to select a suitable set of clusters. Experiments show that it is possible to create clusters that provide a good trade-off between running times and quality.

References

1. Manyika, J., Chui, M., Brown, B., Bughin, J., Dobbs, R., Roxburgh, C., Byers, A.H.: Big Data: The Next Frontier for Innovation, Competition, and Productivity. Technical report, McKinsey Global Institute (2011)
2. Hilbert, M., López, P.: The World's Technological Capacity to Store, Communicate, and Compute Information. Sci. **332**(6025), 60–65 (2011)
3. van der Aalst, W.M.P.: Process Mining: Discovery, Conformance and Enhancement of Business Processes, 1st edn. Springer Publishing Company Incorporated, Heidelberg (2011)
4. van der Aalst, W.M.P., Rubin, V., Verbeek, H.M.W., van Dongen, B.F., Kindler, E., Günther, C.W.: Process mining: a two-step approach to balance between underfitting and overfitting. Softw. Syst. Model. **9**(1), 87–111 (2010)
5. Bergenthum, R., Desel, J., Lorenz, R., Mauser, S.: Process mining based on regions of languages. In: Alonso, G., Dadam, P., Rosemann, M. (eds.) BPM 2007. LNCS, vol. 4714, pp. 375–383. Springer, Heidelberg (2007)
6. Solé, M., Carmona, J.: Process mining from a basis of state regions. In: Lilius, J., Penczek, W. (eds.) PETRI NETS 2010. LNCS, vol. 6128, pp. 226–245. Springer, Heidelberg (2010)
7. Carmona, J.A., Cortadella, J., Kishinevsky, M.: A region-based algorithm for discovering petri nets from event logs. In: Dumas, M., Reichert, M., Shan, M.-C. (eds.) BPM 2008. LNCS, vol. 5240, pp. 358–373. Springer, Heidelberg (2008)
8. van der Werf, J.M.E.M., van Dongen, B.F., Hurkens, C.A.J., Serebrenik, A.: Process Discovery using Integer Linear Programming. Fundam. Inform. **94**(3–4), 387–412 (2009)
9. van der Aalst, W.M.P., Weijters, A.J.M.M., Maruster, L.: Workflow Mining: Discovering process models from event logs. IEEE Trans. Knowl. Data Eng. **16**(9), 1128–1142 (2004)
10. Adriansyah, A., van Dongen, B.F., van der Aalst, W.M.P.: Conformance Checking using Cost-Based Fitness Analysis. In: Chi, C., Johnson, P., eds.: IEEE International Enterprise Computing Conference (EDOC 2011), pp. 55–64. IEEE Computer Society (2011)

11. Muñoz-Gama, J., Carmona, J.: A fresh look at precision in process conformance. In: Hull, R., Mendling, J., Tai, S. (eds.) BPM 2010. LNCS, vol. 6336, pp. 211–226. Springer, Heidelberg (2010)
12. Muñoz-Gama, J., Carmona, J.: Enhancing precision in Process Conformance: Stability, confidence and severity. In: CIDM, pp. 184–191. IEEE (2011)
13. Rozinat, A., van der Aalst, W.M.P.: Conformance checking of processes based on monitoring real behavior. Inf. Syst. **33**(1), 64–95 (2008)
14. van der Aalst, W.M.P.: Decomposing Petri nets for process mining: A generic approach. Distrib. Parallel Databases **31**(4), 471–507 (2013)
15. Verbeek, H.M.W., van der Aalst, W.M.P.: Decomposing Replay Problems: A Case Study. In: Moldt, D., (ed.) PNSE+ModPE. vol. 989 of CEUR Workshop Proceedings, CEUR-WS.org, pp. 219–235 (2013)
16. van der Wiel, T.: Process mining using integer linear programming. Master's thesis, Eindhoven University of Technology, Department of Mathematics and Computer Science (2010). http://alexandria.tue.nl/extra1/afstversl/wsk-i/wiel2010.pdf
17. van Dongen, B.F.: BPI Challenge 2012 (2012). http://dx.doi.org/10.4121/uuid: 3926db30-f712-4394-aebc-75976070e91f

Evaluating the Performance of a Batch Activity in Process Models

Luise Pufahl, Ekaterina Bazhenova$^{(\boxtimes)}$, and Mathias Weske

Hasso Plattner Institute at the University of Potsdam, Potsdam, Germany
{Luise.Pufahl,Ekaterina.Bazhenova,Mathias.Weske}@hpi.uni-potsdam.de

Abstract. The goal of many organizations of today is optimization of business process management. A factor for optimization of business processes is reduction of costs associated with mass production and customer service. Recently, an approach to incorporate batch activities in process models was proposed to improve the process performance by synchronizing a group of process instances. However, the issue of optimal utilization of batch activities and estimation of associated costs remained still open. In this paper, we present an approach to evaluate batch activity performance, based on techniques from queuing theory. Thus, cost functions are introduced in order to (1) compare usual (i.e., non-batch) and batch activity execution and (2) find the optimal configuration of a batch activity. The approach is applied to a real-world use case from the healthcare domain.

Keywords: Process analysis · Batch activity · Cost function · Queuing theory

1 Introduction

Today, business processes are managed by many companies in a process-oriented fashion. This means that they are documented as process models and then often automatized with the help of business process management systems [18]. Traditionally, instances of a business process, the executions of cases, are handled independently of each other in such systems. Along with that, an improved process performance can be reached by synchronizing the execution of a group of instances, as reflected in works dedicated to incorporation of batch activities in business processes [6,11,13,15]. For example, a nurse in a hospital brings multiple blood samples of patients to the laboratory at once to save transportation costs instead of bringing each individually. In contrast, all other activities of the blood analysis process, e.g., the blood taking require an individual instance handling. For use-case specific incorporation of batch routine in processes, a recent approach in [10,11] allows individual batch activity configuration by the process designer with a concrete execution semantic.

Yet until now, the issue of optimal incorporation of batch activities in business processes remained an open question, because the evaluation of parameters, such as optimal batch size, time of batch activation, etc. appeared to be

© Springer International Publishing Switzerland 2015
F. Fournier and J. Mendling (Eds.): BPM 2014 Workshops, LNBIP 202, pp. 277–290, 2015.
DOI: 10.1007/978-3-319-15895-2_24

use-case dependent. In this paper, we present a generic scheme of evaluating the performance of batch activities.

In the mentioned example, the batch activity is used for synchronizing the transport of several blood samples to save transportation costs, i.e., execution costs. However, instances need to wait until a batch is formed. The experienced waiting time by instances is usually also associated to certain costs, e.g., loss in future sales [1] or in our use case, costs of new blood samples due to expiration of sample with too long waiting times. Our approach consists in introducing cost functions depending on waiting and service costs, with the help of which we (1) compare batch execution with usual activity execution (i.e., a non-batch activity) and (2) compare different configurations of a batch activity to find the optimal parameters.

Queuing theory provides different techniques to analyze systems with queues and provide important parameter them, e.g., the average waiting time in a queue [5]. We use queuing theory systems to identify parameters of our introduced cost functions and illustrate this on our running example showing that (i) the batch activity provides here a better performance than the usual one and (ii) an optimal batch activity configuration can be identified.

The rest of the paper is structured as follows, Sect. 2 presents a motivating example and introduces shortly the batch activity concept. In Sect. 3, the two costs function for the evaluation are developed and their input parameters are discussed. It is followed by the presentation of how these costs function can be obtained with queuing theory systems and a concrete application of the health-care use case. Section 4 is devoted to the discussion of related work which is followed by the conclusion.

2   Motivating Example and Batch Activity Concept

As running example, we will use a process from the healthcare domain to introduce shortly the batch activity concept [11] and to motivate why a quantitative analysis of a batch activity is necessary.

Medical experts in a hospital need blood tests to determine the healthcare status of their patients at a ward. The process is denoted as BPMN (Business Process Modeling and Notation) model in Fig. 1. If a blood test is needed, a blood test order is prepared and then the blood sample is taken from the patient. Both are transported to the laboratory by a nurse where the test is conducted. After the test, the results are published in a hospital information system which the medical experts can access and evaluate.

The single blood testing instances are usually conducted completely independent from each other, e.g., the blood test taking. However, as several blood samples are taken at a ward, the nurse does not transport each individually. They are transported in a batch to save transportation time and the corresponding costs. For capturing this behavior, a batch activity can be installed based on the approach in [11] as it was done in Fig. 1 in which the batch activity is represented with a double border. Each batch activity has the configuration parameters *activationRule*, *maxBatchSize* and *isSequential*.

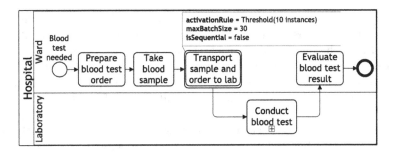

Fig. 1. Blood testing process with a batch activity, represented here with a double border.

The *activationRule* specifies when a batch execution is activated and provided to the task performer. In the example, a threshold rule was selected. It defines that a threshold of 10 instances has to be reached to activate a batch. The maximum batch capacity, defined by the *maxBatchSize*, is 30 instances in the given example. The instances contained in a batch can be executed in parallel (*isSequential = false*) or in sequence (*isSequential = true*). More information regarding the execution semantics of a batch activity can be found in [11].

In the following, the motivation of evaluating the performance of a batch activity is shown on two scenarios with different blood sample arrival rates. In Scenario 1, we assume 5 blood samples being taken in average per hour. In Scenario 2, a low occupied ward is assumed, with 2 blood samples in average per hour (see Fig. 2). In general, the nurse needs 10 min to bring the blood samples to the laboratory and to return back to the ward as shown in Fig. 2. If we assume a nurse salary of 30 EUR per hour, the costs to perform the transportation service are 5.00 EUR. Usually, a certain time frame blood samples can not be used anymore for the analysis, because the blood gets clotted etc. In case of analyzing the coagulation, most blood samples expire the latest after 4 h, some also earlier [9]. The costs of taking a new blood sample are 5.35 EUR[1]. Next, we want to discuss the costs of batch activity execution and the number of expired blood samples for the two scenarios to estimate the performance of the given batch activity in Fig. 1.

For scenario 1, in which 5 samples are taken in average per hour, it can be roughly estimated that a batch is activated in average every two hours. Thus, expired blood samples would be rarely observed. The cost for transporting would account nearly 1.00 EUR per blood sample (5.00 EUR divided by approximately 5 samples in a batch). In contrast, if the nurse brings each blood

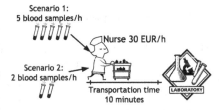

Fig. 2. Illustration of the parameters needed for a batch activity evaluation for scenario 1 and scenario 2

---

[1] Such assumption is based on German Medical Fee Schedule (http://www.e-bis.de/ goae/defaultFrame.htm). According to this document, taking a coagulation blood sample costs 3.35 EUR added with 2 EUR material cost.

sample individually, she would spend a lot of her working time in transporting samples and service costs per blood sample are 5.00 EUR. Intuitively, it can be concluded that the installation of a batch activity is more beneficially then the usual activity execution. However, these statements need a quantitative proof. For scenario 2, in which approximately two samples are processed per hour, it can be estimated roughly that a batch is activated every 5 h. At least, two blood samples would expire resulting in higher costs for waiting then saving transportation costs. Therefore, we can intuitively say that in such scenario the usage of batch will not be beneficial. Here, a usual activity should be installed or the configuration parameters should be changed.

These two scenarios illustrate the importance of evaluating the benefit of a batch activity before installation. However, for this evaluation we need a method to quantify concretely the batch activity performance and compare it to a usual activity. As shown, service costs (e.g., the transportation costs) on the one hand and waiting costs (e.g., costs when a blood sample expires) on the other hand play an important role. In next section, an approach for quantifying the batch activity performance is presented.

3   Cost Functions for Usual and Batch Activity

In the following section, we introduce an approach to measure the performance of usual activity and batch activity. With regards to Dumas et al. in [2], the process performance measures are time, cost, quality and flexibility. The main performance indicator considered in this paper is costs, because the batch activity aim at synchronizing several instances to share execution costs (i.e., service costs) between them. The time performance factor is important as well as instances have to wait for each other until a batch is created. They could experience a higher waiting time, which can be translated into waiting costs. These two aspects are included in a function to provide an use-case independent method. Such a method can be extended in future work by taking into account quality and flexibility performance factors, from which we abstract in the current paper.

Firstly, a cost-function for any activity of a process model is introduced. If a process model is executed, process instances arrive randomly at a certain point at the respective activity as illustrated in Fig. 3. The arrival process can be described by a certain distribution. This leads to the accumulation of instances being ready for the execution of this activity. We assume that the instances are

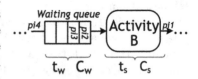

Fig. 3. Evaluation model of an usual activity

organized in the queue according to the first-come first-served (FCFS) queuing discipline. Each process instance in the queue receives the described service of the activity by a task performer (i.e., human resource, non-human resource or software service). The service provision is related to so-called *service costs* C_s (cf. Fig. 3) The task performer needs a certain time to perform the service, i.e., *service time* t_s. If a process instance arrives and the task performer is busy in serving an earlier arrived instance, then it experiences a certain *waiting time* t_w before its processed. The waiting of instances incorporates certain costs, i.e., *waiting costs* C_w.

Examples of waiting costs are the costs to store an item, the costs of paying idle employees, or the costs of lost customers due to long waiting. Especially for the latter, it is a challenge to "assign a monetary value to" it [1]. Davis presents in [1] an approach to monetize waiting costs by calculating the future losses in sales due to waiting times. It is captured by a waiting costs function depended on the waiting time. For each type of waiting a different cost function exists, mostly linear function, but also non-linear functions, e.g., future losses of sales.

Taking into account that waiting and service costs are the most significant costs, we propose the following total costs function for usual activity:

$$C = C_w(t_w) + C_s \qquad (1)$$

Based on 1, the total activity costs C of executing one process instance are composed of the waiting costs C_w of the process instance and the service costs C_s of an activity execution. The waiting costs C_w is the resulted value from the waiting costs function $C_w(wt)$ for the waiting time t_w of the respective process instance.

Let us consider the case of a batch activity. As basis, the function 1 of a usual activity can be taken. However the difference is that process instances are joint in batches and synchronized during the activity execution (cf. batch shown in Fig. 4). The service costs of one execution are shared between the instances of one

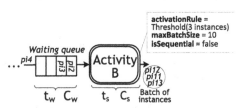

Fig. 4. Evaluation model of a batch activity

batch. Then, the service costs for one instance is calculate by dividing the service costs of an execution by the number of instances in a batch. The following equation can be used to calculate the total batch activity costs:

$$C_b = C_w(t_w) + C_s/Y \qquad (2)$$

From 2, the total batch activity costs C_b of executing one process instance are composed of the waiting costs C_w of the process instance and the service costs C_s of an activity execution divided by the size of its batch Y. The waiting costs C_w is the resulted value from the waiting costs function $C_w(wt)$ for the waiting time t_w of the process instance.

The presented functions can be either obtain analytically based on techniques from the queuing theory or based on a simulation. As shown in Fig. 5, several input parameters are needed being fixed for both functions so that the results can be compared. The *arrival time*, the *service time* and the *number of task performers* available are needed to determine the waiting time. Further, the *waiting cost function* and the *service costs* are needed. These input parameters are discussed in more detail in the following:

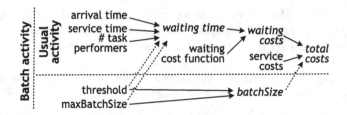

Fig. 5. Schematic representation of calculating the cost functions with needed input parameters.

Arrival time. The arrival time is usually distributed. It is often described by the *Poisson process* [2] providing the interval between the arrival of two instances as a negative exponential distribution with a mean of $1/\lambda$. Thereby, λ describes the mean arrival rate per time unit. This can be identify based on expert knowledge or the analysis of process logs [12].

Service time. The service time can be either a constant value (e.g., blood analysis activity), can be depended on the number of handled instances (e.g., printing activity), or is distributed (e.g., transportation activity). Distributed service time are often described by exponential distribution whereby a mean value is provided. Expert knowledge or analysis of process logs is needed to define the mean service time.

Number of task performers. For an activity, either one or several resources can be available as task performer. The more resources are available, the more instances respectively batches of instances can be handled simultaneously.

Waiting cost function. As stated, for each type of waiting a waiting cost function has to be identified by process experts. In literature, works can be found which discuss different functions for specific domains, e.g. in [14] different linear and non-linear holding cost functions for different types of products are presented.

Service costs. The service costs describe costs of an activity execution. This can be dependent on the service time (e.g., activities which are executed by a human task performer receiving a certain salary per time unit) or can be fixed service costs (e.g., the costs of one machine run).

Relevant input parameters for the second costs function – the total costs of a batch activity – are the selected configuration parameters of the batch activity [11] discussed in Sect. 2. For the sake of simplification, we assume that instances are always handled in parallel (*isSequential* = false) and the threshold rule is used as activation rule. Thus, the following input parameters are further relevant (cf. lower part of Fig. 5):

Maximal batch size. The maximal batch size describes how many instances can by contained by a batch at maximum. It is usually defined by the capacity restriction of the task performer (e.g., machine capacity).

Threshold value. The threshold defines how many instances have to be at least available for batch activation. If the optimal threshold for a batch activity should be identified, this can also be the output by finding for which threshold the most optimal balance between service costs and waiting costs is reached.

In the next section, we present how these functions can be obtained analytically based on techniques from queuing theory and can be used to compare usual and batch execution as well as finding the optimal threshold value to minimize the total costs.

4 Analytical Analysis

4.1 The M/M/1 and the M/M(a,b)/1 System

For evaluating the performance of batch activities in process models, it is beneficial to consider the processing of instances as a queuing system. The queuing system is composed of jobs at a service facility requesting its service. They join a queue if service is not immediately available, and leave when receiving service [7]. Conventionally, the standard approach used to describe and classify a queuing system is Kendall's notation [4]. In our work, we will use the queuing systems which are given by three factors $A/B/s$. Here A is an inter-arrival time distribution, B is a distribution of service times, and s is a number of servers in the system.

The consideration of batch activities as queuing systems served as the prerequisite for taking into account two types of queuing systems. As presented below, they correspond to usual and batch processing based on definitions from the queuing theory [5].

Definition 1 (M/M/1 system). $M/M/1$ represents the queue system with a single task performer, where arrivals are determined by a Poisson process and service time has an exponential distribution.   ⋄

Definition 2 (M/M(a,b)/1 system). $M/M(a,b)/1$ represents the queue system with a single task performer, where arrivals are determined by a Poisson process. With that, the service commences in batches, when the queue size reaches or exceeds a threshold value a, and the capacity of the service is b, so that $1 \leq a \leq b$. As well, the service time is independent of the batch size and has an exponential distribution.   ⋄

It is assumed in both queuing systems that the arrivals are determined by a Poisson process with average inter-arrival rate λ, and the service time distribution is exponential with rate parameter μ. For avoiding the eternal accumulation of unserved arrivals, we also assume that the service rate is faster than the arrival rate, i.e., $\mu > \lambda$.

For comparing the performance of the introduced systems, we fix the input parameters for both system, such as arrival and service rates, and service costs

C_s. The waiting costs of the system are represented by a function $C_w(t_w)$, which depends on the waiting time of an instance in each system correspondingly. In the case of batch processing, an additional parameter of batch size Y is needed.

Under such assumptions, the evaluation of costs can be conducted. A distribution of a variable is commonly defined by its expected value, therefore for identifying the distribution of total costs, we consider the expected (mean) parameters of arrival and service. For variable X, we conventionally denote its mean by $E[X]$.

Characteristic parameters of M/M/1 system. With regards to Formula (1) (Sect. 3), the total expected costs of a usual activity are following:

$$E[C] = E[C_w] + E[C_s] = C_w(E[t_w]) + C_s \qquad (3)$$

In the general case of the M/M/1 system, total expected costs are associated with expected waiting costs and expected service costs. We assume service costs C_s as a constant input parameter, therefore its expected value $E[C_s]$ is equal to C_s. In contrast, as waiting cost function $C_w(t_w)$ depends on the waiting time of an instance in the system, its expected value $E[C_w]$ is equal to its value for the expected waiting time of an instance $C_w(E[t_w])$. The expected time one instance spends in the queue, $E[t_w]$, can be calculated by formula from queuing theory [7] and is equal to:

$$E[t_w] = \lambda/[\mu(\mu - \lambda)]. \qquad (4)$$

Characteristic parameters of M/M(a,b)/1 system. With regards to Formula 2 (Sect. 3), the total expected costs are following:

$$E[C_b] = E[C_w] + E[C_s]]/E[Y] = C_w(E[t_w]) + C_s/E[Y] \qquad (5)$$

Analogously to $M/M/1$ system, we assume expected service costs $E[C_s]$ equal to C_s, with the expected waiting time $E[C_w]$ equal to its value for the expected waiting time of an instance $C_w(E[t_w])$. The expected size of the batch $E[Y]$ is a variable which can be obtained using queuing theory. Algorithm 1 presents the calculation of expected waiting time $E[t_w]$ and expected service batch size $E[Y]$ for an instance in the queue system, with regards to approach described in [7].

In Algorithm 1, the input parameters are characteristics of the queue system, such as threshold value a and batch service capacity b, inter-arrival rate of instances λ and service rate μ. In theory, the differential equation system has to be set up to identify the expected waiting time and batch size. The steady-state solution of this system can be identified by finding the root of a characteristic equation for the system, which is given in step 1, where z is an unknown arbitrary variable. The function $findRoot$ should be implemented in step 2 such that it finds a real root r of the equation $h(z) = 0$. This root should meet the following condition: $0 < r < 1$. It is proved in [7], that this equation has only such root. Based on the input parameters, in steps 3, 4 and 5 of Algorithm 1 the auxiliary parameters w, p and $P_{0,0}$ are calculated. Explanation of this parameters are not provided as we will use them in our research only indirectly for numerical calculation of the goal parameters. Details can be found in [7]. In steps 6 and 7,

Algorithm 1. Calculation of characteristical parameters of M/M(a,b)/1 system

Input: λ, μ, a, b
Output: $E[t_w], E[Y]$
1: $h(z) \equiv \mu z^{b+1} - (\lambda + \mu)z + \lambda;$ $h(z)$ is a characteristic equation, z is an unknown variable
2: $r = findRoot(h(z));$ r is a real root, $0 < r < 1$
3: $w = \lambda/(\lambda + \mu);$
4: $p = \lambda/\mu;$
5: $P_{0,0} = \left[\frac{a}{1-r} + \frac{r^{a+1}-r^{b+1}}{(1-r)^2}\right]^{-1};$
6: $E[t_w] = \frac{P_{0,0}}{\lambda(1-r)}\left[\frac{r^2(1-r^b)}{(1-r)^2} + \frac{a(a-1)}{2} + \frac{r^2(ar^{(a-1)}(1-r)-(1-r^a))}{(1-r)^2}\right];$
7: $E[Y] = a(1 + \frac{(r-w)pP_{0,0}}{wr(1-r)^2} + \frac{(1-w)r^{a+1}pP_{0,0}}{(1-r)^3}[1+r+a-ar] - \frac{(r-w)pP_{0,0}}{w(1-r)^3}[1+2b+(1-2b)r]);$

the expected waiting time $E[t_w]$ and expected batch size $E[Y]$ are calculated according to formulas from queuing theory.

With these two queuing systems, the numerical values of cost functions for the particular cases of usual and batch processing could be calculated. If the costs associated with batch processing are lower than in usual processing, it can be stated that the incorporation of batch activity is reasonable and beneficial. As well, an optimal configuration of batch processing can be found, by fixing the input parameters and changing the threshold value of the M/M(a,b)/1 system. The optimal threshold is the value minimizing the total cost function.

4.2 Application to the Use Case

In this section, we apply our cost functions in the context of our case, presented in Sect. 2. For this sake, we firstly describe the needed input data. Then, we compare total costs in M/M/1 and M/M(a,b)/1 systems. At last, we identify the optimal threshold value in batch processing system.

Input data. We take Scenario 1 from Sect. 2 with following input parameters:

- the arrival time is Poisson process with rate $\lambda = 5$ (samples per hour);
- the service time distribution is exponential with rate $\mu = 6$ (transports of samples per hour a 10 min);
- service costs $C_s = 5$ (EUR per blood test);
- threshold value of a batch $a = 10$ (instances);
- maximum batch capacity $b = 30$ (instances).

For defining the waiting cost function in our case, we take as basis the approach in [3] for calculating the cumulative holding cost for perishable goods in grocery stores. This approach is similar, as the quality of blood tests is also decreasing with the curse of time waiting in the queue.

An often conducted blood test is the coagulation test which have to be undertaken the latest after 4 h according to guidelines [9]. However, the guidelines do not provide statistics of expiration of blood tests. Therefore, for the sake of integrity of our use case, we propose to evaluate the distribution of expiry of blood tests, analogously to the distribution of spoilage of perishable goods [3]. In case of real evaluation, such data should be obtained from expert statistical analysis. As given in Sect. 2, taking a new blood sample for this test costs 5.35 EUR.

The graphic of the resulting waiting costs function with the assumed parameters is shown in Fig. 6. We assume that 1.5 % of blood samples expire after 1 h of waiting, 2 % expire after 2 h and so forth, as shown in the figure. As the costs of taking a new blood test is 5.35 EUR, the cumulative expiration cost per sample is $(0.015) * 5.35$ EUR≈ 0.08 EUR after 1 h; $(0.015 + 0.02) * 5.35$ EUR ≈ 0.19 EUR after 1.5 h, and so forth.

With that, the waiting costs are equal to zero at the time span when the blood test do not expire (less than 0.5 h), and the expiration costs are equal to the maximum value of 5.35 EUR after the recommended stored time (more than 4 h). Thus, as can be seen from Fig. 6, the waiting costs function is a piecewise function. It is constant for the time preceding the start of expiration of blood tests, and exceeding the recommended stored time. For the time span between these two moments, we approximated the waiting cost function with a polynomial function.

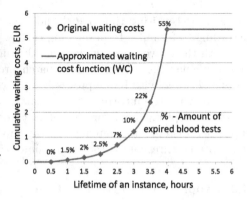

Fig. 6. Piecewise waiting cost function for the blood samples.

Total costs calculation. We return now to our claims mentioned in the introduction.

Firstly, we would like to calculate total expected costs in M/M/1 and in M/M(a,b)/1 systems. For that, we use Formulas 3 and 5, with the corresponding input data. The calculation of total expected costs gives the following results. The average waiting time in M/M/1 system is 49.8 min, and the average waiting time of a blood test in M/M(a,b)/1 system is 54.0 min. However, the total expected costs in M/M/1 are equal to 10.35 EUR, and the total expected costs in M/M/1 are equal to 0.57 EUR.

Thus, we can see that though the average waiting time is a bit higher for the batch activity, but the total expected costs are significantly. Therefore, the first conclusion can be made, that the batch activity significantly improves the processing of blood tests, in comparison with usual processing.

Secondly, the analysis of the optimal threshold value can be done. For that, we fix the input parameters and change the threshold a in the range from 1 to maximum batch capacity of 30. In our use case, it means that we would like to identify the optimal number of blood samples which the nurse should include

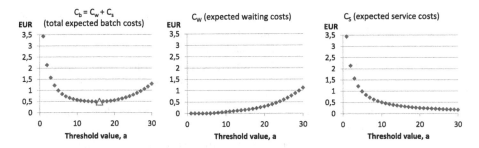

Fig. 7. Total expected costs, waiting costs and service costs for the batch activity for a changing threshold from 1 to maximum batch capacity of 30.

into a batch. The results, depending on different threshold values a, are reflected in Fig. 7.

The left graph in Fig. 7 shows that the function of total expected costs, depending on the threshold value a, is convex and has a minimum (depicted by a white triangle marker). The minimum of the function is equal to 16, with total expected costs per one instance equal to 0.49 EUR. Under such configuration, the average waiting time of an instance is 1.5 h.

The middle and right graphs in Fig. 7 provide a visual explanation for the existence of the minimum, which is a sum of expected waiting and service costs functions. In the first interval, during which the threshold value a is changing from 0 to its optimal value of 16, the expected waiting costs are relatively low, but the expected service costs are decreasing. In the second interval, during which the threshold value a is changing from its optimal value of 16 to the maximum batch capacity of 30, the expected service costs are approaching to zero, but the expected waiting costs are raising. In the context of our use case, an increased percentage of blood samples get expired with the curse of waiting time, so the associated costs get higher. The more blood samples the nurse can bring at once, the lower are the expected service costs per sample. Both, the waiting and service costs function are convex, therefore a minimum of its sum function exists.

Thus, the second conclusion can made, that the optimal threshold value a in case of batch processing system exists and can be found analytically.

5 Related Work

Few approaches, e.g., in [6, 13, 15], exist which consider the integration of batch activities into process models. These approaches are limited in their batch configuration possibility for the process designer. A recent approach in [11] offers with several parameters for the configuration of the batch activity and provides a concrete execution semantics. This was extended in [10] to batch regions enabling the synchronization of instances over a set of activities and the clustering of instances into specific batches based on their data characteristics. However, none of these approaches provides possibilities to evaluate the performance of a batch activity. In this work, a quantitative analysis approach, consisting in introduction of two cost functions for usual and batch activities, was presented.

In [2], different approaches as flow analysis, queuing theory, and simulation for the quantitative analysis of process models in general are discussed. However, batch activities are not considered in their discussion.

The batch service problem is intensively studied by queue theory providing means to determine waiting time, the average queue length etc. [5,7]. Further, different policies for starting a batch service are investigated, e.g., the threshold rule used in this paper was firstly analyzed by Neuts in [8] or the cost-based rule presented in [16]. A quantitative analysis of batch services based on a cost function can be found in [17]. However, this cost function was defined only for infinite capacity batch services with linear waiting costs. Our approach considers infinite as well as finite batch capacities and different types of waiting cost function to apply it for any use case.

6   Discussion and Conclusion

This paper presents an approach to evaluate the performance of a batch activity in a process model. For this sake, two generic cost functions were introduced which allow to calculate the waiting and service costs of usual and batch activities. With these functions, (1) the performance of using a batch activity can be compared to a usual activity and (2) an optimal configuration of a batch activity can be identified. Further, the functions were specified analytically with the help queuing theory. The presented approach was applied on a use case in which the batch activity demonstrated higher performance than the usual one. Additionally, the configuration minimizing the total cost for the batch activity was identified.

The queuing systems under discussion assumed exactly one task performer for the evaluated activity. However, our approach represents a generic scheme which can be applied analogously to the case of $M/M(a, b)/c$ system with c task performers. Further, in the systems under consideration, it was assumed that the type of arrival and service flow are Poisson and exponential correspondingly. Our approach can be applied for distributions of other kinds. In such cases, other queuing theory systems should be used to calculate the average waiting time and batch size.

Despite that the application of queuing theory enabled calculation of the introduced cost functions, there are certain limitations of its usage. If more complex configuration should be evaluated, the equations of queuing theory become more complicated, hardly applicable in practice. Further, not all configuration possibilities can be covered by existing queuing systems. Currently, we focus only on the evaluation of one activity and not on the whole process. For extending it to the whole process, techniques from queuing theory can not be applied anymore. Other techniques, e.g., queuing networks has to be used. However, those become quite complex.

An alternative method for evaluation of the batch activity performance, is simulation which is planned for future research. As well, our plan is to extend our evaluation to the batch regions concept [10] enabling the synchronization of instances with similar data characteristic over a set of activities.

References

1. Davis, M.M.: How long should a customer wait for service? Decis. Sci. **22**(2), 421–434 (1991)
2. Dumas, M., La Rosa, M., Mendling, J., Reijers, H.A.: Fundamentals of Business Process Management. Springer, Heidelberg (2013)
3. Ferguson, Mark E., Jayaraman, Vaidy, Souza, Gilvan C.: Note: an application of the EOQ model with nonlinear holding cost to inventory management of perishables. Eur. J. Oper. Res. **180**(1), 485–490 (2007)
4. Kendall, D.G.: Stochastic processes occurring in the theory of queues and their analysis by the method of the imbedded Markov chain. Ann. Math. Stat. **24**(3), 338–354 (1953)
5. Kleinrock, L.: Queueing Systems. Theory, vol. I. Wiley Interscience, New York (1975)
6. Liu, J., Hu, J.: Dynamic batch processing in workflows: model and implementation. Future Gener. Comput. Syst. **23**(3), 338–347 (2007)
7. Medhi, J.: Stochastic Models in Queueing Theory. Academic Press Professional Inc., San Diego (1991)
8. Neuts, M.: A general class of bulk queues with poisson input. Ann. Math. Stat. **38**(3), 759–770 (1967)
9. Polack, B., Schved, J.-F., Boneu, B.: Preanalytical recommendations of the d'Etude sur l'Hémostase et la Thrombose (GEHT) for venous blood testing in hemostasis laboratories. Pathophysi. Haemost. Thromb. **31**(1), 61–68 (2001)
10. Pufahl, L., Meyer, A., Weske, M.: Batch regions: process instance synchronization based on data. In: Enterprise Distributed Object Computing (EDOC). IEEE (2014, accepted for publication)
11. Pufahl, Luise, Weske, Mathias: Batch activities in process modeling and execution. In: Basu, Samik, Pautasso, Cesare, Zhang, Liang, Fu, Xiang (eds.) ICSOC 2013. LNCS, vol. 8274, pp. 283–297. Springer, Heidelberg (2013)
12. Rozinat, Anne, Mans, R.S., Song, M., van der Aalst, W.M.P.: Discovering simulation models. Inf. Syst. **34**(3), 305–327 (2009)
13. Sadiq, S., Orlowska, M., Sadiq, W., Schulz, K.: When workflows will not deliver: the case of contradicting work practice. In: BIS, Witold Abramowicz, vol. 1, pp. 69–84 (2005)
14. Sazvar, Zeinab, Baboli, Armand, Jokar, Mohammad Reza Akbari: A replenishment policy for perishable products with non-linear holding cost under stochastic supply lead time. Int. J. Adv. Manufact. Technol. **64**(5–8), 1087–1098 (2013)
15. van der Aalst, W., Barthelmess, P., Ellis, C., Wainer, J.: Proclets: a framework for lightweight interacting workflow processes. IJCIS **10**(4), 443–481 (2001)
16. Weiss, H., Pliska, S.: Optimal control of some Markov processes with applications to batch queueing and continuous review inventory systems. The Center for Mathematical Studies in Economics and Management Science, Discussion Paper 214 (1976)

17. Weiss, Howard J.: The computation of optimal control limits for a queue with batch services. Manage. Sci. **25**(4), 320–328 (1979)
18. Weske, M.: Business Process Management: Concepts, Languages, Architectures, 2nd edn. Springer, Heidelberg (2012)

Genetic Process Mining: Alignment-Based Process Model Mutation

M.L. van Eck$^{(\boxtimes)}$, J.C.A.M. Buijs, and B.F. van Dongen

Eindhoven University of Technology, Eindhoven, The Netherlands
{m.l.v.eck,j.c.a.m.buijs,b.f.v.dongen}@tue.nl

Abstract. The Evolutionary Tree Miner (ETM) is a genetic process discovery algorithm that enables the user to guide the discovery process based on preferences with respect to four process model quality dimensions: replay fitness, precision, generalization and simplicity.

Traditionally, the ETM algorithm uses random creation of process models for the initial population, as well as random mutation and cross over techniques for the evolution of generations. In this paper, we present an approach that improves the performance of the ETM algorithm by enabling it to make guided changes to process models, in order to obtain higher quality models in fewer generations. The two parts of this approach are: (1) creating an initial population of process models with a reasonable quality; (2) using information from the alignment between an event log and a process model to identify quality issues in a given part of a model, and resolving those issues using guided mutation operations.

1 Introduction

Over the years, more and more data is recorded and stored in information systems. Process mining aims to *discover, monitor and improve real processes by extracting knowledge from event logs* readily available in today's information systems [1]. Process *discovery* techniques can be used to automatically produce process models from such event logs and different techniques return different process models, with different properties and qualities.

There are four basic quality dimensions, shown in Fig. 1a, that are generally considered when discussing the quality of a process model [1,3]. The *replay fitness* dimension quantifies the extent to which the model can accurately replay the cases recorded in the log. The *precision* dimension measures whether the model prohibits behavior which is not seen in the event log. The *generalization* dimension assesses the extent to which the model will be able to reproduce possible future, yet unseen, behavior of the process. The complexity of the model is captured by the *simplicity* dimension, which operationalises Occam's Razor.

A general approach for genetic process discovery is shown in Fig. 1b. First, a *population* of models is created that are then evaluated according to the four quality dimensions described above. The models in the population are repeatedly changed using random mutation and crossover operations, and then re-evaluated until a stop criteria is satisfied. Finally, the best scoring model will be returned.

© Springer International Publishing Switzerland 2015
F. Fournier and J. Mendling (Eds.): BPM 2014 Workshops, LNBIP 202, pp. 291–303, 2015.
DOI: 10.1007/978-3-319-15895-2_25

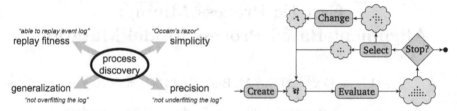

(a) The four quality dimensions used to calculate process model fitness (from [1]).

(b) The different phases of a genetic process discovery algorithm, as given in [3].

Fig. 1. The four quality dimensions and the genetic process discovery approach.

The quality of the models is measured as a weighted average over the four dimensions. Although all quality dimensions are of importance, obtaining a good quality in the dimension of replay fitness is crucial since it relates the observed behavior in the log to the model [3]. The replay fitness is computed using the alignment-based fitness computation defined in [2]. Alignments are explained in more detail in Subsect. 2.2, but basically they provide insights into where exactly the differences are between the behavior observed in the log and the model under consideration.

Unfortunately, genetic algorithms cannot discover models from large logs very efficiently [1]. This is because it is computationally complex to obtain the alignments needed to determine replay fitness [2,5] and alignment calculation is already heavily optimized [2]. Moreover, in every generation of the algorithm, new models have to be aligned with the event log. Therefore, in this paper, our goal is to improve genetic process discovery by evaluating fewer models, i.e. we aim to discover higher quality models in fewer generations.

To reach this goal, we introduce two extensions that each address a particular part of the genetic process discovery lifecycle. The first extension is the guided creation of an initial population of models with a reasonable quality, such that few changes are needed to reach a model with a high quality. The second extension identifies quality issues in a given part of a model, which are then resolved using guided mutation operations instead of making completely random changes. In this paper we do not alter crossover.

We have chosen to use process trees, described in Subsect. 2.1, as the process modelling formalism for our approach. This choice was made because we want to support processes that contain duplicate activities and silent steps, and process trees are guaranteed to represent sound models. Also, we need a modelling formalism for which alignments are defined because they are used to determine the replay fitness of the models. Therefore, our approach has been developed in the context of the Evolutionary Tree Miner (ETM) [3], a genetic process discovery algorithm for process trees.

We explain our approach using a small event log from an example process shown in Fig. 2. The process starts with an A activity, followed by the parallel execution of B with a loop of C and D activities that is stopped after executing E. After this parallel execution, there is the choice to either execute or skip

ABCEG	×11	ABCEFG	×10
ACBEG	×7	ACBEFG	×10
ACEBG	×9	ACEBFG	×8
ACBDCEG	×5	ACDCEBG	×5
ACBCDCEFG	×1	ACDBCEG	×4
ACDBECDEG	×4	*ABCHIG*	×3
ACDBECDEFG	×2	*ACBCEG*	×2
ACDBCDCDEG	×3	ABCDCEFG	×3
ACDCBDCDCDEFG	×2	ACBDCEFG	×4
ACDCDCDBCDCDEG	×1	ACDCBEFG	×6

(a) The example event log. The red italic traces do not fit the modelled process completely.

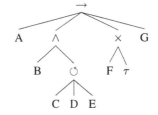

(b) A process tree of the example process.

Fig. 2. The event log and a model of the running example process.

activity F and the process ends after activity G. The event log reflects this behavior, but it also contains traces that do not conform to the process.

The structure of this paper is as follows: Sect. 2 contains an introduction on process trees and alignments. In Sect. 3 we explain how we create an initial population of good quality process trees. In Sect. 4 we show how to identify the parts of a process tree with a low quality and how to modify those parts. The experimental evaluation of our approach is presented in Sect. 5. Related work is discussed in Sect. 6 and we conclude this paper with Sect. 7.

2 Preliminaries

This section contains a short introduction to the process tree model notation and alignments which are used in the rest of the paper.

2.1 Process Trees

There exist many different process model notations and in this paper we use process trees to describe our process models. Process trees are used by the ETM algorithm internally because traditional modelling languages allow the creation of models that are not *sound* [3], i.e. these models contain deadlocks, livelocks and other anomalies. Process trees, however, are guaranteed to represent sound process models, which reduces the ETM algorithm's search space since unsound models do not have to be considered [3].

Figure 3 shows the possible operators that process trees can be composed of, and their translations to BPMN constructs. *Operator* nodes specify the relation between their children. The five available operator types are: sequential execution ($\rightarrow$), parallel execution ($\wedge$), exclusive choice ($\times$), non-exclusive choice ($\vee$) and repeated execution ($\circlearrowright$). Children of an operator node can again be operator nodes or they can be *leaf* nodes that represent the execution of an activity. The order of the children matters for the sequence and loop operators. The order of the children of a sequence operator specifies the order in which the children are executed (from left to right). Nodes can have an arbitrary number of children, except for loop nodes ($\circlearrowright$) that always have three children. The left child is the 'do' part of the loop

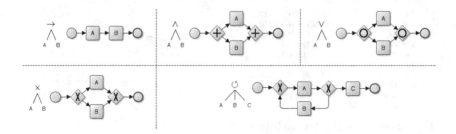

Fig. 3. The process tree operators and their relation to BPMN constructs.

and after its execution either the middle child, the 'redo' part, may be executed or the right child, the 'exit' part, may be executed. After the execution of the 'redo' part the 'do' part is again enabled and the 'exit' part is disabled. Process trees can also contain unobservable activities, indicated with a τ.

2.2   Alignments

Conformance checking techniques can be used to identify exactly where process executions that are stored in an event log deviate from the behavior allowed by a process model [1]. The most robust and state-of-the-art conformance checking technique *aligns* an event log and a process model by relating events in the event log to model elements and vice versa [2]. It does this by constructing an alignment that contains a minimal amount of deviations between the event log and the process model.

Figure 4a shows such an alignment, represented as a sequence of moves relating the trace $l = \langle A, C, B, D, C, E, G \rangle$ from our running example with an execution sequence σ of the model in Fig. 4b. Occurrences of events in l that are matched to activity executions in σ are called *synchronous moves*, e.g. move $\frac{A}{A}$. Events in l that cannot be executed at that point in σ are called *log moves*, e.g. activity B cannot be executed in the model during move $\frac{B}{\gg}$. Similarly, *model moves* are activities in σ for which there is no matching event in l at that point, e.g. moves $\frac{\gg}{B}$ and $\frac{\gg}{F}$. This information can be used to identify which activities should be skipped or inserted, and at what position in the model, to make it conform to the event log, as we show in Subsect. 4.1.

Move	1	2	3	4	5	6	7	8	9
l	A	C	B	D	C	E	$\gg$	$\gg$	G
σ	A	C	$\gg$	D	C	E	B	F	$\gg$

(a) An alignment between the trace $l = \langle A, C, B, D, C, E, G \rangle$ and an execution of the process tree in Fig. 4b.

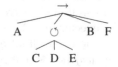

(b) A process tree discovered for the running example process.

Fig. 4. An alignment between a trace and a process tree.

3 Guided Population Creation

The first step in any evolutionary algorithm is the generation of an initial population, or in our case, the generation of an initial set of process trees. Since process trees are structured, sound process models, the generation of a random collection of process trees given a set of activities is rather straightforward. However, the quality of such a population typically leaves much to be desired.

In this section we present an approach that is used to create an initial population of process trees that describe part of the event log. This improves the ETM algorithm's process discovery performance because fewer changes are needed from the initial population to reach high quality models.

Our approach is based on the idea that the main behavior of a process is often captured in the most frequently occurring traces in an event log. Therefore, process trees describing the main behavior of a process can be created by first creating simple process trees that describe a small number of randomly selected individual traces, and then merging these simple trees.

The resulting models will in general have a higher quality than randomly generated process models. Their replay fitness may not be very high, because they only explain a part of the event log, but they will fully describe the selected traces. This means that they score very high on precision and simplicity, and also high on the current generalization metric. This balance of the different quality dimensions is desirable because the guided mutation operations described in Sect. 4 focus mainly on improving replay fitness.

3.1 Trace-Model Creation

Creating a process tree that describes a single trace, i.e. a *trace-model*, is relatively straightforward. The root is a →-operator with all the activities from the trace as its children, arranged in the same order as they occur in the trace, as shown for the trace $\langle A, C, D, B, E, C, D, E, G \rangle$ in the left model in Fig. 5.

When there are duplicate activities in a trace we modify the trace-model slightly to remove the duplicate activities, as shown in Fig. 5, to make it easier to merge the trace-models in the next step. Duplicate activities are detected by counting the number of occurrences of each activity in a trace. If there are

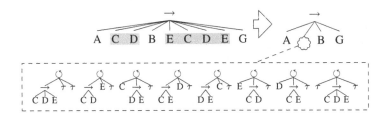

Fig. 5. Trace-model creation for the trace $\langle A, C, D, B, E, C, D, E, G \rangle$. The cloud in the right model is replaced with one of the possible ○-subtrees.

duplicate activities, such as activities C, D and E marked in gray, then the trace-model is parsed and a ↻-operator is inserted at the point where the first activity that occurs multiple times is encountered, which is between A and B in our example. The duplicate activities are removed from the trace-model and divided randomly over the 'do' and 'redo' children of the ↻-operator, while the order of the activities in these children is maintained, resulting in one of the 8 possible ↻-subtrees shown in the dashed rectangle.

Note that the duplicate elimination may result in a model that is unable to fully replay the original trace used to create the trace-model. Activities that are interleaved with duplicate activities, like activity B here, will be executed out of order. However, mutation operations can easily resolve this issue during evolution by putting B in parallel with the ↻-operator. The random choice for the ↻-subtree structure may also cause incorrect replay, but we want to introduce variation in the initial population here because the ETM's mutation operations have difficulties moving activities between the children of ↻-operators.

3.2 Merging Trace-Models

The second step in the guided population creation is merging several trace-models into a process tree that describes multiple traces. This is done iteratively by merging two trace-models and then merging the result with the remaining trace-models. This merging process continues until all randomly selected traces and their trace-models have been merged or until duplicate activities are introduced. Duplicate activities make it difficult to create a mapping of activities to merge two process trees, so if duplicate activities are introduced then the resulting process model is used and the remaining trace-models are discarded.

To merge two process trees without duplicate activities we create a process tree that contains the common behavior from both process trees and a choice between the behavior that is different, which is shown in Fig. 6 using examples. To identify the common behavior and the differences, we create a mapping between the nodes of the process trees being merged. Such a mapping is easily

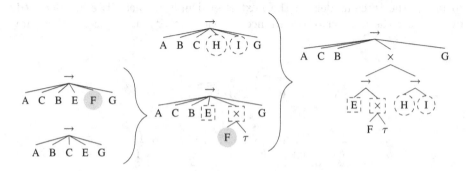

Fig. 6. Merging of trace models with nodes in the original and merged models marked for clarity.

created since each activity occurs at most once in each process tree. The order of activities that can be mapped is ignored because this can be improved later by the mutation operations introduced in Sect. 4. Therefore, the only important difference between the two leftmost models in Fig. 6 is activity F. The resulting merged model contains the mapped nodes from one process tree and a choice to skip the unmapped activity F. Similarly, merging the resulting model and the top right model introduces a choice between the unmapped activity E and ×-subtree from the first model, and the unmapped activities H and I from the second model.

4 Guided Mutation

The ETM algorithm aims to improve the quality of individual process trees in a population through the successive application of mutation and crossover operations that modify randomly selected nodes or subtrees, after which the quality of the resulting model is re-evaluated. We present an alternative approach to modify process trees, which reuses the replay fitness alignments to identify quality issues for a given node that are resolved using guided mutation operations.

In Subsect. 4.1, we introduce the *alignment move mapping* that shows the quality issues and what types of modifications may improve the quality. In Subsects. 4.2, 4.3 and 4.4 we introduce new operations that mutate process trees in a guided way using the mapping. Additional details can be found in [4].

Our approach focusses on replay fitness because it is generally considered to be the most important quality dimension [3,5]. However, while changing process trees we aim to improve the replay fitness without reducing precision. We also take into account generalization and simplicity, by inserting structured process model parts and by relying on the ETM algorithm to balance all four dimensions.

4.1 Identifying Quality Issues

The alignments described in Subsect. 2.2 provide *local* information on the parts of the model that are not conform the event log. Model moves indicate activities that should be able to be skipped in the model, while log moves indicate activities that should be inserted in the model. In order to identify where activities should be inserted or made skippable in the tree, we create a mapping between alignment moves and nodes in the tree for each trace in the event log.

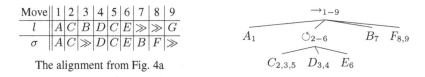

Move	1	2	3	4	5	6	7	8	9
l	A	C	B	D	C	E	≫	≫	G
σ	A	C	≫	D	C	E	B	F	≫

The alignment from Fig. 4a

Fig. 7. A mapping of the moves of the alignment in Fig. 4a on the process tree from Fig. 4b. The subscripts show which moves are mapped onto each node.

An alignment move mapping, as shown in Fig. 7, is created as follows. Synchronous and model moves in an alignment can be easily mapped onto nodes in the process tree because it is known which node was executed during such a move, e.g. move 1 $\left|\frac{A}{A}\right|$ is mapped onto node A and move 7 $\left|\frac{\gg}{B}\right|$ is mapped onto node B. However, no node in the process tree is executed during a log move, so therefore they are mapped onto the node related to the preceding and succeeding synchronous or model move. For example, move 3 $\left|\frac{B}{\gg}\right|$ is mapped onto activities C and D, while move 9 $\left|\frac{G}{\gg}\right|$ is mapped onto activity F. The argument for mapping log moves like this is that there are usually multiple suitable locations to insert activities to eliminate a log move, but including all possibilities makes modifying the process tree too complex.

All moves mapped to the children of a node are also mapped to the node itself. For example, the moves mapped to nodes C, D and E are also mapped to the ↻-operator and all moves are mapped to the root of the process tree. In this way, the alignment move mappings provide an indication of the behavior and the problems of each subtree within a process tree.

We use the information from the alignment move mapping to determine how to incrementally improve a process tree by mutating a given node. Behavior is removed if the given node is a leaf node onto which model moves, but no log moves, are mapped (Subsect. 4.2), behavior is added if the given node is a leaf node onto which log moves are mapped (Subsect. 4.3), and behavior is changed if the given node is an operator node (Subsect. 4.4).

4.2   Removing Behavior

Behavior can be removed from a process tree in two ways: by making activity nodes skippable or by removing them. Activity nodes are only removed from a process tree by the mutation operation if they are never executed as a synchronous move, otherwise they are made skippable.

Activity nodes are made skippable by replacing them with a choice between that node and a τ-node, as shown in Fig. 6 where node F is made skippable. Removing an activity node from a process tree is trivial, and an operator node without non-τ children can be removed as well. However, if a node's parent node is a ↻-operator then the node cannot be deleted because loop operators need to have three children, so the node is then replaced by a τ-node instead.

4.3   Adding Behavior

Behavior can be added to a process tree by inserting additional activity nodes into the tree, as shown in Fig. 8 where an activity is added to node F. First, an activity is randomly chosen from the set of log moves mapped onto the selected node. In this case, G is the only log move activity mapped to F. The old node is then replaced with an operator node joining both activities.

The choice for the operator node's type depends on the relation between the two activities in the event log. For each non-↻-operator type, we check what

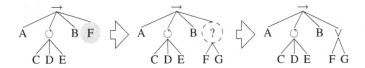

Fig. 8. Adding activity G next to node F in the process tree from Fig. 7.

percentage of the trace alignments where at least one of the two activities is executed, can be correctly replayed by the operator. In our example log, ∨ can replay all traces, while × can replay 54 %, and ∧ and → can replay only 46 % of the traces because activity F is not always executed while G is.

We then choose the most restrictive operator that enables the correct replay in at least a certain percentage of all traces, in order to prevent unnecessary losses in precision. In Fig. 8 the ∨-operator was chosen, but if a replay percentage over 50 % was good enough then the more precise ×-operator would have been chosen. Note that the ×-operator and ∧-operator are more restrictive than the ∨-operator, and the →-operator is more restrictive than the ∧-operator.

An exception to the approach above occurs if the two activities that we want to join together are identical, in which case we have identified a self-loop and instead of the above approach, the leaf node in the process tree is simply replaced with a ↻-operator that can repeatedly execute the activity.

4.4 Changing Behavior

The behavior of a process tree can be changed by adding and removing activities, but it can also be changed by modifying operator nodes. We use an iterative approach to change the type of an operator node, as shown in Fig. 9.

The first step in this approach is the random selection of two children of the operator node being changed, which are joined together with a new operator type chosen using the method discussed in Subsect. 4.3. In this example, the ↻-operator and node B are first joined with an ∧-operator because the activities below the ↻ are interleaved in the traces with B. The next step is randomly taking one of the remaining children and joining this child to the subtree created in the previous step. This is repeated until all children of the original operator

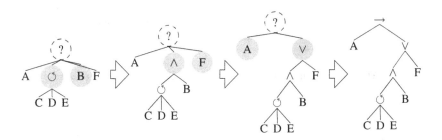

Fig. 9. Changing the behavior of the →-operator in the model from Fig. 7.

are added with an operator to the new subtree. Here, F is randomly selected in the second step and joined to the ∧-subtree with an ∨-operator because F is often missing in traces. Finally, A is selected as the last remaining child and joined with a →-operator because it is always the first activity.

5 Evaluation

The guided population creation and the guided mutations described in the previous sections have been evaluated using the running example log and a real-life event log[1]. The ETM algorithm and the extensions presented in this paper have been implemented in the ETM plug-in for the process mining framework ProM 6 [10]. Additional experimental evaluation can be found in [4].

5.1 Guided Population Creation

The results of the evaluation of the ETM's random initial population creation and the new approach from Sect. 3 are shown in Fig. 10. Both approaches were used to create 100 models that were evaluated in terms of an overall fitness score, calculated as a weighted average of the replay fitness (×10), precision (×5), simplicity (×1) and generalization (×0.1), which generally gives good results [3]. The resulting quality scores are presented as boxplots with the minimal and maximal values as the endpoints.

The results clearly show that guided population creation produces process trees with a higher quality than randomly generated models. For both logs, more than 75 % of the guided creation models are significantly better than the best randomly created model. Guided population creation produces models that have high scores for precision, simplicity and generalization [4], so they are well suited to be improved using guided mutation, as it focusses on improving replay fitness.

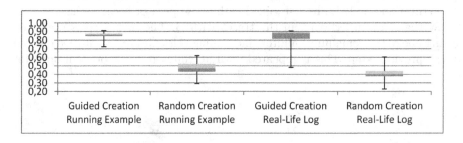

Fig. 10. Evaluation of the results of the initial population creation.

---

[1] The event log is publicly available at http://dx.doi.org/10.4121/uuid:a07386a5-7be3-4367-9535-70bc9e77dbe6.

5.2   Guided Mutation

The guided mutation operator evaluation consisted of multiple runs of 10,000 generations on the example log and 1,000 generations on the real-life event log. In each generation, the quality of the best scoring model was reported. The time required to mutate process trees is negligible compared to the time required to calculate their fitness. Therefore, we measure performance as the number of generations needed to reach a certain overall fitness score, defined as above. There was a 0, 25, 50, 75 or 100 % probability to apply a guided mutation operator instead of a random mutation when modifying process trees, with five runs for each setting. These settings also determined the probability that guided tree creation was used when creating a model for the initial population.

The results of the evaluation on the artificial event log are shown in Fig. 11a. The guided mutation operators are able to quickly improve the high quality initial models to reach quality scores that the original ETM needs many more generations to reach. The 25 %, 50 % and 75 % guided mutation runs also reached a quality score that the original ETM could not. An important observation is that the quality score of the runs with 100 % guided mutation is eventually surpassed by the original ETM. The cause of this is likely the limited exploration of the solution search space when random mutations are not used to modify process trees. Random mutation allows for every possible process tree to be created eventually in an infinite run, but this is not true for guided mutation.

The ETM was also tested with 1,000 generations per run on the real-life event log and the results are shown in Fig. 11b. Again, the results show that the initial population has a higher quality when using guided population creation. The guided mutation operators also improve these models quickly to reach an overall fitness score that takes the original ETM algorithm much longer to reach.

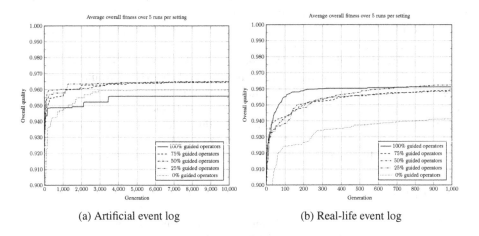

(a) Artificial event log   (b) Real-life event log

Fig. 11. The results of the guided mutation evaluation

6   Related Work

The guided mutation operators presented in this paper are similar to methods that aim to improve the quality of a model by repairing deviations. There exist approaches that repair deviations identified with respect to a known reference model [7], while other approaches use edit distance metrics to find improved models that are most similar to the model being repaired [6,8,9]. However, there are not many approaches that can automatically repair a model based on the deviations identified between a model and an event log [5].

One such repair approach by Fahland et al. [5] features an algorithm that tries to achieve a similar effect as the guided mutation operators introduced here. Their work focusses on repairing deviations between the behavior allowed by a process model and the behavior observed in an event log. These deviations are also detected by the creation of alignments between the process model and traces from the event log. Based on this information, they decompose the event log into several smaller logs containing the nonfitting subtraces. A subprocess is mined for each sublog using a process discovery algorithm and these are then added to the original model at the right location in order to repair the model. A limitation is that the approach cannot handle noise in the event log.

7   Conclusion

In this paper we presented an approach that enables the ETM to make guided changes to models, in order to obtain higher quality models in less time. The approach consists of two parts: (1) creating an initial population of process models with a reasonable quality; (2) identifying quality issues in a given part of a model, and resolving those issues using guided mutation operations.

The approach was evaluated using an artificial and a real-life event log, which showed that our approach can create higher quality models in fewer generations than the original ETM. However, the guided mutation operations are not perfect and random mutation is still required for optimal results.

In future work we plan to improve our approach as follows. The guided population creation can be improved with a more robust algorithm to merge process trees, while guided mutation is lacking when mutating ↺-operators. Furthermore, our approach does not indicate which nodes should be repaired first, while research in this area may help to reduce the dependency on the randomness of the ETM algorithm. Finally, we focussed on improving replay fitness, but similar approaches may be created for the other quality dimensions as well.

References

1. van der Aalst, W.M.P.: Process Mining: Discovery, Conformance and Enhancement of Business Processes. Springer, Heidelberg (2011)
2. Adriansyah, A., van Dongen, B.F., van der Aalst, W.M.P.: Conformance checking using cost-based fitness analysis. In: 2011 15th IEEE International Enterprise Distributed Object Computing Conference (EDOC), pp. 55–64. IEEE (2011)

3. Buijs, J.C.A.M., van Dongen, B.F., van der Aalst, W.M.P.: On the role of fitness, precision, generalization and simplicity in process discovery. In: Meersman, R., et al. (eds.) OTM 2012, Part I. LNCS, vol. 7565, pp. 305–322. Springer, Heidelberg (2012)
4. van Eck, M.L.: Alignment-based process model repair and its application to the Evolutionary Tree Miner. Master's thesis, Technische Universiteit Eindhoven (2013)
5. Fahland, D., van der Aalst, W.M.P.: Model repair - aligning process models to reality. Inf. Syst. **47**, 220–243 (2015)
6. Gambini, M., La Rosa, M., Migliorini, S., Ter Hofstede, A.H.M.: Automated error correction of business process models. In: Rinderle-Ma, S., Toumani, F., Wolf, K. (eds.) BPM 2011. LNCS, vol. 6896, pp. 148–165. Springer, Heidelberg (2011)
7. Küster, J.M., Koehler, J., Ryndina, K.: Improving business process models with reference models in business-driven development. In: Eder, J., Dustdar, S. (eds.) BPM 2006 Workshops. LNCS, vol. 4103, pp. 35–44. Springer, Heidelberg (2006)
8. Li, C., Reichert, M., Wombacher, A.: Discovering reference models by mining process variants using a heuristic approach. In: Dayal, U., Eder, J., Koehler, J., Reijers, H.A. (eds.) BPM 2009. LNCS, vol. 5701, pp. 344–362. Springer, Heidelberg (2009)
9. Lohmann, N.: Correcting deadlocking service choreographies using a simulation-based graph edit distance. In: Dumas, M., Reichert, M., Shan, M.-C. (eds.) BPM 2008. LNCS, vol. 5240, pp. 132–147. Springer, Heidelberg (2008)
10. Verbeek, H.M.W., Buijs, J.C.A.M., van Dongen, B.F., van der Aalst, W.M.P.: XES, XESame, and ProM 6. In: Soffer, P., Proper, E. (eds.) CAiSE Forum 2010. LNBIP, vol. 72, pp. 60–75. Springer, Heidelberg (2011)

Exploring Processes and Deviations

Sander J.J. Leemans$^{(\boxtimes)}$, Dirk Fahland, and Wil M.P. van der Aalst

Eindhoven University of Technology, Eindhoven, The Netherlands
{s.j.j.leemans,d.fahland,w.m.p.v.d.aalst}@tue.nl

Abstract. In process mining, one of the main challenges is to discover a process model, while balancing several quality criteria. This often requires repeatedly setting parameters, discovering a map and evaluating it, which we refer to as *process exploration*. Commercial process mining tools like Disco, Perceptive and Celonis are easy to use and have many features, such as log animation, immediate parameter feedback and extensive filtering options, but the resulting maps usually have no executable semantics and due to this, deviations cannot be analysed accurately. Most more academically oriented approaches (e.g., the numerous process discovery approaches supported by ProM) use maps having executable semantics (models), but are often slow, make unrealistic assumptions about the underlying process, or do not provide features like animation and seamless zooming. In this paper, we identify four aspects that are crucial for process exploration: *zoomability*, *evaluation*, *semantics*, and *speed*. We compare existing commercial tools and academic workflows using these aspects, and introduce a new tool, that aims to combine the best of both worlds. A feature comparison and a case study show that our tool bridges the gap between commercial and academic tools.

Keywords: Process exploration · Multi-perspective process mining · Process deviation visualisation · Conformance analysis

1 Introduction

Process mining, and in particular process discovery, have gained traction as a technique for analysing actual process executions from event data recorded in event logs. Process mining is typically used to learn whether, where, and how a process deviated from the intended behaviour. However, such information is usually not obtained by just running a single algorithm on an event log. A wide variety of (combinations of) algorithms can be used [2, 14, 18–20], typically heavily relying on various parameter settings to reveal and analyse specific aspects and features of a process, depending on the specific interests of the process stakeholder. Here we coin the term *process exploration* which refers to repeated parameter selection and tuning, iteratively performing process discovery, and continuously evaluating the resulting process map [1].

Interestingly, academic and commercial process mining tools support different aspects of process exploration. In this paper, we demonstrate that process exploration can be improved by combining beneficial features of academic

© Springer International Publishing Switzerland 2015
F. Fournier and J. Mendling (Eds.): BPM 2014 Workshops, LNBIP 202, pp. 304–316, 2015.
DOI: 10.1007/978-3-319-15895-2_26

and commercial tools. Existing commercial and some academic tools for process exploration, such as the Fuzzy Miner (FM) [11], Fluxicon Disco (FD) [12], Celonis Discovery (CD) and Perceptive Process Mining (PM), are based on showing directly-follows graphs: nodes are process steps, and in general edges mean that an activity followed another. Thus, one can inspect the process by considering the arrows between them. These visualisations are intuitive, an example is shown in Fig. 1, and some tools allow for extensive log filtering. Although directly-follows graph-based maps are useful for global analysis, they have some limitations. For instance, pure directly-follows based maps do not show parallelism, implying that in a map, the state of the system unrealistically solely depends on the last executed process step. Some tools support parallelism by sacrificing executable semantics, but their maps *cannot be used for automated analysis*; the maps do not show crucial features (e.g., types of splits and joins) and it is impossible to reason over them (e.g., which traces are possible). (In this paper, we refer to a process map with executable semantics as a process *model*.)

To evaluate a model with respect to its event log, several established quality metrics exist, for instance fitness, precision and generalisation [7]. Fitness describes what part of the log is expressed by the model, precision what part of the model is present in the log, and generalisation what part of future behaviour will be expressible by the model. While useful for model comparison, these measures are coarse grained: they provide a number for a model. Using more fine-grained measures and visualisations, *a detailed analysis of where the model deviates from the log and where other problems occur can be performed.* These evaluations require executable semantics and certain guarantees, for instance that

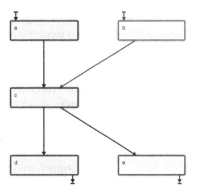

Fig. 1. Example of a process map, discovered by Perceptive.

the model contains no deadlocks, livelocks or other anomalies: that the model is *sound*. On an unsound model, for instance, only an upper bound of fitness can be computed reliably [13]. Only if a discovered process map is sound and has executable semantics, its quality with respect to the event log can be assessed accurately.

Academic tools are usually focused, powerful and the maps produced by them usually have executable semantics. Therefore, deviations and quality metrics can be studied. However, academic tools or plug-ins are often designed for one particular purpose, and combining tools, if possible, challenges usability. The ProM framework [9] streamlines cooperation between tools, as input and output formats of plug-ins of the framework are standardised. However, consider for instance a typical process exploration workflow in the ProM framework: to mine a model from a log using ILP miner and assessing the quality of the model, one has to click through 10 pop-up screens of parameters and options.

In this paper, we aim to bridge this gap between commercial and academic tools by introducing a process exploration tool, *Inductive visual Miner* (IvM), that provides the features of commercial tools and aims to be as user-friendly, while providing maps with semantics and built-in deviation visualisation. We consider some desirable features from both commercial and academic tools, and describe how IvM improves on them. A prototype of IvM has been implemented as a plug-in of the ProM framework and is available for download from http://promtools.org. We perform a feature comparison and a case study on real-life logs.

The remainder of this paper is organised as follows: we first provide some background on process exploration. In Sect. 3 we analyse existing process exploration tools and discuss design decisions for IvM. A high-level feature comparison and a case study are performed in Sect. 4; Sect. 5 concludes the paper.

2   Process Exploration

Process exploration enables users to learn information from an event log. In this section, we first give an example of a process exploration case study, after which four aspects of process exploration are explored: zoomability, evaluation, speed and semantics.

Example. We illustrate process exploration using the winning case study of BPIC12 [4]. In this case study, first a high-level overview was generated to get an initial idea of the complexity of the given event log. The complexity was reduced by applying activity and life cycle filters to the event log. Next, a filter leaving only successful traces was applied and a high-level map was created, showing the 'happy flow' through the process, i.e. the path taken by an average trace. On this happy flow, business impact was measured, i.e. how many traces were successful or rejected with respect to each activity in the happy flow, leading for instance to the conclusion that "Nearly 23 % of the applications that go to validation stage are declined, indicating possibilities for tightening upfront scrutiny at application or offer stage". Further on in the case study, an analysis was made whether the outcome of a trace (successful or rejected) was predictable during execution, which for instance led to the conclusion that "slow moving applications had a less than 6 % chance of getting to approval". The authors note that this analysis, which was performed using decision tree miners, could be repeated at other stages.

This single case study already clearly shows the repeated process of setting parameters, selecting filters, generating process maps and continuously evaluating the results.

Zoomability. In the case study of [4], the log was examined on a high level, and then repeatedly examined in detail for different perspectives, e.g. by applying filters and using both high-level and detailed process maps. Compare it to electronic road maps: users can get a high-level view to see highways, or can zoom in to see alleys. Moreover, different perspectives can be shown, such as bicycle or public transport maps. A process exploration tool should support similar features by enabling a user adjust the level of detail in a process map (e.g. highways and alleys) and to filter it in several ways (e.g. bycicle maps); we refer to this ability as *zoomability*.

As the case study shows, a plethora of filtering options must be available: filters on event name (prefix), frequency, redundancy, data attributes and on resources were all used. Moreover, as used, the tool should be able to provide both a process map showing only the frequent paths of the process, as well as one with the outliers; i.e. maps with several levels of noise filtering. Many more filters are imaginable, however giving an exhaustive list of them is outside the scope of this paper.

Another powerful zoomability parameter is time: using log animation, a user can inspect this time perspective: the event log is visually replayed on the map, which reveals frequent paths and bottlenecks over time, and makes concept drift explicit. If an animation can be paused, it gives a frozen view of the map with the traces that were in the process at a particular point in time.

Evaluation. Given that the quality criteria fitness, precision, generalisation and simplicity compete [7], a perfect model often does not exist. Any process discovery algorithm has to make a trade-off between these criteria, so there may be many Pareto optimal models without there being a clear "best" one. For instance, low fitness could indicate a high-level model that is well-suited for getting the idea, but ill-suited for drawing high-confidence detailed conclusions. High precision indicates that the model closely resembles the behaviour of the event log, while a low precision indicates that the model allows for much behaviour that never happened. A model with bad generalisation has little predictive value (overfits), as it only describes the behaviour of the event log. More specifically, for instance the question whether a violation to the four-eyes principle occurred, i.e. whether two different persons looked at a certain case, should not be answered using a model with 80 % fitness, as roughly 20 % of the behaviour is not shown in it. Another example: a question whether something *could* happen in the future should be answered on a model with high generalisation, rather than an overfitting one.

Thus, conclusions based on discovered models should be drawn carefully while accounting for the quality criteria, and in order to find the best model to answer the question at hand, a process exploration tool should enable a user to evaluate a map.

A quality measure is typically expressed as a number, e.g., a fitness of 0.8. However, a single number for a complete model might be less informative. For example, one half of the process model could have a fitness of 0.6, while the other half might have a fitness of 1.0. A process exploration tool should provide detailed quality indicators, to locate problems in specific parts of the model.

Speed. The speed of process exploration is determined by two elements: the learning curve for users and the responsivity of the tool. Many aspects influence the learning curve of a tool; we highlight two: the map should use a representation that is easy to read by people who are not computer scientists, and the learning curve can be more gradual if the tool invites users to play with its parameters (for which the tool should be responsive).

Responsivity is a challenge that comes with zoomability; exploration requires interaction: a user should neither have to wait long nor have to perform many

actions to adjust the zoom; understanding a process requires a quick and responsive user interface.

Semantics and Guarantees. As described in the introduction, executable semantics and guarantees are essential for evaluation in a process exploration tool. Executable semantics allow for replay, which enables decision point analysis (which
was performed in the BPIC12 case study: for a specific point in the process it
was analysed what made a trace likely to succeed, and the authors note that
they would like to repeat this experiment for other points in the process; using
a model, the decision points would be known, allowing for automation [15]),
enables prediction [22], and enables compliance checking [16].

3   Existing Tools and Design Decisions

In this section, we analyse existing tools
with respect to the requirements discussed
in Sect. 2. Meanwhile, we describe the
design decisions we made for the Inductive
visual Miner (IvM).

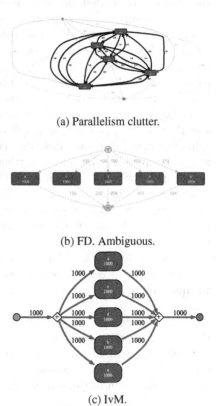

(a) Parallelism clutter.

Tools. In this paper, we consider the following commercial tools: Fluxicon Disco
$(FD)^1$ [12], Celonis Discovery $(CD)^2$ and
Perceptive Process Mining $(PM)^3$. For the
academic tools, we consider three chains
of plug-ins within the ProM framework:
(1) Fuzzy Miner [11] (FM), (2) the chain
$(IMi\text{-}C)$, consisting of Inductive Miner -
infrequent (IMi) [13], followed by PNetReplayer [3] and Project Manifest to Model
for Conformance, and (3) the chain $(ILP\text{-}C)$, consisting of ILP miner (ILP) [21],
followed by PNetReplayer [3] and Project
Manifest to Model for Conformance. We
need to consider chains of plug-ins to allow
for a fair comparison.

(b) FD. Ambiguous.

*Representation and Process Discovery
Technique.* The first choice to make for a
process exploration tool is what discovery
technique and which representation to use.

The existing tools use three categories
of discovery techniques: directly-follows

(c) IvM.

Fig. 2. Examples of tools applied to a
log containing five parallel activities.

---

[1] http://fluxicon.com/disco/; April/May 2014.
[2] http://www.celonis.de/en/discover/our-product; April/May 2014.
[3] http://www.perceptivesoftware.co.uk/products/perceptive-process/process-mining;
fast miner, April/May 2014.

based (FD, CD, PM, FM)[4], inductive mining (IMi) and optimisation problem mining (ILP). Directly-follows based tools either provide no semantics (FD, CD, FM) or do not support parallelism (PM), but are fast and allow for filtering; ILP provides semantics, and guarantees perfect fitness and best-possible precision, but does not guarantee soundness; IMi strikes a balance: it is fast, guarantees soundness, can guarantee fitness, and allows for noise filtering.

The learning curve of a tool is important for the speed aspect. We consider the directly-follows based representations to have the most gradual learning curve, and the Petri net based representations to have the steepest. Therefore, in order to obtain the most gradual learning curve, we design our representation to be as close as possible to the directly-follows based representation, but we add parallelism while keeping semantics.

For logs containing parallelism, directly-follows based tools usually connect all parallel activities, which yields clutter. For instance, the parallel execution of 5 activities yields a clique containing 20 edges (Fig. 2a). A strategy to reduce this clutter is to manually filter out the parallel activities, as done in the BPIC12 case study [4]. Another strategy, used in for instance FD and FM, is to filter these edges (Fig. 2b). However, Fig. 2b looks exactly like the exclusive choice between 5 activities; only the numbers on the edges, denoting the frequency with which an edge was taken, tell the difference. So, while fixing parallelism, ambiguity is introduced.

In IvM, behind the scenes we use a variation of IMi. Internally, IMi and IvM use so-called process trees to ensure sound models. However, the results are shown to the user using a directly-follows based representation to stay close to that representation and its learning curve; we extend it with a start state, an end state and Petri net places to provide semantics, those are drawn very small and can be safely ignored by considering them a way to connect edges; to support parallelism and to avoid parallelism clutter, we extend it with BPMN parallel gateways (Fig. 2c). The complete representation is easily translatable to both BPMN and Petri nets.

Enrichment. The edges and nodes of the map provide an opportunity to enrich the map with information from the event log, such as frequency (FD, CD, PM, FM, IMi-C, ILP-C), performance metrics (FD, CD, PM), data, resources, and deviations (PM, IMi-C, ILP-C) (the latter helping towards evaluation). A perfect process exploration tool would support all of them, and even more, as many measures can provide valuable insight. For now, we demonstrate that these metrics contributing to zoomability can be added, by visualising frequency on the nodes and edges; resources and deviations are visualised using other means.

Zoomabililty. All directly-follows based tools we considered support zoomability by filtering. We discuss a few filtering options here, of which the most common, and basic, are to consider only the most frequent paths (CD, PM, FD), and to consider only the most frequent activities or edges (PM, CD, FD, FM).

---

[4] Some tools (FM) can also take the eventually-follows relation into account.

Another way to filter is on time, for which two options exist: filtering events on timestamp (FD, CD, PM), which results in a map valid for the chosen interval, and animation (FD, CD, PM, FM), which results in a time-based overlay of the overall map. Animation in these four tools is

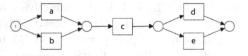

Fig. 3. Map discovered by IMi-C from a log in which b and e were not executed in a single trace, which is not shown.

realised by showing tokens, representing cases, flowing over the edges of the map.

Most tools we considered (PM, CD, FD, FM, IMi-C) have problems discovering and visualising long-distance dependencies, i.e. showing how a choice in the process influences a choice later in the process. For instance, consider the log $L_l = [\langle a, c, e \rangle^{100}, \langle a, c, d \rangle^{100}, \langle b, c, d \rangle^{100}]$, in which b and e are never executed in a single case. This precision information might be interesting, but, as exemplified by Figs. 1 and 3, cannot be derived directly from the output of any tool we considered. In most tools (PM, CD, FD, IMi-C, ILP-C), it is possible to filter all traces not going through b, after which it can be noted that e disappears or is never used. However, some tools make inspecting a *model* difficult by replacing the model with a new one on filtering.

Ideally, a process exploration tool supports as many easily accessible filters as possible. In IvM, we implemented three filters: (1) frequent paths, (2) frequent activities and (3) specific activities. To streamline long-distance dependency inspection, specific activities (3) can be filtered by clicking on nodes in the graph. Moreover, animation was implemented; Fig. 4 shows a screenshot.

Evaluation and Deviations. As explained in Sect. 2, it is important that a process exploration tool enables the evaluation of a model with respect to a log. We analyse evaluation in the existing tools using three levels: model, activity and event. On the model level, there is a single number for an entire model; on the activity level, evaluation is possible on activities or other parts of the model; on the event level, for each event in each trace evaluation is enabled.

The tools CD, FM and FD provide some model level evaluation by means of their parameters. For instance, FD allows to set a percentage of most frequent paths that should be visualised, giving an estimation of fitness. These measures provide little guidance on the quality of the map. Better model-level fitness metrics are given by FM and PM, indicating what percentage of the events in

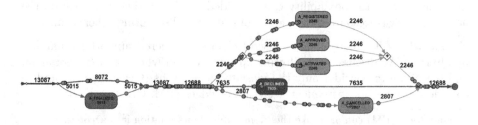

Fig. 4. IvM (excerpt). Log animation on part of the BPIC12 log [8].

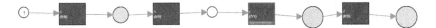

(a) IMi-C. Non-white places contain log moves and their size indicates the frequency. The third activity has model moves as is indicated by a bar and a thick border.

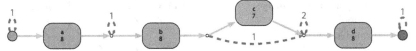

(b) IvM. Dashed edges denote deviations: self-edges are log moves; the bypassing edge is a model move.

Fig. 5. Visualisation of deviations (Color figure online).

the log have a corresponding edge in the map. A detailed event-level view is available (FM) that shows for each event in each trace whether it has such a corresponding edge.

The chains IMi-C and ILP-C first compute a model-log alignment, after which the results are visualised in a plug-in common to both. Such an alignment, given a trace t and a model M, is intuitively a best guess of what run of M could have produced t (minimising the number of deviations between the trace and the path through the model). An alignment consists of *synchronous moves*, in which M and t agree on the step taken; *model moves*, in which M took a step and t did not; and *log moves*, in which the t took a step and M did not. For more information about alignments, please refer to [3]. Both IMi-C and ILP-C provide model level statistics as well as activity-level based aggregations (see Fig. 5a). An event-level visualisation similar to FM's is available in another plug-in.

Instead of using alignments to visualise deviations, they could be used to repair the model [10]. While repairing a model, the model is updated to allow steps at the position of log moves; model moves are accounted for using circumvention constructs. After repair, perfect fitness is guaranteed, but precision can only deteriorate. Given that process exploration should enable a user to find the right balance between quality dimensions, we cannot use model repair directly.

Therefore, in IvM we combine the ideas of model repair and alignment visualisation: we perform a model repair, however do not apply it to the model, but add it to the visualisation of the model in dashed/red edges. (we reduce the information about log moves to frequencies for readability reasons) Fig. 5b shows an example; if all dashed/red edges would be transformed to normal edges, the model would have perfect fitness, which suits a deviations visualisation.

Ideally, a process exploration tool should enable evaluation on all three levels, thereby providing *zoomable evaluation*. We implemented both the event and the activity-level; the event-level visualisation is similar to the one used in FM.

4   Comparison

In this section, we compare IvM to existing process discovery tools in two ways: (1) we summarise the feature comparison of Sect. 3 and (2) perform a case study

Table 1. Feature comparison of process discovery tools.

		FD	CD	FM	PM(4)	IvM	IMi-C	ILP-C
	Log import from XES	✓	✗	✓	✗	✓	✓	✓
	Log import from CSV/XLS	✓	✓	✓	✓	✓	✓	✓
	Map export to vector image	✓	✗(2)	✗(3)	✗(2)	✓	✗(3)	✗(3)
	Local tool	✓	✗	✓	✓	✓	✓	✓
Semantics	Executable semantics	✗	✗	✗	✓	✓	✓	✓
	Guaranteed soundness	-	-	-	✓	✓	✓	✗
	Guaranteed perfect fitness (6)	-	-	-	✓	✓	✓	✓
	Best-possible precision	-	-	-	✗	✗	✗	✓
	Representational bias ∋ parallelism	-	-	-	✗	✓	✓	✓
	Representational bias ≥ ILP-C	-	-	-	✗	✗	✗	✓
	Representational bias ≥ process trees	-	-	-	✗	✓	✓	✗
	Model export to Process Tree	-	-	-	✗	✓	✓	✗
	Model export to Petri net	-	-	-	✗	✓	✓	✓
	Avoid parallelism-clutter	✓	✗	✓	✗	✓	✓	✓
Zoomability	Frequency enrichment	✓	✓	✓	✓	✓	✓	✓
	Performance enrichment	✓	✓	✗	✓	✗	✓(5)	✓(5)
	Path frequency filter	✓	✗(7)	✗	✓	✓	✓	✗
	Activity/edge frequency filter	✓	✓	✓	✓	✓	✗	✗
	Specific activity/edge filter	✓	✓	✓	✓	✓	✓	✓
	Timestamp filter	✓	✓	✗	✓	✗	✗	✗
	Performance filter	✓	✗(7)	✗	✓	✗	✗	✗
	Animation	✓	✓	✓	✓	✓	✗	✗
Evaluation	Model level	✗	✗	✗	✓(1)	✗	✓	✓
	Activity level	✗	✗	✗	✓	✓	✓	✓
	Event level	✗	✗	✗	✗	✓	✓(5)	✓(5)
	Model repair-semantics	✗	✗	✗	✓	✓	✗	✗
Speed	Immediate parameter feedback	✓	✓	✓	✓	✓	✗	✗
	Long-distance dependency filter without model replacement	✗	✓	✗	✗	✓	✗	✗

on two real-life examples. Table 1 contains the feature comparison. Most features were introduced in Sect. 3.[5,6]

Case Study. In this section, we compare the tools used in this paper on two real-life logs: a log of a financial institution (BPIC12) [8], and a log from a building permit approval process of a Dutch municipality (WABO1BB) [5][7]. All tools were applied using their default settings.

---

[5] 'Local tool' denotes whether the tool can run on the machine of the user; 'Representational bias' refers to the class of models that can be discovered with a tool.

[6] Remarks in Table 1: (1) lower bound on fitness (2) vector screenshot export broken; (3) vector screenshot results in embedded bitmap; (4) PM provides a genetic 'thorough' miner, but that does not guarantee termination; we excluded it from the comparison; (5) available in a separate plug-in; (6) perfect fitness until a filter is applied; (7) could possibly be achieved by writing PQL queries.

[7] The WABO1BB log has been published between submission and acceptance or this paper.

The BPIC12 log was filtered to only contain the 23 'complete' activities; Fig. 6 shows the results of process exploration tools applied to it. These figures exemplify problems of tools we tested: Figs. 6c (CD), d (PM) and e (ILP-C) provide little information by their omnipresence of edges; Figs. 6a (FD) and b (FM) could be useful for analysis, but conclusions should be drawn carefully: note that in FD, from only six activities the bottom/end state can be reached, and in both maps it is unclear what the presence or absence of edges actually *means*. As IvM and IMi-C use a similar discovery algorithm and both visualise deviations, their outputs closely resemble one another. However, considering the speed aspect of process exploration, it took 10 screens of parameters/pop-ups to obtain Fig. 6g (IMi-C), and *none* to obtain Fig. 6f (IvM).

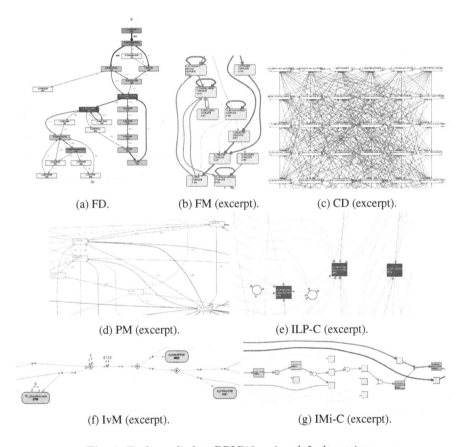

(a) FD.   (b) FM (excerpt).   (c) CD (excerpt).

(d) PM (excerpt).   (e) ILP-C (excerpt).

(f) IvM (excerpt).   (g) IMi-C (excerpt).

Fig. 6. Tools applied to BPIC12, using default settings.

The WABO1BB log was filtered to only contain the 22 'BB' activities. Given the sensitive nature of this log, we were not allowed to upload it to cloud services at time of writing; CD had to be excluded from the analysis. Figure 7 shows the results. Figures 7a (FD) and c (FM) are again useful for analysis, but should be read with care: it is clear that the map deviates from the log as activity 01_BB_730 occurred 13 times and has only 4 outgoing edges in FD, but it is not clear how and where the map deviates. Figure 7b (PM) is a quite readable model, however some of the most-used activities appear to be parallel. The model returned by ILP-C (Fig. 7d) is not a workflow net and replay requires some log and model moves (this could be avoided using the 'empty after completion' parameter). Figures 7e and f show excerpts of the similar models by IMi-C and IvM. The added value of IvM comes when one would like to explore the process and fine-tune the parameters; IMi-C and ILP-C require the user to re-run several plug-ins with each adjustment, IvM does not.

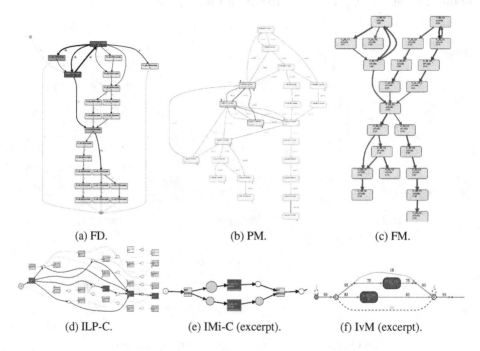

(a) FD.   (b) PM.   (c) FM.

(d) ILP-C.   (e) IMi-C (excerpt).   (f) IvM (excerpt).

Fig. 7. Tools applied to WABO1BB, using default settings.

This small case study shows that on the real-life logs we tried, some commercial tools returned difficult-to-interpret maps and others fail to produce readable maps at all. Probably, fine-tuning the parameters might improve the readability of maps, especially in CD and PM. The FM, while academic and a plug-in of ProM, resembles the commercial tools we considered: no executable model semantics but immediate parameter feedback. As IMi-C and IvM use a similar discovery algorithm, the most notable objective differences between IvM and IMi-C are that IvM provides log animation and immediate parameter feedback: *exploring* a process is easy, while IMi-C and ILP-C require a user to leave the visualisation, call a mining plug-in, set all parameters, call an alignment plug-in, and the visualisation plug-in again.

5   Conclusion

In this paper, we identified a gap between commercial and academic process exploration tools. The commercial tools we considered are easy to use and have many features, such as log animation, immediate parameter feedback and extensive filtering options, but the process maps created either do not show parallelism or have no executable semantics and deviations to the maps cannot be computed. Academic tools often create maps with executable semantics, and deviations can be analysed in detail using replay and alignment techniques. However, features important for the exploration of processes are missing and existing tool chains require many steps, thus making exploration tedious and non-interactive.

We introduced a process exploration tool: the Inductive visual Miner (IvM). It aims to bridge this gap between academic and commercial process exploration tools. IvM immediately discovers an initial model, computes deviations and shows these to the user, using a new visualisation that allows for the animation of the traces of a log. IvM is not as feature-rich or scale-oriented as some of the commercial tools, but shows that it is possible to use powerful academic techniques in a user-friendly package. We hope that IvM will inspire commercial vendors to consider models with executable semantics and support deviation analysis.

For future work, one could consider the fast computation of near-optimal alignments. This paper focused on visualising fitness deviations; precision and generalisation problems could be visualised as well, such as in [17]. Furthermore, the Evolutionary Tree Miner [6] could be integrated to obtain an intuitive interactive guided miner.

Acknowledgement. We thank Robin Wolffensperger for his contributions to the positioning of log moves.

References

1. van der Aalst, W.M.P.: Process Mining: Discovery, Conformance and Enhancement of Business Processes. Springer, Heidelberg (2011)
2. van der Aalst, W.M.P., Weijters, A., Maruster, L.: Workflow mining: discovering process models from event logs. IEEE Trans. Knowl. Data Eng. **16**(9), 1128–1142 (2004)
3. Adriansyah, A.: Aligning observed and modeled behavior. Ph.D. thesis, Eindhoven University of Technology (2014)
4. Bautista, A.D., Wangikar, L., Akbar, S.M.K.: Process mining-driven optimization of a consumer loan approvals process - The BPIC 2012 challenge case study. In: La Rosa, M., Soffer, P. (eds.) BPM Workshops 2012. LNBIP, vol. 132, pp. 219–220. Springer, Heidelberg (2013)
5. Buijs, J.C.A.M.: Environmental permit application process ('wabo'), CoSeLoG project - municipality 1 (2014). http://dx.doi.org/10.4121/uuid:c45dcbe9-557b-43ca-b6d0-10561e13dcb5

6. Buijs, J.C.A.M., van Dongen, B.F., van der Aalst, W.M.P.: A genetic algorithm for discovering process trees. In: IEEE Congress on Evolutionary Computation, pp. 1–8. IEEE (2012)
7. Buijs, J.C.A.M., van Dongen, B.F., van der Aalst, W.M.P.: On the role of fitness, precision, generalization and simplicity in process discovery. In: Meersman, R., et al. (eds.) OTM 2012, Part I. LNCS, vol. 7565, pp. 305–322. Springer, Heidelberg (2012)
8. van Dongen, B.F.: BPI Challenge 2012 Dataset (2012). http://dx.doi.org/10.4121/uuid:3926db30-f712-4394-aebc-75976070e91f
9. van Dongen, B.F., de Medeiros, A.K.A., Verbeek, H.M.W.E., Weijters, A.J.M.M.T., van der Aalst, W.M.P.: The ProM framework: a new era in process mining tool support. In: Ciardo, G., Darondeau, P. (eds.) ICATPN 2005. LNCS, vol. 3536, pp. 444–454. Springer, Heidelberg (2005)
10. Fahland, D., van der Aalst, W.M.P.: Repairing process models to reflect reality. In: Barros, A., Gal, A., Kindler, E. (eds.) BPM 2012. LNCS, vol. 7481, pp. 229–245. Springer, Heidelberg (2012)
11. Günther, C.W., van der Aalst, W.M.P.: Fuzzy mining – adaptive process simplification based on multi-perspective metrics. In: Alonso, G., Dadam, P., Rosemann, M. (eds.) BPM 2007. LNCS, vol. 4714, pp. 328–343. Springer, Heidelberg (2007)
12. Günther, C.W., Rozinat, A.: Disco: discover your processes. In: BPM (Demos). CEUR Workshop Proceedings, vol. 940, pp. 40–44. CEUR-WS.org (2012)
13. Leemans, S.J.J., Fahland, D., van der Aalst, W.M.P.: Discovering block-structured process models from event logs containing infrequent behaviour. In: Lohmann, N., Song, M., Wohed, P. (eds.) BPM 2013 Workshops. LNBIP, vol. 171, pp. 66–78. Springer, Heidelberg (2014)
14. Leemans, S.J.J., Fahland, D., van der Aalst, W.M.P.: Discovering block-structured process models from incomplete event logs. In: Ciardo, G., Kindler, E. (eds.) PETRI NETS 2014. LNCS, vol. 8489, pp. 91–110. Springer, Heidelberg (2014)
15. de Leoni, M., van der Aalst, W.M.P.: Data-aware process mining: discovering decisions in processes using alignments. In: SAC, pp. 1454–1461. ACM (2013)
16. Ramezani, E., Fahland, D., van der Aalst, W.M.P.: Where did I misbehave? Diagnostic information in compliance checking. In: Barros, A., Gal, A., Kindler, E. (eds.) BPM 2012. LNCS, vol. 7481, pp. 262–278. Springer, Heidelberg (2012)
17. Rozinat, A.: Process mining: conformance and extension. Ph.D. thesis, Eindhoven University of Technology (2010)
18. Schimm, G.: Process miner - a tool for mining process schemes from event-based data. In: Flesca, S., Greco, S., Leone, N., Ianni, G. (eds.) JELIA 2002. LNCS (LNAI), vol. 2424, pp. 525–528. Springer, Heidelberg (2002)
19. Solé, M., Carmona, J.: Process mining from a basis of state regions. In: Lilius, J., Penczek, W. (eds.) PETRI NETS 2010. LNCS, vol. 6128, pp. 226–245. Springer, Heidelberg (2010)
20. Weijters, A., Ribeiro, J.: Flexible Heuristics Miner. In: CIDM, pp. 310–317. IEEE (2011)
21. van der Werf, J., van Dongen, B.F., Hurkens, C., Serebrenik, A.: Process discovery using integer linear programming. Fundam. Inform. 94(3–4), 387–412 (2009)
22. Wynn, M., Rozinat, A., van der Aalst, W.M.P., ter Hofstede, A., Fidge, C.: Process mining and simulation. In: Hofstede, A.H.M., van der Aalst, W.M.P., Adams, M., Russell, N. (eds.) Modern Business Process Automation, pp. 437–457. Springer, Heidelberg (2010)

Experimenting with an OLAP Approach for Interactive Discovery in Process Mining

Gustavo Pizarro and Marcos Sepúlveda[(✉)]

Computer Science Department, School of Engineering,
Pontificia Universidad Católica de Chile, Santiago, Chile
marcos@ing.puc.cl

Abstract. Business process analysts must face the task of analyzing, monitoring and promoting improvements to different business processes. Process mining has emerged as a useful tool for analyzing event logs that are registered by information systems. It allows the discovering of process models considering different perspectives (control-flow, organizational, time). However, currently they lack the ability to explore jointly and interactively the different perspectives, which hinder the understanding of what is happening in the organization. This article proposes a novel approach for interactive discovery aimed at providing process analysts with a tool that allow them to explore multiple perspectives at different levels of detail, which is inspired on OLAP interactive concepts. This approach was implemented as a ProM plug-in and tested in an experiment with real users. Its main advantages are the productivity and operability when performing process discovery.

Keywords: Process mining · Business process discovery · OLAP

1 Introduction

During the last decades, the concept of Business Process Management (BPM) has been gradually adopted by organizations worldwide. In many of these organizations, dedicated BPM areas have been created. The key role in these areas is the process analyst, who is responsible for modeling, monitoring and auditing business processes. More recently, the growth of the digital universe has made possible that these activities have an even greater reach, since information systems create event logs that store when the different processes' activities are performed [16, 18]. These logs allow performing a robust analysis about what is actually happening in the organizations through process mining. This discipline enables the automatic analysis of a process using various techniques, including process discovery, conformance checking and process enhancement [18]. Several of them are described in [16] and are sorted out by frequency of use in [5]. In process discovery, a model is created based on an event log without using any a-priori information; see [4, 16, 18, 19, 21], among others.

The current discovery tools allow creating either a control-flow diagram or a social network, but do not allow exploring interactively different process perspectives. We can infer from [2] that understanding the whole process requires an effort that is beyond the capabilities of traditional processes analysts, since the analysis of each perspective:

© Springer International Publishing Switzerland 2015
F. Fournier and J. Mendling (Eds.): BPM 2014 Workshops, LNBIP 202, pp. 317–329, 2015.
DOI: 10.1007/978-3-319-15895-2_27

control-flow, social or time, should be done separately. In addition, the process analyst must choose among a large number of discovery algorithms, each of them having a different representational bias and a set of parameters that must be configured. It is therefore very difficult to achieve a correct multi-perspective understanding of the process in an efficient way using existing tools.

This article proposes a novel approach for interactive discovery aimed at providing process analysts with a tool that allow them to explore a process in several perspectives at the same time, considering different levels of detail, and using dynamic and interactive filtering. Processes can be visualized considering different scenarios, allowing a comparative analysis on the control-flow, organizational or time perspectives. Considering the desired features, and the usability and quality expected, we concluded that such a concept of discovery must be implemented using an OLAP paradigm, providing navigation operations such as drill down, roll up, slice and dice, and pivot, allowing to explore the different perspectives: from groups performing similar tasks or groups that work together to single performers; from all possible paths to variants grouped in clusters; from traces that last little to traces that last long. Pivot views must be available showing control-flow diagrams or social networks that display the relationships between different performers. This approach was implemented as a plug-in in ProM [20] and tested in an experiment with real users.

2 Related Work

In this section related work relevant to the development of this research is discussed.

2.1 The Analyst and His Interactive Exploration Task

Within the process area there are different roles. The most important are: process manager, process owner, process architect and process analyst [7]. Different skills and abilities are required to perform each of them, since they have different responsibilities. According to [1], the process analyst role is to support a holistic view of business processes and to offer the ability to quickly transform the organization. [13] notes that the process analyst should support the BPM life cycle that, among other activities, includes the analysis, design, monitoring and control of business processes. This requires demonstrating knowledge to audit processes, to perform gap analysis, and to support transformational changes in business environments.

In process mining, it has not been cataloged what kind of tool is most appropriate for each type of user. However, in the field of business intelligence, a broader field that includes process mining, different types of users have been identified. According to [8], there are two large categories of users: information consumers and information producers. Within the first group are business analysts and casual users. Casual users include executives, managers, employees and external users; they see reports regularly, but they do not calculate numbers or perform detailed trend analysis on a daily basis. Business analysts can also do more sophisticated analysis. Information consumers, in general, use dashboards, covering query and reporting tools, OLAP, spreadsheets, standard reports and output of statistical models. Within the information producers are report authors that use statistical data mining tools, as well as some business analysts. Some power users can be both information producers and information consumers at the same time. An example of this mixed user is the business analyst. They typically use spreadsheets, pivot tables, simple database queries, and create custom reports. While there is more than one recommended tool for business analysts, most of them are related to dynamic information filtering. Considering the multidimensional approach required in this work and tools that are familiar to business analyst, we decided to implement the OLAP paradigm for processes analysis.

OLAP (Online Analytical Processing) is a solution aimed at speeding up queries to large amounts of data; multidimensional structures are used for this purpose. Some characteristic aspects of this approach are the multidimensional conceptual view, intuitive manipulation of data, and the use of unlimited dimensions and aggregation levels [6]. The different dimensions can be explored using different operations, such as drill down, roll up, slice and dice, and pivot. The relevance of its application to process mining has already been mentioned by [15] and [22], but it is still an open challenge to define what the best way to do it is.

2.2   Process Discovery

In recent years there has been an evolution in the algorithms used for process discovery, but there has been little progress in this task from the process analyst viewpoint [18]. Since 2005, several algorithms have been proposed for control-flow discovery, such as Alpha Mining [19], Heuristic Mining [21] and Region Mining [4], among others. These algorithms have different approaches at the algorithmic level and contribute in different use cases. However, from the process analyst's viewpoint, they do not provide a task-oriented interactive exploration of the event log and do not provide a multidimensional understanding of the process. The first tool aimed at a more complex task than just getting a flow is Fuzzy Mining [10]. Despite being innovative, this proposal only addresses the control-flow perspective and requires process analysts to understand parameters that are algorithmic-centric rather than business-centric.

BPMNAnalysis [2] has as its primary motivations reducing the complexity of dealing with hundreds of algorithms in ProM and getting closer to the business language. It provides a multidimensional discovery by combining different existing tools, considering a holistic view of data, including variants, resources and time dimensions. It is a step forward towards a process analyst oriented discovery, but it does not cover the whole process analyst's viewpoint and it has not been tested on business users.

Recently, there have been a few multidimensional proposals covering the process through different dimensions and incorporating the OLAP concept at the algorithm level. This is the case of Multidimensional [15], which explores what tools are extensible to a multidimensional level, developing, for example, process discovery using HeuristicMiner, considering flows with roles or time. While this work was developed from the algorithmic viewpoint, it contributes to promote the multidimensional approach, incorporating conformance metrics to the multidimensional analysis, and an evaluation of the tool using ISO9126. Another recent proposal is the ProcessCube [12, 22], which allows the comparative analysis of different process models.

It compares different segments of the process (based on subsets of the event logs) or different organizational levels, incorporating a formal description to multidimensional analysis of the event log. These last two works do not focus on the day to day task of process analysts, as BPMNAnalysis and the present investigation do.

3 Proposal – OLAP Discovery

This paper develops a concept of interactive process discovery for process analysts, combining interactive exploration, dynamic filtering, navigation using OLAP operations, and automatic updates. It is also aimed at improving some aspects of usability with respect to existing tools, maintaining currently available discovery functionalities, and achieving a better understanding about what happens in organizations. The type of user (process analyst) and the task to be accomplished (interactive multi perspective discovery) were considered in the design. Already existing discovery tools were used at the algorithmic level.

The OLAP approach allows navigating the process in a similar way to a pivot table found in spreadsheets, exploring the different dimensions of a process, dynamic filtering of some dimensions leaving constant the others, going from a top level view to a detailed one, pivoting from a control-flow view to an organizational view, and comparing different versions. The proposed tool is called OLAPDiscovery, and it is integrated within the ProM framework. The dimensions considered are: social networks using Social Miner [17], variants and trace clustering using Trace Alignment [3], and time based on event timestamps. Results are displayed using the visualization diagrams of Heuristic Miner (control-flow view) and Social Miner (organizational view).

The process analyst must monitor and control processes to promote improvements and to create reports for business managers. Such users are familiar with the BPM approach and have knowledge about business goals, but they are not necessarily experts in data mining or process mining. Complementing this information with the classification of users in the Business Intelligence area, it can be state that in some cases these users are information consumers and in others are information producers. Improve usability for non-experts have been recognized as one of the ten most important challenges in process mining [18]. Furthermore, a recent study indicates that the major drawbacks of current tools are that they are unintuitive and difficult to understand [5]. The desirable discovery tool must allow changing the different variables that influence the process and see dynamically how those changes affect the control-flow and the organizational views.

The OLAP paradigm is useful to implement interactive discovery. The information about the execution of a process contained in an event log fits perfectly to be implemented in an OLAP cube with at least three dimensions: variants, resources and time:

Variant: A process variant is a unique start-to-end trace, a certain sequence of activities in which the process is executed, which has been recorded in the event log at least once. It may be found several times in the event log, representing cases involving different performers at different times. This dimension is composed by clusters of similar variants and it can be explored top-down, from the whole event log to a single variant. The dimension is generated using the Trace Alignment plug-in [3]. Trace Alignment groups variants into clusters based on different criteria. It can be used to explore the process in early stages of analysis, and to answer specific questions in later stages. Therefore, it complements the existing process mining techniques that focus on process discovery and conformance checking. It allows studying the backbone of the process, the critical points that share the variants, to see the gaps between what really happened and what should have happened, to detect patterns and discover variants with minor differences compared to the desired behavior, among others.

Resource: In this dimension, we used the Social Miner plug-in, which allows grouping performers using different criteria. We considered three types of groups: people performing similar tasks, people working together, and handover of work. In addition, the user can change the threshold value that defines when two or more resources are grouped together. The user can also drill down or roll up through the different groups.

Time: A simple criterion was used in this dimension: the duration of each case. The user can filter the log between a minimum and a maximum duration.

Results can be displayed either in a control-flow view or an organizational view, being able to pivot between them at any time. For the control-flow view, the result of the Heuristic Miner was chosen because it describes the main observed behavior and can deal with noise [21]. The resulting view of the Social Miner plug-in is used for the organizational view since this view also allows discovering interactions between performers through visual inspection.

Initially the control-flow view is displayed (see Fig. 1). Buttons in the top right allows pivoting to the organizational view, switching from the comparison view to the single analysis (large) view, resetting the analysis, and saving the current view. In the middle right, a tab is displayed for each dimension (see Fig. 2); by clicking on each of them, the user can filter the event log. Figure 3 shows the two discovery views: the control-flow view and the organizational (resources) view.

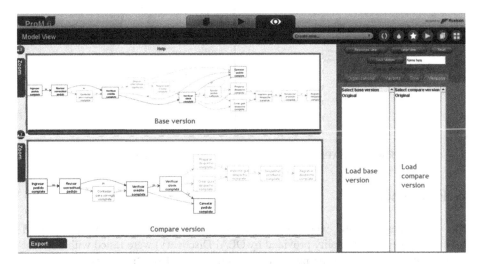

Fig. 1. OLAPDiscovery, comparison view and versions management

The comparison view was included to increase usability. It is possible to view the last view (after different OLAP operations have been applied to the original event log) for a single analysis or a comparison view, where a reference view (at the beginning the one corresponding to the whole event log) can be compared against the last view (see Fig. 1). The user can store a given analysis at any time and later load it for further analysis; it can be loaded in the upper part (as a reference for future comparisons) or at the bottom, for further filtering the recently loaded version.

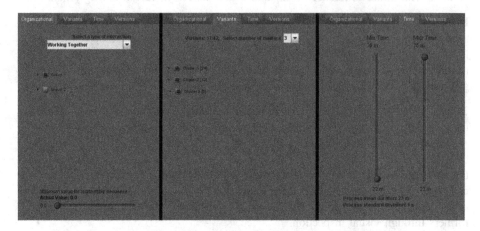

Fig. 2. OLAPDiscovery dimensions

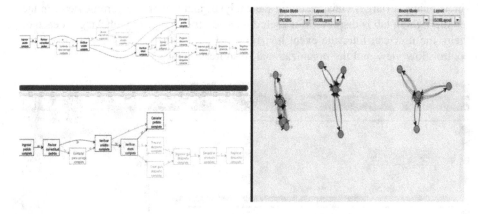

Fig. 3. OLAPDiscovery control-flow and organizational views

4 Experiment

This section describes the experiment, in which OLAPDiscovery, Disco [9] and ProM (without the new functionality provided by OLAPDiscovery) were tested with different users, to analyze what are the perceived advantages of OLAPDiscovery.

4.1 Participants

The sample was composed of 38 people: 16 experts and 22 basic users. Tests were carried out at different times, in groups of 1 to 6 users. Users were students in the last two years from Information Systems or related degrees. We considered as basic users those who have completed a full semester business process modeling course, where student learn BPM concepts and ProM is used in a basic way. On the other hand, we considered as expert users those who have completed a full semester process mining course, where students learn process mining exhaustively based on [16].

4.2 Tasks Performed by the Users

The tasks performed by the users required them to answer two sections of four questions each. The first section was about unidimensional analysis, one for each dimension of the process behavior. Some questions were statements about the process, and the user had to determine if they were true or false; the rest were multiple-choice questions about basic characteristics of the process. The second section consisted of tasks that combined different dimensions. In this case, users had to answer whether some statements were true or false. For answering the statements, users were required to analyze whether in a given scenario (a group of performers executing some variants in a certain time interval) the process behaves or not in a certain way. The user had to complete each unidimensional task in a maximum of 5 min and each multidimensional task in a maximum of 12 min. To reduce learning curve effects, each user received an accurate training about how to perform each task before answering any questions. In addition, each question had a companion explanation that described step by step how to perform the analysis. Every user had to answer three different tests (one for each tool) with eight questions each, based on three different event logs. There was no time limit, but they could finish the task if the recommended time was exceeded. Each tool was evaluated in a different order by each user to evaluate whether using one of the tools before the others might influence the results.

4.3 Description of the Evaluation

We used a simple software quality assessment model based on ISO9126 [11], a. standard that has already been used for evaluating process mining tools [15]. We combined ISO9126-3 and ISO9126-4 techniques [11]. The following attributes from the functionality and usability features of ISO9126-3 were considered: suitability, understandability, learnability and operability. Other attributes were excluded, because they were less relevant to the approach of our tool. From ISO9126-4, effectiveness, productivity and satisfaction were considered; security was left out because it is not the focus of this research.

Both objective and subjective metrics were considered for measuring software quality. Table 1 shows the objective metrics, which are based on users' performance answering all questions. Table 4 shows the subjective metrics, which measure users' perception after completing all activities. A brainstorming was performed to find out the attributes we wanted to measure, creating an initial list of 80 questions. Based on the judgment of BPM experts, we selected the 16 most representative. We did not want an extensive questionnaire, since users were required to answer it for each tool.

Table 1. Objective metrics

Attributes	Metrics
Completed tasks	Tasks completed/Total tasks
Effectiveness	Tasks completed successfully/Total tasks
Unidimensional time	Time needed to complete unidimensional tasks
Multidimensional time	Time needed to complete multidimensional tasks
Productivity	Effectiveness/Time needed to complete tasks

4.4   Results

In this section, we first focus on some objective metrics: effectiveness and productivity, and then we discuss the results for subjective metrics.

Table 2 shows the average number of unidimensional and multidimensional tasks that were correctly completed by the users using the different tools (note that OLAP-Discovery is abbreviated OLAP-D in all figures and tables).

All tools allow users to complete unidimensional tasks. The number of correct answers in ProM and OLAP-D is similar, showing both tools are well suited to answer unidimensional requirements. With Disco more incorrect answers are obtained because this tool has some limitations for analyzing resources. Users could not complete successfully all multidimensional tasks in ProM, showing the need for a tool that can handle multi-perspective tasks. In average, users could not complete or answer wrongly 1 out of 4 tasks in ProM; most of them basic users. On the other hand, only one user could not complete a multidimensional task using OLAP-D; and two, using Disco. These multidimensional tasks are more challenging and therefore the number of incorrect answers is higher for all tools.

Table 2.   Average completed unidimensional and multidimensional tasks.

	Completed unidimensional tasks		Completed multidimensional tasks		
	Correct answers	Incorrect answers	Correct answers	Incorrect answers	Incomplete answers
ProM	4,82	0,18	2,95	0,55	0,50
Disco	4,58	0,42	3,34	0,63	0,03
OLAP-D	4,84	0,16	3,29	0,68	0,03

Not only completing tasks is relevant, but also the time it takes. Table 3 shows the time required to perform unidimensional tasks, multidimensional tasks, and all tasks for the three tools, considering the order in which they were tested by the users; first, second or third. It can be seen the time required to complete both unidimensional and multidimensional tasks is greater in OLAP-D than in Disco and in ProM. The best case in Disco is not less than the slowest case in OLAP-D. Moreover, the best case in ProM requires more than twice the time required in the slowest case in OLAP-D.

Table 3. Time required for performing different tasks, according to the order of testing.

Tool	Order on the testing	Time in unidimensional tasks (minutes)	Time in multidimensional tasks (minutes)	Total time (minutes)
OLAP-D	1	4.5	7.8	12.3
OLAP-D	2	2.9	5.9	8.8
OLAP-D	3	2.4	6.4	8.8
Disco	1	5.9	9.6	15.6
Disco	2	4.3	9.4	13.7
Disco	3	4.2	9.5	13.7
ProM	1	12.5	18.5	31.0
ProM	2	11.2	18.0	29.1
ProM	3	10.0	15.9	25.9

Figure 4 shows the productivity achieved by the users with the different tools. It displays the relationship between effectiveness (tasks completed correctly/total tasks) and the total time required for performing all tasks; it also considers the order in which they were tested by the users. It can be seen that the productivity achieved with OLAP-D is greater; the tasks were performed with greater effectiveness in less time. This figure also shows that with the current sample of users, it is not possible to conclude that the learning curve is smaller with any of the three tools.

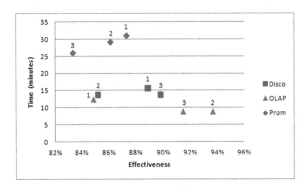

Fig. 4. Productivity represented as the relationship between effectiveness and total time.

Table 4 summarizes the results of the subjective comparison between OLAP-D and the other two tools, ProM and Disco. It is shown the non-parametric Mann-Whitney U test that compares two samples to evaluate if they are the same; both the Mann-Whitney

Table 4. Subjective metrics - statistic tests for comparing the different tools

Attribute - Metric	OLAP-D vs Disco		OLAP-D vs ProM	
	Mann–Whitney U	Significance	Mann–Whitney U	Significance
Effectiveness - I can understand a process as a whole (with all the characteristics that distinguish it)	611,0	0,214	357,0	<0,001
Effectiveness - I can understand a process accurately (and clearly)	682,5	0,666	476,5	0,001
Productivity - The steps required to perform an analysis are adequate	636,0	0,315	225,5	<0,001
Productivity - The time required to perform an analysis is reasonable	511,0	0,017	110,0	<0,001
Satisfaction - I would recommend this software to my colleagues	635,5	0,323	217,5	<0,001
Satisfaction - I would use this software to analyze processes	630,5	0,286	268,5	<0,001
Suitability - The available parameters are suitable	689,0	0,700	481,5	0,007
Suitability - The software is useful for the analysis of my processes	689,0	0,710	470,5	0,006
Suitability - The organization of menus is logical	705,0	0,851	354,0	<0,001
Understandability - The features of this software are easy to understand	639,0	0,348	157,0	< 0,001
Understandability - The information generated is easy to understand	658,0	0,453	316,0	< 0,001
Learnability - It is easy to remember how to do things	555,0	0,050	250,0	< 0,001
Learnability - The tool is simple to use	647,5	0,390	124,0	< 0,001
Operability - It is easy to act based on the information generated	522,5	0,022	272,0	<0,001
Operability - It is easy to combine an analysis of all aspects of a process	409,0	0,001	174,0	<0,001
Operability - It is easy to move from one feature to another one	502,0	0,013	273,5	<0,001

U test and the corresponding significance are displayed. The Mann-Whitney U test [14] was used since distributions were not normal; this method is widely used to study ordinal variables such as Likert scale statements.

When comparing OLAP-D and ProM, the difference in most statements is quite broad. OLAP-D has their mode values between "strongly agree" and "agree" for all statements while ProM has their mode values in "agree" in only seven cases. For all metrics, the significance of the Mann-Whitney U test is less than 0.05, showing OLAP -D is different (better) in all statements compared to ProM.

When comparing Disco and OLAP-D, quite similar results were obtained. However, in some statements OLAP-D was considered to be better than Disco. It is the case of the statement "The time used for the analysis is reasonable" (Productivity) and all statements about Operability. Therefore, according to the users' viewpoint, OLAP-D is as good as Disco, but it is considered to be more productive (which is consistent with the objective metrics discussed above) and having a higher operability.

When results are split by type of users (basics vs. experts), the results show expert users appreciate ProM better than basic users, but still like Disco and OLAP-D better. Expert users evaluate OLAP-D better in Operability and Productivity compared to Disco. On the other hand, basis users do not see any significant difference between OLAP-D and Disco. This might be explained because while OLAP-D offers more advanced functionalities, Disco is friendlier for basic users.

4.5   Experiment Limitations

There are two main limitations of the experiment. First, the tasks designed to measure multidimensional analysis only cover the most common scenarios considered in the development of OLAPDiscovery; ProM and Disco provide additional features that are useful in other scenarios. Second, the size of the sample of users is small.

5   Conclusions

This article introduces OLAPDiscovery, a novel approach for interactive process discovery aimed at providing process analysts with a tool that allow them to explore process perspectives at different levels of detail. This approach was implemented as a ProM plug-in and it was tested in an experiment with real users.

The experiment shows that the dynamic, multi-perspective and interactive discovery provided by OLAPDiscovery offers a better productivity, measures as the relationship between effectiveness and time, in both unidimensional and multidimensional tasks compared to the usage of ProM or Disco. The key is the dynamic interactivity offered to the user, and the ability to filter and automatically get results both in the control-flow and the organizational perspectives. The analysis of subjective metrics allows us to conclude that users think this multi-perspective interactive process discovery is more operational and productive than the one provide with existing tools. It is interesting that for basic users OLAP-D is as good as Disco because both tools have different strengths; while Disco provides a nicer user interface, OLAP-D provides features that allow them to solve multidimensional tasks in a simpler way. The aim of this research is better reflected in expert users; they think OLAP-D provides a better productivity and operability compared to Disco.

This research shows that it is relevant to assess the functionality, usability and quality in use of any process mining tools from the users' viewpoint, since not only the algorithm is relevant, but also how to provide a satisfactory experience for the users.

In the future we visualize several research opportunities. First, we have used specific control-flow and organizational algorithms, but it could be possible to enable users to select their own favorite discovery algorithms. Second, we have only explored some process perspectives; a promising and straight-forward enhancement is to extend the OLAP approach to other data perspectives. Third, the OLAP approach could be extended for conformance analysis, allowing users to verify conformance in a subset of the original event log against a subset of the reference model, proving a better understanding of eventual discrepancies between the observed and the expected behavior.

References

1. Bandara, W., Chand, D.R., Chircu, A.M., Hintringer, S., Karagiannis, D., Recker, J.C., van Rensburg, A., Usoff, C., Welke, R.J.: Business process management education in academia: Status, challenges, and recommendations. Commun. Assoc. Inf. Syst. **27**, 743–776 (2010)
2. Bayraktar, İ.: The Business Value of Process Mining Bringing It All Together. Eindhoven University of Technology, Eindhoven (2011)
3. Jagadeesh Chandra Bose, R.P., van der Aalst, W.: Trace alignment in process mining: Opportunities for process diagnostics. In: Hull, R., Mendling, J., Tai, S. (eds.) BPM 2010. LNCS, vol. 6336, pp. 227–242. Springer, Heidelberg (2010)
4. Carmona, J.A., Cortadella, J., Kishinevsky, M.: A Region-Based Algorithm for Discovering Petri Nets from Event Logs. In: Dumas, M., Reichert, M., Shan, M.-C. (eds.) BPM 2008. LNCS, vol. 5240, pp. 358–373. Springer, Heidelberg (2008)
5. Claes, J., Poels, G.: Process mining and the ProM framework: An exploratory survey. In: La Rosa, M., Soffer, P. (eds.) BPM Workshops 2012. LNBIP, vol. 132, pp. 187–198. Springer, Heidelberg (2013)
6. Codd, E.F., Codd, S.B., Salley, C.T.: Providing OLAP (on-line analytical processing) to user-analysts: An IT mandate, vol. 32. Codd and Date (1993)
7. Doebeli, G., Fisher, R., Gapp, R., Sanzogni, L.: Using BPM governance to align systems and practice. Bus. Process Manage. J. **17**(2), 184–202 (2011)
8. Eckerson, W.W.: Performance Dashboards: Measuring, Monitoring, and Managing Your Business. Wiley, New York (2010)
9. Fluxicon Process Laboratories, Inc. [Download]: Disco version 1.5
10. Günther, C.W., van der Aalst, W.M.: Fuzzy mining – Adaptive process simplification based on multi-perspective metrics. In: Alonso, G., Dadam, P., Rosemann, M. (eds.) BPM 2007. LNCS, vol. 4714, pp. 328–343. Springer, Heidelberg (2007)
11. International Organization for Standardization: ISO 9126: Software Engineering – Product quality. Switzerland, Geneva (2001)
12. Mamaliga, T.: Realizing a process cube allowing for the comparison of event data. Master's Thesis, Eindhoven University of Technology, Eindhoven (2013)
13. Mathiesen, P., Bandara, W., Delavari, H., Harmon, P., Brennan, K.: A comparative analysis of business analysis (BA) and business process management (BPM) capabilities. In: ECIS 2011 Proceedings (2011)

14. Newbold, P., Carlson, W., Thorne, B.: Statistics for Business and Economics. Pearson, New Jersey (2008)
15. Ribeiro, J.T.S.: Multidimensional Process Discovery. Eindhoven University of Technology, Eindhoven (2013)
16. van der Aalst, W.M.: Process Mining. Discovery, Conformance and Enhancement of Business Processes. Springer, Heidelberg (2011)
17. Van der Aalst, W.M., Reijers, H.A., Song, M.: Discovering social networks from event logs. Comput. Support. Coop. Work (CSCW) 14(6), 549–593 (2005)
18. van der Aalst, W., et al.: Process mining manifesto. In: Daniel, F., Barkaoui, K., Dustdar, S. (eds.) BPM 2011 Workshop, Part I. LNBIP, vol. 99, pp. 169–194. Springer, Heidelberg (2012)
19. Van der Aalst, W., Weijters, T., Maruster, L.: Workflow mining: Discovering process models from event logs. IEEE Trans. Knowl. Data Eng. 16(9), 1128–1142 (2004)
20. van Dongen, B.F., de Medeiros, A.K.A., Verbeek, H., Weijters, A., van der Aalst, W.M.: The ProM framework: A new era in process mining tool support. In: Ciardo, G., Darondeau, P. (eds.) ICATPN 2005. LNCS, vol. 3536, pp. 444–454. Springer, Heidelberg (2005)
21. Weijters, A.J.M.M., van der Aalst, W.M., De Medeiros, A.A.: Process mining with the heuristics miner-algorithm. Technische Universiteit Eindhoven, Technical Report, p. 166 (2006)
22. van der Aalst, W.M.: Process cubes: Slicing, dicing, rolling up and drilling down event data for process mining. In: Song, M., Wynn, M.T., Liu, J. (eds.) AP-BPM 2013. LNBIP, vol. 159, pp. 1–22. Springer, Heidelberg (2013)

Merging Event Logs with Many to Many Relationships

Lihi Raichelson[(⊠)] and Pnina Soffer

Department of Information Systems, University of Haifa, 31905 Haifa, Israel
LihiRa0s@gmail.com, Spnina@is.haifa.ac.il

Abstract. Process mining techniques enable the discovery and analysis of business processes, identifying opportunities for improvement. However, processes are often comprised of separately managed procedures that have separate log files, impossible to mine in an integrative manner. A preprocessing step that merges log files is quite straightforward when the logs have common case IDs. However, when cases in the different logs have many-to-many relationships among them this is more challenging. In this paper we present an approach for merging event logs which is capable of dealing with all kinds of relationships between logs, one-to-one or many-to-many. The approach matches cases in the logs, using temporal relations and text mining techniques. We have implemented the algorithm and tested it on a comprehensive set of synthetic logs.

Keywords: Process mining · Multiple instances · Merging log files · End-to-end process

1 Introduction

Process mining techniques are used for discovery and analysis of the actual business processes from the event logs of the systems that support and manage them [1, 2]. However, process mining usually considers a single event log, while different process procedures often use different systems and thus have separate logs. To provide a full analysis, process mining should be applied to a log containing all relevant activities of the end-to-end process flow. Such log can only be obtained after identifying and merging related log files from different distributed systems corresponding to the same process.

Existing methods that compose logs [11] either assume identical case ID or the existence of one log's case ID as an attribute in the other log, and simple relationships between procedures (one-to-one or one-to-many). Often, real-life processes include procedures that stand for multiple instances and hence may have complex relations among them (e.g. many-to-one or many-to-many). In such situations, each procedure employs a different case ID, not necessarily directly corresponding to cases in the other procedures. Merging the logs of these procedures becomes a challenging task, which is still mandatory for an extended analysis of the entire process.

In this paper we present an automatic technique for merging event logs, which does not assume any specific relationship between the procedures and is hence applicable for one-to-one as well as for many-to-many relationships, where no unique identifier

© Springer International Publishing Switzerland 2015
F. Fournier and J. Mendling (Eds.): BPM 2014 Workshops, LNBIP 202, pp. 330–341, 2015.
DOI: 10.1007/978-3-319-15895-2_28

correlates the cases in the logs. To illustrate the problem, consider an example process, where different organizational units can directly place orders for office supplies through an ordering system. Consolidated deliveries are received at a warehouse, where they are registered and distributed to the ordering units. We consider the ordering process as the main process, and the delivery handling as the sub-process. Table 1 shows a simplified log of the main process, while a simplified log of the warehouse procedure is given in Table 2.

Table 1. Simplified log of the main process of ordering goods

Order	Timestamp	User	Activity	Item no	Department
3001	02/02/14 10:12	Ilana	open order	1234 1235	dep. 89
3001	02/02/14 10:13	Tsvi	approve order	1234 1235	dep. 89
3001	02/02/14 13:16	Ilana	check status	1234 1235	dep. 89
3001	03/02/14 16:18	Ilana	receive item	1234	dep. 89
3001	04/02/14 16:35	Ilana	receive item	1235	dep. 89
3001	04/02/14 16:36	Ilana	close order	1234 1235	dep. 89
3002	02/02/14 10:30	Sigal	open order	1234 1236	dep. 79
3002	02/02/14 10:31	Rachel	approve order	1234 1236	dep. 79
3002	02/02/14 15:31	Sigal	check status	1234 1236	dep. 79
3002	03/02/14 16:19	Sigal	receive item	1234	dep. 79
3002	04/02/14 16:35	Sigal	receive item	1236	dep. 79
3002	04/02/14 16:36	Sigal	close order	1234 1236	dep. 79

Table 2. Simplified log of the sub process of delivery handling

Delivery	Timestamp	User	Activity	Item no	Department
5001	03/02/14 11:45	Mosh	receive item	1234	
5001	03/02/14 16:15	Mosh	send to dep.	1234	dep. 89
5001	03/02/14 16:16	Mosh	send to dep.	1234	dep. 79
5002	04/02/14 12:46	Mosh	receive item	1235 1236	
5002	04/02/14 16:30	Mosh	send to dep.	1235	dep. 89
5002	04/02/14 16:31	Mosh	send to dep.	1236	dep. 79

In the example, both processes employ multiple instance procedures. Furthermore, the lower-level instances in both processes refer to ordered items. However, the grouping of items to cases is different for the main and sub-process. In the main process, the grouping is by order (serving as case ID), and in the sub process the grouping is by delivery (case ID), where items ordered by different departments are supplied together. As a result, multiple cases of the main process may correspond to multiple cases of the sub process. Merging the logs would enable mining the end-to-end process, and particularly tracing the low-level instances (ordered items). The unified log would employ a single case ID for all the events that relate to the same order. In the absence of a common case ID, the main challenge is to identify the events in both logs that should be considered related to the same case.

The rest of the paper is structured a follows. Section 2 presents the approach and the log merging algorithm, demonstrating it using the running example; Sect. 3 reports the evaluation performed to a set of synthetic logs; Sect. 4 discusses related work. Finally, conclusions are given in Sect. 5.

2 Merging Event Logs

For the above described challenge we suggest an approach of an automatic merge of log files by finding a match between each case in the main process and corresponding cases in the sub process. To handle many-to-many relationships between the cases of the different logs, we duplicate cases of the sub process and merge them with every relevant case in the main process, revealing the end-to-end process flow.

The overall idea is shown in Fig. 1. An illustration of a main log includes cases which may have multiple instances is presented in Fig. 1(a). Those instances are grouped together in the sub process, so instances from case 1 in the main process are included in case 1 and case 2 of the sub process. Our approach, illustrated in Fig. 1(b), generate new case IDs for the unified log file, were each case of the main process corresponds to a unique new case id, and cases of the sub process can be duplicated (e.g. case 1 of the sub process) in order to reflect the relationships to the cases of the main process.

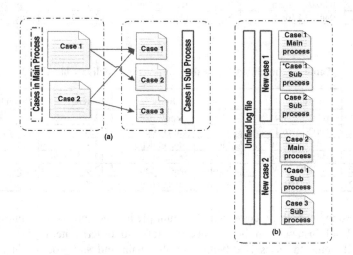

Fig. 1. An illustration of merging cases from different event logs

2.1 Approach Overview

As a preliminary step, the boundaries of the end-to-end process need to be determined and all related procedures identified. As a consequence, a set of logs from various systems can be identified and preprocessed to a uniform format [13]. In this paper we limit ourselves to merging two logs, one related to a main process and the other to a sub-process. However, this can be performed repeatedly to a hierarchy of sub-processes. Note that the identification of a main and sub process might not always be clear. In what follows, we indicate clear temporal relationships that should hold between the process considered as "main" and the one considered as "sub" for the sake of the merging.

As explained, we seek matching cases in the two logs, taking the following assumptions. (1) Both logs are taken from synchronized systems and consist of reliable and comparable timestamps. (2) Both logs might include multiple instances, thus four types of relationships between the logs are possible: one-to-one, one-to-many, many-to-one, and many-to-many. (3) The attribute values in the logs use uniform terms. Note that this assumption can be relaxed by using synonym detecting tools (e.g. Wordnet), but this is not included in our current scope. (4) The attribute values may include free text. The approach should be capable of dealing with logs where the reference to the other log is unstructured and given as free text. (5) The log of the sub process might include cases initiated by other processes. Hence, it is acceptable that not all its cases would be matched to cases of the main process and appears in the unified log file. In other words, the unified log should not necessarily contain all the cases of the sub process log.

Finding a match between log cases is trivial when the logs have a one-to-one relationship and both have the same case ID. In this case, matching is immediate and the logs can be merged directly. For logs whose case ID is not identical, cases are matched based on (i) similarity of *attribute values*, and (ii) appropriate *temporal relations*.

Similarity of attribute values can easily be established if we know in advance which attributes should hold similar values in the two logs. This is often the case, and can rely on domain knowledge. However, according to our assumptions, the logs might contain free-text attributes, and these might contain the information which is relevant for the match.

To accommodate for such situations, we assume that matching cases would have more common words in their attribute values than non-matching cases. For example, consider possible free text in the main log "we wish to order two monitors of models 1234 and 1235", and free text in the sub-process log "ordered by department 89". While generally similar text might appear in many entries across the logs, the specific item ids and department ids - representing the actual case properties - will be common only to the matching cases; hence their common words count is expected to be higher than those of non-matching cases. We hence calculate a similarity score based on the number of common words in the total text associated with the cases. However, some words can be common to all cases (e.g., stop words like "the", or activity names). These should not affect the similarity score. To this end, we use a text mining technique, the Term Frequency-Inverse Document Frequency (tf-idf) [17]. tf-idf relates to the frequency of a word in a given text (case attributes) as compared to its appearance in other texts (other cases). It allows filtering out words that are common to all cases and would not be a good indicator of similarity of two specific cases. The remaining words are extracted to a "bag of words" for each case, and similarity score of two cases is calculated as the count of unique words that are common to them.

In our running example the bag of unique words of the 1st case in the main log (Table 1) would be {3001, Ilana, 1234, 1235, 89} and the bag of unique words of the 1st case in the sub log (Table 2) would be {5001, Mosh, 1234, 89, 79}. The similarity score would hence be 2.

Note that it is common for two logs to include similar but not identical terminology (e.g., concatenation of several attribute values from the other log). This kind of relations can usually be indicated a-priory based on domain knowledge, so the log can be pre-processed accordingly.

Appropriate temporal relations – here we make two requirements. First, since the sub process is triggered by the main process, it should start after the beginning of the main process. Second, we require the sub process to provide some feedback to the main process, and hence it should have some time overlap with the main process and cannot start after the main process has ended. Note that in general it is possible that a sub process will appear in the log as starting after the main process has ended (e.g., recorded

Table 3. The 13 temporal relations with respect to case matching

Case in Main Process Vs. Case in Sub Process	Relation: X=Main; Y=Sub	Match (Y/N)	Illustration	Comments
Main Process takes place *before* Sub Process	X < Y	NO match	X ——— / ——— Y	missing feedback from sub-process (Y) to main process (X)
Sub Process takes place *before* Main Process	Y > X	NO match	Y ——— / ——— X	Main process starts after sub process; No triggering
Main Process *meets* Sub Process	X m Y	NO match	X ——— / ——— Y	Missing feedback
Sub Process *meets* Main Process	Y m X	NO match	Y ——— / ——— X	Main process starts after sub process; No triggering
Main Process *overlaps* with Sub process	X o Y	Positive Match	X ——— / ——— Y	Meets requirements
Sub Process *overlaps* with Main process	Y o X	NO match	Y ——— / ——— X	Main process starts after sub process; No triggering
Main process *starts* with Sub process	X s Y	NO match	X ——— / Y ———	Start at the same time, no triggering
Sub process *starts* with Main process	Y s X	NO match	Y ——— / X ———	Start at the same time, no triggering
Main process start-end *during* Sub process	X d Y	NO match	X / Y ———	Main process starts after sub process; No triggering
Sub process start-end *during* Main process	Y d X	Positive Match	Y / X ———	Meets requirements
Main process start *during* and *finishes* with Sub process	X f Y	NO match	X / Y ———	Main process starts after sub process; No triggering
Sub process start *during* and *finishes* with main process	Y f X	Positive Match	Y ——— / X	Meets requirements
Main process *equal* to Sub process	X = Y	NO match	X / Y ———	Start at the same time no triggering

manually, mistakenly closed cases). Those cases are exceptions and not considered as correct matches in our automatic solution.

To formalize these requirements in terms of temporal relations we rely on Allen's interval algebra [4]. Table 3 specifies for each of Allen's temporal relation types whether it meets the requirements and can be considered a match.

2.2   Algorithm

Following the above discussion the algorithm takes two logs, one of the main process and the other of the sub process, and generates a unified log file. The algorithm, depicted in Listing 1, addresses only situations where the main process and the sub process have different case IDs (*ncasesinmain* log, *mcasesinsub*log). The algorithm uses the following main variables and functions:

Word_Set (case): a set holding all the values of attributes in all events of a case (bag of unique words).

**Function *Match_time* (case1, case2): checks the temporal relation between case1 and case2 and returns TRUE if they meet temporal requirements

***Function *check_Match_Score* [word_set(case 1), word_set(case 2)]: returns an integer value Match_Score($MS_{n,m}$) – the calculated similarity score of attribute values between the cases.

The algorithm generates a new case ID for each case of the main process, and calculates match scores for every case combination that meets the temporal requirements. For every case of the main process (and corresponding New_Case ID) it selects the sub-process cases whose match score is maximal (and above zero), possibly creating duplications of sub-process cases. Finally, it merges the logs accordingly.

Algorithm. Check match score between cases in cross logs for potential merging
1:    Set *word_set {main log(case_id)}* == extract all unique values for every case id in main log
2:    Set *word_set {sub log(case_id)}* == extract all unique values for every case id in sub log
3:
4:    **For all** *case_id* ∈ *main log* **do**
5:        **For all** *case_id* ∈ sub *log* **do**
6:            **If** ** *match_time {case1 (main_log); case2 (sub_log)}* **then**
7:                *** $MS_{n,m}$ == check_Match_Score {word_set (case1);word_set (case2)}
8:            **end if**
9:        **end for**
10:    **end for**
11:
12:    **For all** *case_id* ∈ *main log* **do**
13:      **Generate** new_case_id
14:        **For all** *case_id* ∈ sub *log* **do**
15:          **Return** case_id {$MS_{n,m}$ > 0 && Max($MS_{n,m}$)}
16:          **merge** {case_id(main_log),case_id(sub_log)}
17:        **end for**
18:    **end for**
19:    **return** *UnifiedLogFile*

2.3 Running Example

A merged log of one New Case for our running example (Tables 1 and 2) is given in Table 4. While being related to a New ID, the events keep record of the reference log where they originated and the respective original case ID. The new case relates to an end-to-end process of one order (3001) placed by one department (89) for two items (1234 and 1235). Since handling the delivery of these items is grouped at the warehouse with items ordered by another department (79), the new case of the merged log includes the respective events as well.

Table 4. Illustration of the merged log of the running example.

New ID	Ref log	ID	Timestamp	User	Activity	Item no	Department
3001-A	main log	3001	02/02/14 10:12	Ilana	open order	1234 1235	dep. 89
3001-A	main log	3001	02/02/14 10:13	Tsvi	approve order	1234 1235	dep. 89
3001-A	main log	3001	02/02/14 13:16	Ilana	check status	1234 1235	dep. 89
3001-A	sub log	5001	03/02/14 11:45	Mosh	receive item	1234	
3001-A	sub log	5001	03/02/14 16:15	Mosh	send to dep.	1234	dep. 89
3001-A	sub log	5001	03/02/14 16:16	Mosh	send to dep.	1234	dep. 79
3001-A	main log	3001	03/02/14 16:18	Ilana	receive item	1234	dep. 89
3001-A	sub log	5002	04/02/14 12:46	Mosh	receive item	1235 1236	
3001-A	sub log	5002	04/02/14 16:30	Mosh	send to dep.	1235	dep. 89
3001-A	sub log	5002	04/02/14 16:31	Mosh	send to dep.	1236	dep. 79
3001-A	main log	3001	04/02/14 16:35	Ilana	receive item	1235	dep. 89
3001-A	main log	3001	04/02/14 16:36	Ilana	close order		dep. 89

3 Evaluation

The proposed algorithm has been implemented and evaluated in a controlled experiment using synthetic logs. The use of synthetic logs for evaluating the algorithm enables a fully controlled experiment, since (a) the correct match between cases is known in advance, allowing an accurate measurement of precision and recall [9, 14] of the results, (b) when generating the logs, a full coverage of relationship types (one-to-one up to many-to-many) and temporal relations between the logs can be ensured, and (c) it is also possible to control the amount of text-related noise (additional irrelevant text) in the attribute values.

We generated event logs specifying a process model for each of the introduced relationships (i.e. one-to-one, one-to-many, many-to-one, many-to-many) as shown in Table 5. As a result, four logs of a main process (similar to the running example) and corresponding logs of sub processes were generated. The logs includes up to 260 cases, each case consisting of 3–7 events. The generated synthetic logs included the following mandatory fields (possibly with multiple instances): case ID (order number vs. delivery number), timestamp, user, department number, item number, and activity. The logs were generated by simulating the end-to-end process with the three possible temporal relations between the main and the sub-process, namely (1) sub process during main process (2) main process overlaps with sub process (3) sub process finishes main process (see Table 3).

Note that the logs included cases of the end-to-end process with similar attribute values. The corresponding cases in the main and sub log could have a relatively high match score, but should not be candidate for merging due to inappropriate temporal relations (e.g., main process before sub process or sub process before main process).

Table 5. Synthetic logs generated for the evaluation

Logs Relationship	Main Log – number of cases	Sub Log – number of cases	Unified log – expected number of cases
One-To-One (OTO)	130	130	130
One-To-Many (OTM)	130	260	260
Many-To-One (MTO)	260	130	260
Many-To-Many (MTM)	260	260	520

Applying the algorithm to all four versions of log combinations resulted in a perfect unified log with 100 % recall and precision. Recall was calculated as the proportion of correctly matched cases from all the positives matches, and precision was calculated as the proportion of correctly identified matched cases from the total identified matches.

Yet, the investigated logs included only fully structured data with no free text. To evaluate the ability of the algorithm to handle noisy free text, we relied on the structure and context of real-life logs, with a 200 words free text attribute in the main log and three five - words free text attributes in the sub-log. Following this, we (1) added to the main logs a free text attribute of up to 200 words, and (2) added to the sub logs three free text attributes with up to five words each. The text for the attributes in all logs was randomly selected from the free text attributes of the real-life log. Note that the additional free text attributes served as noise, and were not supposed to determine the match. The results obtained by applying the algorithm to the logs that include free text are given in Table 6 and graphically presented in Fig. 2.

In general the results indicate that the algorithm performs well, with recall of at least 94 % and precision of at least 89 %. Recall was higher than precision in most cases (except for MTO, where they were equal). It should also be noted that no substantial trade-off was observed between precision and recall, and that no relationship type was identified as "easier match" with superior performance over the others, with insignificant differences of F measure values: 92 % to 96 %.

Note that despite the encouraging results, this evaluation is still too limited to draw general conclusions, but it is reasonable to believe based on these results that the performance of the algorithm is not sensitive to the type of relationship between the logs.

Table 6. The table present recall and precision calculations vs. relationship types.

Logs relationship	True positives (*tp*) - correctly identified	False positives (*fp*) - incorrectly identified	False negative (*fn*) - incorrectly rejected	Recall	Precision	F-measure
OTO	126	16	4	97 %	89 %	93 %
OTM	244	28	16	94 %	90 %	92 %
MTO	239	11	10	96 %	96 %	96 %
MTM	501	35	15	97 %	93 %	95 %

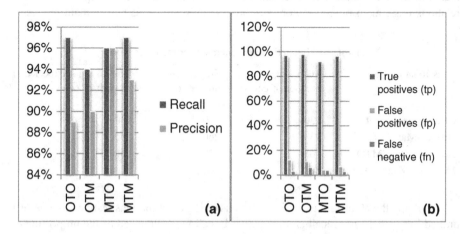

Fig. 2. Evaluation results: (a) precision/recall for all types of relationships (b) true positives/false positives/false negatives for all types of relationships

Sensitivity to the amount and distribution of free text in the logs is yet to be tested. Last, the ability of the algorithm to handle real life complexity should be tested using a real-life log. To obtain an initial indication of the scalability of the algorithm and the required processing time when handling realistically large logs, we applied it to real-life logs taken from the 2014BPI challenge. The main process log contains 26,876 instances and the sub process log contains 21,960 instances. With this data, a unified log was obtained in 1 minute and 54 seconds. With a real-life log, however, precision and recall would only be estimated, as the real matches would not be known a priori.

4   Related Work

Process mining uses event logs data in order to discover, monitor and improve the actual processes in an organization from an event log commonly available in information systems [1]. However, it should be applied to a single event log [1, 3]. In case the addressed business processes are conducted at different systems, the pre-processing of the log, which usually aims at obtaining a "clean" and uniformly formatted dataset [17], should also combine the logs of the systems into a single one.

Merging logs as a preparatory step to process mining has not been widely addressed. The work which is closest to the one we propose is presented in [11], whose approach for matching the cases in the different logs is based on genetic algorithms. The main difference in the problem addressed is that they assume that each case in the sub-process relates to exactly one case in the main process, thus many-to-many relationships are not addressed. Another difference is that free-text data is not addressed by [11]. Another closely related work is [8], which addresses conformance checking of processes comprised of various sub-processes (proclets), each possibly having a separate log. Differently than our work, their basic assumption is that the connection between the sub-processes is known. Rather than merging the logs before mining, they mine each sub-process separately and then combine the process models.

The problem we address is related to mining hierarchical process models, since our aim is to facilitate the discovery of an end-to-end process comprised of sub-procedures. Mining hierarchical models has received research attention [6, 10, 12, 19] In most of these works, mining applies to a single log, and various approaches are taken to determine the hierarchy and to overcome abstraction challenges [6, 10, 19], attempting to cluster events into sub-processes [8, 9]. In our case, we only lay the ground for mining by providing a unified log that can be mined. Since we keep the information of the original log each event is taken from, hierarchical mining would be easier and would not need techniques for discovering this information.

Process hierarchy is an inherent part of artifact-centric processes [5, 7, 18]. Artifact-centric processes are centered around an artifact, which encompasses data and life-cycle models. Artifact lifecycle is modeled by a Guard-Stage-Milestone (GSM) model [18], which provides a natural hierarchy of the model. Artifacts also enact and trigger other artifacts in a hierarchical manner, often including multiple instances. The triggered artifacts might be managed separately by different information systems and have separate logs. Following this, mining artifact lifecycle is of much relevance. Indeed, [16] and [15] address the possibility of many-to-may relationships between artifacts, and hence they abandon the case as a basis for mining. Yet, they assume a single log where all events are recorded. With this log, the effort is to relate each event to a relevant artifact so artifact-related logs are created, and then mining can produce a GSM model of these artifacts.

In summary, to the best of our knowledge the problem of merging logs with many-to many relationships in preparation for process mining has not been addressed so far. Additionally, while text processing has received much attention is various areas, process mining mostly does not currently relate to free text data in logs.

5 Conclusions

Process mining techniques, which are useful for discovery and analysis of actual processes, rely on a single case ID that classifies all events into process cases. Hence, in common situations where processes include separately managed procedures with separate logs, some preprocessing is required for producing a unified log with unique case IDs. Existing techniques are able to do this only when the main and sub-process have one-to-one or one-to-many relationships. This paper proposes an algorithm which can produce a unified log for all relationship types and specifically for the many-to-many case, where each log has non-matching case IDs. Another unique feature of the proposed algorithm is its ability to handle logs that contain unstructured and free-text data by using text mining techniques.

These capabilities enable mining complex and distributed processes that often exist in organizations and analyzing their flow. Process improvement opportunities that would emerge from such analysis would address the end-to-end flow rather than local views that relate to the individual sub-processes comprising the overall one. In particular, lack of coherence, correlation and synchronization among the different parts of the process can be identified. However, while the unified log provides a good support to overall flow analysis, it is less suitable for other analysis types. In particular since it includes duplicate sub-process activities that are associated with several main cases, it does not support analysis of activity frequencies and resource load.

Two other limitations of the algorithm are the assumption of comparable terminology and attribute values across logs, and the assumption of synchronized systems, producing timestamps along one time-line (as opposed to, e.g., systems in different time zones). The former can be overcome by using synonym-detection tools like Wordnet; the latter can be overcome if the lack of synchronization is consistent (different time zones). Then timestamps can be modified consistently as a preparatory step, to provide a uniform time-line for all logs. However, if lack of synchronization is not consistent and the time-gap between the systems might unexpectedly change, temporal relations between cases cannot be determined and the algorithm will not produce correct results.

Future research includes a number of directions. First, additional evaluation on real-life logs would be beneficial in order to better test the performance of the developed algorithm. Second, using the merged logs for the end-to-end process discovery might require some specialized visual representation. Visualizations used by current process discovery techniques are not fully supportive of the many-to-many relationship along process hierarchy, and might not provide the full benefits of process visualizations that apply to simply structured processes. Last, match results can be improved through interaction with the user, who can evaluate the matching of specific cases based on domain knowledge. Based on the user feedback, machine learning techniques can be used for improving the match results.

Acknowledgment. This research was partly supported by the Israel Science Foundation, grant 856/13.

References

1. Van der Aalst, W.M.P.: Discovery, Conformance and Enhancement of Business Processes. Springer, Heidelberg (2011)
2. Van der Aalst, W.M.P., et al.: Process mining manifesto. In: Daniel, F., Barkaoui, K., Dustdar, S. (eds.) Business Process Management Workshops. LNBIP, vol. 99. Springer, Berlin Heidelberg (2012)
3. Van der Aalst, W.M.P., Weijters, T., Maruster, L.: Workflow mining: discovering process models from event logs. IEEE Trans. Knowl. Data Eng. 16(9), 1128–1142 (2004)
4. Allen, J.F.: Maintaining knowledge about temporal intervals. Commun. ACM 26(11), 832–843 (1983)

5. Nigam, A., Caswell, N.S.: Business artifacts: an approach to operational specification. IBM Syst. J. **42**(3), 428–445 (2003)
6. Baier, T., Mendling, J.: Bridging abstraction layers in process mining by automated matching of events and activities. In: Daniel, F., Wang, J., Weber, B. (eds.) BPM 2013. LNCS, vol. 8094, pp. 17–32. Springer, Heidelberg (2013)
7. Cohn, D., Hull, R.: Business artifacts: A data-centric approach to modeling business operations and processes. Bull. IEEE Comput. Soc. Tech. Comm. Data Eng. **32**(3), 3–9 (2009)
8. Ferreira, D., Zacarias, M., Malheiros, M., Ferreira, P.: Approaching process mining with sequence clustering: experiments and findings. In: Alonso, G., Dadam, P., Rosemann, M. (eds.) BPM 2007. LNCS, vol. 4714, pp. 360–374. Springer, Heidelberg (2007)
9. Günther, C.W., Rozinat, A., Van Der Aalst, W.M.: Activity mining by global trace segmentation. In: Rinderle-Ma, S., Sadiq, S., Leymann, F. (eds.) Business Process Management Workshops. LNBIP, vol. 43, pp. 128–139. Springer, Heidelberg (2010)
10. Greco, G., Guzzo, A., Pontieri, L.: Mining hierarchies of models: from abstract views to concrete specifications. In: van der Aalst, W.M.P., Benatallah, B., Casati, F., Curbera, F. (eds.) BPM 2005. LNCS, vol. 3649, pp. 32–47. Springer, Heidelberg (2005)
11. Claes, J., Poels, G.: Integrating computer log files for process mining: a genetic algorithm inspired technique. In: Salinesi, C., Pastor, O. (eds.) CAiSE Workshops 2011. LNBIP, vol. 83, pp. 282–293. Springer, Heidelberg (2011)
12. Li, J., Bose, R.P.J.C., van der Aalst, W.M.P.: Mining context-dependent and interactive business process maps using execution patterns. In: zur Muehlen, M., Su, J. (eds.) BPM 2010 Workshops. LNBIP, vol. 66, pp. 109–121. Springer, Heidelberg (2011)
13. Raichelson, L., Soffer, P.: Unifying event logs to enable end-to-end process mining. In: Proceeding of the 7th Israel Association for Information Systems (ILAIS) Conference, July 2013
14. Moghnieh, A., Blat, J.: The potential of Recall and Precision as interface design parameters for information retrieval systems situated in everyday environments (2011)
15. Nooijen, E.H.J., van Dongen, B.F., Fahland, D.: Automatic discovery of data-centric and artifact-centric processes. In: La Rosa, M., Soffer, P. (eds.) BPM 2012. LNBIP, vol. 132, pp. 316–327. Springer, Heidelberg (2013)
16. Popova, V., Fahland, D., Dumas, M.: Artifact lifecycle discovery. arXiv:1303.2554 (2013, preprint)
17. Rajaraman, A., Ullman, J.D.: Mining of Massive Datasets. Cambridge University Press, Cambridge (2012)
18. Hull, R., Damaggio, E., De Masellis, R., Fournier, F., Gupta, M., Heath III, F.T., Vaculin, R.: Business artifacts with guard-stage-milestone lifecycles: managing artifact interactions with conditions and events. In: Proceedings of the 5th ACM international conference on Distributed event-based system, pp. 51–62. ACM (2011)
19. Yzquierdo-Herrera, R., Silverio-Castro, R., Lazo-Cortés, M.: Sub-process discovery: Opportunities for process diagnostics. In: Poels, G. (ed.) Enterprise Information Systems of the Future. LNBIP, vol. 139, pp. 48–57. Springer, Heidelberg (2013)

Process Model Realism: Measuring Implicit Realism

Benoît Depaire[1,2][✉]

[1] Faculty of Business Economics, Hasselt University,
Agoralaan Bldg D, 3590 Diepenbeek, Belgium
[2] Research Foundation - Flanders (FWO),
Egmontstraat 5, 1000 Brussels, Belgium
benoit.depaire@uhasselt.be

Abstract. Determining the quality of a discovered process model is an important but non-trivial task. In this article, we focus on evaluating the realism level of a discovered process model, i.e. to what extent does the model contain the process behavior that is present in the true underlying process and nothing more. The IR Measure is proposed which represents the probability that a discovered model would have produced a log that is missing a certain amount of behavior observed in the discovered model. This measure expresses the strength of evidence that the discovered process model could be the true underlying model. Empirical results show that the Measure behaves as expected. The IR value drops when the discovered model contains unrealistic behavior. The IR value decreases as the amount of unrealistic behavior in the discovered model increases. The IR value increases as the amount of behavior in the underlying process increases, ceteris paribus.

Keywords: Process model quality · Process model realism · Implicit realism measure

1 Introduction

When process models are discovered from event logs, it is important to determine the quality of the discovered model. Originally, most focus was on process fitness [1], but over time other quality measures were introduced [2,3]. Nowadays, process quality is considered a multidimensional concept with fitness, precision, generalization and simplicity as the most common dimensions. As others have indicated, a trade-off exists between the different quality dimensions [4] and to determine the relative importance of each dimension one must take the context and goals of the process mining analysis into account.

This paper focusses on the specific goal to capture the true underlying process and to learn a model which describes the AS-IS situation. Note that the true process refers to the way work is done and not necessarily to an explicit or normative model. To assess the quality of the discovered model, one must ask whether the model is a realistic reflection of the underlying process. This kind

© Springer International Publishing Switzerland 2015
F. Fournier and J. Mendling (Eds.): BPM 2014 Workshops, LNBIP 202, pp. 342–352, 2015.
DOI: 10.1007/978-3-319-15895-2_29

of quality assessment is among others relevant in an auditing context, where one needs a depiction of the true process to evaluate its conformance to a set of rules and its exposure to certain risks.

The next section will elaborate on the quality concept of process realism and will illustrate that it has to be decomposed in several pieces. This paper will focus on one of these puzzle pieces, i.e. to what extent does the discovered process model contain unobserved behavior that is unlikely to be part of the underlying process. In a subsequent section, a statistical approach and implementation are presented which makes it possible to provide an informed answer to this question. Finally, empirical results are provided to illustrate the new quality measure and conclusions for future research are drawn.

2 Process Model Realism

Process model realism is a quality measure that quantifies to what extent the discovered model represents the true underlying process. Note that we assume the event log to be free from measurement errors, i.e. all process behavior in the event log did actually happen. While in reality event logs might contain measurement errors, its removal belongs to the data clean-up stage and not the process discovery stage, similar to fields as statistics and knowledge discovery. Secondly, it is important to realize that the goal is to learn the AS-IS situation, even if this contains illogical or prohibited behavior.

To understand process model realism one must make a distinction between observed and unobserved process behavior. By (un)observed behavior we refer to any behavior which is (not) observed in the event log. To be a realistic model, all observed behavior should be present in the model. We refer to this as explicit realism, which can be quantified by existing fitness measures.

As for all possible behavior which is not observed in the event log, the model should only model the behavior that is part of the true underlying process, which is referred to as implicit realism. Obviously, implicit realism is harder to measure since the true underlying process is unknown and there is no direct way to distinguish between unobserved realistic behavior and unobserved unrealistic behavior.

If one assumes that unobserved realistic behavior exists, i.e. the event log is incomplete, the implicit realism measure holds close connections to the concepts of generalization and precision [3,5–7]. A common definition of precision is the extent to which a model does not contain too much behavior nor underfits reality. This implies that a precise model does not contain unrealistic unobserved behavior. A common definition of generalization is the extent to which a model does not contain too little behavior nor overfits reality, which implies that a model contains realistic unobserved behavior.

However, almost every existing precision and generalization implementation actually follows the definitions provided by Weidlich et al. [8]: *Precision is the degree to which the process model is restricted to the observed behavior* and *Generalization is the degree to which the process model allows for additional behaviour.*

These definitions are much less related to implicit realism as they only quantify the amount of unobserved behavior in the model, without distinguishing between unobserved realistic behavior and unobserved unrealistic behavior. As a consequence, these measures cannot be used to evaluate the level of implicit realism.

An approach that is related to measuring implicit realism can be found in [6], which implements generalization using the probability that given a process state, the next event will correspond to a new activity. In their work, a low generalization value implies a high likelihood that new events will exhibit unmodelled behavior for a given process state, which implies that the realistic unobserved behavior was not modelled. However, this approach has several limitations such as the fact that non-local dependencies, based on the order of previous activities, are not taken into account. Furthermore, the suggested approach defines the probability of a new unobserved activity equal to 1 when the number of different activities observed in a specific state s is equal to the number of times the state is visited. This implies that the number of different activities for that state would theoretically be infinite.

In the next section we will focus on the different side of implicit realism, i.e. to what extent does the process model not contain unrealistic unobserved behavior. To our knowledge, this aspect of process model realism has not yet been studied and no measure exists to quantify it yet.

3   An Implicit Realism Measure

3.1   Preliminaries

The problem we are facing deals with a discovered process model M which is assumed to consist of a finite number of execution paths $p_i \in \{p_1, \ldots, p_m\}$. This model is discovered from an event log $L = \{c_1, \ldots, c_n\}$ of size n. For the time being, we assume that all cases in the event log can be perfectly replayed by the model, which allows us to rewrite the log as a multiset of execution paths $L = \{p_1^{x_1}, \ldots, p_m^{x_m}\}$ where x_i refers to the number of occurrences of a certain path in the log, such that $\sum_i^m x_i = n$. In the remainder of the text, the shorter notation $L = \{x_1, \ldots, x_m\}$ will be used. The number of cases in the log will be denoted as $|L| = n$, the number of execution paths in the model will be denoted as $|M| = m$ and the number of execution paths of model M observed in log L will be denoted as $\|L\|_M$. This allows us to define the number of modelled but unobserved execution paths as $\tau_M(L) = m - \|L\|_M$.

Let $\mathcal{L}_{M,n}$ be the set of all possible logs L_i of size n generated by M, then we can define the following subsets of $\mathcal{L}_{M,n}$:

$$\mathcal{L}_{M,n}^u = \{L_i \in \mathcal{L}_{M,n} | \tau_M(L_i) = u\} \tag{1}$$

$$\mathcal{L}_{M,n}^{u \to} = \{L_i \in \mathcal{L}_{M,n} | \forall i \in [1, u] : x_i = 0\} \tag{2}$$

$$\mathcal{L}_{M,n}^{u \to |} = \{L_i \in \mathcal{L}_{M,n}^u | \forall i \in [1, u] : x_i = 0\} \tag{3}$$

$$\mathcal{L}_{M,n}^{u \to k} = \{L_i \in \mathcal{L}_{M,n}^{u \to} \mid \|\{x_u + 1, \ldots, x_m\}\|_M = m - (u + k)\} \tag{4}$$

$\mathcal{L}_{M,n}^{u}$ is the set of logs with exactly u unobserved execution paths, whereas $\mathcal{L}_{M,n}^{u\rightarrow}$ denotes the set of logs where at least the first u paths in model $M = \{p_1, \ldots, p_m\}$ are unobserved. Furthermore, $\mathcal{L}_{M,n}^{u\rightarrow|}$ denotes the set of logs where only the first u paths are unobserved, and $\mathcal{L}_{M,n}^{u\rightarrow k}$ is the set of logs where the first u paths are unobserved, followed by k additional unobserved paths.

3.2   General Approach

At first sight, it seems impossible to measure implicit realism since the true process is unknown and therefore no basis for distinguishing between realistic and unrealistic unobserved behavior seems to exist. However, instead of stating whether the model contains unrealistic unobserved behavior and to what extent, one can also try to estimate the probability that the modeled unobserved behavior is in fact realistic unobserved behavior. As we will show, the latter is in fact possible.

The key to implementing this approach lies in the field of statistics. More specifically, we use the Null Hypothesis Significance Testing (NHST) approach as introduced by Sir Ronald Fisher [9,10]. The outcome of Fisher's NHST approach is a p-value that measures the *strength of evidence* that the null hypothesis is supported. To implement this approach, the following four steps should be translated to the problem at hand:

1. Specify a statistic that summarizes the data in a single number.
2. Define a null hypothesis.
3. Calculate the probability of a value equal or larger than the test statistic if the null hypothesis would hold.
4. Reject the null hypothesis if the probability is too low.

Our approach to quantify implicit realism is by measuring the probability that the model contains too much unobserved behavior. Following Fisher's NHST approach, we identify the event log as the data and select the number of unobserved execution paths in the model $\tau_M(L)$ as the test statistic. Next, the null hypothesis is defined as the fact that the model M does not contain too much unobserved execution paths. To determine the level of implicit realism, we must estimate the probability that an event log would have $\tau_M(L)$ or more unobserved execution paths if model M was indeed the true process.

To determine this probability, first define $P(p_i)$ as the probability that path $p_i \in M$ is executed and is observed in log L. We can then regard a log file of size n as the outcome of a multinomial experiment described by the following distribution:

$$\text{Multinom } (\{x_1, \ldots, x_m\}, n, \{P(p_1), \ldots, P(p_m)\}) \tag{5}$$

The multinomial distribution is typically used to determine the probability for a specific result in an experiment of n independent trials, with m possible outcomes for each trial and fixed probabilities $P(p_i)$ for each outcome. In our situation, each trial represents a process execution and each outcome corresponds to a possible execution path in the model M.

Given the multinomial distribution in Eq. 5, the probability for a specific log file becomes $P(L|M,n) = \frac{n!}{x_1!...x_m!} p_1^{x_1} ... p_m^{x_m}$. The probability that a log file of size n with u missing execution paths is generated by M can then be defined as $P(\tau_M(L) = u|M,n) = \sum_L^{\mathcal{L}_{M,n}^u} P(L)$, which results in the following formula for the Implicit Realism (IR) measure:

$$IR(L,M) = P(\tau_M(L) \geq u|M,n) \tag{6}$$

$$= \sum_{z=u}^{m} P(\tau_M(L) = z|M,n) \tag{7}$$

$$= \sum_{z=u}^{m} \sum_L^{\mathcal{L}_{M,n}^z} P(L) \tag{8}$$

The Implicit Realism measure now quantifies the probability that if model M were the true underlying model, a log of size n with u or more unobserved execution paths would be observed. If this probability is too low, one rejects the model M on the basis of insufficient implicit realism.

3.3   Implementation

Equation 8 shows that the IR measure can be computationally expensive since one has to sum over all possible event logs generated by a model with at least u missing execution paths. This problem can be tackled by assuming that every execution path p_i in M has equal probability of occurring $P(p_i) = \frac{1}{m}$. While this is a naive assumption, it should be noted that currently such information is not provided by most process discovery algorithms. Also, this 'trick' is only required when computation time becomes unacceptably long.

A first advantage of the assumption $P(p_i) = \frac{1}{m}$ is that the probability that at least the first u paths are unobserved in an event log, $P(L \in \mathcal{L}_{M,n}^{u \rightarrow}|M,n)$, becomes fairly easy to calculate. A log file of size n with at least the first u paths missing is in fact the outcome of a binomial experiment with n trials and n successes, where a trial is a process execution and a success is achieved when that trace does not correspond to any of the first u execution paths. The probability of success is $P(\text{Success}) = 1 - \sum_i^u P(p_i)$, which results in

$$P(L \in \mathcal{L}_{M,n}^{u \rightarrow}|M,n) = \left(1 - \frac{u}{m}\right)^n \tag{9}$$

This probability is important because it allows the calculation of the probability that only the first u paths are unobserved in the event log.

$$P(L \in \mathcal{L}_{M,n}^{u \rightarrow |}|M,n) = P(L \in \mathcal{L}_{M,n}^{u \rightarrow}|M,n) - \sum_{i=1}^{m-u} P(L \in \mathcal{L}_{M,n}^{u \rightarrow i}) \tag{10}$$

The idea behind this calculation is that $\mathcal{L}_{M,n}^{u \rightarrow |} \subset \mathcal{L}_{M,n}^{u \rightarrow}$ and the difference between these two sets are all logs with more than the first u paths missing. If one inspects Eq. 10, it shows that the second term actually calculates the joint probability for all the logs with more than the first u paths missing. Because of our assumption $P(p_i) = \frac{1}{m}$, the probability that a log file is missing a number of i paths in addition to the first u paths is independent of the selection of i additional missing paths. Therefore, we can rewrite Eq. 10 as Eq. 11, where the binomial coefficient expresses the number of ways one can select i additional paths from $m - u$ remaining paths.

$$P(L \in \mathcal{L}_{M,n}^{u \to |}|M, n) = P(L \in \mathcal{L}_{M,n}^{u \to}|M, n) - \sum_{i=1}^{m-u} \binom{m-u}{i} P(L \in \mathcal{L}_{M,n}^{u+i \to |}) \quad (11)$$

Next, one can calculate the probability that exactly u paths are missing, irrespective of their position. Again, the assumption $P(p_i) = \frac{1}{m}$ ensures that the probability is independent from the specific set of u missing execution paths. Considering that $\binom{m}{u}$ represents the number of combinations of drawing u paths from m original paths, we get

$$P\left(\tau_M(L) = u|M, n\right) = \binom{m}{u} P(L \in \mathcal{L}_{M,n}^{u \to |}|M, n), \quad (12)$$

from which we can easily derive $\mathrm{IR}(L, M)$.

The different steps are summarized in Algorithm 1. Note that due to the recursive nature of Eq. 11, one must start by calculating $P(L \in \mathcal{L}_{M,n}^{u \to |}|M, n)$ for $u = m - 1$, considering the fact that $P(L \in \mathcal{L}_{M,n}^{m \to |}|M, n) = 0$.

Algorithm 1. Efficient Calculation of the Implicit Realism Measure

---

$m \leftarrow |M|$
$P(L \in \mathcal{L}_{M,n}^{m \to |}|M, n) \leftarrow 0$
for $j \leftarrow m - 1, u$ **do**
 $P(L \in \mathcal{L}_{M,n}^{j \to |}|M, n) \leftarrow \left(1 - \frac{j}{m}\right)^n - \sum_{i=1}^{m-j} \binom{m-j}{i} P(L \in \mathcal{L}_{M,n}^{j+i \to |})$
end for
$P\left(\tau_M(L) = u|M, n\right) \leftarrow \binom{m}{u} P(L \in \mathcal{L}_{M,n}^{u \to |}|M, n)$
$\mathrm{IR}(L, M) \leftarrow \sum_{u=||L||_M}^{m} P(\tau_M(L) = u|M, n)$

---

4 Empirical Analysis

4.1 Interpretation of the IR Measure

The IR measure is substantially different from other quality measures and their implementations because of the fact that it has a statistical foundation and a very precise interpretation. A clear understanding of the IR Measure is crucial for its proper use and to this end the next paragraph provides an academic example to illustrate the use of the IR Measure.

Imagine a researcher who received a log file L and uses process mining to discover process model M^d. The goal of his analysis is to find a realistic representation of the underlying process M^r that produced L and he notices that M^d allows for certain behavior that he did not witness in the log. More specifically, he notices that 2 % of the behavior in M^d is not represented in L. He wonders if this is possible, i.e. if it is likely that a log L of a certain size n is missing 2 % of the behavior of its underlying process M^r.

This is exactly the kind of question the IR Measure can answer. In fact, the value the IR Measure produces in this scenario is the exact probability that M^r would have produced a log of size n with 2 % or more of its behavior missing. Note that if this probability is low, the researcher has reasonable evidence to believe M^d is not the underlying process M^r which produced L and he can decide to discard the model and learn a different model. However, the opposite is not true. If the probability expressed by the IR Measure is high, the researcher has little evidence to question the validity of M^d, but this is not the same as having reasonable evidence that $M^d = M^r$.

This interpretation of the IR Measure follows directly from the statistical properties underlying the IR Measure and are valid by definition under the assumption made by the statistical implementation. Therefore, any empirical evaluation of the IR Measure is simply an empirical reflection of its theoretical foundations, and in particular the multinomial distribution. Therefore, the goal of the empirical evaluation in the next subsection is not to empirically prove statistical concepts that have been developed and validated a long time ago, but rather to illustrate the behavior of the IR Measure and to illustrate its sensitivity to different elements of the log and the discovered model.

4.2 Empirical Illustration

The purpose of this empirical section is to illustrate how different elements influence the probability that a model produces a log file with a certain amount of missing process behavior. More particularly, we will focus on the following elements: log size, amount of process behavior in the model and the amount of behavior in the model which is not part of the true underlying model.

The setup of our experiments is as follows. First a model M^r is defined which will act as the true underlying model. Next, a set of 100 log files of size n are generated from this M^r. Subsequently several models M_p^d are created by extending M^r with a varying amount p of process behavior that is not part of the underlying process. These models M_p^d represent the discovered models whose implicit realism needs to be tested. If $p > 0$, M_p^d contains unrealistic unobserved behavior and lacks implicit realism.

Note that the results from these experiments hold irrespective of the process discovery algorithm used, since the models which act as the discovered models are constructed artificially. Furthermore, since the IR measure treats a process model as a set of execution traces, the actual process model structure has no impact on the result. Therefore, the actual process model structure used for M^r is irrelevant for the behavior of the IR Measure.

In total, two hypothetical models M^r were created, a first one M_{60}^r with 60 possible execution paths and a second one M_{2520}^r with 2520 different execution paths. M_{60}^r was constructed by taking randomly 50 % of all possible execution paths from a model with a parallel construct of 5 different activities. M_{2520}^r was constructed by taking randomly 50 % of all possible execution paths from a model with a parallel construct of 7 different activities. For each model M^r, 100 log files were generated of respectively 10, 50, 100, 500 and 1000 cases. For each model M^r, 5 models M_p^d were constructed with p equal to respectively 0 %, 5 %, 10 %, 50 % and 75 %. Each model M_p^d was constructed by adding $p\%$ of the execution paths which were not selected for the construction of M^r. These models represent the discovered models which do or do not contain unrealistic behavior.

The IR Measure was calculated for each combination of a model M_p^d and the corresponding log files, i.e. the log files generated from the related M^r. The results of these experiments are presented in Table 1. The reported values for the IR Measures are the IR values averaged over the 100 log files.

Table 1. Empirical analysis of IR measure behavior

$|M^r|$	Log size	p				
		0 %	5 %	10 %	50 %	75 %
60	10	0.73	0.72	0.71	0.66	0.64
	50	0.52	0.45	0.38	0.10	0.05
	100	0.59	0.41	0.26	0.00	0.00
	500	0.98	0.00	0.00	0.00	0.00
	1000	1.00	0.00	0.00	0.00	0.00
2520	10	0.96	0.96	0.96	0.96	0.96
	50	0.75	0.75	0.75	0.72	0.72
	100	0.57	0.55	0.53	0.42	0.37
	500	0.47	0.37	0.28	0.03	0.01
	1000	0.49	0.30	0.16	0.00	0.00

First we will evaluate how the IR Measure relates to the log size. As Table 1 illustrates, a distinction must be made between the IR Measure for the model M_0^d which perfectly reflects the true underlying model M^r and the models M_p^d where $p > 0$ and which represent models that contain unrealistic (unobserved) behavior. For the latter type of models, we can clearly see how the IR Measure drops as the log size increases. This makes perfect sense as increasing log sizes provide increasing amount of evidence that the null hypothesis is not true and thus rejects M_p^d as the true underlying model.

However, the relation between the log size and the IR Measure is not that clear for the models M_0^d in which case the null hypothesis is actually true and the discovered model does not contain unrealistic behavior that is not part of the underlying true process. As one can observe in Table 1, the IR Measure first drops as the log size increase, but seems to have a turning point after which it increases again towards an IR value of 1. This pattern is most clear for the true model M_{60}^r.

However, for both M_{60}^r and M_{2520}^r, it is apparent that, irrespective of the log size, the discovered models which correspond to the true underlying model, i.e. $p = 0\,\%$, yields a higher IR Measure than the discovered models which contain unrealistic behavior. Table 1 also shows that the differences in IR values increase as the log size increases. These results make perfect sense. It is obvious that discovered models with increasingly unrealistic behavior are increasingly less likely to have generated the log files at hand and thus the probability that the null hypothesis holds decreases likewise. Furthermore, as the log files increase in size, the evidence against the null hypothesis increases.

Finally, the relationship between the size of the true underlying model $|M^r|$ and the IR Measure can be studied. The results in Table 1 illustrate that as the number of real execution paths increase, the evidence required to reject the null hypothesis in case of a discovered model with unrealistic behavior also increases. For example, if the true process only has 60 execution paths, a discovered model with 90 execution paths, i.e. $p = 50\,\%$, has an average IR value of 0.66 for log files of size 10. In other words, there is a 66 % probability on average that this discovered model has produced the observed log files of size 10. In contrast, when the true process has 2520 execution paths, a discovered model with 3780 execution paths, i.e. $p = 50\,\%$, still has an average IR value of 0.96 for log files of size 10. Again, this result is rather intuitive. One can expect that more evidence, which means larger log files, is required in order to correctly reject the null hypothesis when the true process allows for more behavior and more diverse log files.

Overall, the IR Measure behaves as expected, which is not that remarkable since the empirical behavior is a mere reflection of its theoretical foundation. However, the results of this section do provide useful insights to understand the behavior of the IR Measure.

5   Conclusions and Future Research

This paper focusses on the context of discovering the true underlying process model and representing the AS-IS situation. The concept of process realism, i.e. to what extent the discovered model reflects reality, can be decomposed into explicit and implicit realism. Explicit realism refers to the amount of observed behavior reflected in the discovered model, while implicit realism refers to the amount of unobserved but realistic behavior reflected in the discovered model. More specifically, in this paper we developed a new quality measure that focusses on the amount of behavior in the discovered model which is not part of the underlying model.

We introduce a measure which is based on the statistical NHST approach from Fisher and expresses the probability that the discovered model has produced the observed event log which lacks a certain amount of observed behavior from the model. This probability relies strongly on the multinomial distribution and can be calculated exactly. However, the latter can be computationally expensive and to that end a more efficient implementation was developed, which relies on the assumption that each execution path in the model has equal probability of occurrence.

The empirical analysis of the IR Measure illustrated several relationships between the IR Measure itself and properties of the log files and the discovered model. Firstly, as the log file increases, the IR value will drop when the discovered model contains unrealistic behavior. Secondly, irrespective of the log size, the IR value decreases as the amount of unrealistic behavior in the discovered model increases. Thirdly, as the amount of behavior in the underlying process increases, larger log files are required to prove that a discovered model with unrealistic behavior is not the true underlying process.

The IR Measure has several practical advantages. Firstly, it has a statistical foundation which makes its behavior predictable and sound. Secondly, the IR Measure is a probability, which turns it into a measure with an intuitive and straight-forward interpretation. While the IR Measure promises to be an interesting new approach for measuring process model quality, the current version has many opportunities for improvements.

Firstly, the current approach assumes a perfect fit between the event log and model, which is seldom the case. One approach to tackle this can be found in [11], where the log file is first aligned to fit the model. A second assumption is the fact that the number of execution paths should be finite, which implies the absence of unlimited loops. This can be approached by transforming all infinite loops to finite loops such that the model is still capable of replaying the event log.

Thirdly, the suggested implementation assumes that the probability of all execution traces are equal. While this might seem reasonable for parallel constructs, it might be too restrictive for other process constructs such as choice. Therefore, future research is needed to evaluate the implication of this assumption in situations where it does not hold. Furthermore, ways to drop this assumption while keeping the IR Measure computationally feasible is also worth investigating. Finally, an interesting research avenue could be the study of other test statistics to implement Fisher's NHST approach in the context of process realism or process quality in general.

References

1. van der Aalst, W., Weijters, T., Maruster, L.: Workflow mining: discovering process models from event logs. IEEE Trans. Knowl. Data Eng. **16**(9), 1128–1142 (2004)
2. Rozinat, A., de Medeiros, A.A., Günther, C.W., Weijters, A., van der Aalst, W.M.: Towards an evaluation framework for process mining algorithms. Beta, Research School for Operations Management and Logistics (2007)

3. De Weerdt, J., De Backer, M., Vanthienen, J., Baesens, B.: A multi-dimensional quality assessment of state-of-the-art process discovery algorithms using real-life event logs. Inf. Syst. **37**(7), 654–676 (2012)
4. Buijs, J., van Dongen, B.F., van der Aalst, W.M.P.: Discovering and navigating a collection of process models using multiple quality dimensions. In: Ninth International Workshop on Business Process Intelligence (2013)
5. Leemans, S.J.J., Fahland, D., van der Aalst, W.M.P.: Discovering block-structured process models from event logs - a constructive approach. In: Colom, J.-M., Desel, J. (eds.) PETRI NETS 2013. LNCS, vol. 7927, pp. 311–329. Springer, Heidelberg (2013)
6. van der Aalst, W., Adriansyah, A., van Dongen, B.: Replaying history on process models for conformance checking and performance analysis. Wiley Interdisc. Rev. Data Min. Knowl. Disc. **2**(2), 182–192 (2012)
7. Rozinat, A., van der Aalst, W.M.: Conformance checking of processes based on monitoring real behavior. Inf. Syst. **33**(1), 64–95 (2008)
8. Weidlich, M., Polyvyanyy, A., Desai, N., Mendling, J., Weske, M.: Process compliance analysis based on behavioural profiles. Inf. Syst. **36**(7), 1009–1025 (2011)
9. Fisher, R.A.: Statistical Methods For Research Workers. Cosmo Publications, New Delhi (1925)
10. Fisher, R.A.: Statistical methods and scientific inference. Hafner Press, New York (1973)
11. Adriansyah, A., Munoz-Gama, J., Carmona, J., van Dongen, B.F., van der Aalst, W.M.P.: Measuring precision of modeled behavior. Inf. Syst. e-Bus. Manag. **13**, 1–31 (2014)

Analyzing a TCP/IP-Protocol with Process Mining Techniques

Christian Wakup[1] and Jörg Desel[2]([⊠])

[1] rubecon information technologies GmbH, Düsseldorf, Germany
[2] Fakultät für Mathematik und Informatik,
FernUniversität in Hagen, Hagen, Germany
joerg.desel@fernuni-hagen.de

Abstract. In many legacy software systems the communication between client and server is based on proprietary Ethernet protocols. We consider the case that the implementation and specification of such a protocol is unknown and try to reconstruct the rules of the protocol by observation of the network communication. To this end, we translate TCP/IP-logs to appropriate event logs and apply Petri net based process mining techniques. The results of this contribution are a systematic approach to mine client/server protocols, an according tool chain involving existing tools and new tools, and an evaluation of this approach, using a concrete example from practice.

1 Introduction

Since the 1980s, many software solutions for business software in various application domains have been based on proprietary hardware for a client/server-architecture, and often also on proprietary operating systems. Since this software is highly mature and dependable, emulation software was used in the 1990s for migration to the Windows- or to the UNIX-world. This is still today's situation at many places. Communication between client and server is often based on proprietary protocols which respect the requirements of the original terminals. These protocols are determined by fixed rules for the interaction behavior between their respective partners or system components [7]. However, often neither these rules nor a precise definition of the resulting behavior is known today. Substitution of an interface involved in a protocol may cause rule violations, resulting in severe consequences. Therefore, conformance to the protocol definition is highly desirable when interface software is newly implemented. To this end, identification of this definition is an obvious first prerequisite for protocol implementation substitution. So we aim at reconstructing specification models of a protocol from its behavior.

According to the *Process Mining Manifesto* [3], process mining aims at discovering, monitoring and improving real processes by extracting knowledge from event logs. The considered processes are mainly business processes, and the event

---

Based on the thesis [14] of the first author, supervised by the second author.

© Springer International Publishing Switzerland 2015
F. Fournier and J. Mendling (Eds.): BPM 2014 Workshops, LNBIP 202, pp. 353–364, 2015.
DOI: 10.1007/978-3-319-15895-2_30

logs are sequences of observed and recorded occurrences of business process activities. These activities typically involve the considered information system and human interaction, but they also can be automatized activities. There exists a large variety of mining techniques and tools as well as suggestions how to systematically choose and apply these techniques, based on the given application.

In our setting, we apply process mining techniques to event logs generated from automatized activities only. The underlying process is more a technical protocol than a business process. So we aim at discovering *protocols* instead of processes from logs. Our core research question is whether process mining techniques are useful in this context as well, and if so, how to adapt existing mining techniques to this application area. The result is quite positive, as the case study at the end of the paper will show.

This case study is based on a real industrial challenge: recover an existing legacy interface protocol without known definition. A new version of this protocol had been implemented in an ad-hoc way, and this implementation has subtle differences to the original one. So the task was not only to recover the original protocol definition, but also to compare it to the new one and find out precisely the differences between both. In this sense, this work can also be seen as a study in *conformance checking*, another main objective of process mining (up to which delta is the new protocol conform to the original protocol definition?).

The protocols to be discovered in our approach describe the interface behavior of clients and servers that communicate via TCP/IP. So this setting does not offer event logs that can immediately be used by process miners. Instead, the only way to acquire information about behavior is to record traffic data from the involved network. Actually, this is the first step of our approach. We apply the *Wireshark* network protocol analyzer [11] which is able to observe and record transmitted packets in the network. Moreover, this program offers useful filtering capabilities that are used to create logs for single communications between specific clients and specific servers.

These logs are not immediately suitable for process mining algorithms. Based on published requirements for event logs for process mining, we develop an approach and introduce a tool to transform them into event logs. To this end, information is gathered from different layers of the network protocol, and from information added by the *Wireshark* tool. Since the information about the performed activity type is not achievable this way, we add a semi-automatic technique to derive this information. This technique is supported by our tool, too.

Finally, the event logs are transformed in the XES standard format [6] so that mining algorithms such as provided by ProM [12] can be applied. We select a collection of algorithms that are promising for this application area and compare their respective results. We apply the techniques described above to a practical example and thus evaluate these techniques and the developed tool. In this case study, process miners are not only applied for generating protocol models, but also to check whether models can be viewed as sub-models of other models which are generated from additional use cases. Finally, the protocol derived from mining is compared to a protocol generated in an ad-hoc way.

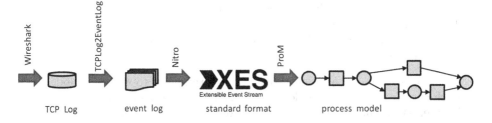

Fig. 1. The complete tool chain of our approach

The complete sequence of steps of our procedure, together with supporting tools, is summarized in Fig. 1.

The topic of this paper has strong relations to *service mining* [1], which is also based on more technical events, but aims at the identification of web services. Service mining can be viewed as a sub-discipline of the more general *protocol mining*, which is, however, not yet an established field. In particular, mining of protocols is usually not covered by *protocol engineering* [7]. Thus, our contribution also suggests a new research area combining mining techniques and engineering techniques for more general protocols.

The paper is structured as follows. In Sect. 2 we report about the generation of logs from the network and the pre-processing necessary to use these logs for process mining. In particular, we introduce our tool *TCPLog2EventLog*. Section 3 is devoted to process mining approaches applied to our logs. We recall characteristics of different miners and select miners that appear to be capable of delivering useful results in our setting. In Sect. 4 we describe our case study in more detail and show results for particular use cases. Section 5 recapitulates the findings of this study.

2   From Network Traffic to Logs

Network protocols are defined on messages between the protocol partners. For mining purposes, these messages have to be observed and logged in an appropriate way. For service mining, [5] suggests an HTTP-listener for the generation of event logs, i.e., runs of web services. This listener precisely filters out and records the relevant data traffic of the web server. The situation in our client/server setting is quite similar to the data exchange between services. Hence we follow the above suggestions for service mining, but adapt the logs and the generation mechanism where appropriate or necessary. To this end, we developed a new software tool, *TCPLog2EventLog*, that supports the construction of event logs from packet-based network protocol data.

In this section, we show how to come from network traffic to logs, where each log contains all relevant data for the later process mining. For the latter, we refer to [2], which characterizes the requirements for data entries in event logs. These requirements distinguish different cases of processes. Usually, entries of event logs can refer to different cases, which have interleaved actions. Since each run of the process to be mined belongs to a single case, each entry has to refer to its respective case. This, and other requirements of [2], are summarized in the following list:

– Each entry refers to an event at one point in time, not to a time period.
– Each entry refers to one single event, which is uniquely identifiable.
– Each entry should include a description of the respective event.
– Each entry refers to a single process case.
– Each process case refers to a specific process definition.

Since our approach is not based on HTTP, as in the case of web services, we apply the software *Wireshark*, a tool for analyzing network traffic [11]. This tool allows a complete recording of data exchange between two devices and offers several filtering features. The recorded data is stored on the server, which ensures that the recorded traffic between the server and *all* clients is complete, and that it is available at one place.

This recorded data contains communication information relevant for the protocol of interest, but also the complete further data exchange that happened in the same time interval. Data items might refer to the establishment of TCP connections and even to duplicated packets in case of retransmission. This additional information complicates the further construction of correct event logs, or it can result in noise. Using the filtering functions provided by Wireshark, we therefore filter this data as follows:

1. Each TCP connection uses a single port of a network. Each network-based communication which is relevant for our purposes uses a particular port. By filtering out all data which does not refer to this port, we get rid of additional traffic from other applications
   (*Wireshark* filter: `tcp.port==<port number>`).
2. The establishment and deletion of a connection uses particular flags. In an existing connection, usually these flags are `SYN` or `ACK`
   (*Wireshark* filter: `tcp.flags==0x18`).
3. Repeatedly sent packets should only be recorded once. *Wireshark* also offers a filter support for that: `!tcp.analysis.retransmission`.

This recorded and filtered packet data is logged in a text file by *Wireshark*. Each entry contains the original data of the network packets plus a time stamp representing the time the packet was observed. We will call these files *TCP logs* in the sequel.

TCP logs are not yet suitable for process mining, because important characteristics of the entries, namely case identifier, resource and activity, are still missing [4]. Moreover, TCP logs store data in hexadecimal form which requires translation to suitable ASCII character strings.

For completion of the data, we (i.e., our tool *TCPLog2EventLog*) refer to the different layers of the TCP/IP protocol: Ethernet-Frame, IP-packet, TCP segment and application, see Fig. 2. All this information, and additionally a time stamp representing the recording time, is available in TCP logs and will be used for generating suitable log entries for process mining.

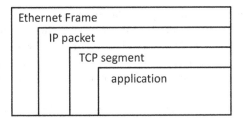

Fig. 2. Schematic structure of an internet packet

32 Bit							
0	4	8	12	16	20	24	28
Version		IHL		TOS		Total Length	
Identification				Flags		Fragment Offset	
TTL		Protocol (IP)		Header Checksum			
Source Address							
Destination Address							
Options and Padding (optional)							

Fig. 3. IPv4 header

32 Bit												
0		4	8		12	16		20		24		28
Source Port						Destination Port						
Sequence Number												
Acknowledgement Number												
Data		Reserved			U	A	P	R	S	F	Window	
Checksum						Urgent Pointer						
Options												
Data												

Fig. 4. TCP header

- As *time stamps* of event logs, we take the time stamp (recording time) of the TCP log.
- The *resource* is taken from the Source Address of the IPv4 header (IP protocol according to RFC 791, see Fig. 3).
- The TCP header (TCP protocol according to RFC 793, see Fig. 4) contains, among others, a Sequence Number, an Acknowledgment Number and a Data Field. According to the TCP protocol, Sequence and Acknowledgment Numbers ensure safe transmission of packets between sender and receiver as follows: The first Sequence Number is chosen arbitrarily by the respective host. Each subsequent packet of the same communication uses as Sequence Number the Sequence Number of the previous packet, increased by the length of the Data Field of the previous packet (in bytes). When the receiver answers to a packet,

the Acknowledgment Number equals the Sequence Number of the subsequent message of the sender, calculated as above. Using these numbers, we uniquely assign each entry of the TCP log to a conversation between a particular client and a particular server. These conversations receive subsequent, and hence distinct, numbers in our approach. Each conversation number constitutes the *case id* of the respective log entries.

- To obtain *activities* in event logs we use the Data Field of the IP protocol, as discussed below.

As a result of the decision to use the Data Field entries as activity names, very similar tasks might be represented by different activity names. For example, registration activities of different users are not recognized as the same task. This is not desirable. Moreover, this data, taken directly from the TCP header definitions, is unreadable for humans. Therefore, in a further step we group and classify similar activities (such as all registration activities), and give these groups readable names that eventually should appear in the process model. To this end, *TCPLog2EventLog* uses activity patterns, each with a semantics and an appropriate name. These patterns are obtained by a previous procedure: We perform atomic user activities within the application and thus within the protocol to be mined (pressing single keys, moving the mouse etc.). The resulting traffic is recorded as described above. Since the obtained logs only refer to the atomic activity, we can deduce which bit strings in the Data Field describe certain single activities, and we assign an appropriate name to this pattern. This pre-processing is supported by *TCPLog2EventLog*, too. The derived patterns are collected in a template file for further processing.

More technically, the output data of *TCPLog2EventLog*, i.e., the event log without activity classification, is stored and will later be used to identify activity classes. Therefore, each record receives a class name so that this pattern file has the following format: <data of the packet>; <name of the activity class>.

Whereas the classification of the activities might contain errors, there is one important attribute of each activity that is easily derived from the data, namely the respective sender of a message (server or client). To capture this information, each class name receives the prefix `Server:` or `Client:`.

The following table summarizes the preliminary transformation of TCP logs to event logs.

TCP log	event log
time stamp	time stamp
sequence number/acknowledgement number	process ID
source IP-address	resource
abstracted user data via template identified class	activity

After creation of activity class names, it remains to assign single activities to according classes. This is done using the template file mentioned above. Since the Data Field entry of a packet is not identical to the previously found patterns for known activities in general, we implemented the Levenshtein Algorithm [8], which studies similarities between strings of characters, in *TCPLog2Eventlog*. If the Data Field entry of a TCP log entry is recognized to be similar to a known Data Field then the respective activity is assigned to the class of this known Data field, and the existing array is extended by the new name. If no assignment is possible, then the result will be a new activity class `Answer xx`, where `xx` is a consecutive number. Obviously, it is desirable to have not too much of these exceptional activities. Finally, the program *TCPLog2Eventlog* outputs the data for process ID, time stamp, resource and activity as a CSV file.

The above mentioned prerequisites for event logs (for process mining) have been standardized in form of the *Meta Models Mining eXtensible Markup Language (MXML)* in [4]. The *eXtensible Event stream (XES)* standard [6], developed by the IEEE task Force on Process Mining, can be viewed as a successor approach that better supports extensibility. Both approaches are supported by today's process mining tools, and both are based on XML.

So our pre-processing ends with a conversion of the event log to the XES format, which will serve as an input format for mining tools such as *ProM* [12]. This conversion is done by the commercial tool *Nitro* developed by *Fluxicon*.

3   Mining of Event Logs

There is no *best* process miner, each miner and each mining algorithm has particular advantages and drawbacks. The selection of a process miner primarily depends on the goal of mining. For our purposes, the following mining algorithms (all available via ProM[1]) seem to be suitable. In this list, we refer to the *ProM Tips* provided in [13].

- **Alpha Miner.** A simple algorithm based on dependency relations between events which needs ideal event logs without noise. Improved by the α^+-miner, that also handles "short loops", i.e., mutual dependencies between events. The output is a Petri net. This algorithm is not recommended in [13] for real logs, because highly sensitive w.r.t. quality of logs.
- **Heuristics Miner.** Based on the mechanisms of the Alpha Miner, but additionally takes the number of identified relations into account and is therefore more robust against noise. Produces so-called Heuristic Nets, which can easily be transformed in a normal Petri net. Its use is recommended for real data with a limited amount of different activities, in particular if a Petri net is desired [13].
- **Fuzzy Miner.** Good if behavior shows little structure and has many different activities. Can simplify very complex data or a very complex model. The output is a so-called Fuzzy Model, which is not easily transformed in another language.

---

[1] Our study is based on ProM 6.2.

- **Multi Phase Miner.** Aims at constructing event-driven process chains with logical connectors, as used by the ARIS tools. Needs noise-free input.
- **Genetic Miner.** Based on genetic algorithms, can cope with incomplete logs and noise. The output is a Petri net or a Heuristic Net.

The Process Mining Manifesto [3] defines five maturity levels of event logs, from the highest level 5 of excellent quality (correct and complete) to the lowest level 1 (missing events, wrong events). Before selecting process miners to be considered further, we classify the event logs of our setting. The maturity of our event logs can be assumed to be on level 3 (automatic recording, missing completeness, little noise). The Multi Phase Miner seems inappropriate for our setting because it results in an event driven process chain whereas other miners construct Petri nets and are thus better comparable. Moreover, the Multi Phase Miner assumes a particularly high quality of the input event logs which we cannot guarantee. The Fuzzy Miner has the advantage to provide an abstraction of activities dynamically, i.e., distinct activities that always appear in the same context, are embraced. Since in our procedure this step was done just before mining, it is not helpful after mining again. So we apply the mining algorithms Alpha Miner, Heuristic Miner and Genetic Miner in the sequel and will compare the respective results in the next section.

4   Case Study

This work was motivated by a real application. The software company *rubecon information technologies GmbH* [9] is specialized on software solutions for the printing industry. One of its products is the software *hd-druckdialog* which is based on the CDIX Business Application Framework. This product was migrated to Windows. The precise implementation of the windows client is unknown, and so is the protocol. Recently, a new software client for the CDIX protocol was developed, called *SmartClient*. Its behavior is *not* based on the mining approach of this paper. Tests showed that it slightly differs from the original protocol.

The current aim is to reconstruct the original protocol from observed behavior and to formalize it by means of a model, compare this model with a model of the *SmartClient* implementation and to identify and explain differences.

For the sake of this case study, we derive a model for a particular use case. This has the advantages that the model is not too complex and that we have a better chance to assign activities to classes correctly. A disadvantage is that the usable input data for mining is comparably small. If the mining procedure is successful, the use case (and thus the model) can be extended.

The simple use case in our experiment is given as follows: The software *hd-druckdialog* is started; then the user authenticates herself, and finally the software is terminated. Its extension opens after successful authentication the customer management windows, which requires navigation in the menu structure of the software. Also in this use case, the software is subsequently terminated.

These use cases were performed a number of times, using the classical protocol implementation. In doing so, possible variants of the user interface were chosen, such as a wrong password or different navigation paths, so that this part of the communication protocol is captured as complete as possible. The traffic was recorded and the steps described in the previous sections were performed, leading to a minable event log.

The software *TCPLog2EventLog* determines the number of use cases that appear in the present event log. The further considerations only make sense, if this number coincides with the real number (two in our case). If this number deviates, the log is too faulty and can not be used. A further criterion for the quality of the log is the appearance of xx-activities, i.e., of activities that were not mapped to an activity class. In this case, either the generation of the template file was insufficient or the event log contains activities not known before, which can also be due to non-conformity reasons.

In our case study, we have a comparable small amount of use cases and hence can assume that the event logs are incomplete. Since we constructed the event logs carefully manually, we assume lack of noise. So we tried the Alpha Miner first, yielding the model shown in Fig. 5. All server activities are located in the upper part of the figure, all client activities in the lower one.

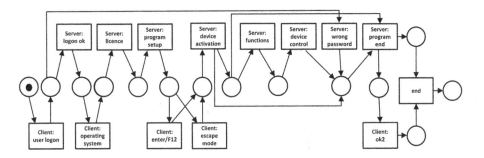

Fig. 5. The registration process of the original windows client

The transitions of this (Petri net) model are inscribed by the sender of a message, followed by the content type. We checked completeness of this model, i.e., found out that all use case activities are possible. Subsequently, we did the same for the extended use case and checked whether the new model is in fact an extension of the first one. This model is shown in Fig. 6. It turned out to be complete as well. A conformance check by ProM additionally confirmed that in fact the first model is included in the second, because the log of the first example can be played on the second model, too (the inclusion of the first model is depicted in Fig. 6).

This example already shows that in principle process mining is applicable to recover protocols from network traffic. We also tried other mining algorithms, with the following results: The Heuristic Miner yields a structure shown in Fig. 7, which is semantically equivalent to the result of the Alpha Miner. The Genetic Miner derives a considerably different model, shown in Fig. 8 (the differences are depicted). This model is not conform to the event log.

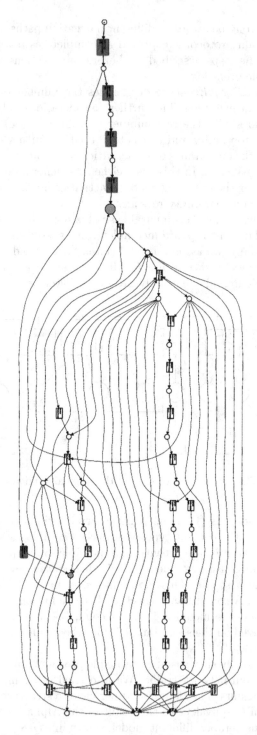

Fig. 6. The extended use case (in grey: replay of the event log of the simple use case)

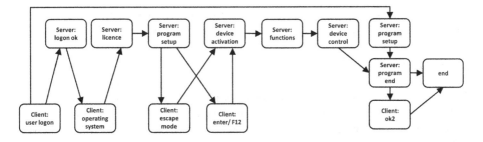

Fig. 7. Result of the Heuristic Miner

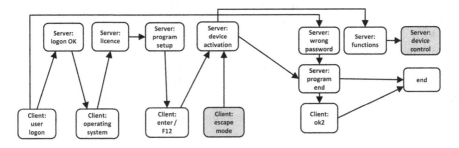

Fig. 8. Result of the Genetic Miner

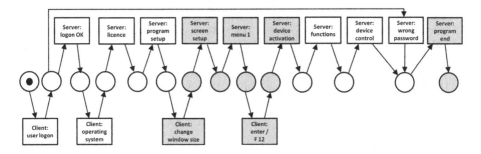

Fig. 9. Model of the communication process of the simple use case of *SmartClient*

A final step of our case study is the comparison of the obtained model derived from the classical protocol with the new protocol *SmartClient*. To this end, we constructed a model of this new protocol (shown in Fig. 9) for the single use case in the same way as for the classical protocol. Both protocols have obvious differences, depicted in the figure, and they also behave differently:

- After the program start, SmartClient maximizes the window size.
- The classical client distinguishes three possibilities to terminate the program, SmartClient has only one such possibility.
- Only SmartClient sends no confirmation after program termination.

We finally checked whether SmartClient is still conform to the classic client. Since also the classical protocol allowed to change window size, this behavioral derivation does not spoil correctness. The other differences, however, are more serious although they do not lead to any misbehavior observable by the user.

5 Conclusion

This paper developed a concept to derive event logs from network traffic, which makes it possible to apply process mining techniques and tools for protocol mining. The concept has several steps, many of them supported by a novel software program. A use case from practice proved the concept to work in general.

A different approach would have been to view clients and servers of our setting as respective loosely coupled services. Then many already existing tools for services could have been applied, such as *FIONA, WENDY, LOLA* or *BPEL-2OWFN* [10]. The underlying formalism, *Open Petri Nets*, would have been an ideal language for protocol definitions. However, all these tools, as well as the underlying techniques, start with services modeled in the *Business Process Execution Language (BPEL)*. Since we could neither derive service definitions formulated in BPEL nor open workflow nets with defined message exchange activities by application of the mining tools, this approach was not (yet) viable.

References

1. van der Aalst, W.M.P.: Service mining: using process mining to discover, check, and improve service behavior. IEEE Trans. Serv. Comput. **6**(4), 525–535 (2013)
2. van der Aalst, W.M.P., van Dongen, B.F.: Discovering Petri nets from event logs (2013). http://wwwis.win.tue.nl/wvdaalst/publications/z2.pdf. Accessed 10 May 2013
3. van der Aalst, W.M.P.: Process mining manifesto. In: Daniel, F., Barkaoui, K., Dustdar, S. (eds.) BPM Workshops 2011, Part I. LNBIP, vol. 99, pp. 169–194. Springer, Heidelberg (2012)
4. van Dongen, B.F., van der Aalst, W.M.P.: A meta model for process mining data. In: EMOI-INTEROP (2005)
5. Dustdar, S., Gombotz, R.: Discovering web service workflows using web services interaction mining. Int. J. Bus. Process Integr. Manage. **1**(4), 256–266 (2006)
6. Günther, C.W., Verbeek, E.: Xes standard definition (2012). http://www.xes-standard.org/meida/xes/xesstandarddefinition-1.4.pdf. Accessed 26 April 2013
7. König, H.: Protocol Engineering. Springer, Heidelberg (2012)
8. Levenshtein, V.I.: Binary codes capable of correcting deletions, insertions and reversals. Dokl. Akad. Nauk SSSR **163**(4), 845–848 (1965)
9. rubecon information technologies GmbH. hd-druckdialog (2013)
10. Service technology.org (2013). http://service-technology.org/tools/start. Accessed 10 May 2013
11. Wireshark Foundation. Wireshark version 1.6.3. http://www.wireshark.org
12. ProM. Process Mining Workbench. http://www.promtools.org
13. Rozinat, A.: ProM tips - which Mining Algorithm sould you use (2012). http://fluxicon.com/blog/2010/10/prom-tips-mining-algorithm. Accessed 28 April 2013
14. Wakup, C.: Konzeption und Evaluation eines Verfahrens zur Ermittlung der internen Funktionsweise eines TCP/IP-basierten Kommunikationsprotokollsmit Hilfe von Process-Mining. Bachelorarbeit, FernUniversität in Hagen (2013)

BPMC 2014

YAWL in the Cloud: Supporting Process Sharing and Variability

D.M.M. Schunselaar[(✉)], H.M.W. Verbeek, H.A. Reijers,
and Wil M.P. van der Aalst

Eindhoven University of Technology,
P.O. Box 513, 5600 MB Eindhoven, The Netherlands
{d.m.m.schunselaar,h.m.w.verbeek,h.a.reijers,w.m.p.v.d.aalst}@tue.nl

Abstract. The cloud is at the centre of attention in various fields, including that of BPM. However, all BPM systems in the cloud seem to be nothing more than an installation in the cloud with a web-interface for a single organisation, while cloud technology offers an excellent platform for cooperation on an intra- and inter-organisational level. In this paper, we show how cloud technology can be used for supporting different variants of the same process (due to "couleur locale"), and how these organisations can aid each other in achieving the completion of a running case. In this paper we describe how we have brought a BPM system (YAWL) into the cloud that supports variants.

Keywords: BPM · Cloud · YAWL · Process variability · Process cooperation · Configurable process models

1 Introduction

In the CoSeLoG project[1], 10 Dutch municipalities collaborate to see how cloud technology can be used to share resources and exchange knowledge. Of course, by bringing these municipalities into the cloud, we gain well-accepted benefits associated with the cloud. First, instead of having to buy and administer their own servers, the municipalities can simply use the cloud and focus more on their core processes. The municipalities still have to administer their own processes, but at least they do not have to administer the hardware these processes are running on. Second, by using the cloud, they can dynamically scale the required hardware up or down, depending on the current need. For example, if due to a change of legislation getting a building permit will become more difficult, then one can expect a rise in the number of applications for a building permit before the new building permit legislation comes into place. One can scale up the amount of hardware required before the bulk of applications arrives. When

---

The installation manual and files can be downloaded from http://www.win.tue.nl/coselog/wiki/yawlinthecloud.

[1] This research has been carried out as part of the Configurable Services for Local Governments (CoSeLoG) project (http://www.win.tue.nl/coselog/).

© Springer International Publishing Switzerland 2015
F. Fournier and J. Mendling (Eds.): BPM 2014 Workshops, LNBIP 202, pp. 367–379, 2015.
DOI: 10.1007/978-3-319-15895-2_31

the volume of applications drops, one can scale down again. Furthermore, during peaks, a municipality can be aided by staff of another municipality. As a result, using the cloud will be cheaper and more flexible for a municipality, in a way that is similar to the advantages that the cloud brings to other organisations.

What sets the municipalities apart from many organisations, though, is that they are not competing with each other. For example, a citizen of Eindhoven cannot go to the Amsterdam municipality to apply for a building permit. Clearly, this citizen has no other choice than to come the Eindhoven municipality to apply for this building permit. As such, every municipality has its own, exclusive, collection of customers.

This presents us with a setting which is quite different from a regular cloud setting. As the municipalities are not competing with each other, they are quite willing to exchange ideas, to learn from each other, and to share insights with each other. As a result, when bringing municipalities into the cloud, there is no need to assume that they, as cloud tenants, are to be kept strictly separated. As a result of this, in the CoSeLoG project, we can model the similar processes of different municipalities using a single *configurable process model*. All municipalities share this single configurable process model, but they all have configured the model at deploy-time to cater for their own "couleur locale". Using such a configurable process model, one can capture common behaviour while still leaving room for some differences. As a result, all municipalities use a process model that is based on the same model (the configurable process model), but they all may run different process models.

In this paper, we assume that the cloud tenants are using variants of some super process model, are willing to cooperate, and are willing to disclose information about their processes. How can cloud technology then be best used to their advantage? This paper will show that advantages include *deploy-time* advantages, *run-time* advantages, and *post-run-time* advantages. To showcase the feasibility of a cloud implementation, we provide a proof-of-concept implementation that supports configurable process models and demonstrates these advantages.

The remainder of this paper is organised as follows: Sect. 2 explains configurable process models and lists the deploy-time, run-time, and post-run-time advantages. In Sect. 3, we present our proof-of-concept implementation. The proof-of-concept implementation is showcased by means of a scenario in Sect. 4. Relevant related work is discussed in Sect. 5. Finally, the conclusions are presented in Sect. 6.

2   Advantages of Cloud Technology

By combining configurable processes and cloud technology, we can achieve advantages in three areas: deploy-time, run-time, and post-run-time. Prior to going into these advantages, we first explain configurable process models as these are on the basis of some of the advantages.

Configurable Process Models. Configurable process models describe a family of process models using variation points. Variation points are locations in the process model which can be modified by the user. In other words, the municipality can select to remove that part from the model or substitute that part of the model with a model fragment from a predefined set of model fragments. When the user has set all the variation points, we have a process model that can be executed by a BPM system.

In the configurable process model (Fig. 1), we have the option to *hide* certain parts (orange curved arrow) and we have the option to *block* certain parts (no-entry sign). When a certain part is hidden, that part is substituted by an automatic task. Blocking a certain part results in the removal of that part from the model. Taking Fig. 1 as an example, hiding "Toetsenontvangekijkheid (adviseur RO)" entails replacing that activity with an automatic task. Blocking "Verzoeken om aanpassing van aanvraag" means that the exclusive choice "Weigeren vergunning" will always evaluate to "Versturen weigering". Note that activities do not vary from model to model, i.e., the presence of an activity can be changed but not the contents of the activity. In case of the configurable process model in Fig. 1, the activity "Toetsenontvangekijkheid (adviseur RO)" can be hidden in a model but if it is not hidden then it is the same as "Toetsenontvangekijkheid (adviseur RO)" in any other obtainable model.

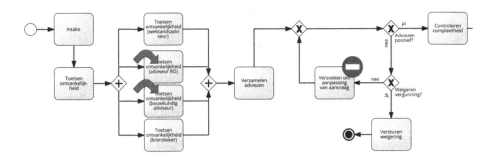

Fig. 1. Part of the configurable process model from the scenario.

Deploy-time Advantages. A municipality that wants to deploy a process model in this cloud setting does not have to create a model from scratch. Instead, it only needs to configure an existing model from a configurable process model.

In the classical setting, each municipality maintains its own process models and IT infrastructure. This means that every change in legislation has to be incorporated by every municipality. When moving to the cloud using configurable process models, changes mainly have to be incorporated in the configurable process model. Municipalities might have to change their configuration. In Fig. 2, the old situation is compared to a hypothetical cloud situation. Although the maintenance efforts for the configurable process model are larger than for the individual models (it is more complex), the total maintenance effort is smaller than the sum of maintenance efforts of each of the municipalities.

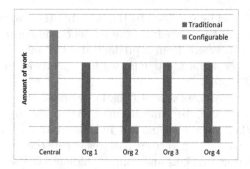

Fig. 2. The expected benefit in maintenance when municipalities move to the cloud using a configurable process model.

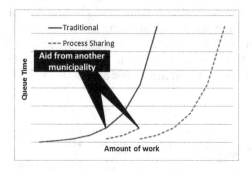

Fig. 3. In the traditional situation, the queue time increases significantly when the amount of work increases. Using Process Sharing, we expect that employees from other municipalities can aid to postpone the significant increase in queue time.

Run-time Advantages. Next to the deploy-time advantages, the municipalities can also expect run-time advantages. Some of the run-time advantages are directly related to the use of the cloud, i.e., scalability, availability, reliability, cost reduction, etc. Other advantages during run-time, however, amount to an increase in the flexibility and robustness of the organisation.

The expected increase in flexibility is achieved by the fact that municipalities are capable of allocating work to resources from another municipality. In the traditional situation (Fig. 3), we have the well-known curve related to the PASTA property, i.e., when the amount of work increases this results in the utilisation rate approaching 1 yielding a queue time which goes to infinity. By sharing the execution of the process between municipalities, other municipalities can offer staff when the queue time becomes too long (until there are no resources left). Next to this, municipalities can also share an expert to aid them in their executions. The addition of an expert means that part of the execution of a case is partly outsourced. This flexibility has as added advantage that the robustness increases. For instance, in case of disasters (flooding, power failure, etc.), staff of other municipalities can aid. One can argue that the process models are different between municipalities and thus aiding another municipality requires learning

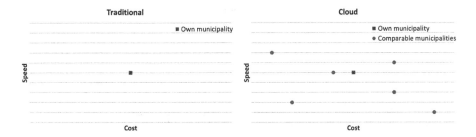

Fig. 4. In the traditional situation, a municipality can only compare itself to itself. With the use of a single cloud service and a configurable process model, we expect a graph similar to the right one where municipalities can benchmark.

the other's process model. However, as mentioned with the configurable process model, the process models might be different but the individual activities do not differ with respect to content. This means that if a municipality also executes a particular activity, then that municipality can aid in executing that activity.

Post-run-time Advantages. Traditionally, municipalities are only able to look at themselves. By having comparable executions, municipalities can benchmark themselves with respect to others (see Fig. 4 for a hypothetical graph). The comparability of the executions comes forth from the fact that all models are deduced from a configurable process model and the use of a single cloud service which guarantees uniform naming conventions, same level or granularity, and comparable data structures.

3   Proof-of-Concept Implementation

To be able to show the advantages sketched earlier, we made a proof-of-concept implementation. For our proof-of-concept implementation we have chosen YAWL as our BPM system since YAWL has the following advantages: components are decoupled making them ideal to be run in distributed mode, and native support for configurable process models [1]. For the cloud provider, we have chosen Microsoft Azure. Finally, YAWL in the cloud runs on the PaaS (Platform as a Service) layer.

We managed to make YAWL available in the Azure cloud without making changes to YAWL itself. This has the advantage that updates of YAWL can be used and there is no need to maintain a special YAWL version. Furthermore, by not changing YAWL itself, we maintained the look and feel people are familiar with; removing the need to learn a new system. Finally, we created a component to control the cloud allowing administrators to, amongst others, upload configurable process models.

YAWL [1] is a workflow system based on Petri net semantics. YAWL has an architecture which is service-oriented. Part of the architecture of YAWL is depicted in Fig. 5. The individual components, e.g., the engine, resource service, etc., are independent components which are coupled using different interfaces.

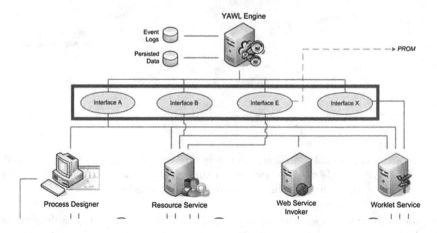

Fig. 5. Part of the architecture of YAWL. Figure taken from [1].

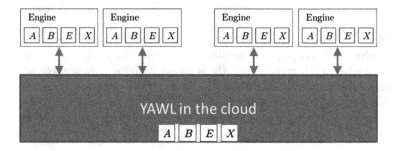

Fig. 6. The high-level architecture for YAWL in the Cloud.

In this paper, we "cloudify" the engine, therefore, we briefly touch upon the interface A, B, E, and X (highlighted in the red rectangle in Fig. 5). Interface A is used for, amongst others, loading and unloading process specifications. Interface B is used for most of the handling of work items and creating new process instances. Interface E is used for the retrieval of process logs. Finally, interface X is used for exception handling.

As mentioned, YAWL consists of components which communicate with each other using different interfaces. In a non-cloud based YAWL installation, there is a single engine. This engine receives requests on its interfaces and acts accordingly. With bringing YAWL into the cloud, we want to allow for multiple engines running concurrently. In order to be able to scale up and down, we want to use a dynamic amount of engines. Furthermore, the other components within YAWL expect to communicate with a single engine. Therefore, within YAWL in the cloud, we have created an abstraction from the engines allowing for multiple engines to be used and at the same time offer a single set of interfaces (A, B, E, and X) to the outside world to communicate with. This results in the high-level architecture shown in Fig. 6.

By using this architecture, we do not need to make any changes to YAWL. Furthermore, by offering the same set of interfaces to the outside world, there is no change noticeable, i.e., one cannot see the difference between a single engine or the entire cloud. However, since we do not make any changes to YAWL, the YAWL engines are oblivious of each other. This means that, for instance, the case identifiers are unique per engine, but not amongst engines. Furthermore, engines might now be used for multiple organisations resulting in cases running in different contexts for a single engine (engines normally run within a single context). To accommodate for this, we propose the more detailed architecture shown in Fig. 7.

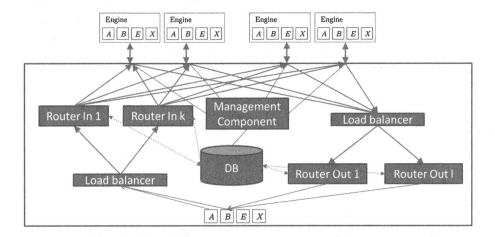

Fig. 7. The detailed architecture for YAWL in the Cloud.

As shown in Fig. 7, there is a central cloud based database which is used to transform case identifiers etc. from the local context of an engine, to the global context of the cloud and vice versa. By using a cloud based database, all scalability challenges are handled by the cloud. Furthermore, we have introduced routers to route the various requests to the correct engine(s), e.g., when an organisation wants to know all the cases currently running for that organisation, the router performs a lookup to see which engines to contact. After contacting the various engines, the router combines each of their responses into a single response as this is expected by the environment. Finally, since we have distributed the engines, we also want to distribute the routers for the same reasons, therefore, we can use a cloud based load balancer to automatically forward requests to the least busy router. This cloud based load balancer scales automatically up and down without any involvement.

In the centre of the detailed architecture, we have a management component. This management component can query the database for information on the various engines. Furthermore, it can be used to add/remove available engines; the enablement and disablement of engines is handled by the cloud.

Most notably for the implementation is the fact that YAWL in the cloud, similar to YAWL, is implemented in java. Furthermore, we use Hibernate[2] as abstraction layer from the database. Both java and Hibernate make YAWL in the cloud largely platform independent. Unfortunately, YAWL did not work properly with the cloud based version of MSSQL, therefore, we have used a virtual machine with MySQL. The implementation and an installation manual can be downloaded from http://www.win.tue.nl/coselog/wiki/yawlinthecloud.

4   Proof-of-Concept Scenario

We evaluate our implementation by means of a hypothetical scenario. In this hypothetical scenario, all the CoSeLoG municipalities want to cooperate with each other in the cloud. To reap the deploy-time benefits, they obtain a configurable process model capable of supporting their processes (part of this model is depicted in Fig. 1). Next to the configurable process model, the municipalities use the Synergia toolset [2] to define their configurations. The configurable process model and configurations are uploaded to the cloud (Fig. 8).

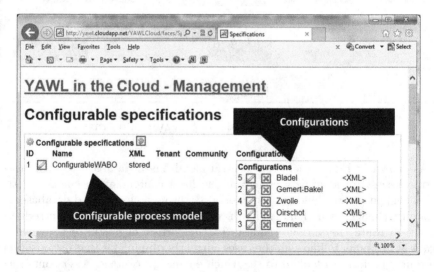

Fig. 8. A configurable process model in the cloud with the configurations for the various municipalities.

Using the Synergia toolset, the configuration can be projected on the configurable process model to obtain an executable process model. These are added to the set of loadable specifications (Fig. 9).

To give the municipalities the possibility to work on their cases, virtual machines are created in Microsoft's Azure cloud (Fig. 10 contain the virtual machines for Emmen and Gemert-Bakel). Each municipality is offered a slightly

---

[2] http://hibernate.org.

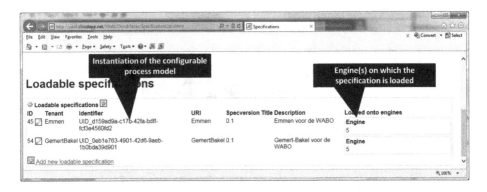

Fig. 9. Specifications for some municipalities have been uploaded to a (shared) engine.

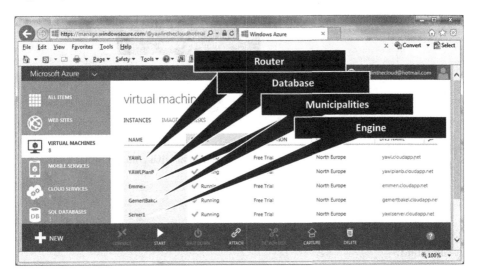

Fig. 10. The various virtual machines for the municipalities, a router, an engine, and a database server.

customised portal to YAWL in the cloud where already some of their cases are present (Fig. 11).

Assume all employees able to handle the process in Gemert-Bakel get ill. Luckily, we have the run-time benefits of the cloud and promptly employees from Emmen are logging in to aid Gemert-Bakel in the execution of their processes (Fig. 12).

A similar scenario like this has been presented to the participating municipalities of the CoSeLoG project in our yearly meeting. The contact persons were subdivided into municipalities and got some hands-on experience with YAWL in the cloud. The various contact persons were enthusiastic about the presented implementation. However, this was not a real evaluation but more a small showcase to show the work conducted in the project.

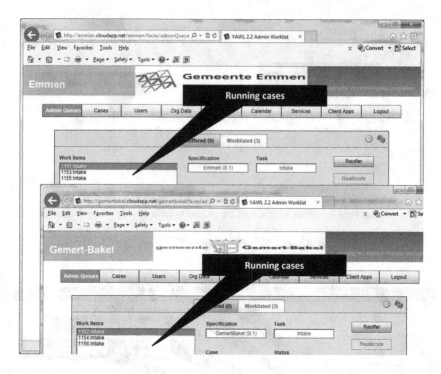

Fig. 11. The portal for Emmen and Gemert-Bakel with some running cases.

5 Related Work

Both in academia and industry, there has been a lot of interest in BPM/WFM in the cloud.

Academic publications. In [3], the authors bring BPEL to the cloud. The authors extensively discuss different considerations for bringing BPEL to the cloud using different levels, i.e., infrastructure, platform, and software, and security considerations. The authors state that they are busy with modifying an open-source BPEL engine to be used in the cloud. In [4], the authors add configurability to BPEL in an extension called *VxBPEL*. In [5], configurable BPEL is presented. However, for both approaches there is no graphical editor making it cumbersome to maintain the models.

In [6], ARIS in the cloud is presented where resources can be shared amongst different locations around the world. It is unclear whether this is based on a single process model being used for all the branches. Although this approach is not directly applicable to the municipality setting, the approach can be beneficial for companies with multiple branches, e.g., Hertz.

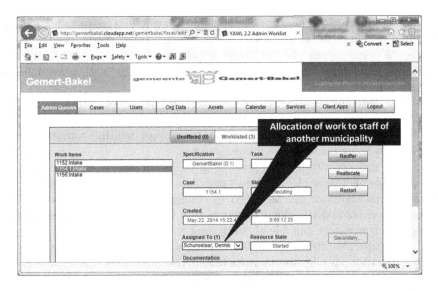

Fig. 12. An employee from Emmen (Dennis Schunselaar) is executing cases for Gemert-Bakel.

The workflow engine CPEE[3] [7] offers a cloud based workflow engine. This workflow engine has been built from scratch and allows for run-time modifications of the process model. It is designed with a single organisation in mind.

Industrial solutions. As mentioned, there exist a multitude of cloud solutions from the industry. However, most of these solutions seem nothing more than a web-based interface to a classical BPM system running on the servers of the vendor or outsourced to a third party. We list the cloud based BPM systems based on Gartners Magic Quadrant for Intelligent Business Process Management Suites [8]. We do not list all of the companies but mention only the ones where there is a strong cloud platform according to Gartner.

Kofax [9] offers a cloud platform called TotalAgility. One of the features of Kofax is the use of "process skins". Process skins allow the user to manage multiple versions of the same process type. Whenever there is an update to the process all skins are updated accordingly. This seems to be similar to configurable process models, but the expressive power and capabilities are not specified. Finally, TotalAgility reasons with a single organisation in mind.

Other solutions mentioned do not support configurable process models, these include: Appian [10], OpenText [11], PNMSoft [12], and Software AG [13].

6   Conclusion

We have sketched the added benefits of bringing non-competing organisations like municipalities, court houses, ministries, etc. into the cloud. These benefits

---
[3] www.cpee.org.

include well-known cloud benefits like: scalability, availability, cost reduction etc. But these benefits can be extended towards deploy-time advantages (by using configurable process models), run-time advantages (increase in flexibility and robustness), and post-run-time advantages (benchmarking with other municipalities).

Next to sketching the benefits, we have provided an implementation where we brought YAWL into the cloud. Within YAWL in the cloud, we support multiple organisations, and we offer the possibility to support multiple variants of the same process using configurable process models.

To show process variability is possible in the cloud, we presented a proof-of-concept implementation of YAWL in the cloud. In this proof of concept implementation, we show we did not need to change YAWL. Furthermore, in the evaluation, we showed the cloud infrastructure is invisible. Finally, we showed parts of the component capable of controlling the cloud.

In this paper, we focussed on the setting of non-competitive organisations working together, specifically municipalities. Also, note that this approach can be beneficial within a single organisation as well. Take for instance Hertz, which has numerous branches in numerous countries. Instead of having an installation per branch, there can now be a centralised BPM system in the cloud in which the various branches can cooperate.

Acknowledgements. The authors would like to thank T.F. van der Avoort for his work on the implementation of YAWL in the cloud as part of his master thesis [14].

References

1. Hofstede, A.H.M., Aalst, W.M.P., van der Adams, M., Russell, N. (eds.): Modern Business Process Automation: YAWL and Its Support Environment. Springer, Heidelberg (2010)
2. La Rosa, M., Gottschalk, F.: Synergia - comprehensive tool support for configurable process models. In: de Medeiros, A.K.A., Weber, B. (eds.) BPM (Demos), CEUR Workshop Proceedings, vol. 489 (2009). CEUR-WS.org
3. Anstett, T., Leymann, F., Mietzner, R., Strauch, S.: Towards BPEL in the cloud: exploiting different delivery models for the execution of business processes. In: SERVICES I, pp. 670–677. IEEE Computer Society (2009)
4. Koning, M., Ai Sun, C., Sinnema, M., Avgeriou, P.: VxBPEL: supporting variability for web services in BPEL. Inf. Softw. Technol. **51**(2), 258–269 (2009)
5. Gottschalk, F.: Configurable Process Models. Ph.D. thesis, Eindhoven University of Technology, The Netherlands (2009)
6. Scheer, A.-W., Klueckmann, J.: BPM 3.0. In: Dayal, U., Eder, J., Koehler, J., Reijers, H.A. (eds.) BPM 2009. LNCS, vol. 5701, pp. 15–27. Springer, Heidelberg (2009)
7. Stuermer, G., Mangler, J., Schikuta, E.: Building a modular service oriented workflow engine. In: SOCA, pp. 1–4. IEEE (2009)
8. Jones, T., Schulte, W.R., Contara, M.: Magic Quadrant for Intelligent Business Process Management Suites. Gartner G00255421 (2014)

9. Kofax: TotalAgility. http://www.kofax.com/smart-process-application-platform/. Last accessed 4 Apr 2014

10. Appian: Appian. http://www.appian.com/bpm-software/cloud-bpm.jsp. Last accessed 4 Apr 2014

11. OpenText: OpenText Cordys. http://www.opentext.com/What-We-Do/Products/Business-Process-Management/Process-Suite-Platform/BPM-in-the-Cloud. Last accessed 4 Apr 2014

12. PNMSoft: Cloudworks. http://www.pnmsoft.com/technology/cloud-bpm/. Last accessed 4 Apr 2014

13. SoftwareAG: webMethods BPMS. http://www.softwareag.com/corporate/products/wm/bpm/products/bpms/overview/default.asp. Last accessed 4 Apr 2014

14. van der Avoort, T.F.: BPM in the Cloud. Master's thesis, Eindhoven University of Technology,The Netherlands (2013)

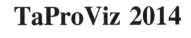

TaProViz 2014

A Generic Approach for Calculating and Visualizing Differences Between Process Models in Multidimensional Process Mining

Carsten Cordes, Thomas Vogelgesang[(✉)], and Hans-Jürgen Appelrath

University of Oldenburg, 26129 Oldenburg, Germany
{carsten.cordes,thomas.vogelgesang}@uni-oldenburg.de, appelrath@offis.de

Abstract. Process mining automatically generates process models from event logs. In multidimensional process mining, these models can be analyzed from various viewpoints by clustering event traces according to their attributes, e.g. age or region of the patient for a healthcare process. For each cluster, a distinct process model is calculated. Since these models are supposed to be identical in most parts, differences between them are hard to spot. Therefore, a tool for emphasizing these differences is needed. To face the different challenges presented by multidimensional process mining like the representational bias, such an approach has to be customizable to support different modeling languages and different layout and differencing algorithms. This paper presents a generic approach to calculate and visualize differences between process models which can be used to compare models in multidimensional process mining.

Keywords: Visualization · Differencing · Multidimensional process mining

1 Motivation

Process models are important for analyzing and optimizing business processes. While traditional process management makes use of manually created process models, *process mining* [7] allows for the automatic generation and analysis of process models based on *event logs*. Event logs are collections of real process data collected by process aware information systems (PAIS). Whenever an event takes place, it is recorded by the PAIS. These records can be summarized into event logs. Entries in event logs normally contain at least information about the process and the *process instance* they belong to, where an instance describes an actual case (for example the consulting of a particular client). Process mining consists of three different activities:

Process discovery automatically creates a process model from an event log that consists of events recorded during the execution of the process. In the event log, the time-ordered events are grouped by their process instance. While mined models should be as precise as possible, they should also allow for traces which

© Springer International Publishing Switzerland 2015 •
F. Fournier and J. Mendling (Eds.): BPM 2014 Workshops, LNBIP 202, pp. 383–394, 2015.
DOI: 10.1007/978-3-319-15895-2_32

are not in the event log. This is because in general, event logs do not contain all possible traces of a process, but only example behavior (open-world-assumption).

Process conformance determines the compliance of a given process model by comparing it to an event log. Usually, this is done by replaying event sequences on the model.

Process enhancement improves an existing model with information from an event log to add further *perspectives*. In the time perspective for example, time-stamps from the event log are mapped to the model to analyze execution times of activities and identify bottlenecks in the process. The organizational perspective focuses on the actors of a process, e.g. to identify social networks while the case perspective examines a single instance of a process e.g. to identify decision rules.

On the one hand, process mining leads to more realistic models, because real data is used instead of assumed workflows. On the other hand, calculated models also tend to be more complex than planned models and can contain a lot of unnecessary detailed or even wrong information due to noise. In general this makes automatically generated process models harder to analyze. Because of that, the decision which modeling language to use and which information to display in the model are very important in the process mining context.

Multidimensional process mining can be used to analyze a given process in relation to particular attributes, for example the patient's age, gender, or region in the domain of health services research (HSR). Reference [24] proposes to use OLAP-techniques to cluster event-logs by relevant attributes and to mine a separate process model for each cluster. When looking at age groups and regions in HSR for example, this approach allows to mine different process models for each age group and region as outlined in the left part of Fig. 1. To identify problems like inappropriate healthcare, an analyst could be interested if there are deviations in the treatment process for a particular illness between the young (<50) and the old patients (>69) in the region *East*. By comparing these models, as shown in the right part, differences in the healthcare process between these age groups can be identified, indicating possible problems.

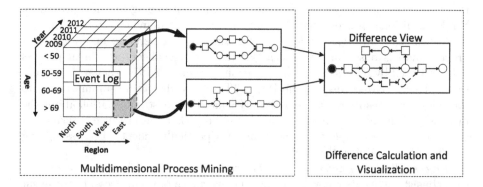

Fig. 1. Difference calculation and visualization in multidimensional process mining.

Without additional tools however, the differences between these process models representing variants of the same process can be very difficult to find: First of all, these models can be very complex and big, depending on the analyzed process and the mining method. Additionally, when looking at process variants, the resulting models tend to be very similar in large parts, making it even harder to find the differences. The goal of difference calculation in multidimensional process mining is to simplify the analysis of differences between two or more different variants of the same process.

While there are already approaches to compare graphical models, none of them takes into account the special problems in multidimensional process mining. For example, the modeling language of the process variants depends on the used discovery algorithm. Due to this, the difference calculation and visualization should be independent from the modeling language to avoid limitations to particular process mining algorithms. Most existing approaches however, support only a particular modeling language. Therefore, we propose a novel approach to compare model variants in process mining which calculates the differences and visualizes them accordingly. It is kept as generic as possible to be suitable for multidimensional process mining, e.g. by using arbitrary difference calculation algorithms that are independent of a specific modeling language.

This paper presents the challenges for differencing process models in multidimensional process mining and proposes a generic approach to deal with these challenges. Section 2 explains the specific problems in comparing models of process variants and Sect. 3 presents how these problems can be solved in a generic way. Section 4 describes a prototypical implementation of our approach. The appropriateness of our approach to the problem is discussed in Sect. 5. Related work is presented in Sect. 6. Finally, Sect. 7 concludes the paper.

2   Problem Description

In most approaches, calculating differences between graphical models serves as a method to transform models between different versions, for example in a version control system. Enhancing existing methods like textual diff helps software engineers to keep track of their previous work. In contrast to this, in multidimensional process mining there is typically no need to transform between model variants, e.g. the treatment of old and young patients. Therefore, different use cases have to be considered to support the analyst in result interpretation.

Calculating differences could be done either syntactically or semantically. In syntactic analysis only the structure of the models is compared. In semantic analysis, the meaning of different models is compared. In the context of process mining, semantic analysis is normally done by comparing the possible traces between two models, for example all possible variations of the treatment process for old patients with all variations for young patients. When two models produce the same traces, these models represent the same process. Because both approaches are useful when analyzing a process, a software to compare process variants in multidimensional process mining should be able to do semantic as well as syntactic analysis.

A lot of algorithms used in software engineering assume an implicit parent-child relation between the different process models and rely on previously recorded change logs between the different versions. In general, there are no such relationships between process variants, e.g. the treatment processes of old and young patients are mined independently. Furthermore, there is no version control system to record the differences between these variants in multidimensional process mining, hence these algorithms do not work properly here. As a consequence, a differencing tool for process variants should be able to compare models without any model-specific additional information, such as change logs.

In process mining, different modeling languages, for example Petri nets [18], causal nets [21] and BPMN [25] are applied. Each language has its own set of structures which cannot be modeled properly due to restrictions of the language's syntax. In Petri nets, for example, there is no possibility to model a logical OR, only XOR is supported [19]. This problem is referred to as representational bias.

In process mining, where algorithms are used to mine the models, most of these algorithms depend on a specific modeling language. For example the α-algorithm [22] only generates Petri nets. If Petri nets are not able to represent the best fitting model, the algorithm cannot find it either. This is why different languages are used in process mining to represent all types of processes in the best way possible. Because of this, an approach to calculate differences between models in process mining needs to be adjustable to different modeling languages. On the one hand, this means, that the method for calculating differences needs to be independent of the modeling language, while on the other hand it should be able to visualize the model in the corresponding modeling language.

In process mining, models are often enriched with additional information in perspectives, for example how long a patient usually has to wait for an examination. An approach for comparing models in multidimensional process mining should be able to display and to compare this additional information to make process analysis easier, e.g. to find optimization potentials. In the following section, we will present our approach, which addresses the identified problems.

3   Generic Diff Concept

Figure 2 gives an overview of the general workflow, where ellipses denote customizable parts in the process. To be able to deal with different types of process models, a language specific mapping must be present when loading a model. With such a mapping, each process model is transformed into an intermediate model. The mapping itself contains transformation rules between the modeling language and the intermediate data model used throughout the application. Both, the mapping and the models can be provided as XML-files.

Using an intermediate model allows for the comparison of a wide variety of modeling languages with generic algorithms. Without an intermediate model, each modeling language would need its own set of algorithms. To make implementing generic algorithms easier, the intermediate model should be as simple as possible on the one hand. On the other hand, the intermediate model must

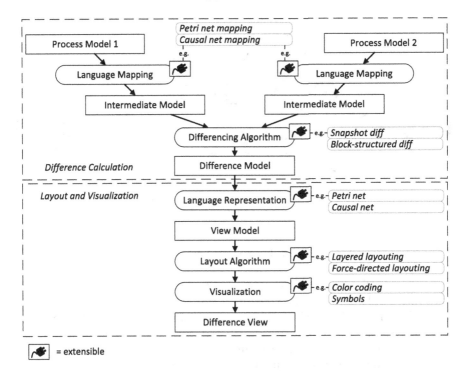

Fig. 2. Overview of differencing workflow and its extensible parts.

not lose any information contained in the original model. Compared models in a single comparison have to be in the same modeling language. This is due to semantic and syntactic differences between different modeling languages, for example events in BPMN which cannot be properly modeled in Petri nets.

The structure of the intermediate model is based upon TGraphs [4]: TGraphs in general consist only of linked nodes. While there is no distinction between different node types or between nodes and edges, these nodes can contain additional information, e.g. provided as key-value-pairs.

Each element of the original model is mapped to a node in the TGraph, nodes like transitions and places of a Petri net as well as edges like the arcs of a Petri net. The original model's structure is retained by linking these nodes accordingly. In doing so, each process model can be transformed into a simple structured intermediate model, regardless of the original model's language. The usage of TGraph simplifies the difference calculation, as the algorithms only have to consider nodes for comparison.

Since language or model specific information is not contained in the intermediate model's structure, this information should be annotated in the according node by providing appropriate key-value-pairs. For example, a node can be marked as a transition by saving the value "transition" for the key "type".

Differencing algorithms can now compare intermediate models, resulting in a difference model. By making these algorithms interchangeable, generic algorithms,

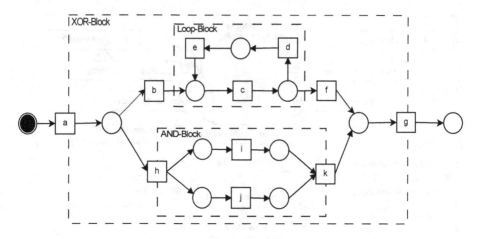

Fig. 3. Logical block model.

as well as specialized algorithms for a certain modeling language can be used. The resulting difference model is generated as an intermediate model itself where the nodes are marked, e.g. as *unchanged*, *added*, *deleted* or *changed*. Depending on the analysis' goals, additional semantic and syntactic differencing algorithms can also be implemented. Some semantic algorithms, e.g. [14], however need information about the logical structure of the process model instead of the syntactical structure. One way to provide this information is a logical block model as shown in Fig. 3: The process model (e.g. a Petri net) is interpreted as a set of nested logical blocks, e.g. XOR-blocks, LOOP-blocks or AND-blocks.

Our approach allows to define simple logical patterns, for example XOR-splits and XOR-joins, in a modeling language's mapping. These patterns are described in the corresponding modeling language to avoid a representational bias between the model and the patterns. Logical blocks in a process model can be identified by searching for these patterns and deriving the block model.

After calculating a difference model, this model is visualized. To maintain an individual look for each modeling language, a view model is generated from the difference model. The view model's structure is analogous to the difference model but instead of similar nodes, the view model contains different kinds of representation nodes. These depend on the respective modeling language and are defined in the mapping. To differentiate between different node types, e.g. transitions, places and arcs in a Petri net, each node in the intermediate model contains the representation type used for drawing this node. Depending on the situation and goals of an analysis, representations can be changed (e.g., using different colors or changing the size of labels in the Visualisation). By customizing the representation, additional information stored in the internal model can also be displayed. For example, this allows to add the time perspective by storing timestamps in the intermediate model and changing the appearance of a node dependent on these timestamps. Before drawing the model, the view model is laid out. Layout algorithms are interchangeable to allow for generic as well as specialized algorithms.

Sometimes it is desirable to consider more than two models in comparison, e.g. an analyst wants to find the differences of all age groups (indicated in Fig. 1) in relation to the young patients. Our approach allows to compare more than two models by relating them to a selected model serving as a reference. All changes are marked in relation to this reference model. While the comparison of more than three process models is possible, the results are harder to visualize with each additional model, due to the exponential growth of possible states a single node can have. A node could have been added to the second model and been deleted in the third, for example. When trying to highlight these different states by coloring them, the visualization's complexity increases. Hence, to our experience, visualizing differences between more than three models is not useful.

4   Implementation

We implemented our approach as described in Sect. 3 in a prototype. As a proof-of-concept, three modeling languages have been implemented in the prototype: Petri nets, causal nets and process trees [12]. They represent different types of process visualization and are widely used in process mining. Moreover, a tool processing Petri nets should also be able to process similar structured languages, like BPMN with little additional effort.

For difference calculation, three different approaches were implemented: A simple snapshot-diff algorithm [11] provides a way to compare the structure of two process models without considering the models' semantics. This algorithm can be used for additional modeling languages without adapting it or the models in any way as long as both models contain corresponding unique identifiers for each model element in both models. An extended snapshot-diff algorithm distinguishes between edges and nodes. While nodes are compared by their identifier as in the first algorithm, edges are considered equal when the identifiers of their previous and following nodes match. By doing so, only node identifiers need to be equal, but edge identifiers can differ between the two models. This is important for multidimensional process mining where edge ids are typically automatically generated and do not match between different models. The block-structured algorithm explained in [14] has also been implemented in combination with the algorithm in [13], to allow for a semantic analysis. As these algorithms need a process model to be structured as logical blocks, pattern templates for different logical splits and joins were defined for petri-nets.

To be able to easily identify differences between two models, a proper layout and visualization is needed. To layout a model, the layered layout algorithm by Sugiyama et al. [17] is used. This algorithm lays out the model's nodes in layers and then tries to minimize crossing edges by reordering these layers. To minimize crossings, nodes in each layer are positioned as close as possible to the median of their previous nodes' positions. By doing so, the node placement is fast and deterministic. This is necessary because similar process models should be drawn as similar as possible to avoid confusion. Furthermore, the drawing needs to be as fast as possible to be suitable for large models.

To visualize the differences between two models, their difference model is visualized using different colors by default. Elements marked as deleted are drawn in red, elements marked as added are drawn in green and changes are drawn in yellow. However, the view model can be easily adapted to alternative visualization concepts (e.g. dashed lines, symbols etc.). Figure 4 shows the difference model of two process trees from the healthcare domain. The differences are highlighted using color coding and dashed lines. By coloring different parts of an element instead of the same part, the complexity of comparing more than two process models can be slightly reduced. Which part of the according model element (e.g. the background or the border) is colored depends on the definition of the element's representation and can be customized as needed.

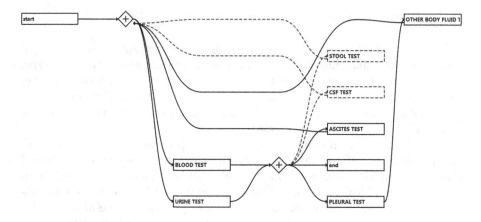

Fig. 4. Visualization of the differences between two process models.

5   Discussion

In the following, we discuss our approach and show how it addresses the challenges in multidimensional process mining. As pointed out in Sect. 2, difference calculation in multidimensional process mining must not require additional, model-specific information, such as change logs. While our approach requires a language-specific mapping, it does not need any additional information besides the compared models.

To deal with the problem of representational bias, the approach supports different modeling languages by transforming these languages into an intermediate model. Thus the user can deal with representational bias (as long as the compared models are in the same language) by properly configuring the modeling language. Differencing algorithms are interchangeable, thus specialized algorithms, as well as generic algorithms are possible. To allow for semantic analysis, patterns can be defined which help identifying logical blocks in the model which can be utilized by semantic algorithms. Hence, syntactical and semantic analysis are supported.

Once compared, differences are marked according to the kind of difference, e.g. addition, deletion or change. In doing so, common structures in the compared models are unobtrusive, whereas differences between these models are emphasized. To maintain a specific appearance for each modeling language, each language's representation can be customized as needed and it is possible to represent additional information (e.g. perspectives) in the model. To ensure a clear visualization, the layout algorithm can be exchanged, e.g. to minimize crossings at the cost of run-time performance.

6   Related Work

Process mining in general is summarized in [7] and explained in detail in [20].

While calculating differences between process models is not often necessary in normal process mining, it is very useful in multidimensional process mining. Reference [24] explicitly motivates the use of difference models to emphasize differences between model variants. This work also suggests different kinds of visualizations for these differences, including the one used in this approach.

In software engineering, a lot of research has already been done about comparing graphical models in the context of software evolution, for example in [5,8,26]. However, these approaches focus on differences between different versions of one model. Furthermore, they mostly rely on previously recorded change logs which are not available when comparing models mined from event data.

A simple method to compare the structure of two models is a Snapshot differential analysis, shown for example in [11]. Although this method is normally used to calculate differences in data warehousing, it can also be applied for comparison of process models. Model elements are matched by their identifiers and differences are annotated. This algorithm is easy to implement and only requires model element identifiers to be equal in both models. The comparison itself however is not very powerful and thus not suitable for advanced (e.g. semantic) analysis. Furthermore, unique identifiers cannot be guaranteed in multidimensional process mining. Apart from that, some specialized algorithms for comparing process models in a non-software-engineering context exist:

References [2,3,23] provide and evaluate different metrics and algorithms to determine the degree of similarity between two process models (e.g., to search for a model in a repository). In contrast to this, we focus on identifying and highlighting the differences between process models.

Reference [1] introduces a method to compare process models in scientific workflows. First, these workflows are transformed into series-parallel graphs. Then basic operations, such as path insertion and path deletion are used to calculate the minimal edit distance between these graphs and a specification containing all possible workflows. This algorithm can be used to find differences between process variants by assuming the overall process model as process specification. However, it only identifies structural differences and lacks support of semantic analysis. Besides, it implies that a complete specification of the analyzed process exists which contradicts the open world assumption. This could be a problem in the context of multidimensional process mining.

Reference [14] is a semantic approach, where different process models are compared by the traces they allow. This is done by creating an order matrix (as explained in [13]) for the intersection of each model and comparing these matrices. Their differences are minimized, resulting in a minimal set of changes between the models. This method however needs a model to consist of semantic structures like logical splits and joins to create the order matrix. In most cases, mined process models do not provide these structures by themselves.

References [15, 16] demonstrate a method to mine the changes between different process variants directly from the event log and treat these variants as differences to a calculated reference model. This reference model and the differences change dynamically with each new trace added to the model. However, this method cannot always be applied to other multidimensional process mining approaches, for example [24], since it relies on the output of the presented mining algorithm.

Reference [10] introduces a method to merge different process models into a configurable workflow model [6]. A configurable workflow model is a process model, where paths can be enabled and disabled as needed. This allows to merge two models while keeping the original models' information. However, this work focuses on the merging algorithm itself. Hence, no advice on visualizing differences and commonalities in a generic way is given.

Reference [9] presents a visualization concept for displaying differences between process models which supports different modeling languages. Compared models are merged and differences colored accordingly. By showing instance traffic in the difference model, this method intends to find optimization potentials in a process. As opposed to this, the approach presented in this paper focuses on identifying the differences between process models in multidimensional process mining. Therefore, we chose a more generic approach to be adaptable to different circumstances, e.g. to allow for semantic and syntactic analysis of a process. Furthermore, our approach is extendable to allow for comparing and visualizing different process mining perspectives, while [9] focuses on the control-flow perspective.

7   Conclusion

In process mining, process models are automatically mined from event logs. While these models are normally more realistic than manually designed models, they also tend to be much more complex. In multidimensional process mining, multiple process models are mined from clustered sets of traces. Differences between these models can help to identify problems in the process. In addition to their complexity, they are supposed to be identical in most parts which makes finding differences between them very difficult. Thus, a tool to compare these models and emphasize their differences can significantly ease the analysis.

In this paper, we presented a generic approach for calculating and visualizing differences between process model variants in the context of multidimensional process mining. As the application implies several challenges like the representational bias, our approach supports arbitrary modeling languages by mapping the original language to an intermediate representation based on TGraphs. Apart from the modeling language's mapping, no additional model-specific information (such as change logs) is required. This allows the comparison of not hierarchically related models as required in multidimensional process mining. Furthermore, the concept also allows for syntactic and semantic differentiation between models and additional, specialized algorithms can be added as needed.

By using a layered layout, models are neatly arranged and colors are used to emphasize differences. To be suitable for different analytical purposes, the visual representation of each model element can be changed and additional layout algorithms can be provided. Additional perspectives can be visualized, too. Hence, by using a suitable configuration, the complexity of difference analysis in multidimensional process mining can be reduced significantly. Thus, the presented approach provides a highly customizable method for comparing different process models in the context of multidimensional process mining.

To further improve our approach, a method to visualize differences between multiple models in a more user friendly way would be useful. This would allow for the comparison of even all mined process model variants at once. Furthermore, our approach should be evaluated in a user case study.

References

1. Bao, Z., et al.: Differencing provenance in scientific workflows. In: Proceedings of the 25th International Conference on Data Engineering (ICDE), pp. 808–819. IEEE (2009)
2. Dijkman, R., Dumas, M., García-Bañuelos, L.: Graph matching algorithms for business process model similarity search. In: Dayal, U., Eder, J., Koehler, J., Reijers, H.A. (eds.) BPM 2009. LNCS, vol. 5701, pp. 48–63. Springer, Heidelberg (2009)
3. Dijkman, R., et al.: Similarity of business process models: metrics and evaluation. Inf. Syst. **36**(2), 498–516 (2011)
4. Ebert, J., Franzke, A.: A declarative approach to graph based modeling. In: Mayr, E.W., Schmidt, G., Tinhofer, G. (eds.) WG 1994. LNCS, vol. 903, pp. 38–50. Springer, Heidelberg (1995)
5. Gerth, C., et al.: Precise mappings between business process models in versioning scenarios. In: IEEE SCC, pp. 218–225. IEEE (2011)
6. Gottschalk, F., van der Aalst, W., Jansen-Vullers, M.H., La Rosa, M.: Configurable workflow models. Int. J. Coop. Inf. Syst. **17**(2), 177–221 (2008)
7. van der Aalst, W., et al.: Process mining manifesto. In: Daniel, F., Barkaoui, K., Dustdar, S. (eds.) BPM Workshops 2011, Part I. LNBIP, vol. 99, pp. 169–194. Springer, Heidelberg (2012)
8. Jacobsen, E.E., Kristensen, B.B., Nowack, P., Worm, T.: Software evolution: prototypical deltas. In: TOOLS (31), pp. 14–30. IEEE Computer Society (1999)
9. Kriglstein, S., Wallner, G., Rinderle-Ma, S.: A visualization approach for difference analysis of process models and instance traffic. In: Daniel, F., Wang, J., Weber, B. (eds.) BPM 2013. LNCS, vol. 8094, pp. 219–226. Springer, Heidelberg (2013)

10. La Rosa, M., Dumas, M., Uba, R., Dijkman, R.: Merging business process models. In: Meersman, R., Dillon, T.S., Herrero, P. (eds.) OTM 2010, Part I. LNCS, vol. 6426, pp. 96–113. Springer, Heidelberg (2010)
11. Labio, W.J., Garcia-molina, H.: Efficient snapshot differential algorithms for data warehousing. In: Proceedings of VLDB, pp. 63–74 (1996)
12. Leemans, S.J.J., Fahland, D., van der Aalst, W.M.P.: Discovering block-structured process models from event logs - a constructive approach. In: Colom, J.-M., Desel, J. (eds.) PETRI NETS 2013. LNCS, vol. 7927, pp. 311–329. Springer, Heidelberg (2013)
13. Li, C., Reichert, M., Wombacher, A.: Representing block-structured process models as order matrices: basic concepts, formal properties, algorithms. Technical report, University of Twente, Enschede, The Netherlands, December 2009
14. Li, C., Reichert, M., Wombacher, A.: On measuring process model similarity based on high-level change operations. In: Li, Q., Spaccapietra, S., Yu, E., Olivé, A. (eds.) ER 2008. LNCS, vol. 5231, pp. 248–264. Springer, Heidelberg (2008)
15. Li, C., Reichert, M.U., Wombacher, A.: Discovering process reference models from process variants using clustering techniques, March 2008
16. Li, C., Reichert, M., Wombacher, A.: Mining process variants: goals and issues. In: IEEE SCC (2), pp. 573–576. IEEE Computer Society (2008)
17. Sugiyama, K., Tagawa, S., Toda, M.: Methods for visual understanding of hierarchical system structures. IEEE Trans. Syst. Man Cybern. 11(2), 109–125 (1981)
18. van der Aalst, W.: The application of petri nets to workflow management. J. Circ. Syst. Comput. 8, 21–66 (1998)
19. van der Aalst, W.: On the representational bias in process mining. In: WETICE, pp. 2–7. IEEE Computer Society (2011)
20. van der Aalst, W.: Process Mining: Discovery, Conformance and Enhancement of Business Processes, 1st edn. Springer, Heidelberg (2011)
21. van der Aalst, W., Adriansyah, A., van Dongen, B.: Causal nets: a modeling language tailored towards process discovery. In: Katoen, J.-P., König, B. (eds.) CONCUR 2011. LNCS, vol. 6901, pp. 28–42. Springer, Heidelberg (2011)
22. van der Aalst, W., Weijter, A.J.M.M., Maruster, L.: Workflow mining: discovering process models from event logs. IEEE Trans. Knowl. Data Eng. 16, 2004 (2003)
23. van Dongen, B.F., Dijkman, R., Mendling, J.: Measuring similarity between business process models. In: Bellahsène, Z., Léonard, M. (eds.) CAiSE 2008. LNCS, vol. 5074, pp. 450–464. Springer, Heidelberg (2008)
24. Vogelgesang, T., Appelrath, H.-J.: Multidimensional process mining: a flexible analysis approach for health services research. In: Proceedings of the Joint EDBT/ICDT 2013 Workshops, pp. 17–22. ACM (2013)
25. White, S.A.: Introduction to BPMN. IBM Cooperation, pp. 2008–2029 (2004)
26. Xing, Z., Stroulia, E.: UMLDiff: an algorithm for object-oriented design differencing. In: Proceedings of ASE 2005, pp. 54–65. ACM (2005)

Enabling a User-Friendly Visualization of Business Process Models

Markus Hipp[1]([✉]), Achim Strauss[2], Bernd Michelberger[3],
Bela Mutschler[3], and Manfred Reichert[2]

[1] Group Research and Advanced Engineering, Daimler AG, Stuttgart, Germany
markus.hipp@daimler.com
[2] Institute of Databases and Information Systems, University of Ulm, Ulm, Germany
{achim.strauss,manfred.reichert}@uni-ulm.de
[3] University of Applied Sciences Ravensburg-Weingarten, Weingarten, Germany
{bernd.michelberger,bela.mutschler}@hs-weingarten.de

Abstract. Enterprises are facing increasingly complex business processes. Engineering processes in the automotive domain, for example, may comprise hundreds or thousands of process tasks. In such a scenario, existing modeling notations do not always allow for a user-friendly process visualization. In turn, this hampers the comprehensibility of business processes, especially for non-experienced process participants. This paper tackles this challenge by suggesting alternative ways of visualizing large and complex process models. A controlled experiment with 22 subjects provides first insights into how users perceive these approaches.

Keywords: Process visualization · User experiment · Visual design

1 Introduction

Enterprises are facing increasingly complex business processes [1]. Engineering processes in the automotive domain [2], for example, may comprise hundreds or thousands of process tasks.

Consider Fig. 1 showing a BPMN model of a (simplified) requirements engineering process from the automotive domain. Note that the example only serves for illustration purposes. The process involves roles *E/E Development* (*R*1), *Component Responsible* (*R*2), *Expert* (*R*3), *Project Responsible* (*R*4), and *Decision Maker* (*R*5). It further comprises 9 tasks (*T*1-*T*9), related to the preparation, writing and validation of a requirements specification, and 12 data objects (*D*1-*D*12) associated with them. Even this simplified process model reveals significant weaknesses regarding its visualization:

- **Positioning of data objects:** Usually, data objects are positioned right next to process tasks or between them [3]. However, such positioning might mislead

This research was conducted in the niPRO project funded by the German Federal Ministry of Education and Research (BMBF) under grant number 17102X10.

F. Fournier and J. Mendling (Eds.): BPM 2014 Workshops, LNBIP 202, pp. 395–407, 2015.
DOI: 10.1007/978-3-319-15895-2_33

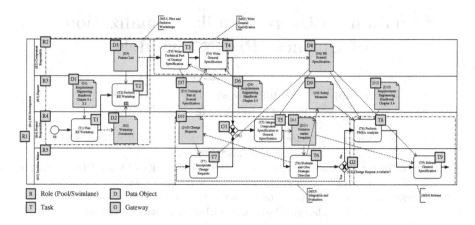

Fig. 1. Example of a requirements engineering process.

users; e.g., $D7$ is positioned within swimlane $R3$ although $D7$ is not related to $R3$. Note that $D7$ is only linked to $T3$ and $T4$ contained in $R2$.

- **Data object relations:** Data objects can be related with more than one process task. In turn, this might lead to "long distance" data relations (i.e., dotted arrows) decreasing model comprehensibility [4]. For example, $D8$ is related to five process tasks, resulting in five data relations.
- **Intersections:** Sequence and data flows might overlap. Furthermore, data objects and process tasks may be overlapped by data relations (see $D11$ in Fig. 1). In general, such intersections affect the model's comprehensibility [5].

Regarding large process models, these drawbacks might significantly affect a model's *comprehensibility* [5] and *aesthetic appearance* [6]. To remedy this drawback, this paper presents four different concepts aiming at a user-friendly visualization of process models. Section 2 discusses requirements for visualizing process models. Section 3 then presents four visualization concepts and Sect. 4 related results from a controlled experiment. Section 5 discusses related work and Sect. 6 concludes the paper with a summary.

2 Requirements

This section summarizes major requirements regarding the comprehensibility as well as aesthetic appearance of process models. These requirements were derived in the context of two case studies in the automotive and healthcare domain [7,8]. Their generalizability was confirmed by a literature study [9]. Finally, Table 1 summarizes the derived requirements.

2.1 Process Model Comprehensibility

Process model comprehensibility is crucial with respect to the quality of process models [5]. Important factors influencing the comprehensibility of process models include its size as well as the degree of sequentiality, concurrency, density, and structure [10,11]. Concerning large and complex process models, two requirements are particularly relevant.

Sequence Flow. The sequence flow determines the order of process tasks in a process model and should be visualized in a comprehensible manner.

Clarity. Users should be able to get a quick overview of a process model. In particular, its visualization should enhance the clarity of process models.

2.2 Aesthetic Appearance

Humans are confronted with a continuously growing amount of visual information and, therefore, tend to become more intolerant to non-aesthetic one. Hence, aesthetic appearance significantly influences the acceptance of user interfaces [12]. Our case studies and literature study confirm the importance of aesthetic process model visualizations, especially with respect to two issues:

Interest. To increase their aesthetic appearance, process models must be visualized in an interesting manner as humans are more attracted to visualizations being different from what they already know [13].

Stimulation. People always grasp at developing personal knowledge and skills [13]. The aesthetic appearance of process models should stimulate these goals.

2.3 Further Requirements

Simplicity. The complexity of a process model has a significant negative influence on its comprehensibility [10] as well as its aesthetic appearance [12]. Therefore, the visualization of process models must be intuitive and simple.

Appeal. The graphical representation of a process model should support the user's perception of the entire process. In particular, users should feel comfortable when working with process models in order to foster their willingness to reuse the models later on [13]. To achieve this goal, the visualization of process models should be appealing.

Structure. Mendling et al. [5] state that small variations in process models might lead to significant differences in respect to their comprehensibility. Amongst others, the structuring of a process model was identified as a factor positively influencing comprehensibility and aesthetic appearance [6].

3   Process Visualization Concepts

This section presents and discusses different concepts for visualizing process models: the *Bubble*, *BPMN3D*, *Network*, and *Thin Line* concepts [14]. In order to ensure same conditions and foster readability, the visualization concepts are presented along an abstract process model (cf. Fig. 2) including nine tasks (A-I). Due to space limitations, this process model is rather simple. In our evaluation (cf. Sect. 4), participants deal with models of different sizes and complexity.

Table 1. Overview on requirements.

Req #	Name	Requirement
Req #1	Sequence Flow	The sequence flow of a process model must be *comprehensible*
Req #2	Clarity	The visualization of a process model must be *clear*
Req #3	Interest	The visualization of a process model must be *interesting*
Req #4	Stimulation	The visualization of a process model must be *stimulating*
Req #5	Simplicity	The visualization of a process model must be *simple*
Req #6	Appeal	The visualization of a process model must be *appealing*
Req #7	Structure	The visualization of a process model must be *structured*

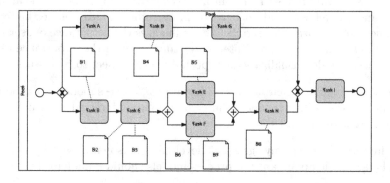

Fig. 2. Running example.

3.1   Bubble Visualization Concept

The first visualization concept, called *Bubble*, does not use common shapes like rectangles and hexagons. Instead, it is inspired by a node-oriented network representation. Figure 3 shows *Bubble* as applied to our running example. Unit-size circles are used to represent process tasks in an appealing, but simple manner (Req #6). In particular, circles are graphically better distinguishable from rectangular document icons representing data objects [6]. Thus, data objects can be easier identified in the process model providing a better overview (Req #2) and structure (Req #7). In turn, data objects are presented using document icons. Arrows are used to model both the sequence and data flow (Req #1). The concept uses symbols for gateways and events that are similar to the ones known from BPMN. Task labels are added to the task's edge. Finally, additional information may be accessed using the plus and gearwheel buttons, e.g., to detail task descriptions.

3.2   BPMN3D Visualization Concept

BPMN3D aims to use standard BPMN elements, but "outsources" the visualization of data objects into a third dimension (cf. Fig. 4). This concept is inspired by

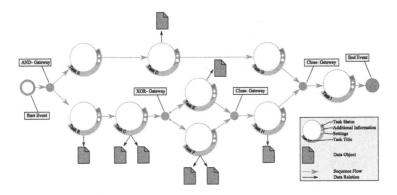

Fig. 3. Bubble visualization concept.

already existing approaches, e.g., provided in [15]. In particular, process tasks, events and sequence flows are represented through common BPMN elements on a common two-dimensional plain, whereas the presentation of data objects requires a third dimension. More precisely, *BPMN3D* extends every process task with a *pole*, pointing to the third dimension, which is then mapped to the 2-dimensional visualization. Data objects are aligned to these poles in terms of circles. In turn, icons indicate the type of the data objects (e.g., pdf files, office files, images). Applying this concept, data objects appear to be more independent from the actual sequence flow. This improves the structure of the process model (Req #7) and its overview (Req #2).

3.3 Network Visualization Concept

Like *Bubble*, the *Network* concept constitutes a network representation (cf. Fig. 5) (cf. Reqs #3 and #4). Each process task is represented through a *node* and comprises a small, centered circle (called *core*) as well as the *galaxy*. The latter offers space for *references*, which may be used to connect a node to other nodes, data

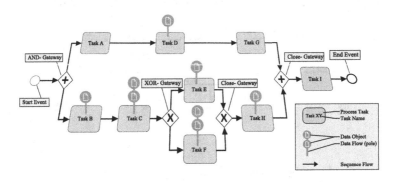

Fig. 4. BPMN3D visualization concept.

objects, or roles. To reduce complexity of the visualized process as well as mental load of the user, this concept focuses on single process tasks, i.e., single nodes. Only one node is dynamically emphasized as shown in Fig. 5 (Task E in the example). Other nodes and corresponding references, data objects and roles are greyed out. *Network* provides a new way of visualizing process models (Req #8).

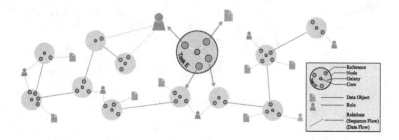

Fig. 5. Network visualization concept.

3.4   Thin Line Visualization Concept

The goal of *Thin Line* is to better structure the information displayed. The basic idea is to separate process tasks and sequence flows from data objects. This increases the overview of the process model and facilitates its comprehensibility (cf. Req #2 and Req #7). On one hand, users can focus on the sequence flow of the model. On the other, data objects are easily accessible in an explicit area below the sequence flow visualization (cf. Fig. 6). This approach can be considered as a minimalistic one with respect to process visualization. Both process tasks and sequence flow are represented through arrows, which results in a significant reduction of the amount of information displayed (Req #5). The title of a process task is displayed on top of each arrow. Further, additional elements for gateways and events are introduced. Finally, vertical lines guide the user to the area the related data objects are displayed. Table 2 shows the requirements addressed by each of the four visualization concepts.

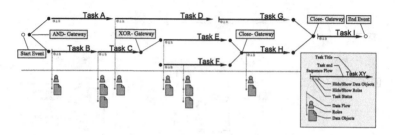

Fig. 6. Thin Line visualization concept.

Table 2. Requirements met by the visualization concepts.

Concept	Req #1	Req #2	Req #3	Req #4	Req #5	Req #6	Req #7
Bubble	++	++	+	+	+	++	+
BPMN3D	++	++	+	-	+	+	++
Network	-	+	++	++	-	++	+
Thin Line	+	-	++	++	++	+	++

++: addressed; +: partially addressed; -: not addressed

4 Evaluation

We evaluate the four visualization concepts through a controlled experiment involving 22 subjects; 9 of them are students, 5 are working in academics, and 8 subjects stem from industry. In the experiment, all four visualization concepts are presented along various process models of different complexity. A questionnaire is then used to collect data about the perception of the concepts. Part 1 of this questionnaire comprises questions concerning the subjects' modeling experience. In part 2 the subjects must rate each concept with respect to different variables using a five step Likert-scale. Possible answers range from *"I totally agree (5)"* to *"I totally disagree(1)"*. Finally, in part 3 subjects must evaluate each concept with an overall rating between 0 and 10. Table 3 summarizes the evaluated variables, which are derived from the presented requirements.

Table 3. Measured variables.

Research Questions	Variables	Source
Comprehensibility	*Overall Comprehensibility*	–
	Sequence Flow	Req #1
	Clarity	Req #2
Aesthetic Appearance	*Interest*	Req #3
	Stimulation	Req #4
Other Variables	*Simplicity*	Req #5
	Appeal	Req #6
	Structure	Req #7

4.1 Comprehensibility

BPMN3D is perceived as the most *comprehensible* concept ($mean = 4.14$; *std dev* = .834) with $p = 0.047$*[1] (cf. Fig. 7a), followed by Bubble (3.64/.790) and Thin Line (3.36/1.177). With (2.00/.926), Network performs worst. According

---

[1] Significant based on a 5 % significance level. Significant results are marked with a *.

to [5], this result is traceable since BPMN3D is most similar to BPMN. In turn, Network introduces new ideas to visualize process models.

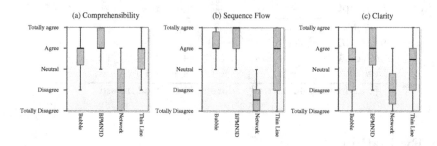

Fig. 7. Experiment results concerning comprehensibility.

Concerning the *sequence flow* (cf. Fig. 7b), again, BPMN3D is perceived as most comprehensible (4.59/.590) with $p = 0.012^*$. In turn, Bubble is rated with (3.91/1.065), followed by Thin Line (3.36/1.497) and Network (1.68/.945).

The *clarity* of the visualization concepts shows similar results (cf. Fig. 7c). Again, BPMN3D obtains significantly better ratings (4.05/.090) with $p = 0.011^*$ compared to Bubble (3.18/1.053) and Thin Line (3.18/1.181). Finally, Network (2.09/1.921) performs worst.

Altogether, BPMN3D is rated significantly better than the other concepts. The ratings for *comprehensibility* ($p = 0.047^*$), *sequence flow* ($p = 0.012^*$), and *clarity* ($p = 0.011^*$) are significant. Thus, process models visualized with BPMN3D are perceived as significantly better comprehensible.

4.2 Aesthetic Appearance

Interestingly, Bubble is perceived as the most *interesting* concept (4.14/.834), although the difference to the other concepts is not significant with $p = 0.109$ (cf. Fig. 8a). BPMN3D receives the second highest rating (3.73/.827). Whether a visualization concept *stimulates* the subjects has been answered with similar ratings (cf. Fig. 8b). Our evaluation with respect to aesthetic appearance, therefore, does not allow for general conclusions.

4.3 Other Variables

As can be seen in Fig. 9a, BPMN3D is perceived as the most *simple* concept (4.0/.873) with $p = 0.090$, followed by Bubble (3.55/.858). Concerning *appeal*, we receive similar results (cf. Fig. 9b). Again, BPMN3D is perceived as the most appealing concept (4.18/.795) with $p = 0.185$, followed by Bubble (3.86/.774). BPMN3D is also perceived as the best *structured* concept (4.41/.734) (cf. Fig. 9c), while Bubble (3.59/.908) and Thin Line (3.55/1.057) are rated second and third best in this category. Results are significant ($p = 0.02^*$).

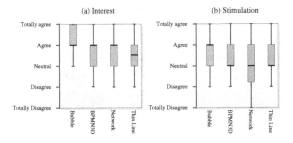

Fig. 8. Experiment results concerning aesthetic appearance.

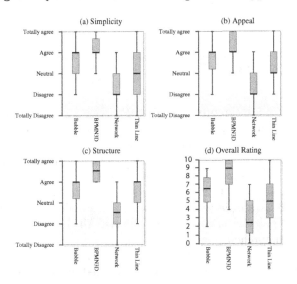

Fig. 9. Experiment results concerning other variables.

4.4 Overall Rating

Subjects are asked to rate each concept concerning its overall impression (cf. Fig. 8d). BPMN3D is rated with 9.18 out of 10 points (*std dev* = 1.868) and significantly better than the other concepts ($p = 0.004^*$). For 7 out of 9 variables, BPMN3D received the highest rating (with 5 significant results; cf. Table 4).

4.5 Discussion

Experimental results underline that the subject's expertise might influence their opinion; e.g., [5] confirms that the amount of theoretical modeling knowledge influences the comprehensibility of process models. As Bubble also uses BPMN-like structures, its second highest overall rating fosters this assumption. Note that this paper focuses on visualization aspects, whereas interaction methods, which

Table 4. Results.

Variable	Best Rating	p-Value
Comprehensibility	BPMN3D	0.047*
Sequence Flow	BPMN3D	0.012*
Clarity	BPMN3D	0.011*
Interest	Bubble	0.110
Stimulation	Bubble	0.879
Simplicity	BPMN3D	0.089
Clearness	BPMN3D	0.185
Structure	BPMN3D	0.021*
Overall Rating	BPMN3D	0.004*

* significant based on a 5 % significance level.

might also influence the comprehensibility of process models, are not discussed[2]. Visualization concepts for process models should combine well-known elements and structures from process model notations with few new ideas.

Our experiment further shows that distinguishing process tasks from data objects increases the comprehensibility of process models. BPMN3D, for example, uses a third dimension to visualize data objects. In turn, Thin Line displays process tasks and data objects in different areas. Finally, Bubble uses different visualizations for process tasks and data objects. All three concepts are considered being well comprehensible.

To improve the *internal validity* of the experiment, the visualization concepts are presented the same way. All concepts are applied to the same process model, i.e., the resulting visualizations present the same amount of information. In particular, the visualization itself is the only varying factor. Finally, to all subjects, all visualization concepts are introduced in the same way. Regarding *external validity*, the chosen process model might be too small. Further, the fact that all subjects are experienced with BPMN might have influenced results.

5   Related Work

Personalized views on business processes are provided, for example, in [17–19] based on abstraction and reduction techniques. In turn, [20] presents a visualization concept facilitating the management of large business process models through views with reduced complexity. All these approaches focus on technical issues, whereas issues related to the graphical representation of process artifacts (e.g., process tasks or data objects) are factored out. Various visualization concepts are provided in [21], which focus on visualizing traffic in process models, whereas [22] presents visualization concepts for time-aware process models.

---

[2] Research on process interaction can be found in [16].

Finally, niPRO enables advanced interactions based on a sophisticated navigation concept [16,23,24]. The 3D visualization of process models is addressed by [25,26], which enable collaborative process modeling in a 3D environment based on 3D avatars. In turn, [27,28] pick up a 2D process visualization as a starting point and derive a 3D visualization from it. Note that we applied this idea in the context of BPMN3D as well. Finally, [29] make use of process hierarchies to visualize complex process models on a small canvas, facilitating the presentation of information on different semantic levels.

6   Summary and Outlook

Enterprises use process model notations for visualizing business processes. However, visualizations like BPMN tend to be not user-friendly, especially when process models become large and complex. This paper presented novel visualization ideas focusing on comprehensibility and aesthetic appearance of process models. We further evaluated these concepts in a controlled experiment. Results show that BPMN3D is considered being the most appealing visualization concept, since it combines well-known elements from BPMN with fresh ideas (e.g., a third dimension for data-objects). In future work, we will refine our visualization concepts and apply them in case studies in the automotive domain.

References

1. Weber, B., Reichert, M., Mendling, J., Reijers, H.A.: Refactoring large process model repositories. J. Comput. Indus. **62**, 467–486 (2011)
2. Müller, D., Herbst, J., Hammori, M., Reichert, M.: IT support for release management processes in the automotive industry. In: Dustdar, S., Fiadeiro, J.L., Sheth, A.P. (eds.) BPM 2006. LNCS, vol. 4102, pp. 368–377. Springer, Heidelberg (2006)
3. Recker, J.C.: Opportunities and constraints : the current struggle with BPMN. J. Bus. Process Manag. **16**(1), 181–201 (2010)
4. Miers, D., White, S.A.: BPMN Modeling and Reference Guide - Understanding and Using BPMN. Future Strategies Inc., Lighthouse Point (2008)
5. Mendling, J., Reijers, H.A., Cardoso, J.: What makes process models understandable? In: Alonso, G., Dadam, P., Rosemann, M. (eds.) BPM 2007. LNCS, vol. 4714, pp. 48–63. Springer, Heidelberg (2007)
6. Norman, D.A.: The Design of Everyday Things. The MIT Press, London (1988)
7. Hipp, M., Mutschler, B., Reichert, M.: On the context-aware, personalized delivery of process information: viewpoints, problems, and requirements. In: ARES 2011, pp. 390–397 (2011)
8. Michelberger, B., Mutschler, B., Reichert, M.: On handling process information: results from case studies and a survey. In: Daniel, F., Barkaoui, K., Dustdar, S. (eds.) BPM Workshops 2011, Part I. LNBIP, vol. 99, pp. 333–344. Springer, Heidelberg (2012)
9. Michelberger, B., Andris, R.-J., Girit, H., Mutschler, B.: A literature survey on information logistics. In: Abramowicz, W. (ed.) BIS 2013. LNBIP, vol. 157, pp. 138–150. Springer, Heidelberg (2013)

10. Mendling, J., Moser, M., Neumann, G., Verbeek, H.M.W.E., van Dongen, B.F., van der Aalst, W.M.P.: Faulty EPCs in the SAP reference model. In: Dustdar, S., Fiadeiro, J.L., Sheth, A.P. (eds.) BPM 2006. LNCS, vol. 4102, pp. 451–457. Springer, Heidelberg (2006)
11. Reijers, H.A., Mendling, J.: A study into the factors that influence the understandability of business process models. J. IEEE Trans. Syst. Man Cybern. Part A **41**(3), 449–462 (2011)
12. Birkhoff, G.D.: Aesthetic Measure. Harvard University Press, Cambridge (1933)
13. Wright, C.P.: Funology - From Usability to Enjoyment. Human-Computer Interaction Series, vol. 3. Springer, Netherlands (2003)
14. Strauss, A.: Information visualisation in process-oriented semantic information networks. Diploma thesis, Ulm University (2012)
15. Effinger, P., Spielmann, J.: Lifting business process diagrams to 2.5 dimensions. In: VDA 2010, vol. 7530, p. 75300 (2010)
16. Hipp, M., Michelberger, B., Mutschler, B., Reichert, M.: Navigating in process model repositories and enterprise process information. In: RCIS 2014, IEEE (2014, accepted for publication)
17. Bobrik, R., Reichert, M., Bauer, T.: View-based process visualization. In: Alonso, G., Dadam, P., Rosemann, M. (eds.) BPM 2007. LNCS, vol. 4714, pp. 88–95. Springer, Heidelberg (2007)
18. Kolb, J., Kammerer, K., Reichert, M.: Updatable process views for user-centered adaption of large process models. In: Liu, C., Ludwig, H., Toumani, F., Yu, Q. (eds.) ICSOC 2012. LNCS, vol. 7636, pp. 484–498. Springer, Heidelberg (2012)
19. Reichert, M.: Visualizing large business process models: challenges, techniques, applications. In: La Rosa, M., Soffer, P. (eds.) BPM Workshops 2012. LNBIP, vol.132, pp. 725–736. Springer, Heidelberg (2013)
20. Streit, A., Pham, B., Brown, R.: Visualization support for managing large business process specifications. In: van der Aalst, W.M.P., Benatallah, B., Casati, F., Curbera, F. (eds.) BPM 2005. LNCS, vol. 3649, pp. 205–219. Springer, Heidelberg (2005)
21. Kriglstein, S., Wallner, G., Rinderle-Ma, S.: A visualization approach for difference analysis of process models and instance traffic. In: Daniel, F., Wang, J., Weber, B. (eds.) BPM 2013. LNCS, vol. 8094, pp. 219–226. Springer, Heidelberg (2013)
22. Lanz, A., Kolb, J., Reichert, M.: Enabling personalized process schedules with time-aware process views. In: Franch, X., Soffer, P. (eds.) CAiSE Workshops 2013. LNBIP, vol. 148, pp. 205–216. Springer, Heidelberg (2013)
23. Hipp, M., Michelberger, B., Mutschler, B., Reichert, M.: A framework for the intelligent delivery and user-adequate visualization of process information. In: SAC 2013 Symposium, pp. 1383–1390. ACM (2013)
24. Hipp, M., Mutschler, B., Reichert, M.: Navigating in complex business processes. In: Liddle, S.W., Schewe, K.-D., Tjoa, A.M., Zhou, X. (eds.) DEXA 2012, Part II. LNCS, vol. 7447, pp. 466–480. Springer, Heidelberg (2012)
25. Poppe, E., Brown, R., Recker, J., Johnson, D.: Improving remote collaborative process modelling using embodiment in 3D virtual environments. In: APCCM 2013, vol. 143, pp. 51–60. ACS (2013)
26. Brown, R., Recker, J., West, S.: Using virtual worlds for collaborative business process modeling. J. Bus. Process Manag. **17**(3), 546–564 (2011)
27. Schönhage, B., van Ballegooij, A., Eliëns, A.: 3D gadgets for business process visualization. In: WEB3D-VRML 2000 Symposium, pp. 131–138 (2000)

28. Effinger, P.: A 3D-Navigator for business process models. In: TAProViz 2012 Workshop, pp. 737–743 (2012)
29. Seyfang, A., Kaiser, K., Gschwandtner, T., Miksch, S.: Visualizing complex process hierarchies during the modeling process. In: La Rosa, M., Soffer, P. (eds.) BPM Workshops 2012. LNBIP, vol. 132, pp. 768–779. Springer, Heidelberg (2013)

Lights, Camera, Action! Business Process Movies for Online Process Discovery

Andrea Burattin[1]([✉]), Marta Cimitile[2], and Fabrizio Maria Maggi[3]

[1] University of Padua, Padua, Italy
burattin@math.unipd.it
[2] Unitelma Sapienza University, Rome, Italy
marta.cimitile@unitelma.it
[3] University of Tartu, Tartu, Estonia
f.m.maggi@ut.ee

Abstract. Nowadays, organizational information systems are able to collect high volumes of data in event logs every day. Through process mining techniques, it is possible to extract information from such logs to support organizations in checking process conformance, detecting bottlenecks, and carrying on performance analysis. However, to analyze such "big data" through process mining, events coming from process executions (in the form of event streams) must be processed on-the-fly as they occur. The work presented in this paper is built on top of a technique for the online discovery of declarative process models presented in our previous work. In particular, we introduce a tool providing a dynamic visualization of the models discovered over time showing, as a "process movie", the sequence of valid business rules at any point in time based on the information retrieved from an event stream. The effectiveness of the visualizer is validated through an event stream pertaining to health insurance claims handling in a travel agency.

Keywords: Online process discovery · Dynamic process model visualization · Event stream analysis · Declarative process models · Concept drifts · Operational decision support

1 Introduction

Process innovation and optimization is a crucial step of the business process management lifecycle of an organization. In addition, nowadays, high volumes of data are available and can be used for process improvement. In this scenario, process mining techniques [1] may support analysts in extracting useful information from data recorded during process executions in the so-called event logs that can provide valuable insights for process enhancement. In particular, the goal of one of the main branches of this discipline, process discovery, is to build process models representing the process behavior as recorded in the logs. However, one of the challenges that exist when several gigabytes of data need to be analyzed is to process the data on-the-fly through techniques that work at runtime and analyze the data as soon as it becomes available. Unfortunately, traditional process

F. Fournier and J. Mendling (Eds.): BPM 2014 Workshops, LNBIP 202, pp. 408–419, 2015.
DOI: 10.1007/978-3-319-15895-2_34

discovery techniques are limited to the off-line analysis of event logs and require several iterations on the data for discovering a process model. For this reason, these techniques cannot be used in an online setting with the consequence of a reduced capability to support real-time process comprehension and monitoring.

In [15], we propose an approach to automatically discover declarative process models from streams of data, at runtime. A declarative process model is a set of business rules that describe the process behavior under an open world assumption, i.e., everything that is not forbidden by the model is allowed. These models can be used to express process behaviors involving multiple alternatives in a compact way and are very suitable to be used in changeable and instable environments with respect to the conventional procedural approaches. In [15], an online process discovery technique is proposed to automatically construct, from an event stream, a representation of complex business processes in the form of business rules, without using any a-priori information and processing the events on-the-fly, as they occur. In addition, this approach is able to detect concept drifts, i.e., changes in the process execution due to periodic/seasonal phenomena that are vital to be detected and analyzed to deeply understand how the process adapts its behavior over longer periods of time.

Even if this approach has been implemented in the process mining tool ProM [19], its previous implementation was able to cope only with "static" objects and a graphical visualization of the evolution of the process model over time was missing. In this work, we try to address this limit by presenting a graphical visualizer for process models extracted from an event stream through the declarative process discovery approach presented in [15]. The visualizer has been developed using a client-server architecture in which the stream source is the server and a number of miners, modeled as clients, can be connected to the source using TCP connections. When a new event is emitted, a log fragment is encoded only containing that event and sent to the clients. The reconstruction of the complete final process instance (by grouping together events belonging to the same case) is delegated to the miners. The output models are visualized in the form of an animated "process movie" that dynamically shows how the behavior of the process that produces the event stream changes over time. The process models are represented using Declare [2] a declarative process modeling language to describe process behaviors through business rules. The added value provided by the visualizer to the process stakeholders is to have continuously updated "de facto" models showing the real behavior of the process as recorded in the stream.

The paper is structured as follows. Section 2 introduces the characteristics of event stream mining as well as some basic notions about Declare. Here, we also give a short description of the online process discovery technique underlying the proposed visualizer. Section 3 introduces the visualizer and describes its implementation. In Sect. 4, the tool is applied to an event stream pertaining to health insurance claims handling in a travel agency. Finally, Sect. 5 reports some conclusion and final remarks.

2   Preliminaries

This section provides a general introduction to the basic elements we are going to use throughout the paper. In particular, we introduce the notion of event stream and we give a quick overview of the Declare language. Also, we introduce the approach for the online discovery of Declare models that we use to produce the process movies presented in this paper.

2.1   Event Streams

Several works in the data mining literature, such as [3,4,12], agree in defining a *data stream* as a fast sequence of data items. It is common to assume that: *(i)* data has a small, typically predefined, number of attributes; *(ii)* mining algorithms are able to analyze an infinite number of data items, handling problems related to memory bounds; *(iii)* the amount of memory that the learner can use is finite and much smaller than the memory required to store the data observed in a reasonable span of time; *(iv)* each item is processed within a certain small amount of time (algorithms have to linearly scale with respect to the number of processed items): typically the algorithms work with one pass on the data; *(v)* data models associated to a stream (i.e., the "underlying concepts") can either be stationary or evolving [20].

An event stream is a potentially infinite sequence of events. It is possible to assume that sequence indexes comply with the time order of events (i.e., given the sequence S, for all indexes $i \in \mathbb{N}^+$, $\#_{\text{time}}(S(i)) \leq \#_{\text{time}}(S(i+1))$). Starting from a general data stream (not necessarily a stream of events), it is possible to perform different analysis. The most common are clustering, classification, frequency counting, time series analysis, and change diagnosis (concept drift detection) [3,10,20].

2.2   Declare: Some Basic Notions

In this paper, the process behavior as recorded in an event stream is described using Declare rules. Declare is a declarative process modeling language originally introduced by Pesic and van der Aalst in [2]. Instead of explicitly specifying the flow of the interactions among process events, Declare describes a set of rules that must be satisfied throughout the process execution. The possible orderings of events are implicitly specified by rules and anything that does not violate them is possible during execution. In comparison with procedural approaches that produce "closed" models, i.e., all what is not explicitly specified is forbidden, Declare models are "open" and tend to offer more flexibility for the execution.

A Declare model consists of a set of rules applied to events. Declare rules, in turn, are based on templates. Templates are patterns that define parameterized classes of properties, and Declare rules are their concrete instantiations. Templates have a user-friendly graphical representation understandable to the user and their semantics can be formalized using different logics [17], the main one being LTL, making them verifiable and executable. Each rule inherits the graphical representation and semantics from its templates. The major benefit of using templates is that analysts do not have to be aware of the underlying logic-based formalization to understand the models. They work with the graphical representation of templates, while the underlying formulas remain hidden. Table 1 summarizes some of the Declare templates (we indicate template parameters with capital letters and concrete activities in their instantiations with lower case letters). For a complete overview on the language the reader is referred to [18].

Table 1. Graphical notation and meaning of the Declare templates.

Template	Meaning	Notation
Responded Existence(A,B)	if A occurs then B occurs before or after A	A •——— B
Co-Existence(A,B)	if A occurs then B occurs before or after A and vice versa	A •———• B
Response(A,B)	if A occurs then eventually B occurs after A	A •——▶ B
Precedence(A,B)	if B occurs then A occurs before B	A ——▶◀ B
Succession(A,B)	for A and B both precedence and response hold	A •——▶◀ B
Alternate Response(A,B)	if A occurs then eventually B occurs after A without another A in between	A ⇒ B
Alternate Precedence(A,B)	if B occurs then A occurs before B without another B in between	A ⇒◀ B
Alternate Succession(A,B)	for A and B both alternate precedence and alternate response hold	A •⇒◀ B
Chain Response(A,B)	if A occurs then B occurs in the next position after A	A ■——▶ B
Chain Precedence(A,B)	if B occurs then A occurs in the next position before B	A ——■▶ B
Chain Succession(A,B)	for A and B both chain precedence and chain response hold	A ■——■▶ B
Not Co-Existence(A,B)	A and B cannot occur together	A •‖— B
Not Succession(A,B)	if A occurs then B cannot eventually occur after A	A •‖▶ B
Not Chain Succession(A,B)	if A occurs then B cannot occur in the next position after A	A ■‖■▶ B

Consider, for example, a *response* rule connecting activities a and b. This rule indicates that if a *occurs*, b must eventually *follow*. Therefore, this rule is satisfied for traces such as $t_1 = \langle a, a, b, c \rangle$, $t_2 = \langle b, b, c, d \rangle$, and $t_3 = \langle a, b, c, b \rangle$, but not for $t_4 = \langle a, b, a, c \rangle$ because, in this case, the second instance of a is not followed by a b. Note that, in t_2, the considered response rule is satisfied in a trivial way because a never occurs. In this case, we say that the rule is *vacuously satisfied* [14]. In [6], the authors introduce the notion of *behavioral vacuity detection* according to which a rule is non-vacuously satisfied in a trace when it is activated in that trace. An *activation* of a rule in a trace is an event whose occurrence imposes, because of that rule, some obligations on other events in the same trace. For example, a is an activation for the *response* rule between a and b, because the execution of a forces b to be executed eventually.

An activation of a rule can be a *fulfillment* or a *violation* for that rule. When a trace is perfectly compliant with respect to a rule, every activation of the rule in the trace leads to a fulfillment. Consider, again, the response rule connecting activities a and b. In trace t_1, the rule is activated and fulfilled twice, whereas, in trace t_3, the same rule is activated and fulfilled only once. On the other hand, when a trace is not compliant with respect to a rule, an activation of the rule in the trace can lead to a fulfillment but also to a violation (at least one activation leads to a violation). In trace t_4, for example, the response rule between a and b is activated twice, but the first activation leads to a fulfillment (eventually b occurs) and the second activation leads to a violation (b does not occur subsequently). An algorithm to discriminate between fulfillments and violations for a rule in a trace is presented in [6].

2.3   Online Discovery of Declare Models

In this section, we describe how to discover, at runtime, a Declare model out of a stream of events. The approach for online discovery of Declare models we use in this paper is based on three algorithms. The first algorithm is called *Sliding Window* [11]. The basic idea of this algorithm is to keep the latest observed events and consider them as a static event log. The other two approaches are called *Lossy Counting* [16] and *Lossy Counting with Budget* [9]. The basic idea of these approaches is to consider aggregated representations of the latest observations, i.e., instead of storing repetitions of the same event, to save space, they store a counter keeping trace of the number of instances of the same observation. As presented in [15], we use these algorithms for memory management in combination with algorithms for the online discovery of Declare rules referring to different templates.

Algorithm 1. Online discovery scheme

Input: S: event stream, *conf*: approximate algorithm configuration (either LC or LCB, with the corresponding configuration: ϵ or $\mathcal{B}$), *update model condition*

```
 1  R ← ∅                                              /* Set of template replayers */
 2  foreach Declare template t do
 3      Add a replayer for t (according to conf) to R
 4  end
 5  forever do
 6      e ← observe(S)
 7      if analyze(e) then
 8          foreach r ∈ R do
 9              r(e, conf)                              /* Replay e on replayer r */
10          end
11      end
12      if update model condition then
13          model ← initially empty Declare model
14          foreach r ∈ R do
15              Update model with rules in r
16          end
17          Use model                  /* For example, update a graphical representation */
18      end
19  end
```

Algorithm 1 presents a general overview of our online discovery approach. Here, we keep a set R of *replayers*, one for each template we want to discover (line 3). Note that replayers for different templates implement different discovery algorithms each one developed based on the characteristics of the corresponding template. Then, when a new event e is observed from the stream S, if it is necessary to analyze it, the algorithm replays e on all the template replayers of R (line 9). Periodically (the period may depend either on the number of events observed, or on the actual elapsed time), it is possible to update the discovered Declare model, by querying each replayer for the set of satisfied rules (line 15). These models are used in our visualizer as "frames" to build the process movies.

The candidate rules to be included in the discovered Declare model can be selected based on the percentage of activations that leads to a fulfillment (event-based rule support) or based on the percentage of cases in which the rule is satisfied (trace-based support). Of course, in this latter case, the event stream should provide not only information about the case to which each event belongs but also an indication on the exact point in which each trace starts and ends.

3   The Visualizer

The visualizer described in this paper has been implemented as plug-in of the process mining tool ProM.[1] In the following sections we describe the tool and its characteristics.

3.1   The Event Streamer

The current implementation of ProM is able to cope only with "static" objects, e.g., log files and process models. Instead, as previously stated, an event stream cannot be fit into a static object, because of its dynamic nature. In particular, when someone queries an event stream for the "next" event, the provided answer will depend on the "query time".

In order to achieve our goal, we decided to model event streams using TCP connections [7,8]. In particular, we employed a client-server architecture in which the stream source acts as a server and several miners, modeled as clients, can be connected to the same source. Figure 1 reports a graphical representation of such idea: the stream source forwards each event, represented as a box, to all the connected miners (clients) via TCP connections.

When a new event is emitted, a log fragment is encoded only containing that event and sent to the clients. Specifically, the log fragment contains only one trace which contains only the event emitted and is encoded in XML, using the XES standard [13]. It is important to note that, differently from what happens with static log files, events are not grouped anymore by process instance. Instead, each event is wrapped into different trace elements which have the same value for the "case id" attribute. The reconstruction of the complete trace is delegated to the clients.

---

[1] See http://www.processmining.org for more information.

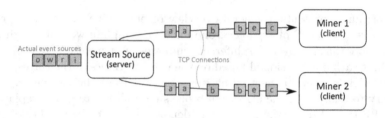

Fig. 1. Graphical representation of the stream architecture: the stream source is a *server*, and each miner is a *client* connected via TCP. Each square box represents an event. The background color of a box corresponds to the case id of the event.

```
1   <log openxes.version="1.0RC7" xes.features="nested-attributes"
        xes.version="1.0" xmlns="http://www.xes-standard.org/">
2       <trace>
3           <string key="concept:name" value="7235124248-6934584346" />
4           <event>
5               <string key="concept:name" value="Activity A" />
6           </event>
7       </trace>
8   </log>
```

Listing 1.1. Log fragment streamed over the network and encoded using XES.

The log fragment reported in Listing 1.1 represents an example of data written through the network connection.

We opted for this architecture since it is an extremely flexible solution and allows different computational nodes to communicate easily. Moreover, it is extremely easy, for an existing information system, to emit events to be analyzed using our implemented solution. In order to simulate specific stream scenarios, we use an *event streamer*, which takes as input a (finite) event log and simulates an event stream using the events contained in the log. Specifically, all the events of the log are sorted according to their timestamp. Then, each event is sent through the network. The time passing between two consecutive events is a parameter of the streamer. Clearly, the stream generated using this tool is not infinite, but it is still useful for testing purposes.

Figure 2 reports a screenshot of the ProM implementation of the *event-streamer*. On the right hand side of the screenshot there is a graphical representation of the stream: each colored point represents an event of the stream (green dots represent sent event whereas blue dots represent the events that still need to be sent). The x axis represents the time, the y axis has no specific semantic (simultaneous events are vertically distributed for readability purposes). The left hand side of the screenshot contains some configuration panels. In particular, it is possible to configure the network port that is used to accept incoming miners, the time passing between the emission of two consecutive events, and the control buttons to start and to stop emitting events on the network channel. Few other controllers are available as well. For example, it is possible to assign different colors to the events visualization according to the activity name or according to the case id.

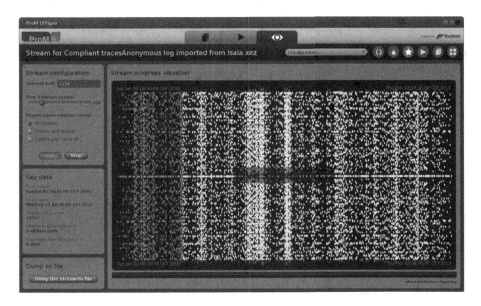

Fig. 2. Screenshot of the streamer interface.

3.2   The Declare Stream Miner

The ProM implementation of the Declare stream miner is fundamentally based on the "observer pattern": every time the stream receives a new event, different replayers update their internal status with the new observation. With a certain periodicity, either with respect to the number of events received or with respect to the time passed, the Declare model is updated, taking into account the new status recorded by each replayer.

Since the mined model is not static (it evolves over time), it is not possible to generate one model to be added to the ProM workspace. Therefore, we decided to implement a *dashboard* in the ProM toolkit. This dashboard (Fig. 3) shows the current status of the stream, together with some general historical information. The current behavior as detected from the event stream is shown in the form of a list of Declare rules that change over time. While the stream progresses, the visualization in the dashboard is periodically updated showing the currently valid Declare rules. The dashboard is composed of several parts: the bottom panel contains some general controllers, to turn on and off the miner, together with some general information about the number of received events. The main panel is vertically splitted: the left hand side part reports a graphical representation of the top 10 rules currently valid (the ones with the highest fulfillment ratio). In this panel, the value of the fulfillment ratio is encoded using different colors: brighter blue indicates the lowest values, darker blue indicates the highest values. The same panel contains two more controllers: one to export the currently displayed Declare model into the ProM workspace, and another one to attach the rule name to each connector in the model. The right hand side

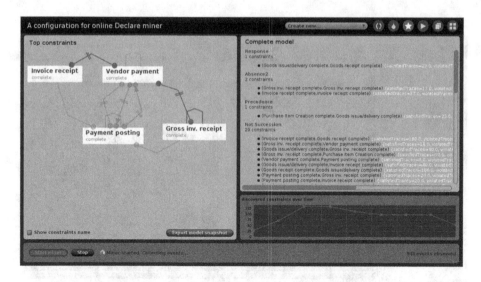

Fig. 3. Screenshot of the stream miner dashboard.

of the dashboard contains two panels: the one on the top contains a list with the complete set of discovered rules (with the corresponding statistics), the panel on the bottom part contains a line chart with some historical information. In our specific case, the chart shows the trend of the number of rules discovered over time, but several other statistics can easily be added as well (e.g., the average fulfillment ratio of the rules).

4   Case Study

For our experiment,[2] we have generated two synthetic logs ($\mathcal{L}_1$ and $\mathcal{L}_2$) by modeling two variants of the insurance claim process described in [5] in CPN Tools[3] and by simulating the models. The following characteristics are common to both process variants. Upon registration of a claim, a general questionnaire is sent to the claimant. In addition, a registered claim is classified as high or low. A cheque and acceptance decision letter is prepared in cases where a claim is accepted while a rejection decision letter is created for rejected claims. In both cases, a notification is sent to the claimant. Three modes of notification are supported, i.e., by email, by telephone (fax) and by postal mail. The case should be archived upon notifying the claimant. The case is closed upon completion of archiving task.

$\mathcal{L}_1$ contains 14,840 events and $\mathcal{L}_2$ contains 16,438 events. We merged the logs (four alternations of $\mathcal{L}_1$ and $\mathcal{L}_2$) using the *Stream Package*, publicly available

---

[2] The entire process movie generated in our experiment can be found at http://youtu. be/9gbrhkSfRTc.

[3] See http://cpntools.org.

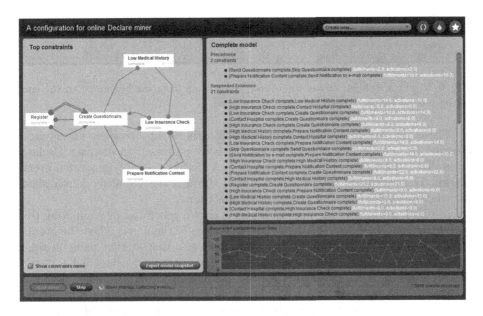

Fig. 4. Screenshot of the visualizer (frame from $\mathcal{L}_1$).

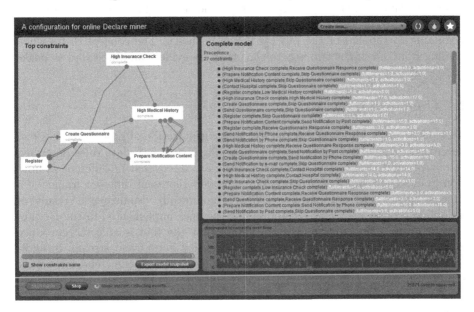

Fig. 5. Screenshot of the visualizer (frame from $\mathcal{L}_2$).

in the ProM repositories. The same package has been used to transform the resulting log into an event stream. The event stream contains 250,224 events and has three concept drifts (one for every switch from $\mathcal{L}_1$ to $\mathcal{L}_2$).

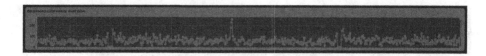

Fig. 6. Trend of the number of discovered constraints from the beginning to the end of the process movie.

The event stream has been simulated with the event streamer. The events, received by the Declare stream miner has been processed to discover Declare rules that hold with a fulfillment ratio of 1. A Declare model is generated every 100 ms, i.e., every 100 ms the model shown through the visualizer is refreshed and the process movie progresses with a new frame.

In Fig. 4, a frame of the process movie is shown generated by simulating the event stream. The figure shows one of the frames of the movie when the events from $\mathcal{L}_1$ are sent to the miner. The frame indicates that at that point in time during the stream evolution the Declare rules involving claims classified as "low" are prevalent in terms of fulfilment ratio. As already mentioned, this view can be exported to create a snapshot of the process behavior at that point in time during the stream progression. Figure 5 shows one of the frames of the movie when the events from $\mathcal{L}_2$ are sent to the miner. In this case, the Declare rules involving claims classified as "high" correspond to a higher fulfilment ratio.

In Fig. 6, the entire trend of the number of discovered constraints from the beginning to the end of the process movie is shown. The concept drifts when passing from one of the two logs to the other are evident and indicated as peaks in the curve.

5   Conclusion

This paper proposes a tool for the dynamic visualization of process models discovered through a technique for the online discovery of Declare rules described in our previous work. The different models are discovered in different evaluation points from an event stream. These models represent different frames of a process movie. A process movie is a way of dynamically visualizing the results of an online process discovery technique like the ones implemented in the Declare stream miner. Our experimentation shows that the tool is able to reproduce graphically the evolution of process cases encoded in an event stream. In addition, concept drifts are also graphically captured through the trend line representing the number of discovered Declare rules over time.

Acknowledgment. The work of Andrea Burattin is supported by the Eurostars-Eureka project PROMPT (E!6696).

References

1. van der Aalst, W.: Process mining: overview and opportunities. ACM Trans. Manage. Inf. Syst. **3**(2), 7:1–7:17 (2012)

2. van der Aalst, W., Pesic, M., Schonenberg, H.: Declarative workflows: balancing between flexibility and support. Comput. Sci. R&D **23**, 99–113 (2009)
3. Aggarwal, C.: Data Streams: Models and Algorithms, Advances in Database Systems, vol. 31. Springer, Boston (2007)
4. Bifet, A., Holmes, G., Kirkby, R., Pfahringer, B.: MOA: massive online analysis learning examples. J. Mach. Learn. Res. **11**, 1601–1604 (2010)
5. Bose, R.J.C.: Process Mining in the Large: Preprocessing, Discovery, and Diagnostics. Ph.D. thesis, Eindhoven University of Technology (2012)
6. Burattin, A., Maggi, F., van der Aalst, W., Sperduti, A.: Techniques for a posteriori analysis of declarative processes. In: EDOC. pp. 41–50 (2012)
7. Burattin, A., Sperduti, A., van der Aalst, W.: Heuristics Miners for Streaming Event Data. CoRR abs/1212.6383 (2012)
8. Burattin, A., Sperduti, A., van der Aalst, W.: Control-flow discovery from event streams. In: Proceedings of the IEEE Congress on Evolutionary Computation. IEEE (2014). (to appear)
9. Da San Martino, G., Navarin, N., Sperduti, A.: A lossy counting based approach for learning on streams of graphs on a budget. In: Proceedings of the Twenty-Third International Joint Conference on Artificial Intelligence, pp. 1294–1301. AAAI Press (2012)
10. Gaber, M.M., Zaslavsky, A., Krishnaswamy, S.: Mining data streams: a review. ACM SIGMOD Rec. **34**(2), 18–26 (2005)
11. Gama, J.A.: Knowledge Discovery from Data Streams, Chapman and Hall/CRC Data Mining and Knowledge Discovery Series, vol. 20103856. Chapman and Hall/CRC, Boca Raton (2010)
12. Golab, L., Özsu, M.T.: Issues in data stream management. ACM SIGMOD Rec. **32**(2), 5–14 (2003)
13. Günther, C., Verbeek, H.: XES Standard Definition (2009). http://www.xes-standard.org/
14. Kupferman, O., Vardi, M.: Vacuity detection in temporal model checking. Int. J. Softw. Tools Technol. Transfer **4**, 224–233 (2003)
15. Maggi, F.M., Burattin, A., Cimitile, M., Sperduti, A.: Online process discovery to detect concept drifts in LTL-based declarative process models. In: Meersman, R., Panetto, H., Dillon, T., Eder, J., Bellahsene, Z., Ritter, N., De Leenheer, P., Dou, D. (eds.) ODBASE 2013. LNCS, vol. 8185, pp. 94–111. Springer, Heidelberg (2013)
16. Manku, G.S., Motwani, R.: Approximate frequency counts over data streams. In: VLDB, pp. 346–357 (2002)
17. Montali, M., Pesic, M., van der Aalst, W.M.P., Chesani, F., Mello, P., Storari, S.: Declarative specification and verification of service choreographies. ACM Trans. Web **4**(1), 1–62 (2010)
18. Pesic, M.: Constraint-Based Workflow Management Systems: Shifting Controls to Users. Ph.D. thesis, Beta Research School for Operations Management and Logistics, Eindhoven (2008)
19. Verbeek, E., Buijs, J., van Dongen, B., van der Aalst, W.: Prom 6: the process mining toolkit. In: Demo at the 8th International Conference on Business Process Management (BPM 2010) (2010)
20. Widmer, G., Kubat, M.: Learning in the presence of concept drift and hidden contexts. Mach. Learn. **23**(1), 69–101 (1996)

Towards a Generalized Notion of Audio as Part of the Concrete Syntax of Business Process Modeling Languages

Jens Gulden[✉]

University of Duisburg-Essen, 45141 Essen, Germany
jens.gulden@uni-due.de

Abstract. The considerations presented in this position paper provide a starting point for incorporating model representations on additional perception channels, e. g., by using audio, into the concrete syntax specification of modeling languages. As it turns out, this cannot be done inside the frameworks of existing concrete syntax specification approaches, but first means to question the state-of-the-art of treating concrete syntax definitions as static mapping structures, and subsequently requires to widen the understanding of what concrete syntax is to an operative view on how humans interact with models.

Keywords: Model perception · Modeling language · Domain specific modeling · Concrete syntax · Business process modeling

1 A General Perspective on Business Process Modeling with Multiple Perception Channels

Especially for business process modeling languages [1,2], which express a high degree of domain specific semantics, the potentials of using additional perception channels besides vision for exploring and editing models are attractive objects of interest for scientic investigations. From a language design perspective, it is desirable to provide language specification options that allow to equip business process modeling languages and other domain specific languages with representations for multiple perception channels, without each time having to individually specify the way how audio and other media on the one hand, and conceptual model content on the other hand, could potentially be linked together. A generic framework for incorporating variant channels of perception into the specification of a concrete syntax for modeling languages [3] would allow to efficiently produce research prototypes, that operate with model representations on diverse perception channels. Having such tools at hand would allow for examining practical applications in those fields, where the use of different perception channels for model representation appears suitable. However, elaborating such a generic approach demands for prerequisite research about what it means to represent model concepts as part of a concrete syntax in general.

© Springer International Publishing Switzerland 2015
F. Fournier and J. Mendling (Eds.): BPM 2014 Workshops, LNBIP 202, pp. 420–425, 2015.
DOI: 10.1007/978-3-319-15895-2_35

Business process models incorporate rich domain specific semantics [4]. The degree of semantics is intentionally higher than that of general purpose modeling languages, because domain specific modeling languages incorporate an invariant body of knowledge about the domain they have been developed for. Due to richer semantics attached to the modeling concepts used in business process modeling, human modelers require more imaginative capabilities for understanding the model concepts they operate with. This puts the question into focus, how modeling languages can be equipped to offer more efficient cognitive means for humans to grasp the notions of complex model concepts.

For specific usage scenarios, such as modeling on devices with limited display capabilities, monitoring in security-relevant environments, or when people with inabilities are operating with models, it makes especially sense to ask if cognitive access to business process models can be provided by additional concrete syntax elements from other perception channels, that support or complement the visual perception of a model.

As a prerequisite for answering this question, an understanding has to be established of what it means to include, e. g., audio, and other sensual impressions, into the concrete syntax of modeling languages. The work at hand asks initial questions that arise when trying to establish such a notion of specifying modeling languages, as an extension to the well-known idea of using network-structured concrete visual syntax elements for visual representations. As it will turn out, this requires a reconceptualization of concrete syntax as an interaction process between a tool and a user.

Research related to these questions is discussed in the following section. In Sect. 3, fundamental differences between various perception channels are identified, and, as a result, the need for widening the expressiveness of concrete syntax description is discussed. Section 4 sketches how such a widening with regard to incorporating operational events and states during modeling can look like on an abstract level. A conclusion from the overall discussion is drawn in the final Sect. 5.

2   Related Work

Most of the existing research body about using alternative perception channels for modeling deals with how to apply audio representations of model content in specific use-cases.

Approaches for incorporating audio into data analysis and modeling have been suggested by a number of publications, especially from the research community around the "auditory display" [5,6]. Early considerations about performing data analysis with audio support have already been published by the end of the past century [7]. Some of the existing works specifically focus on sonification techniques for process monitoring [8–10].

As it turns out in the considerations undertaken in this paper, an attempt to formalize language specifications including concrete audio syntax will have to deal with the procedural nature of events and states while modifying and/or exploring models. Such procedural aspects of modeling language use have been examined especially for the purpose of merging and detecting conflicts among multiple branches of concurrently modified models by [11,12].

With regard to handling the technical aspects of audio data, e. g., specifying playback pitch and volume, or marking segments of waveforms, no scientific challenges are expected to be faced. Specification approaches for handling audio on this technical level already exist, e. g., [13], and can be applied as is.

3   Audio as Part of the Concrete Syntax of Modeling Languages

For the following considerations, questions of incorporating audio into a modeling language's concrete syntax are sketched. The ideas presented here with respect to audio can be expected to be generalizable to other non-visual perception channels, too, e. g., force-feedback reactions of input/output devices, or modifications of the environmental settings of the modeler's workspace (light, temperature, possibly even olfactory impressions). Unlike visual perception, these perception channels have in common that humans are more passively exposed to them, and can much less actively decide which sensual impression to perceive or not. As a consequence, the use of these channels requires to structure sensual impressions over time, to make them perceivable as information. This is not inherently necessary for visual perception channels, because in visual perception, the recipient can actively contribute to these structuring activities.

When reasoning about timely structured audio representations for models, several questions come into mind which need to be dealt with before starting to design a description mechanism for the inclusion of audio and other non-visual perception channels into concrete syntax definitions.

Among these questions are:

- In which situations should the occurrence of audio be actively caused by actions carried out by modelers during modeling?
- Which model elements should make sound without prior interaction, and how is the point in time determined at which the sound occurs?
- Is audio representation to be used at design time of models, e. g. business process models, and/or should it be used at model instantiation time, e. g. during the actual execution of a business process model?
- When used at design time, how can the set of actions be conceptualized, that are possibly carried out during modeling, and which types of events can be derived from them to be associated with audio?
- Can a unified view be taken for the purpose of concrete syntax specification, that combines the notion of events occurring during design time, and events occurring during the execution of models?

Besides representing individual events that occur during language use, a generic approach for specifying concrete syntax should also incorporate the representation of entire model states. As a consequence, it also has to be taken into account:

- Are there generic states (like emptiness of a model, or error states), which should be associated with audio?
- Which other states of a model (e. g. described by invariant constraints) are suited for audio representation?
- How can an understanding of patterns (e. g., spatial constellations among multiple visualized model elements) be expressed via other perception channels?

Most of the above questions are not concerned with simply relating audio to elements of a modeling language, but they ask about the relationships between specific events and states during modeling, and non-visual sensual impressions for their representation.

These considerations suggest, that limiting the expressiveness of a concrete syntax declaration to only static mappings between perceivable impressions and modeling language elements can not be sufficient. A concrete syntax description should rather be understood in an operative sense, describing the space of possibile interactions that a human modeler can perform with a tool, relative to a given current state of a model instance described in a modeling language. This idea is further laid out in the next section.

4 Need for an Operative Notion of a Concrete Syntax

From the previous considerations, a demand for widening the range of expressiveness when specifying concrete syntax definitions has become clear.

In visual concrete syntaxes, model concepts can be displayed by the same graphical representation at any time during the process of using a model. For traditional visual concrete syntax specifications, it thus appears sufficient to restrict the specification of a modeling language's concrete syntax to be a set of ternary relation specifications, applicable to individual model elements such as objects or relationship:

$$(\text{Type, Instance}) \rightarrow \text{Symbol}$$

A little degree of dynamics can still be realized with this approach, by making the symbol representation dependent on states of the represented instance, e. g., setting a symbol's size or color according to an attribute value in the model. In contrast to this, as audio impressions are perceived over time, the occurrence of audio is bound to specific points in time during modeling. These points in time are determined by events and states that occur during modeling performed by a human modeler, or during the instantiation of models at execution time.

Including the occurrence of time-based audio and other media into modeling language specifications means to anticipate and specify these events and states, that can occur and can be reached during creating, modifying, or exploring models. A modeling language in this sense is not solely a description means for statically storing knowledge. Instead, the use of a modeling language needs to be taken into consideration as an inherent part of the language specification. The specification of the language should be "aware" of the actions applied to the representation of its instances, and should include descriptions of actions that may occur during its use.

Consequently, the notion of specifying a concrete syntax for a modeling language is to be widened by incorporating the idea of operatively acting on model instances, expressed through events that characterize the dynamics of the use of a modeling language. This abstract view on a modeling language's concrete syntax specification for representing model elements results in a quarternary relationship, that associates a three-tuple of a model element's type, its instance, and an event in time, to the occurrence of sound or other sensual impressions:

$$(\text{Type}, \text{Instance}, \text{Event}) \rightarrow \text{Sound}$$

Accordingly, a mapping for associating model states that occur during modeling, to non-visual representations, needs to be provided.

5   Conclusion

The previously discussed thoughts take an initial perspective on how to integrate additional perception channels into concrete syntax specifications for modeling languages. It quickly turns out that these questions cannot be answered by monotonically extending existing conceptualizations of visual concrete syntax specifications to be used with additional perception channels. Two main reasons for this have been identified, which at first are the inherent linear nature of audio and other sensual perception, and an underspecified notion of what concrete syntax is in traditional concrete syntax specification approaches. A wider approach for providing cognitive access to models should include aspects of active language use into concrete syntax specifications. These are not covered by state-of-the-art conceptualizations, which treat concrete syntax mainly as a mapping between an abstract syntax structure and a diagram representation structure.

This position paper has sketched how additional research can be expected to base on existing work originating from the auditory display community, as well as on work about distributed model synchronization. Putting these lines of argument together to develop a generalized understanding of concrete syntax specification is subject to further investigations.

References

1. Weske, M.: Business Process Management: Concepts. Languages, Architectures. Springer, Heidelberg (2012)
2. van der Aalst, W., Desel, J., Oberweis, A.: Business Process Management: Models, Techniques, and Empirical Study. Springer, Heidelberg (2000)
3. Kelly, S., Tolvanen, J.-P.: Domain Specific Modeling - Enabling Full Code Generation. Wiley, Hoboken (2008)
4. Frank, U.: Outline of a Method for Designing Domain-Specific Modelling Languages, ICB Research Report, Institute for Computer Science and Business Information Systems, University of Duisburg-Essen, No. 42 (2010)

5. Hermann, T.: Taxonomy and definitions for sonification and auditory display. In: Proceedings of the 14th International Conference on Auditory Display, ICAD2008, Paris, France (2008)
6. Beilharz, K., Ferguson, S.: An interface and framework design for interactive aesthetic sonification. In: Aramaki, M.A., Kronland-Martinet, R., Ystad, S., Jensen, K. (eds.) Proceedings of the 15th International Conference on Auditory Display, ICAD 2009. New – Digital Arts Forum, Copenhagen (2009)
7. Hermann, T., Ritter, H.: Listen to your data: model-based sonification for data analysis. In: Lasker, G.E. (ed.) Advances in Intelligent Computing and Multimedia Systems, pp. 189–194. International Institute for Advanced Studies in System Research and Cybernetics, Baden-Baden (1999)
8. Vickers, P.: Sonification for process monitoring. In: Hermann, T., Hunt, A., Neuhoff, J.G. (eds.) The Sonification Handbook, pp. 455–492. Logos, Berlin (2011)
9. Hildebrandt, T., Kriglstein, S., Rinderle-Ma, S.: On Applying Sonification Methods to Convey Business Process Data, CAiSE 2012 Forum. Gdansk, Poland (2012)
10. Hildebrandt, T.: Towards enhancing business process monitoring with sonification. In: Lohmann, N., et al. (eds.) Business Process Management Workshops, BPM 2013 International Workshops. Springer, Berlin (2013)
11. Bartelt, C.: Consistence preserving model merge in collaborative development processes. In: Proceedings of the 2008 international workshop on Comparison and Versioning of Software Models, CVSM 2008. ACM, New York (2008)
12. Reiter, T., Altmanninger, K., Bergmayr, A., Schwinger, W., Kotsis, G.: Models in conflict - detection of semantic conflicts in model-based development. In: Proceedings of the 3rd International Workshop on Model-Driven Enterprise Information Systems, MDEIS 2007, pp. 29–40. INSTICC Press (2007)
13. Gulden, J., Rutz, H.: Proposal for an XML format representing time, positions and parts of audio waveforms. In: Baalman, M., Schampijer, S. (eds.) Proceedings of the Linux Audio Conference 2007, LAC 2007, pp. 1–12, Berlin (2007)

BPMS2 2014

Tagging Model for Enhancing Knowledge Transfer and Usage during Business Process Execution

Reuven Karni and Meira Levy[(✉)]

Department of Industrial Engineering and Management,
Shenkar College of Engineering and Design,
12 Anna Frank Street, 52526 Ramat-Gan, Israel
{rkarni,lmeira}@shenkar.ac.il

Abstract. Tagging mechanisms allow users to label content, which mainly resides in Internet resources or Web 2.0 social tools, with descriptive terms (without relying on a controlled vocabulary) for navigation, filtering, search and retrieval. The current paper presents two tagging models. The first combines structured, automatically generated metadata, with manually inserted unstructured tagging labels, to facilitate annotation of content that enhances knowledge transfer and usage; and embeds tagging capabilities within a business process model for activation during execution. The second describes a tagged knowledge cycle that allows process performers to create and tag their knowledge and experiences as the process is carried out, and have it transferred for use by an associated stakeholder. The benefits of the models are discussed in the context of service processes, using an illustrative scenario of an inbound telesales process workflow with embedded Web 2.0. social tools.

Keywords: Tag · Tagging system · Business process execution · Web 2.0 · Business process modelling (BPM) · Knowledge management · Service processes

1 Introduction

In the current knowledge era, organizations are required to exploit their explicit knowledge assets, and in addition the tacit knowledge gained by their employees, encompassing skills and experiences. Specifically, the usage and capture of knowledge during business process *execution* can improve performance and enable learning processes – both from previous and current experiences [1]. Social systems, known as Web 2.0 tools, have the potential to enhance knowledge intensive business processes as Web 2.0 processes are characterized by an underlying "architecture of participation" that supports crowd-sourcing as well as a many-to-many broadcast mechanism [2]. Web 2.0 tools are realized as bottom-up *lightweight* information systems, because their setup time, use and maintenance require less time and effort; and they do not impose a pre-defined structure, but rather one that evolves over time according to the users' usage and interest, compared with traditional *heavyweight* organizational information

© Springer International Publishing Switzerland 2015
F. Fournier and J. Mendling (Eds.): BPM 2014 Workshops, LNBIP 202, pp. 429–439, 2015.
DOI: 10.1007/978-3-319-15895-2_36

systems such as Computer Aided Design (CAD), Product Data Management (PDM), or Product Lifecycle Management (PLM) systems) [3, 4].

Classical Business Process Modeling (BPM) targets the modeling of business processes designed to deliver products or services for external or internal customers [5]. Workflow systems, that normally implement heavyweight, structured BPM, can benefit from integrating lightweight Web 2.0 tools to enable both knowledge and insight capture and flexibility and adaptation to exceptions to the normal workflow. "The process does not need to be completely specified in the sense that it is allowed that activities not pre-specified occur in some of its instances. This allows the instantaneous adaptation of process instances to the emergence of new organizational needs" [6].

Social BPM adds social networking applications to traditional business process (BP) practices, so that external stakeholders (e.g., suppliers and customers, and the process performer) can participate in the design and regulation of the process model [3]. The BPM4People project [7], for example, does this by extending classical specification techniques with the aid of specific notations that enable the addition of social processes such as web applications along public or private Web social networks [3]. By integrating social channels, the project seeks to boost process execution through exploitation of weak ties and implicit knowledge; decision process transparency; extension of process engagement by various stakeholders; enabling more people to be active in process execution; and disseminating decisions to relevant recipients [7]. Their attitude follows other studies that foster the emergent requirement for flexible, knowledge intensive business process models; "[f]or many organizations, well-defined and ill-defined [often knowledge-intensive] processes coexist and should be handled in the final enterprise model" [8, 9]. Other research addresses the collaboration opportunities that social software enables. "The lack of formal barriers also tears down psychological barriers. Resistance is supposed to be lower due to a low entrance barrier. Instead, due to the immediate effects of employee action, their involvement and commitment may be increased. Therefore, social software has the potential to enhance collaborative and knowledge intensive business processes by improving the exchange of knowledge and information to speed up decisions and to improve the global reactivity of the enterprise" [10].

While social media provide means to capture knowledge, there are challenges to the knowledge management life cycle, which includes phases of share, create, access, use and maintain [11, 12]. Tagging systems allow annotation of content without relying on a controlled vocabulary, thus facilitating knowledge organization for further navigation, filtering, search and retrieval; and so provide opportunities for techniques such as data mining [13]. Former studies discuss the importance of tagging systems in general [13, 14] and in the context of BPM in particular [3, 8, 9]. However, they do not provide any specific model concerning the tagging of service processes, which addresses both tagging content and tagging processes.

The research described in this paper contributes to and provides means for tagging content posted within social systems during service process design and execution. Based on the studies regarding tagging [13, 14], it is proposed to embed a tagging mechanism in the service process workflow, combining structured, automatically generated metadata, as well as manually inserted unstructured tags. The model facilitates annotation of content that enhances knowledge transfer and usage. The tagging system enables various stakeholders to gain knowledge either in a "pull" manner – when searching for a specific tag – or by a "push" manner – when the knowledge is annotated with an *urgent* tag. Thus, the proposed tagging model enhances knowledge transfer across the enterprise – specifically, that created and captured during the enactment of service processes.

The contributions of this paper are:

- A tagging lifecycle model
- A tagged-knowledge lifecycle model from creation to use
- Illustration of knowledge creation, tagging, capture, transfer and usage through a detailed analysis of an inbound telesales service process
- Discussion of the opportunities and benefits provided by social software and tagging systems for the design and operation of business processes

The rest of the paper is organized as follows: The next section elaborates the tagging mechanism which enables knowledge transfer and usage within the organization. In Sect. 3 we detail our two tagging models that embed a tag creation process and a tag usage process within BPM, and suggest a preliminary structure that organizations can employ and further develop. Section 4 illustrates the application of the model principles to the design and execution of an inbound telesales process [15], followed by a discussion and future research plans in Sect. 5.

2 Web 2.0 and Tagging

Recently, research approaches related to "social BPM" have arisen. These aim to augment traditional BPM with Web 2.0 and social software using applications such as blogs, wikis, and social networks for knowledge capturing and social tagging [1]. "Tagging" refers to marking content with descriptive terms, also called keywords or tags, for future navigation, filtering, search and retrieval [16]. Silva et al. [3] define tagging as creating folksonomies around generic instances in order to add semantic value to their content and foster business process model evolution. A collaborative form of this process is termed social tagging, which has no predefined taxonomic structure, and is created by shared and emergent social structures and behaviors, as well as related conceptual and linguistic structures of the user community [13]. For business process performers, tagging allows them to label actions and decisions, and to participate in the creation of ontologies for the business process.

While the potential of social tools to enhance business process is well acknowledged, there are still barriers to overcome before the full potential of these tools are explored [17]. In particular, there are knowledge-sharing barriers that include self-censorship behaviors, lack of commitment and reward, inability to access knowledge, lack of time for organizing the needed knowledge, lack of awareness, communication difficulties (language and formats) and trust [17]. Hence, the incentives and motivations for users also play a significant role in affecting the tags that emerge from social tagging systems, which may stem from personal needs, sociable interests or willing to contribute to a collective process [13].

In our research we argue that while tagging has a communicative nature, wherein users attempt to express, through the tags they choose, themselves and their opinions [13], the tagging process should be handled as a business process of its own. In the next section we propose our tagging model in the organization, in the context of BPM.

3   Tagging Models in BPM

The tagging models presented in the following sections complement each other. The first model presents the tagging perspective when designing a business process; the second model deals with the knowledge perspective, hence, how tagging enables capture, transfer and usage of knowledge and insight gained during process execution.

3.1   Model 1: Tagging Lifecycle

The first tagging lifecycle model (Fig. 1) deals with *tagging content*, which addresses the structured and unstructured tags that can be added to any knowledge captured during execution of the business process model; *tagging processes* that concern adding tag-related activities during BPM development, including the design of automatic and manual activities while designing BP workflows; and *tagging dimensions* that define the architecture of a tagging system.

Tagging Content. BPM-related tagging content handles both structured and unstructured tags. *Structured tags* ("top down"), also termed metadata, are added automatically to the post content captured during process execution. They include terms such as workflow name, business unit, execution date, customer, product and any further structured information residing in information systems that interact with the workflow and that the organization wishes to tag. *Unstructured tags* ("bottom up") resemble the shared vocabulary that emerges in the organization and creates its folksonomy [13]. We suggest arranging them in several dimensions such as: business, urgency, and routing. *Business tags* are terms that concern business intent, outcome or customer relations, which capture the essence of the post. *Urgency tags* necessitate automatic dissemination of knowledge when the post is urgent so that the relevant stakeholders can become aware of it in real time. *Routing tags* define tags that can be specific persons, roles, organizational units or other stakeholders targeted by the post.

Tagging Process. The BPM-related tagging process is concerned with tag design and workflow performance. The designer defines (1) what information should be added as automatic metadata to content posted by the process performer; and (2) what are further initial tags that reflect that area of the organization taxonomy associated with the specific process or process activity. Then, as part of designing a business process workflow, the designer attaches a special tagging process in places where knowledge is captured, which enable the workflow performer both (3) to add "free" tags according to his/her simple or multiple categorization of the post, and also (4) to choose a-priori tags from an existing "tag cloud" constituting the shared folksonomy. Workflow processes are also needed (5) to handle approval of new tags and maintenance of the organizational "tag cloud"; and (6) to analyze tag usage as a component of business intelligence regarding customer behavior or business outcome. These processes are described in Fig. 1 which presents the life-cycle of tagging within the organization.

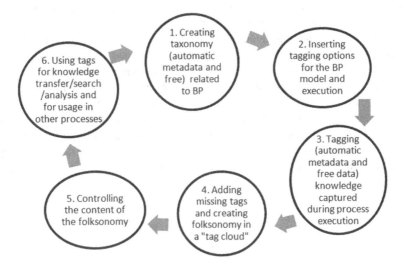

Fig. 1. Tagging lifecycle

Tagging Dimensions. Marlow et al. [13] express the architecture of a tagging system in terms of seven dimensions: tagging rights (self-tagging, permission based), tagging support (blind, suggested, viewable), aggregation model (bag, set), object type (textual, non-textual), source of material (user contributed, system, global), resource connectivity (links, groups, none), and social connectivity (links, groups, none). For a tagging system linked to business process activities the following structure is appropriate, as exemplified by the illustrative example detailed in the next section:

1. *Tagging rights:* permission-based (stakeholders in the process, especially the process performer and the process owner (e.g., sales))
2. *Tagging support:* suggested tags (stakeholders in the process, especially the process performer and the process owner (e.g., sales, logistics and warehousing))
3. *Aggregation:* bags (multiplicity of tags from different stakeholders for the same process or process activity (e.g., sales, logistics and warehousing))
4. *Type of object:* textual (written-down response to two types of process-related events: reaction to an unfavorable decision (decision nodes), and reaction to an unusual event (action nodes))
5. *Source of material:* system (events during process execution (e.g., telesales))
6. *Resource connectivity:* links (actions and decisions of the process) and groups (e.g., organizational IT relating to the specific process)
7. *Social connectivity:* groups (organizational departments and business functionalities concerned with the business goal of the process (e.g., sales to customers)).

3.2 Model 2: Tagged Knowledge Usage

The second tagging model deals with the life-cycle of tagged knowledge flow accompanying the execution of the associated business process (Fig. 2). Each element of the process is either an action or a decision (see Fig. 3). When the performer takes a decision, an unfavorable outcome will prompt him/her to explain why this happened and what could have been done to avoid it. When the performer is evoking an action, and some unusual event or deviation from the norm has happened, this will prompt him/her to record this and suggest how it could be prevented or exploited. This results in a post ("created knowledge"). The performer then adds free tags and the system adds metadata; the post becomes "tagged knowledge" and is retained in a repository of tagged posts. It is also transferred to and captured by the indicated stakeholder ("captured knowledge"). Reflection on this knowledge, together with other similarly tagged knowledge from the repository, results in enrichment of the knowledge ("learned knowledge") which is then applied by the stakeholder for the benefit of the enterprise ("applied knowledge"). Details of the usage are also passed to the general knowledge bank.

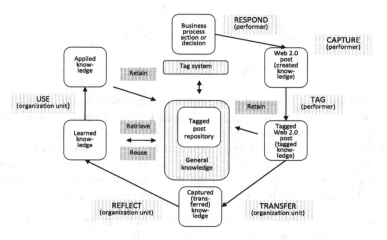

Fig. 2. Tagged knowledge capture, transfer and usage

4 Illustrative Example: Receipt of a Customer Order Incorporating Web 2.0 Activities

We study the application of the two models to the operation of an inbound telesales process for a wholesale firm [15] (Fig. 3). It describes how a particular item is ordered and sold through an incoming telephone call, provided the order meets several customer-determined conditions regarding price and delivery time. Several strategies are employed to maximize the likelihood of making a sale: persuading the customer to accept a delivery date and product price; and negotiating a satisfactory delivery date if persuasion fails.

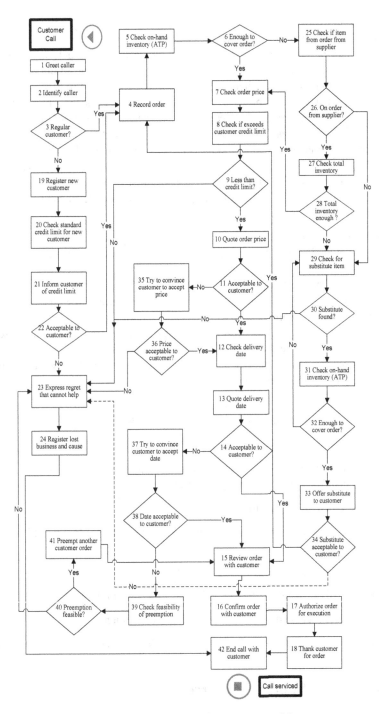

Fig. 3. Inbound telesales process model

In accordance with the first model (Fig. 1), the BPM designer specifies automatic metadata (e.g., *process, activity, product, customer*) as well as initial tags (e.g., *price change, customer notification, credit limit*). Then the designer adds activities during the process that enable adding tags from the original created tags, or additional free tags (e.g., *call wait time*), in places where knowledge may be captured (e.g., activity # 9 ⇒ activity # 23). In a separate process the organization controls the "tag cloud" and enables analysis and search capabilities of tags for learning purposes (e.g., how many times the tag *"call wait time"* has been used during the past month).

In accordance with the second model (Fig. 2), we simulate the following stages: (1) knowledge creation (reactions to unfavorable outcomes generated at decision junctions and spontaneous reactions to events occurring during process execution); (2) automatic and performer ("free") tagging; and (3) knowledge transfer, capture and use by organizational units.

1. Knowledge creation
   Illustrative Web 2.0 activities posted by the sales agent during the call are detailed in Appendix 1.
2. Automatic and process performer tagging
   Tags attached to the posts are detailed for each activity in Appendix 1.
3. Knowledge transfer, capture and use by organizational units
   Channeled by the tags, the posted responses come to the attention of several organizational departments: marketing, sales, customer relationships, the sales team and business process management (process improvement). The departments can make immediate use of this knowledge.

   (a) Marketing

   - Notify customers of price changes (Example 1)

   (b) Sales

   - Introduce an extended payment agreement to encourage the customer to accept the organization's price (Example 2)

   (c) Customer relationship management

   - Use personalized greetings to well-known customers (supported by CRM) (Example 4)

   (d) Sales team

   - Investigate ways to reduce call wait time (Example 4)

   (e) Business process management (process improvement)

   - Provide delivery date flexibility (scheduled or special, with/out surcharges) (Example 3)

5 Discussion and Future Research

Social systems provide the means to create social networks that produce collective intelligence [2, 19] and transform economic and production systems [20]. In particular, social BPM systems allow integration of knowledge from various stakeholders during business process execution [3, 7]. However, while there are social systems that enable social interactions during business process execution, we lack models that address the usage of knowledge which resides in these systems. The current paper fosters the embedding of a versatile tagging mechanism within business process design and activation. To this end, two models are presented. The first defines the tagging lifecycle in the organization (tag management perspective); the second shows how knowledge can be transferred and used throughout the organization through the application of the tagging mechanism (knowledge management perspective).

Our models and illustrative example afford many variegated insights as to how tagged knowledge can add value to the enterprise: (a) employees and end users can provide innovations regarding the outputs of the enterprise ("allow the sales agent to provide product advice to customers"); (b) brand building can be enhanced ("deal with customer awareness of competitive products"); (c) the enterprise can sense market forces and respond to nuances hint at unarticulated needs ("deal with customer awareness of competitive products"); (d) product development can be aided ("deal with customer awareness of competitive products"); (e) business processes can be improved through richer, socially enabled software interactions ("the customer was unaware that the item price had been raised; we should modify the process model to handle changes in product prices"); and (f) mechanisms for the human agents within the enterprise can be created to add value to the knowledge of the company ("we should offer a fast delivery with a surcharge"); (g) it is invaluable in creating and sustaining customer loyalty ("I always give a special extra greeting to a regular customer"); (h) it enables real-time feedback regarding process alignment [18] ("we need to discuss new ways to reduce call wait time"); and (i) it provides the opportunity to reveal when employee empowerment would greatly improve process performance ("why can't I suggest an extended payment agreement to encourage the customer to accept our price?").

Future research will deal with validating and examining these models, and investigating the organizational insights obtainable through their application, in real and variegated settings, while learning about people's perceptions about these models.

Appendix 1: Illustrative interactions between telesales process and Web 2.0

(a) Dealing with unfavorable decisions
Example 1: Order price exceeds credit limit (activity # 9 ⇒ activity # 23) (Fig. 3)

- Post *The customer was unaware that the item price had been raised. Maybe we should modify the process model to handle changes in product prices and also add a notification to the customer regarding the new prices.*
- Tags *meta (decision, product, customer, urgent, marketing); free (price change, customer notification, credit limit)*

Example 2: Order price unacceptable to customer (# 36 ⇒ # 23)

- Post *The "price convince" script is bad – it should be targeted on payment and not price. Why can't I suggest an extended payment agreement to encourage the customer to accept our price?*

- Tags *meta (decision, product, customer, not urgent, marketing); free (price, script, payment agreement)*

  Example 3: Delivery date unacceptable to customer (# 14 ⇨ # 37)

- Post *The item is very popular and the customer (retailer) has run out of stock. We should offer a fast delivery with a surcharge.*
- Tags *meta (decision, product, customer, urgent, logistics); free (delivery, surcharge)*

(b) Dealing with unusual occurrences
  Example 4: The customer is a regular customer (# 3 ⇨ # 4)

- Post 1 *The customer complained that he waited too long for the call to be answered. We need to discuss new ways to reduce call wait time.*
- Tags 1 *meta (action, customer, urgent, customer relations); free (call wait time, team social network)*
- Post 2 *I always give a special extra greeting to a regular customer.*
- Tags 2 *meta (action, customer, not urgent, customer relations); free (greeting, customer loyalty, team social network)*

  Example 5: The customer order is recorded (# 4)

- Post 1 *The customer spoke about our competitor's product and said he hoped ours would be as good or better. In future it is worthwhile comparing our product with the competing products via the organization social network.*
- Tags 1 *meta (action, product, customer, not urgent, marketing); free (competition, competitor specifics; competing product specifics)*
- Post 2 *Can I offer some advice to the customer about using the item – especially a new product?*
- Tags 2 *meta (action, product, customer, not urgent, marketing); free (product usage, product usage wiki, product promotion).*

References

1. Balzert, S., Fettke, P., Loos, P.: A framework for reflective business process management. In: 45th Hawaii International Conference on System Sciences (HICSS), Maui, Hawaii, pp. 3642–3651 (2012)
2. O'Reilly, T.: What is web 2.0: Design patterns and business models for the next generation of software. http://www.oreilly.com/web2/archive/what-is-web-20.html
3. Silva, A.R., Meziani, R., Magalhães, R., Martinho, D., Aguiar, A., Flores, N.: AGILIPO: Embedding social software features into business process tools. In: Rinderle-Ma, S., Sadiq, S., Leymann, F. (eds.) BPM 2009. LNBIP, vol. 43, pp. 219–230. Springer, Heidelberg (2010)
4. Larsson, A., Ericson, Å., Larsson, T., Randall, D.: Engineering 2.0: Exploring lightweight technologies for the virtual enterprise. In: Proceedings of International Conference on the Design of Cooperative Systems (2008)
5. Smart, P.A., Maddern, H., Maull, R.S.: Understanding business process management: implications for theory and practice. Br. J. Manage. **20**(4), 491–507 (2009)

6. Lincoln, M., Gal, A.: Content-based validation of business process models. Working Paper, Faculty of Industrial Engineering, Technion IIT (2011)
7. Brambilla, M., Fraternali, P., Vaca, C., Butti, S.: Combining social web and BPM for improving enterprise performances: the BPM4People Approach to Social BPM. In: Proceedings of the 21st World Wide Web Conference, Lyon, France, 223–226 (2012)
8. Bruno, G., Dengler, F., Jennings, B., Khalaf, R., Nurcan, S., Prilla, M., Sarini, M., Schmidt, R., Silva, R.: Key challenges for enabling agile BPM with social software. J. Softw. Maintenance Evol. Res. Pract. 23(4), 297–326 (2011)
9. Erol, S., Granitzer, M., Happ, S., Jantunen, S., Jennings, B., Koschmider, A., Nurcan, S., Rossi, D., Schmidt, R., Johannesson, P.: Combining BPM and social software: Contradiction or chance? J. Softw. Maintenance Evol. Res. Pract. 22, 449–476 (2010)
10. Levy, M., Karni, R.: A Web 2.0 Platform for Product-Service Systems: Serviceology for Services. Springer, New York (2014)
11. Hooff, B.V., Vijvers, J., De Ridder, J.: Foundations and applications of a knowledge management scan. Eur. Manage. J. 21(2), 237–246 (2003)
12. O'Dell, C., Grayson, J.C.: Identifying and transferring internal best practices. In: Holsapple, C.W. (ed.) Handbook on Knowledge Management, vol. 1, Chapter 31. Springer, New York (2003)
13. Marlow, C., Naaman, M., Boyd, D., Davis, M.: Tagging paper, taxonomy, flickr, academic article, to read. In: Proceedings of the Seventeenth ACM Conference on Hypertext and Hypermedia, pp. 31–40. ACM Press, New York (2006)
14. Wu, H., Zubair, M., Maly, K.: Harvesting social knowledge from folksonomies. In: Proceedings of the Seventeenth ACM Conference on Hypertext and Hypermedia, pp. 111–114. ACM Press, New York (2006)
15. Shtub, A., Karni, R.: ERP: the Dynamics of Supply Chain and Process Management. Springer Science + Business Media, The Netherlands (2010)
16. Golder, S.A., Huberman, B.A.: The structure of Collaborative Tagging Systems. HP Labs, Technical Report. http://www.hpl.hp.com/research/idl/papers/tags/
17. Levy, M.: Web 2.0 implications on knowledge management. J. Knowl. Manage. 13(1), 120–134 (2009)
18. Morrison, E.D., Ghose, A.K., Dam, H.K., Hinge, K.G., Hoesch-Klohe, J.: Strategic alignment of business processes. In: 7th International Workshop on Engineering Service-Oriented Applications, Paphos, Cyprus (2011)
19. Surowiecki, J.: The Wisdom of Crowds. Anchor, New York (2005)
20. Benkler, Y.: The Wealth of Networks: How Social Production Transforms Markets and Freedom. Yale University Press, New Haven (2006)

Classification Framework for Context Data from Business Processes

Michael Möhring[1(✉)], Rainer Schmidt[2], Ralf-Christian Härting[1],
Florian Bär[2], and Alfred Zimmermann[3]

[1] Aalen University, Beethovenstr. 1, 73430 Aalen, Germany
`Michael.Moehring@htw-aalen.de`
[2] Munich University of Applied Sciences, Lothstr. 64, 80335 Munich, Germany
`{Rainer.Schmidt,Florian.Baer}@hm.edu`
[3] Reutlingen University, Alteburgstr. 150, 72762 Reutlingen, Germany

Abstract. New business concepts such as Enterprise 2.0 foster the use of social software in enterprises. Especially social production significantly increases the amount of data in the context of business processes. Unfortunately, these data are still an unearthed treasure in many enterprises. Due to advances in data processing such as Big Data, the exploitation of context data becomes feasible. To provide a foundation for the methodical exploitation of context data, this paper introduces a classification, based on two classes, intrinsic and extrinsic data.

Keywords: Context data · BPM · Intrinsic data · Extrinsic data · Business processes

1 Introduction

Enterprise 2.0 is a business concept used by more and more enterprises and organizations in order to quickly adapt to changing customer requirements and to exploit the innovative potential of customers and suppliers [1]. A core concept of Enterprise 2.0 is the use of social production [2] in addition to classical tayloristic [3] organizational approaches. By using social software employees are empowered to create data in the context of business processes, that means outside of predefined procedures and transactional information systems such as ERP systems [4]. This context data is mostly semi- and unstructured. It is estimated that more than 85 % of all relevant business data are unstructured [5].

Unfortunately these context data is a still unearthed treasure in many companies. Although information systems provide very elaborate means for managing structured information such as accounting and transactions, such a broad processing support lacks for context data. The reason is, that, context data are difficult to exploit with traditional means [6]. In most cases, human beings have to transform context data into the input for business process management. In effect, large amounts of context data are not used because the effort to prepare it is too high [7].

The contribution of this paper is to prepare the methodological exploitation of context data by introducing a classification. There are two basic classes of context data,

F. Fournier and J. Mendling (Eds.): BPM 2014 Workshops, LNBIP 202, pp. 440–445, 2015.
DOI: 10.1007/978-3-319-15895-2_37

intrinsic and extrinsic context data. Intrinsic data has been created from within the business process lifecycle (e.g. a comment on a process model). Extrinsic paper originate from outside, such as a blog entry by a customer.

The paper is structured as follows. In the following section, a classification of business process context data into extrinsic and intrinsic data is introduced. Related work is analyzed in the following section. Finally, an outlook and the conclusion is given.

2 Classification of Business Process Context Data

Context data associated with business processes can be differentiated whether the data has been created extrinsically or intrinsically as shown in Fig. 1. Extrinsic data is created independently from the business process lifecycle [8]. Intrinsic data of a business process is created during the business process lifecycle.

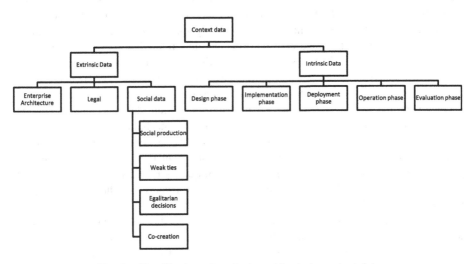

Fig. 1. Classification of extrinsic and intrinsic context data

2.1 Extrinsic Data

Extrinsic data is differentiated into data describing enterprise architecture, legal documents and data created by social software, so-called social data [9, 10].

Enterprise architecture. Enterprise architecture [11, 12] is a static view on the enterprises defining the relationship of business units and IT-components. It also describes how to align business and IT in order to realize the company's goals and implement the company's strategy. Therefore, defining enterprise architecture is a crucial task of management. Enterprise architecture is connected with Taylorism [13] that means dividing up larger tasks into smaller, assigning them to individuals and controlling the execution of the tasks. Nevertheless a large amount of semi-and unstructured data associates these formal models (e.g. in TOGAF [14]).

Legal data. Legal data [15] shall be defined as data given by the lawmaker. It contains laws, regulatory status and implementation comments that influence the design of the business process and their operation.

Social data. Enterprise 2.0 and social software replace the Taylorism [16] -oriented production of goods and provisioning of services by a bottom-up organized, egalitarian and co-creation oriented one. The four key concepts weak ties [17], social production [2] egalitarian decision-making [18] and co-creation [19] imply the creation of vast amounts of unstructured data. By analyzing these data, valuable information influencing one or more perspectives of business processes may be gathered. These perspectives are the organizational, operational, control, data and functional perspective.

Weak ties [17] are informal relationships across the formal organization of enterprises and organizations. They are created to exchange knowledge and to combine competencies in order to handle tough problems. Weak ties can be identified by analyzing the competencies, the areas of work of the employees and by created artifacts. Especially artifacts may be helpful to discover hitherto unknown colleagues working on the same themes. By analyzing weak ties the organizational perspective of business process models can be enriched both by organizational relationship and competencies.

Social production [2] inverses the product design of tayloristic approaches. Instead, a top-down-approach a bottom-up approach is used. The product is created by the number of individual contributions. Instead of realizing the master-plan of the top-management, the individual stakeholders may introduce their ideas and thoughts on the design of the product. Social production uses an inverse mechanism of quality control. Instead of pre-defining rules for measuring the quality of contributions it uses an a posteriori and holistic approach. Each contribution of an individual is visible to the public. Therefore, the individuals strive for a high quality in order to avoid damage to their social reputation. Social production provides information for the operational and functional perspective.

Enterprise 2.0 and social software [1] also change the way decisions are made within enterprises. Instead of hierarchy based decisions, more egalitarian decisions are made. This implements concepts such as the wisdom of the crowds that prefer combining the opinions many stakeholders instead of relying on the decisions of a few specialists.

The co-creation of products [20] is replacing the separation of consumer and producer and unidirectional, limited interaction by a bidirectional, more frequent interaction between a producer and prosumer. A prosumer [21] is a consumer actively participating in the design of a product. During the interaction of producer and prosumer, a lot of valuable information is exchanged to improve products and services. It may influence the operational control and functional perspective (Table 1).

2.2 Intrinsic Data

Intrinsic data is created during the business process lifecycle [8]. It may be attached directly to a process element, e.g. an explanation of a task in a process graph, or it may refer to larger parts or the whole process or even process group. Often overlooked, but

Table 1. Social data and its impact on business process perspectives

	Organizational	Operational	Control	Data	Functional
Weak Ties	+				
Social production		+			+
Egalitarian decision making			+		
Co-production				+	

nevertheless of increasing importance are semi- and non-structured data associated with structured process definitions. Business process models using notations (e.g. BPMN [21]) and are often accompanied by non-structured data such as text files, in order to give further explanations. Text files contain explanations of business models. Furthermore comments of users contain suggestions for improving business processes and governance documents (like rules for the process design). During process design, interviews and questionnaires deliver both semi- and unstructured data. This data also embraces comments and suggestions for improving an existing process. In the implementation phase, documentation describing the relationship between the abstract process model and its implementation in the company's organization and software systems is created. Also, documents created during the deployment phase, that means the workflow to put the process into operation, may contain valuable data for other phase, e.g. the operation phase. In the operations phase, huge amounts of semi-structured data is collected by tracing the process execution in log files. These log files contain data about the history of the process executions consisting of execution time, duration, resource consumptions, etc. In the evaluation phase, evaluations and questionnaires are made in order to collect data how to improve the business process.

3 Related Work

There are a number of approaches for exploiting context data. A first approach to automatically extract extrinsic information from policy documents is described in [22]. In [7, 23] approaches for process models from/to natural language text is described. The extraction of workflow models from maintenance manuals is described in [24]. Process mining [25] uses semi-structured information from event-logs in order to discover processes, verify the compliance of process execution etc.

4 Conclusion and Outlook

Data in the context of business processes is a valuable source of information for business process management. Context data may be extrinsic or intrinsic and is often unstructured. Advances in data processing allow to use context data to a far broader extent than before. Therefore, this paper showed how to leverage context data for business process management. Academics can improve from a new classification of context data from business processes and can so adopt and improve current approaches.

For instance techniques of quality management of BPM and integration of social software can be improved. Practitioners can use e.g. the classification to evaluate and improve current BPM implementations. Future research can explore approaches for automatic context data analytics (e.g. with Text Mining methods) as well as industry sector specific adoptions of the classification and Big Data [26] based approaches.

References

1. McAfee, A.P.: Enterprise 2.0: the dawn of emergent collaboration. MIT Sloan Manag. Rev. **47**, 21–28 (2006)
2. Benkler, Y.: The Wealth of Networks : How Social Production Transforms Markets and Freedom. Yale University Press, New Haven (2006)
3. Taylor, F.W.: The principles of scientific management, vol. 202. Harper, N.Y. (1911)
4. Chang, W.Y., Abu-Amara, H., Sanford, J.F.: Introduction to Enterprise Services and Cloud Resources1. In: Transforming Enterprise Cloud Services. Springer, Netherlands, pp. 1–42 (2011)
5. Blumberg, R., Atre, S.: The problem with unstructured data. DM Rev. **13**, 42–49 (2003)
6. Herbst, J., Karagiannis, D.: An inductive approach to the acquisition and adaptation of workflow models. Proc. IJCAI **99**, 52–57 (1999)
7. Friedrich, F., Mendling, J., Puhlmann, F.: Process model generation from natural language text. In: Mouratidis, H., Rolland, C. (eds.) CAiSE 2011. LNCS, vol. 6741, pp. 482–496. Springer, Heidelberg (2011)
8. Weske, M.: Business Process Management: Concepts, Languages, Architectures. Springer, Heidelberg (2007)
9. Schmidt, R.: Social Data for Product Innovation, Marketing and Customer Relations. Presented at the BPMS2, Tallinn, Estonia, March 09, 2012
10. Brambilla, M., Fraternali, P., Vaca, C.: BPMN and design patterns for engineering social BPM solutions. In: Daniel, F., Barkaoui, K., Dustdar, S. (eds.) BPM Workshops 2011, Part I. LNBIP, vol. 99, pp. 219–230. Springer, Heidelberg (2012)
11. Ross, J.W., Weill, P., Robertson, D.: Enterprise Architecture as Strategy: Creating a Foundation for Business Execution. Harvard Business School Press, Watertown (2006)
12. Schmidt, R., Möhring, M., Zimmermann, A., Wissotzki, M., Sandkuhl, K., Jugel, D.: Towards a framework for enterprise architecture analytics. In: Proceedings of the 18th IEEE International Enterprise Distributed Object Computing Conference Workshops (EDOCW), Ulm/Germany, Ulm, Germany (2014, in press)
13. Guest, R.H., Aitken, H.G.J.: Taylorism at watertown arsenal: scientific management in action 1908–1915. Technol. Cult. **2**(2), 191 (1961)
14. Josey, A.: TOGAF Version 9 A Pocket Guide. Van Haren Pub., England (2009)
15. Governatori, G., Milosevic, Z., Sadiq, S.: Compliance checking between business processes and business contracts. In: 10th IEEE International Enterprise Distributed Object Computing Conference, EDOC 2006, pp. 221–232 (2006)
16. Taylor, F.W.: The Principles of Scientific Management. General Books LLC, Tennessee (2010)
17. Granovetter, M.: The strength of weak ties. Am. J. Sociol. **78**(6), 1360–1380 (1973)
18. Surowiecki, J.: The Wisdom of Crowds: Why the Many Are Smarter Than the Few and How Collective Wisdom Shapes Business, Economies, Societies and Nations. Anchor, London (2005)

19. Prahalad, C.K., Ramaswamy, V.: Co-creating unique value with customers. Strategy Leadersh. **32**(3), 4–9 (2004)
20. Vargo, S., Maglio, P., Akaka, M.: On value and value co-creation: A service systems and service logic perspective. Eur. Manag. J. **26**(3), 145–152 (2008)
21. Klein, S., Totz, C.: Prosumers as service configurators-vision, status and future requirements1. In: E-Life Dot Com Bust., p. 119 (2004)
22. Li, J., Wang, H.J., Zhang, Z., Zhao, J.L.: A policy-based process mining framework: mining business policy texts for discovering process models. Inf. Syst. E-Bus. Manag. **8**(2), 169–188 (2010)
23. Leopold, H., Mendling, J., Polyvyanyy, A.: Generating natural language texts from business process models. In: Ralyté, J., Franch, X., Brinkkemper, S., Wrycza, S. (eds.) CAiSE 2012. LNCS, vol. 7328, pp. 64–79. Springer, Heidelberg (2012)
24. Schumacher, P., Minor, M., Schulte-Zurhausen, E.: Extracting and enriching workflows from text. In: 2013 IEEE 14th International Conference on Information Reuse and Integration (IRI), pp. 285–292 (2013)
25. Van der Aalst, W.M., Weijters, A.: Process mining: a research agenda. Comput. Ind. **53**(3), 231–244 (2004)
26. Schmidt, R., Möhring, M., Maier, S., Pietsch, J., Härting, R.-C.: Big data as strategic enabler - insights from central european enterprises. In: Abramowicz, W., Kokkinaki, A. (eds.) BIS 2014. LNBIP, vol. 176, pp. 50–60. Springer, Heidelberg (2014)

Business Processes in Connected Communities

Nick Russell[(⊠)] and Alistair Barros

School of Information Systems, Science and Engineering Faculty,
Queensland University of Technology, Brisbane 4000, Australia
{n.russell,alistair.barros}@qut.edu.au

Abstract. The notion of *Connected Communities* is evolving from widespread use of social media and networks and represents an emerging paradigm for online connectivity, collaboration and information usage where the basis of interaction is between individual human participants with shared motives in a specific context. Traditional BPM practices operate on the basis of a common frame of reference with regard to overall business strategy and the constituent activities, and makes similar assumptions with respect to human participants in those processes. This paper reviews the implications of digital connectedness between human actors in a process-oriented context, surveys potential community archetypes and outlines core characteristics of connected communities and their significance in a broader BPM context.

Keywords: Connected communities · Digital connectedness · Social groups · Value exchange

1 Introduction

The emergence of social technologies has been the most rapid of IT phenomena and its impact is set to be the most significant. In recent years, its different manifestations (social networks, microblogs, status updates, social bookmarks, video and photo sharing and commenting) have dominated activity on the Internet, exceeding the use of search engines and other forms of online transactional services. A recent McKinsey Global Institute report [1] predicts that between $900 billion and $1.3 trillion of annual value could be unlocked by social technologies in just four sectors (consumer packaged goods, consumer financial services, professional services and advanced manufacturing).

While individuals are already directly benefitting from their participation in social communities, businesses are only just beginning to understand how the digitized connectedness of individuals can boost productivity and drive up new innovation. Individuals - on the basis of the social communities into which they are forming and their connections within and across these communities – are radically reshaping how organisations deliver services. In other words, services must now orient themselves to individuals, not the other way around as has traditionally been the case. In order to understand how new transformations and innovations can proceed in this setting, an enriched understanding is required of

© Springer International Publishing Switzerland 2015
F. Fournier and J. Mendling (Eds.): BPM 2014 Workshops, LNBIP 202, pp. 446–451, 2015.
DOI: 10.1007/978-3-319-15895-2_38

how individuals connect to each other and form social communities. Compelling examples are available from diverse organisations and industries, however our reference of understanding remains anecdotal. Of particular significance is the scant understanding of how existing BPM practices should embrace and integrate communities of digitally connected individuals.

Current conceptions of social technology [2] identify four significant patterns which underpin it: weak ties, social production, egalitarianism and value-co-creation. When we consider the nexus between BPM and social technology, effective integration of the weak ties between connected individuals within business processes is the pattern that has the most immediate impact on current BPM design formalisms and deployment technologies. In this position paper, we explore this nexus in more detail, examining it in the context of indicative use cases and identifying opportunities for extending the existing basis for resource characterisation in business processes to embrace connected communities.

2   Weak Ties in Connected Communities

The notion of communities mediated through digital capabilities have evolved in social structure and sophistication over the last thirty years. The earliest forms of virtual communities [3] in news groups and email lists, have fostered basic provisions for social exchange through information sharing utilities: wider awareness and cognizance beyond individual interactions and value exchange of conventional systems, open and opt-in grouping, peer-to-peer and unstructured communication, open social production and minimal regulation, among others. ECommerce systems have retrofitted virtual communities for extended interactions of transactional value exchanges, for example, for supply, price bidding, information solicitation and group communication. Social media and networks, now the convergent platforms for virtual communities, have introduced greater flexibility of social groups through arbitrary, multi-level connections of their underlying networks (e.g. likes, follows, friends connections). As described through the McKinsey report [1], the sheer growth of digitized connections and social contexts of people around the globe is leading to greater use of virtual communities in public and private sector service delivery.

We refer to *connected communities*, as a form of understanding of communities, through enhanced insight into individual connections, as weak ties, transcending online and real-world settings, that are meaningful for value exchanges of utilities (goods and service delivery). These ties or connections can symbolise a range of potential relationships between community members including family ties, employment history, dwelling location, skills and expertise, recreational activity, cultural profile, travel patterns, or simply being at the same place and time in relation to some adverse event. They can have different social strengths, in different contexts, given the degree of certainty (probability), transience or granularity that they represent. They range from tight, long-lasting and static relationships (e.g., family) to temporary relationships of different durations (e.g., colleagues, patients with same symptoms) to location-specific connections (e.g., all citizens attending an event).

While utilities provide a particular focus for value-exchanges, peer-to-peer interactions take place through particular groups, which provide practical social contexts through which individuals request and share information, exchange value and form deeper bonds. Social groups are formed through common interests (e.g. cultural), imperatives (e.g. political), alignments with other structures (e.g. organisational groups) and utilitarian goals (e.g. frequent travellers sharing similar journeys). As understood through classical sociology [4], the social identity of individuals and the strength of value exchanges is tied in social groups. Specifically, social groups provide the social bonding and trust, which in online settings complements that traditionally cultivated through face-to-face, real-world associations. We contend that, explicitly understood and transparent connections between individuals are crucial for social identity and social groupings that ensure trustful value exchanges, especially in utilities which raise uncertainties and risks for individuals.

3   Indicative Use Cases

In this section, we describe key use cases which we are currently investigating as part of our connected communities research [5]. Each exemplifies a distinct type of community both in terms of the nature of connections/relationships between participants, the service utilities concerning participants, and the weak ties of individual connections, groups and trust factors that are instrumental for value exchanges between community members.

Connected employee: The traditional organisational recruitment process relies heavily on validation and evaluation of various forms of social connections between individuals and various entities (previous employers, endorsing managers, educational institutions etc.). This is a time-consuming and potentially error-prone activity which in many cases often does not add value beyond the knowledge that is embodied in social links which already exist between prospective employees and current staff within the organisation. It has been estimated that up to 75 % of applicants for an advertised position turn out to have connections with the organisation through its staff or activities [5]. The challenge lies in identifying the various weak ties that already exist (eg. LinkedIn connections to staff, common universities or professional societies, similar patterns of conference attendance) and developing means of exploiting them for ranking candidates and matching them to prospective vacancies and needs within the organisation. Furthermore, active connections through shared professional interactions between workers, inside and outside the organisation, can provide insights for the formation of professionally meaningful and highly trusted groupings across these. Professional bodies, meetings and forums, and third-party activities (e.g. writing papers) are ways in which active connections and groupings can be fostered. A connected community, as such, could equally apply to employees already within the organisation, providing an enriched and complementary understanding of how weak ties can play out for organisational understanding and decision-making, compared to formal organisational structures.

In this case study, the utilities of recruitment, team formation and professional development, are largely anchored in the organisation, with connected communities providing enhanced intelligence for corporate activities.

Connected commuter: The high reliability and efficiency levels established through Internet ECommerce services are leading to greater sensitivity of online offerings entailing C2C interactions in community settings. A prominent example is in the area of personal mobility, resulting from increased urbanisation of major cities, increased expectations of utilising underused third-party resources for alternative transportation and the prospect of driver-less cars. Supporting a diverse range of on-demand journey solutions on the basis of the weak ties that exist between commuters with similar objectives has proven to be effective in a number of distinct forms. The two most prominent of these are *ridesharing* which involves a driver sharing space in their vehicle with other commuters making similar journeys (cf. Lyft, Ridester) and *carsharing* which involves a vehicle owner making it available on a short term basis for other commuters to utilise (cf. Zipcar). A number of community characteristics directly underpin the effectiveness of a connected commuter solution: the ease of identifying potential rideshare partners or carshare providers via the weak ties which characterise the community, the ability to establish the identity of potential partners and establish trust in them on the basis of the community network, and the practical bearing of groups within the online community which mirror those in real life particularly where the utility provided by the community is of direct applicability. In this case study, we have found that the social identity of influential users and social cohesiveness and perception of value exchanges through subgroups are of crucial importance for mitigating the risks that users perceive in using rideshare and carshare services. An understanding of connections, along different categories, can help shape lead user profiles and social groups in different settings. In contrast to the *connected employee*, this case study entails a service orchestrated within an open, Internet-enabled, community setting.

Connected customer: The rise of topic-centric online virtual communities has significantly changed the nexus of control in the Business-to-Consumer (B2C) relationship. Customers are now more empowered than ever with real-time information on potential product purchases, suppliers and terms of trade shared by other community members. More significantly, participation in these groups leads to a new class of C2C interaction where the group itself can both initiate and fulfill both sides of a transaction via its members (cf. eBay). Furthermore the collective aggregation of community members can result in their participation in a group-based transaction. Many examples are emerging from the financial sector, where utilities supported through a company are offset by community. Friendsurance, for instance, supports insurance policies for group insurance where members in the group cover small claims of other group members, while Friendsurance covers larger claims, reducing the cost of premiums due to the reduced risk of fraudulent claims occurring (due to trust established within groups). Key community considerations include the ability to profile the identity and trustworthiness of potential partners on the basis of connections within the community, the ability of the community to facilitate C2C interactions between community participants and support value exchanges as a consequence of these interactions. In contrast to the *connected employee* and *connected commuter* case studies, this entails utilities and value exchanges in a company as well as a community, through complementary delivery models which are available concurrently. It provides an insight as to how companies can play a mediation role in trust guarantees through community-based interactions.

4   Weak Ties Through BPM in Connected Communities

Contemporary notions of resource integration within business processes remain relatively simplistic. Resources are represented as individual entities with roles, groups and organisational hierarchies used for the purposes of work distribution amongst them. The *Workflow Resource Patterns*[1] provide a canonical overview of resource representation and utilisation considerations in the context of current BPM modelling formalisms and enactment systems. When these patterns are considered in the context of connected communities, it becomes clear that the closed world view on which they are founded is insufficient to deal with the dynamic, open-ended realities of resources as they exist in connected communities and in other online and virtual contexts. Two significant issues that arise when considering resources in these contexts are: (1) identification of individual resources and their capabilities becomes more challenging in a dynamic work environment where there is not necessarily a complete central view of the resource pool and (2) there is no longer a uniform notion of trust and the extent of confidence and assurance that can be expected to exist between resources. The weak ties that exist between individual resources in a community context become more significant when attempting to address these challenges. We consider how two resource patterns can be extended to accommodate these needs. These patterns have applicability to each of the use cases discussed in Sect. 3.

Pattern 8 (Capability-Based Distribution)

Description: The ability to distribute work items to resources based on specific capabilities that they possess. Capabilities (and their associated values) are recorded for individual resources as part of the organisational model.

Necessary Extensions: Traditional BPM notions assume a single view or directory of resource identities and capabilities. These notions can no longer be relied upon in community contexts where the identity of individual resources is based on their participation in multiple communities and their capabilities relevant for work distribution purposes are multi-faceted in nature and recorded in various distributed repositories. To accommodate this shortfall, the ability to dynamically surface and assess a range of viewpoints (cf. distributed resource directories, assessments of known associates, crowd-sourced opinions) is required when determining resource capabilities.

---

[1] See www.workflowpatterns.com for comprehensive details.

Pattern 27 (Delegation)

Description: The ability for a resource to allocate an unstarted work item previously allocated to it (but not yet commenced) to another resource.

Necessary Extensions: In a dynamically changing community context, increasingly the best arbiter of a suitable delegate for a work assignment will be the resource seeking to pass on the activity, where the actual delegate is someone to whom they likely are already connected either directly or indirectly and who they know they can trust. An increased range of supporting utilities will be required to enable such resources to identify and profile other suitably trustworthy resources both within and beyond the community.

5   Conclusion

In this paper, we have provided insights into the evolving sophistication of technology-mediated social networks, shaping a strategic research direction, in connected communities, with major implications for the way conventional, closed world, business processes are understood and orchestrated. While a comprehensive and systematic insight into empirical developments and an impact analysis for BPM are beyond the scope of the paper, we have focussed on a key consideration: weak ties through individual relationality and groupings in communities, and how these impact new ways of delivering services otherwise controlled through strong ties and strict regulation and governance through enterprises. We have provided an emergent understanding of semantic connections that individuals have and how these relate to group formation and trust influential in delivering services through companies, communities and jointly through both. Accordingly for BPMS, we have reconceived two workflow resource patterns which relate to group coordination, further loosening strong ties assumptions, with digitized individual connections manifesting weak ties and, we contend, a new class of value exchanges.

References

1. Chui, M., Manyika, J., Bughin, J., Dobbs, R., Roxburgh, C., Sarrazin, H., Sands, G., Westergren, M.: The social economy: Unlocking value and productivity through social technologies, July 2012. http://www.mckinsey.com/insights/high_tech_telecoms_internet/the_social_economy

2. Bruno, G., Dengler, F., Jennings, B., Khalaf, R., Nurcan, S., Prilla, M., Sarini, M., Schmidt, R., Silva, R.: Key challenges for enabling agile BPM with social software. J. Softw. Maintenance Evol. Res. Pract. **23**(4), 297–326 (2011)

3. Rheingold, H.: The Virtual Community: Homesteading on the Electronic Frontier. MIT Press, London (2000)

4. Giuffre, K.A.: Communities and Networks : Using Social Network Analysis to Rethink Urban and Community Studies. Polity Press Cambridge, Malden (2013)

5. Barros, A., Russell, N., Dulleck, U.: Connected communities: A research agenda for conceptualisation and realisation. Technical Report, QUT (2014)

Social-Software-Based Support for Enterprise Architecture Management Processes

Rainer Schmidt[1](✉), Alfred Zimmermann[2], Michael Möhring[3],
Dierk Jugel[2,4], Florian Bär[1], and Christian M. Schweda[5]

[1] Munich University of Applied Sciences, Munich, Germany
{rainer.schmidt,florian.baer}@hm.edu
[2] Reutlingen University, Reutlingen, Germany
{alfred.zimmermann,
dierk.jugel}@reutlingen-university.de
[3] Aalen University, Aalen, Germany
michael.moehring@htw-aalen.de
[4] University of Rostock, Rostock, Germany
[5] LeanIT42 GmbH, Garching bei München, Germany
christian.schweda@leanit42.de

Abstract. Modern enterprises reshape and transform continuously by a multitude of management processes with different perspectives. They range from business process management to IT service management and the management of the information systems. Enterprise Architecture (EA) Management seeks to provide such a perspective and to align the diverse management perspectives. Therefore, EA Management cannot rely on hierarchic - in a tayloristic manner designed - management processes to achieve and promote this alignment. It, conversely, has to apply bottom-up, information-centered coordination mechanisms to ensure that different management processes are aligned with each other and enterprise strategy. Social software provides such a bottom-up mechanism for providing support within EAM-processes. Consequently, challenges of EA management processes are investigated, and contributions of social software presented. A cockpit provides interactive functions and visualization methods to cope with this complexity and enable the practical use of social software in enterprise architecture management processes.

Keyword: Enterprise architecture management processes

1 Introduction

Modern business models indispensably rely on information processing and a well-operated information economy [1] in the enterprise. Nevertheless, the complexity of a typical information economy has increased in the last two decades, in particular, with the advent of modern technologies supporting more complex business models. The management of enterprise information processing [2, 3] has become increasingly complicated and consequently, different disciplines have developed, each targeting a particular characteristic of the information economy. Business process management,

F. Fournier and J. Mendling (Eds.): BPM 2014 Workshops, LNBIP 202, pp. 452–462, 2015.
DOI: 10.1007/978-3-319-15895-2_39

for example [4], targets the key activities of business execution, whereas IT service management [5] is concerned with the reliable and cost-efficient operation of the IT infrastructure.

Enterprise architecture (EA) Management [2, 3, 6, 22] aims at the alignment of enterprise strategy, business processes, information system landscapes, and IT services. The integrated perspective of the EA provides a base for communication and coordination between the different management processes. EA Management processes seek to optimize the handling of information in the enterprise taking a holistic point of view, and to infuse these optimizations to the related management processes. Traditionally, such overarching planning relies on hierarchic coordination within enterprises, applying a top-down approach. Unfortunately, this approach is not able to cope with the speed and complexity of EA Management in today's economy. Furthermore, hierarchic coordination cannot exploit all potential contributions from the other management processes to find the optimal solution.

EA Management processes are intrinsically knowledge-intensive processes [6]. As such, they are characterized not by a strict execution order. With the growing complexity of management objects, the responsibilities in the EA Management processes are frequently revisited, and more and more roles are defined in response to the increasing complexity and size. This adds complexity to the management and decision processes, as not only the knowledge relevant for holistic decisions become largely dispersed, but also the underlying information.

Social software [7, 8] is a widely used-mechanism for supporting bottom-up, decentralized decision processes. Social Software provides four mechanisms: social production [9], weak ties [10], value-co-creation [11] and egalitarian decision processes [12]. Social production inverses the top-down planning of changes and replaces it with a bottom-up approach. Social software also leverages weak ties for spotting individuals owning important knowledge for EA Management. Value-co-creation complements the tayloristic organization of the specific management processes, like business process management, with a cooperative EA Management. This allows integrating contributions of users hitherto ignored. Egalitarian decision processes replace expert-based decisions and leverage the wisdom of the crowd for EA Management.

The contribution of this paper is therefore to analyze the challenge of EA management processes and to demonstrate the contribution of social software. It introduces interactive visualization-based techniques into social software and enables the use of social software in EA Management processes. By this means, social software shall be capable to cope with the complexity of EA Management.

The paper proceeds as follows. First EA Management is introduced, and its requirements to a bottom-up organization are identified. We revisit the coordinative nature of EA Management, discuss the characteristics of information-centered coordination processes, and outline the challenges and opportunities of tool support in the given environment. Then, the features of social software to support bottom-up and decentralized decisions processes are described. The following section describes the use of social software for decision support in EA Management processes by applying appropriate interactive and visualization-based techniques.

2 Enterprise Architecture Management Processes

Diverse approaches for EA Management for EA Management exist [1–3, 13–15] and amongst them, The Open Group Architecture Framework (TOGAF) [2] has become a widely appreciated de facto standard. TOGAF defines different areas-of-interest in the management object of the EA, namely the business architecture, the information architecture, the information systems architecture, and the technology architecture. As TOGAF further outlines, for each of these architectures, dedicated management processes may be in place in an organization, but only the alignment of plans is able to leverage potential synergies.

The ESARC – Enterprise Services Architecture Reference Cube [16, 17] (see Fig. 1) provides a holistic perspective on the aforementioned different areas-of-interest in the EA, and the activities of EA Management and Architecture Governance targeting the transformation of the EA.

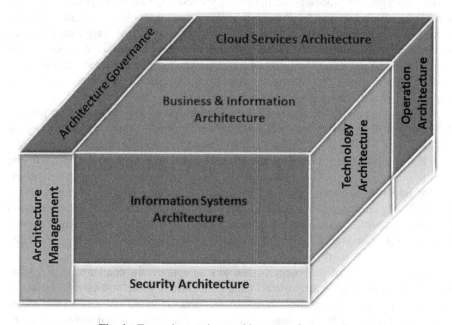

Fig. 1. Enterprise services architecture reference cube

The ESARC further displays the ties on the one hand, between the different areas-of-interest, and on the other hand, between the overall architecture, the management and the governance processes [1, 13]. Taking into account that for the different areas-of-interest also dedicated management processes exist in an enterprise, the challenges of EA Management become apparent immediately:

- Involve stakeholders with diverse concerns in differing but interrelated areas-of-interest.
- Provide a base for a holistic documentation of the EA and the development of enterprise transformations.

– Ensure that envisioned transformations are analyzed accounting for the impact in the different areas-of-interest to leverage synergies and avoid local optimizations.
– Facilitate the communication of enterprise transformations and take actions to promote stakeholder buy-in to the decision taken.

EA Management is a knowledge-intense process relying on complex and densely meshed models of the different components of an enterprise. In particular, size and complexity of these models, make tool support for EA Management indispensable [18]. A majority of prevalent tools does not account for existing management activities targeting selected areas-of-interest in the EA. Only a few tools are promoting an "integration approach" by focusing on integration models to describe the state of these areas-of-interest. These tools do not discuss mechanisms for supporting collaborative decision processes involving stakeholders from different management disciplines in the enterprise.

Enterprise Architecture Management processes are composed of EA Management activities [14]. Buckl et al. in-line with prevalent management literature identify three categories of EA Management activities:

– Develop and Describe: In activities of these categories, the as-is state of areas-of-interest in the EA is described, and planned as well as target states for areas-of-interest are developed.
– Analyze and Evaluate: In activities of these categories, states of the EA are analyzed with respect to optimization potential, and the ongoing transformation of the EA is reflected against the planned states.
– Communicate and Enact: In activities of these categories, views on the EA are communicated to stakeholders from different management processes, and actions are taken to ensure that architectural decisions are adhered to.

Activities of former three categories are complemented by activities characterized as "configure and adapt", which pertain to the management process itself. Thereby, they constitute the Architecture Governance, which as in [1] sets the frame for performing architecture management activities. A key aim of Architecture Governance is to set rules for architecture compliance to internal and external standards. Architecture Governance sets rules for the empowerment of people, defining the structures and procedures of an Architecture Governance Board, and setting rules for communication.

3   Social Software in EAM-Processes

Although concepts such as Business Process Management [4] introduced a customer-oriented perspective, it still contains many concepts following the ideas developed already in [19]. These are the division of larger tasks into defined, smaller tasks and the assignment of individual responsible to accomplish these tasks. Therefore, it does not surprise, that a plenty of approaches such as [20, 21] tried to develop support for cooperation beyond strictly structured business processes as almost all WFMSs and most of the BPMSs, but also some groupware and case management systems. However, these approaches become not as successful as expected.

When supporting EA management processes, one has to meet a number of challenges. The first challenge is the lack of a pre-defined workflow. Similar to adaptive case management [21], the control-flow of EA management processes cannot be pre-defined in most situation. Instead, the control-flow is defined "on-the-fly" during execution of the EA management process.

The second challenge is organizational integration [22]. Many early approaches addressing the support of EA management processes limited the participation of stakeholders. E.g. although classical groupware abstained from pre-defining a strict control flow, specific access rights to documents had been assigned. Thus, the group of possible contributors had been limited. In this way, an apriori-decision had been made deciding who may contribute and who may not. Some stakeholders were not able to contribute.

The third challenge is semantic integration [22]. Due to the involvement of a multitude of stakeholders, semantic frictions such as homonyms and synonyms create misunderstandings between the process participants. These semantic frictions may delay the EA management process or even worse, cause a wrong enterprise architecture.

Social software is based on four basic principles: social production [9], weak ties [10], collective decisions [23], and value co-creation [11]. Each of these principles supports EA management processes by addressing one or more challenge addressed above. These relationships are depicted in Fig. 2.

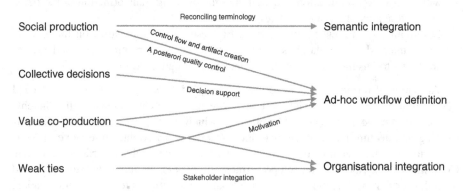

Fig. 2. Social software contributions to EA process challenges

Social production is the creation of artifacts without a top-down created plan but by combining the suggestions and decisions from independent contributors. By abstaining from tayloristic top-down planning, new and innovative contributions outside the original scope can be identified and added. Due to these properties, social production matches the requirements of EA management processes. The control flow of EA management processes can be defined in an ad hoc manner. During execution of the EA process, artifacts as architecture models can be created in a cooperative way. Using social software the model is created by the collaborative effort of all stakeholders instead of some experts. The stakeholders themselves are empowered to design the process. Social production also assures the quality of the created artifacts by using an a posteriori approach. By publishing all steps and results, a multitude of stakeholder is able to evaluate the quality of the artifacts created. By this visibility, contributors strive for an optimum quality not only according to predefined sets of measure, but in the best possible way according to their competence. Furthermore, social production fosters also semantic integration by supporting the collaborative reconciliation of terminology.

Collective decisions provide a new way in EA management processes to make decisions. They provide statistically better results than experts do, if the decision cannot be made using scientific means, and the participants decide independently. Surowiecki describes in [12] the approach of the so-called the wisdom of crowds. He argues that a decision made by several persons often leads to better results, because each person has a specific knowledge. Bringing together the knowledge of each person leads to a superior knowledge than the knowledge of each alone. Surowiecki describes four prerequisites for his these:

– Each person has different information.
– Each person has his own specific knowledge.
– Each person's opinion is independent.
– There are mechanisms to put the person's information and knowledge together.

Collective decisions are important to de-correlate errors by aggregating a large number of independent judgements. This is of particular importance for EA management processes, because decisions have often to be made in areas with not defined rules. A possible procedure is as follows. Past (human) decisions can be used for prediction as well as for further analytics, as shown in Fig. 3. Therefore, new decisions based on similar conditions of past decisions can be prepared or applied. Prediction algorithms for linear-data (e.g. linear Regression ARIMA Models [24, 25]) or non-linear data (e.g. Neuronal networks [26]) can be used for preparation new decisions. At the first, past decision of enterprise specialists must be analyzed. Generally, decisions situations are defined in different possible states (e.g., high usage of the EA; low usage of the EA) and possible actions (e.g. using an SOA EA; using non-SOA EA) as well as in different decision criteria (uncertainty, certainty, under risk) [27, 28].

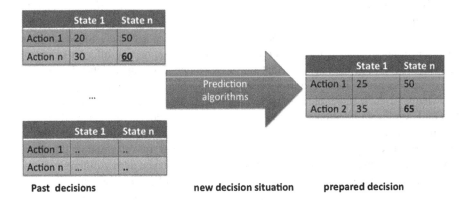

Fig. 3. Decision prediction

EAM specialists can provide and discuss information of different enterprise architecture variants via social software. This information can be used for preparing new decisions (and prediction algorithms) for EA as well as business processes. If this information are not in a structure form (e.g. score of each EA variant) an approach for analyzing unstructured data is needed. In case of text data (e.g. from social networks or blogs), a text mining approach can be applied [29]. Therefore, text data can be analyzed with different text-preprocessing steps like tokenization, stemming, etc. [30] and results based on an implemented enterprise architecture dictionary interpret.

Value-co-production is also supporting the definition and execution of EA management processes by integrating contributions from the business side. By abolishing the separation between artifact producer and consumer, a better adaptation to the individual requirements can be achieved. Furthermore, value co-production enhances the organizational integration. Before the use of social mechanisms, enterprise architecture management has been strongly driven by experts. However, already in the past, this approach was criticized. The knowledge and opinions of many stakeholders had been ignored by this approach. In the consequence, it was not possible to enforce permanently the enterprise architecture designed by the experts. Instead, often some time after the end of enterprise architecture design projects, the stakeholders returned to their old architecture.

Whereas value co-creation strive for the integration of stakeholders already identifier, weak ties help to identify persons with valuable knowledge. Weak Ties are connections between persons not implied by a formal organization. Weak ties may be defined by competencies and experiences but not in a top-down manner by management. Their use in enterprise architecture management changes the binary organization model used so far. Weak ties allow identifying competencies in organizations across department borders. E.g. people who are experts for a certain kind of process task may be distributed to different organizational units. Evaluating the weak ties between helps to solve problems more thoroughly. Capturing weak ties is a supplement to organizational modelling, which is contained in many enterprise architecture tools.

In the following, we want to consider the prerequisites and look how they are fulfilled using an EA cockpit [31]. Each stakeholder who takes place in a cockpit meeting has his own information because each stakeholder can say which views are relevant for him, and all these views are displayed simultaneously. Each stakeholder has his own specific knowledge because the stakeholders have different roles like Application Architect, Business Process Owner or Technology expert and come from different areas of the enterprise. Each role implies a very specific knowledge. Since each stakeholder comes from another area of the enterprise, have a different knowledge and his own goals, it is ensured that the stakeholders have an independent opinion about the decision. Lastly, Surowiecki urges mechanisms to put information and knowledge of each stakeholder together. The approach of Jugel et al. has the premise that all EA relevant information is part of an enterprise-wide EA repository. It has to be ensured that all EA Management relevant information is documented in the EA repository. The views displayed in the cockpit consist of information out of the EA repository. Thus, the consistency of information displayed across different views is made sure. The prerequisite of an integrated information base for the participants of a decision is fulfilled be the EA repository. A meeting moderator can put together the relevant stakeholder's knowledge by discussion.

4   Related Work

The approaches depicted so far follow more or less a tayloristic approach. On the one hand, this is intended to limit the complexity of the individual management processes. On the other hand, this increases complexity and makes un-aligned and potentially conflicting management decisions more likely. The resulting issue calls for bottom-up coordination mechanisms to facilitate the EA Management processes. Different approaches, like the ones of [14, 32–34] seek to apply such mechanisms. These approaches are information-centered and provide a decentralized coordination mechanism and decision making regarding the organization's information processing. Tool support for EA Management does, nevertheless, not embrace such mechanisms, but presents means for hierarchic coordination, if any.

Jugel et al. [31] describe an approach for interactive and visualization-based techniques. The approach gathers the idea of multiple-perspectives and refines it by applying the concept of cockpits in the context of EA planning. Cockpits are well established for e.g. controlling power plants or space missions and typically consist of several screens that simultaneously display necessary information for stakeholders. The information displayed are architecture views defined by viewpoints [35]. EA Visualizations like landscape or cluster diagrams are often used for EA analysis. Jugel et al. enhance such visualizations by interactive functions. These functions support stakeholders in the EA analysis and planning decision-making process. We exemplarily want to describe the interactive functions Graphical Highlighting and Annotating in the following. By applying the Graphical Highlighting, function stakeholders can visually highlight architecture elements that are particular of interest. Thus, all displayed architecture elements are part of an EA model that is part of an enterprise-wide EA Repository a highlighted element will be updated on any view in the cockpit. The annotating function enables a stakeholder to annotate an architecture element with descriptive text. The descriptive text can be used to document analysis results or decisions.

General discussions of social software in the field of business process management are described in [7, 8, 22, 36, 37]. Holden and Wilhelmij [38] describe base aspects of decision making via human resource integration business process factors in health care. Enterprise architecture research and principles are defined in [39]. Research on enterprise architecture and IT manager decisions are explored in [40–42].

5   Conclusions and Future Work

Modern enterprises need Enterprise Architecture Management to assure the alignment of business strategy, business processes and IT resources. EA management cannot rely on hierarchic management processes but has to apply bottom-up, information-centered coordination mechanisms. Social software provides such a bottom-up mechanism for providing support within EAM-processes. Challenges of EA management processes are the ad hoc definition of control flow and artifact creation and both organizational and semantic integration. This paper shows the application of social-software-based support for Enterprise architecture management processes. It is important to create architectures and business processes based on versatile human knowledge form a multitude of stakeholders trough social software. Without doing this, decisions might be non optimal, because of a smaller assessment and discussion of EA and BPM experts. A cockpit provides interactive functions and visualization methods to cope with complexity and enable the practical use of social software in enterprise architecture management processes.

This research shows both, practical and academic implications. First EAM managers can benefit from new knowledge about decision making trough social software. Therefore, the enterprise architecture as well as business processes can be improved in the dimension of time, cost, and quality. Academic implications are in the field of information systems and social science. The research on social-software decision based enterprise architecture is just taking off. Therefore, our paper shows general aspects and methods as well as foundations of the use of social software in this context. There are some limitations to discuss. Social-software based decision processes are not in every case the best decision-making method. Decisions are mostly dependent from the involved specialists. Further research should investigate industry specific differences on the use of decisions via social software, e.g. highly complaint industry sectors.

References

1. Weill, P., Ross, J.W.: It Governance: How Top Performers Manage It Decision Rights for Superior Results. Harvard Business School Press, Boston (2004)
2. Haren, V.: TOGAF Version 9.1. Van Haren Publishing, Amersfoort (2011)
3. Haren, V.: Archimate 2.0 Specification. Van Haren Publishing Series. Van Haren Publishing, Amersfoort (2012)
4. Weske, M.: Business Process Management: Concepts, Languages, Architectures. Springer, Heidelberg (2007)
5. The Stationery Office: The Official Introduction to the ITIL 3 Service Lifecycle: Office of Government Commerce. The Stationery Office Ltd., London (2007)
6. Johnson, P., Lagerström, R., Ekstedt, M., Österlind, M.: IT Management with Enterprise Architecture. KTH, Stockholm (2014)
7. Schmidt, R., Nurcan, S.: BPM and social software. In: Ardagna, D., Mecella, M., Yang, J. (eds.) Business Process Management Workshops. LNBIP, vol. 17, pp. 649–658. Springer, Heidelberg (2009)
8. Schmidt, R., Nurcan, S.: Augmenting BPM with social software. In: Rinderle-Ma, S., Sadiq, S., Leymann, F. (eds.) BPM 2009. LNBIP, vol. 43, pp. 201–206. Springer, Heidelberg (2010)
9. Benkler, Y.: The Wealth of Networks: How Social Production Transforms Markets and Freedom. Yale University Press, New Haven (2006)
10. Granovetter, M.: The strength of weak ties. Am. J. Sociol. **78**(6), 1360–1380 (1973)
11. Vargo, S.L., Maglio, P.P., Akaka, M.A.: On value and value co-creation: a service systems and service logic perspective. Eur. Manag. J. **26**(3), 145–152 (2008)
12. Surowiecki, J.: The Wisdom of Crowds: : Why the Many Are Smarter Than the Few and How Collective Wisdom Shapes Business, Economies, Societies and Nations. Anchor, New York (2005)
13. Ross, J.W., Weill, P., Robertson, D.C.: Enterprise Architecture as Strategy, vol. 1. Harvard Business School Press, Boston (2006)

14. Buckl, S.M.: Developing organization-specific enterprise architecture management functions using a method base. Dissertation, Technische Universität München, München (2011)
15. Schweda, C.M.: Development of organization-specific enterprise architecture modeling languages using building blocks. Dissertation, Technische Universität München, München (2011)
16. Zimmermann, A., Buckow, H., Groß, H.-J., Nandico, O.F., Piller, G., Prott, K.: Capability diagnostics of enterprise service architectures using a dedicated software architecture reference model. In: 2011 IEEE International Conference on Services Computing (SCC), pp. 592–599 (2011)
17. Zimmermann, A., Pretz, M., Zimmermann, G., Firesmith, D.G., Petrov, I.: Towards service-oriented enterprise architectures for big data applications in the cloud. In: 2013 17th IEEE International Enterprise Distributed Object Computing Conference Workshops (EDOCW), pp. 130–135 (2013)
18. Matthes, F., Buckl, S., Leitel, J., Schweda, C.M.: Enterprise Architecture Management Tool Survey 2008. Technische Universität München (2008)
19. Taylor, F.W.: The Principles of Scientific Management, vol. 202. Harper and Brothers, New York (1911)
20. Bruno, G.: requirements elicitation as a case of social process: an approach to its description. In: Rinderle-Ma, S., Sadiq, S., Leymann, F. (eds.) BPM 2009. LNBIP, vol. 43, pp. 243–254. Springer, Heidelberg (2010)
21. Swenson, K.D.: Mastering The Unpredictable: How Adaptive Case Management Will Revolutionize The Way That Knowledge Workers Get Things Do. Meghan-Kiffer Press, Tampa (2010)
22. Bruno, G., Dengler, F., Jennings, B., Khalaf, R., Nurcan, S., Prilla, M., Sarini, M., Schmidt, R., Silva, R.: Key challenges for enabling agile BPM with social software. J. Softw. Maint. Evol. Res. Pract. **23**(4), 297–326 (2011)
23. Tapscott, D., Williams, A.: Wikinomics: How Mass Collaboration Changes Everything. Penguin, New York (2006)
24. Montgomery, D.C., Peck, E.A., Vining, G.G.: Introduction to Linear Regression Analysis, vol. 821. Wiley, New York (2012)
25. Prybutok, V.R., Yi, J., Mitchell, D.: Comparison of neural network models with ARIMA and regression models for prediction of Houston's daily maximum ozone concentrations. Eur. J. Oper. Res. **122**(1), 31–40 (2000)
26. Hagan, M.T., Demuth, H.B., Beale, M.H., et al.: Neural Network Design. PWS Pub., Boston (1996)
27. Dumitru, V., Luban, F.: On some optimization problems under uncertainty. Fuzzy Sets Syst. **18**(3), 257–272 (1986)
28. G. S. die erste B. für diesen A. ab. Research Methodology and Statistical Analysis for M.Com. V K Publications (2008)
29. Tan, A.-H.: Text mining: the state of the art and the challenges. In: Proceedings of the PAKDD 1999 Workshop on Knowledge Disocovery from Advanced Databases, pp. 65–70 (1999)
30. Tan, P.-N., Blau, H., Harp, S., Goldman, R.: Textual data mining of service center call records. In: Proceedings of the Sixth ACM SIGKDD International Conference on Knowledge Discovery and Data Mining, pp. 417–423 (2000)
31. Jugel, D., Schweda, C.M.: Interactive functions of a cockpit for enterprise architecture planning. Presented at the TEAR 2014, Ulm, Germany, 1–5 September 2014
32. Hauder, M., Roth, S., Schulz, C., Matthes, F.: Agile enterprise architecture management: an analysis on the application of agile principles. In: International Symposium on Business Modeling and Software Design BMSD 2014, Luxemburg (2014)

33. Hanschke, I.: Strategisches Management der IT-Landschaft. Auflage Hanser, München (2010)
34. Mueller, T., Schuldt, D., Sewald, B., Morisse, M., Petrikina, J.: Towards inter-organizational Enterprise Architecture Management-Applicability of TOGAF 9.1 for Network Organizations (2013)
35. Emery, D., Hilliard, R.: Every architecture description needs a framework: expressing architecture frameworks using ISO/IEC 42010. In: Joint Working IEEE/IFIP Conference on Software Architecture, 2009 & European Conference on Software Architecture. WICSA/ECSA 2009, pp. 31–40 (2009)
36. Koschmider, A., Song, M., Reijers, H.A.: Social software for business process modeling. J. Inf. Technol. 25(3), 308–322 (2010)
37. Erol, S., Granitzer, M., Happ, S., Jantunen, S., Jennings, B., Johannesson, P., Koschmider, A., Nurcan, S., Rossi, D., Schmidt, R.: Combining BPM and social software: contradiction or chance? J. Softw. Maint. Evol. Res. Pract. 22(6–7), 449–476 (2010)
38. Holden, T., Wilhelmij, P.: Improved decision making through better integration of human resource and business process factors in a hospital situation. J. Manag. Inf. Syst. 12(3), 21–41 (1995)
39. Stelzer, D.: Enterprise architecture principles: literature review and research directions. In: Dan, A., Gittler, F., Toumani, F. (eds.) ICSOC/ServiceWave 2009. LNCS, vol. 6275, pp. 12–21. Springer, Heidelberg (2010)
40. Pulkkinen, M.: Systemic management of architectural decisions in enterprise architecture planning. Four dimensions and three abstraction levels. In: Proceedings of the 39th Annual Hawaii International Conference on System Sciences, 2006, HICSS 2006, vol. 8, p. 179a (2006)
41. Simonsson, M., Lindström, A., Johnson, P., Nordström, L., Grundbäck, J., Wijnbladh, O.: Scenario-based evaluation of enterprise architecture - a top-down approach for chief information officer decision making (2005)
42. Riempp, G., Gieffers-Ankel, S.: Application portfolio management: a decision-oriented view of enterprise architecture. Inf. Syst. E-Bus. Manag. 5(4), 359–378 (2007)

oBPM – An Opportunistic Approach to Business Process Modeling and Execution

David Grünert[(⊠)], Elke Brucker-Kley, and Thomas Keller

ZHAW School of Management and Law, Institute for Business
Information Management, 8401 Winterthur, Switzerland
{grud, brck, kell}@zhaw.ch

Abstract. Traditional workflow management systems are suited to automate well-structured processes based on a strict sequence of user tasks and a top-down approach to model creation. Such a conventional approach does not comply with the bottom-up philosophy of social software and therefore makes it difficult to incorporate its strengths in process modeling and automation. Opportunistic Business Process Modeling (oBPM) aims to overcome these limitations by introducing a new paradigm for modeling and executing business processes that is both user- and document-centric, adequate for bottom-up modeling, agile process modification, opportunistic task scheduling and process mining.

Keywords: Obpm · Content-oriented workflow models · Bottom-up model creation · Artifact-centric workflow models · Document-oriented workflow models

1   Introduction

Automation projects are traditionally modeled in a top-down approach and within two consecutive project phases [13, 14]. In the first phase, a model is created on a business level by business analysts, who are domain experts themselves or who gather insights from domain experts. In the second phase, the model is translated by software engineers into a technical and executable model. Although the two models might be created within the same BPM suite, there is no automated translation from the business to the technical model and no manual translation without profound technical know-how.

In the two phases of the automation project, the creation of the process model and the creation of the technical model, knowledge workers typically only have a consultative role. On the one hand, the reason might be hierarchical acting and thinking within the company, but on the other hand, separation is also caused by the process model itself. The complexity of the models and the required specific know-how of modeling semantics and syntax make it difficult to integrate knowledge workers [16]. Furthermore, most models show the processes from a top-down perspective that covers the activities of many roles. This perspective is not adequate for knowledge workers to develop or change the process because they are only familiar with their own tasks, but often do not know the overall process [16].

Also the granularity of processes typically created in today's automation projects is a problem in the context of social software. Social production as described in [11]

© Springer International Publishing Switzerland 2015
F. Fournier and J. Mendling (Eds.): BPM 2014 Workshops, LNBIP 202, pp. 463–474, 2015.
DOI: 10.1007/978-3-319-15895-2_40

requires a model adequate for agile development that allows combining the input from independent contributors [15]. This is only possible if changes to the model have limited or at least determinable side effects for the overall process and simultaneously applied process modifications.

Applying social software patterns [17] to "ground" traditional top-down business process management is not an easy task. The two-level approach during modeling and the separation of modeling and process execution conflicts with the idea of egalitarianism that intends to handle all contributors of a business process equally in order to get the best solution [12, 16]. The exclusion of business users from hands-on process definition and improvement is not primarily an organizational problem, but caused by the fact that conventional BPM methods and technologies are simply not designed for business users. Business process modeling notations were introduced to provide a common ground for business analysts, who create top-level process models, and software engineers, who turn them into executable processes. BPMN and BPEL may successfully foster the consistent top-down traceability through multiple levels of processes and sub-processes (see [14]). However, they are targeted at BPM specialists and do not empower the business user, who executes the process, to influence the design or to change the execution of the process. Leaving this top-down perspective is a challenge with today's BPM tools and practices. To achieve a user-centric model, business processes must be cut into small sequences that cover activities of only one role. A common approach for this is to define short user-centric processes triggered by ad hoc events. Unfortunately, this model lacks an overall process perspective, making it difficult to define dependencies between such processes. Therefore, modeling with ad hoc triggered user-centric mini-processes within today's BPM suites is rather a workaround than a real modeling paradigm.

Another challenge is agile development and continuous improvement of business processes. If there is more than one model involved, or if the model is not understood by all users including knowledge workers, the development cycle becomes longer compared to an approach with a single model understood by everyone [18].

Another aspect related to egalitarianism is the strict execution order for tasks. The strict task order that is typical for process automation patronizes knowledge workers even if there is no need for such restrictions and makes the task execution not only less efficient but prevents knowledge workers from leveraging their expertise to effectively handle a diverse set of cases. However, modeling opportunistic scheduling using today's process automation frameworks and tools is far more complex than implementing a task with strict order. Hence, it is very challenging to come up with a convincing business case for automating business processes that require a high degree of flexibility.

Opportunistic BPM (oBPM), as outlined in the following chapter, addresses these problems with a model that is simpler and closer to the daily working experience of business users, allowing them to understand and contribute to the model. Furthermore, oBPM includes a top-down as well as a bottom-up perspective that both allow seamless modification to the very same model. This approach makes it unnecessary to synchronize multiple models, while still combining the advantage of the two model perspectives.

In contrast to simple user-centric ad hoc processes modeled with BPMN, oBPM defines the dependencies between all these user-centric processes without making the model complicated. This results in a fine-grained model adequate for agile and simultaneous modification. oBPM also allows opportunistic task scheduling where users can decide what to do first.

All of the challenges mentioned above originate in the lack of a bottom-up perspective and flexibility. Social software enables participation and a dynamic approach to problem solving. But in order to make use of those advantages, a more opportunistic approach to business process modeling and execution is required.

2   Business Process Modeling with oBPM

Opportunistic BPM stands for designing processes with a minimum of control flow by modeling the states of artefacts involved in business processes. The rationale behind this approach is outlined in Sect. 1 and can also be found in [16] *"The participation of end users on the collaborative design of business process models is particularly challenging because they do not master the existing formal business process modeling languages, and they regard business processes on a case-by-case perspective."* or in [18] *"There is much to gain in supporting users to come up with better models in a shorter time-frame."* or in [19] *"Embed processes in a social context. In many BPMSs, users have a very limited view of the processes in which they participate, often only seeing an in-tray as the interface. Instead, users should be given access to a wider context of the processes including information about other people that may contribute to the processes as well as histories of previous process executions."* However, oBPM is not meant to support unstructured communication and knowledge/information sharing as is the focus of pure social software.

The oBPM model is both user- and document-centric[1] and has two different perspectives. The first perspective shows the top-down view based on standard UML diagrams (see also BPM lifecycle [22]). This perspective is useful for process owners or system administrators. The second perspective is used for the bottom-up model creation and allows knowledge workers to read, change and define their own processes as suggested in [17]. The following section introduces the top-down perspective while the bottom-up perspective is introduced in Sect. 3.1.

2.1   The oBPM Model from Top-Down Perspective

This section defines all key elements of the oBPM process model and introduces a sample application. The workflow for any business process modeled with oBPM can be defined with:

- one use case diagram,
- one class diagram and
- as many finite state machine diagrams as there are documents or artefacts used in the workflow.

---

[1] We use the term <document> as a synonym for any kind of artefact.

The following three sections describe these diagrams and their usage in oBPM for a sample application. The sample application supports a process for refunding bills. The process starts when the administration receives bills and ends with the bill being either accepted or rejected. Bills that are accepted are refunded to the submitter by the finance department. Rejected bills are not refunded but the submitter is allowed to file an objection that must be judged by a lawyer. The validation of a bill consists of two independent checks: the check of the submitter for being a valid sender and the subject of the bill for being in line with the respective regulations. In addition, it must be possible to stop the validation process in case of death of a submitter at any time.

Use Case Diagram for Role, Task and Document Associations. The oBPM model uses roles, tasks and documents and defines dependencies between these elements. First, the oBPM model associates every role with tasks that can be executed by this role. This association is directed and the direction defines whether the task is triggered by the role or the system. In the example shown in Fig. 1, users with role <Administration> can initiate the task <File objection>, while the task <Judge bill> is always triggered by the system. Second, the model associates each task with one or more documents used to execute the task. In the example shown in Fig. 1, lawyers need documents of the type <Bill>, <Objection> and <Message> to handle an objection. The role <System> is used to identify automated tasks that do not require user interaction.

Class Diagram for Case and Document Associations. The use case diagram in Fig. 1 only identifies the type of document being used in tasks. It does neither say anything about the number of these documents nor about their dependency with a case. Therefore, the oBPM makes use of an additional model formatted as class diagram that defines the number of documents possibly used in a case as well as their associations. In the example shown in Fig. 2, each case can have an unlimited number of bills with one objection and up to two messages. This information is needed by the oBPM system when new cases are opened and when documents are added to a case. It is also needed to maintain cross references between documents.

State Machine Diagram for Document States. The last diagram used to complete the oBPM model is a state machine diagram. This diagram is the key element of oBPM. It exists once for each document type being used in the use case and in the class diagram. The purpose of the state machine diagram is to define all possible states and state transitions of a document and it also identifies the roles that can initiate these transitions. Figures 3 and 4 show an example of such a state machine for the document named <Bill>. The state machine diagrams can make use of composite state and state hierarchy to model ad hoc events. In addition, state transitions must be labeled with a guard and an event. The guard identifies the role that is allowed to initiate the transition. The event refers to the respective use case.

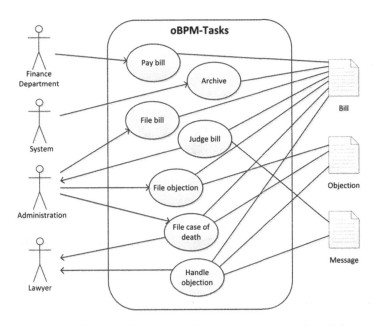

Fig. 1. Use case diagram defining associations between roles, tasks and documents

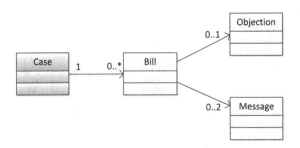

Fig. 2. Class diagram defining dependencies between documents and case

3   Benefits of oBPM

oBPM supports bottom-up model creation, agile process definition, opportunistic task scheduling and process mining. How these benefits are achieved is described in Sects. 3.1 to 3.3.

3.1   Bottom-up Model Perspective and Agile Process Definition

The three diagrams introduced in chapter 2 show the top-down perspective of the oBPM model. This perspective is useful for process owners and system administrators but not for knowledge workers. On one hand, these diagrams require specific know-how of the respective diagram syntax, and on the other hand, the diagrams show many

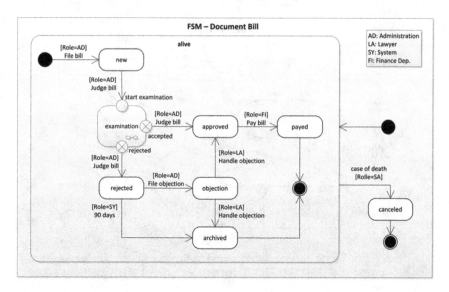

Fig. 3. State machine diagram defining possible state transitions for document <Bill>

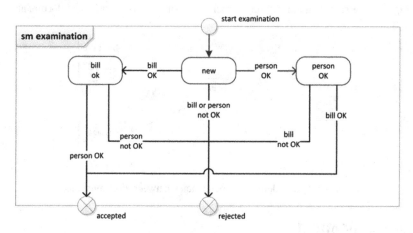

Fig. 4. State machine diagram for sub state <examination>

details not relevant for a specific user role. In the bottom-up perspective of the oBPM model, only tasks relevant for a selected role are shown. From this perspective, the following three questions must be answered:

1. Which tasks can I execute and who is responsible to trigger them?
2. Which documents or artefacts do I need to execute these tasks?
3. What are the possible state transitions for these documents during a task?

This information can be shown in a simple table. Table 1 shows all model information relevant for the role <Administration> as defined in the diagrams in Figs. 1, 2, 3, 4.

It is important to mention that this bottom-up perspective is not a local model. In opposite to the solution proposed in [20], where a type view containing the global model and an instance view containing local variations of the model is defined, oBPM uses a single model with two perspectives. Any modification made in bottom-up perspective alters the global model. Thus is no need to synchronize local and global models as it is the case in [20]. The interface used by end-users to define and change the workflow requires the following functionality:

- Adding, changing and deleting tasks for the user's role.
- Adding and deleting documents to all of the user's tasks.
- Adding, changing and deleting possible state transitions for every document.

By defining the required tasks incrementally, it is possible to specify the overall process in an agile way. Thereby the model remains executable, even if it is incomplete, as described in [20]. Deleting tasks, documents and transitions requires special handling for active cases. For instance, it must be considered that cases don't end up in a dead lock. A dead lock can occur when state transitions are altered in such a way that there is no set of transitions possible leading to an end state. Most other modifications of the model can be applied to active cases without restrictions. Defining new document types might be restricted to system administrators in order to achieve proper linking of the documents to the case as required by Fig. 2.

Table 1. Model summary for role <Administration>

My tasks	Trigger	Document	Start states	End states
File bill	I do	Bill	–	new
Judge bill	System	Bill	new, bill OK, person OK	bill OK, person OK
			bill OK	accepted, rejected
			person OK	accepted, rejected
		Message	–	new
File objection	I do	Bill	rejected	objection
		Message	–	new
Case of death	I do	Bill	any	canceled

3.2 Model Execution and Opportunistic Task Scheduling

In the previous sections, we introduced the modeling aspect of oBPM. We will now address the question how a system can process this information and how the workflow is finally presented to the user.

The system executing oBPM needs to manage the state of all documents and implement a fine-grained access control. This access control is based on document types, roles and on the current state of documents. By applying the model, the executing system is able to derive a role-dependent task list from these states. How this can be done is shown in the following example.

Assuming the system needs to evaluate if users with role <Administration> are currently allowed to file an objection. The system therefore searches the content of Table 1 for required documents and their states. The result of this search is that the documents <Message> and <Bill> are both required. Table 1 also defines that document <Bill> must be in state <rejected>, while for document <Message> no initial state is defined. Having no initial state means that the document can be created "on the fly". Such documents do not define any prerequisites for a task. The system can now apply this rule to all cases and allow the action <File objection> for all cases having a document <Bill> in state <rejected> (see Fig. 5).

Finally, the result of this operation must be visualized for users. A possible solution is a role-dependent task list in combination with a filter. The filter defines which tasks are shown in the list and allows choosing between all tasks and the tasks for a selected case. The tasks shown in the list are grouped according to the categories introduced in Table 2 and can be started directly from there. For illustration, Table 3 assigns the tasks from the example workflow for role <Administration> to the defined categories.

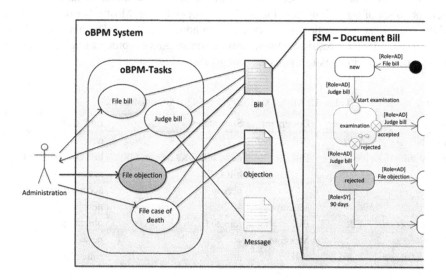

Fig. 5. Example for execution of an oBPM

The way how oBPM is executed by the system also shows how the opportunistic behavior is achieved:

- The tasks do not appear in the task list based on a predefined sequence. Tasks appear as soon as all preconditions in terms of document states are fulfilled.
- In tasks modeled by sub states as shown in Fig. 4, the user is free to choose any execution path within the sub state machine.
- Also in tasks without sub states, users are allowed to partially complete a task by editing only selected documents. The remaining documents can either be edited by users with access to the same task or even by any other role that is allowed to modify these documents. Therefore it is not even required that all users involved have access to the same task!

Table 2. Types of user tasks

Category	Description
Possible actions	Contains all ad hoc actions that can be initiated by the user. Such actions do not need a document as input and the user has to select the case he wants to work on
Tasks for groups	Contains all tasks that can be executed by multiple roles including the role of the user. The system locates these tasks by searching for documents that are in a state where the next transition can be triggered by different roles
Tasks for role	Contains all tasks that can be executed by the user's roles and no other. The system locates these tasks by searching for documents that are in a state where the next transition can only be triggered by the user's role

Table 3. Types of user tasks

Category	Description
Possible actions	File bill: This task is shown because the only document associated is created during this activity
	File case of death: This is an ad hoc task. It can be executed for any case that is in the state <alive>
Tasks for groups	File objection: A separate task is shown for every case where the document Bill is in the state rejected. From this state, the next state transition can either be triggered by the role <Administration> or, when the deadline is reached, by the system
Tasks for role	Judge bill: A separate task is shown for every case where the document Bill is in one of the states <new>, <bill OK> or <person OK>

3.3 Process Mining

oBPM allows to execute a business case in various ways and it even supports continuous improvement of the processes with bottom-up model creation and editing. However, it seems likely that not all execution paths are equal in terms of overall effort, throughput or other performance indicators. By logging the execution path of all cases, oBPM can offer a rich data set to identify the best execution paths for cases. This data set can even be aggregated with externally collected data like customer satisfaction and other performance data to further improve the selection of execution paths. That collected information is richer and more structured than using just e-Mail logs [16], since all the activities follow the rules set up in the state charts for the artefacts and therefore have a well-defined context.

As a result of such an execution path analysis, the system may suggest the most efficient execution paths to the users during execution. The result may also lead to a restriction of model execution to preferred paths by applying rules based on the above mentioned process mining results. With such restrictions, such a process model evolves from oBPM to a traditional well-structured business process. A sophisticated tool could even automate this transition by generating well-structured business processes in BPMN or other tool-specific modeling languages from the collected data sets.

4 Related Work

From an application perspective, oBPM combines Enterprise Content Management (ECM) with Business Process Management (BPM) and a variety of modeling techniques (see Fig. 6). All of these techniques and the approach to combine ECM and BPM applications, for example in document-centric workflow solutions, are nothing new, but there is no product or consulting practice that combines all of these aspects. The Blueprinting Framework, for instance [10] also combines ECM and BPM but does not implement object and state orientation like oBPM. There is also no other approach known for process modeling that is both user- and document-centric with the possibility for bottom-up model creation, agile model adaptation, opportunistic task scheduling and ability for process mining.

A concept closely related to oBPM is the so called content- or data-oriented workflow model. The term "content-oriented" first appeared in [1] and is used as an umbrella term for several scientific workflow approaches, namely "data-driven", "resource-driven", "artifact-centric", "object-aware" and "document-oriented" (see [8]). Common to all of these models is the definition of workflows based on documents, data records or other objects containing process data. Content-oriented workflow models are a topic of ongoing research and numerous publications are available ([2, 3, 6]).

Similar to oBPM, most content-oriented workflow models allow multiple execution paths of a business case similar to the opportunistic task order of oBPM. However, only few approaches make the linking of the document state machines as explicit as oBPM. Because of the content-centric approach, content-oriented workflow models are typically well suited for modeling ad hoc events. What is new in oBPM is the combination of these aspects with the ability for bottom-up model creation, process mining and the definition of a formalized process model in UML.

Several sample implementations of content-oriented workflow models have been made for scientific purpose and could demonstrate their capabilities ([4, 5]). However, most of these implementations are addressing specific application domains like the health sector or the automotive industry. So far, there is no general purpose business process modeling tool implementing a content-oriented workflow model, but there are software providers doing research on artifact-centric workflow models (see [7]).

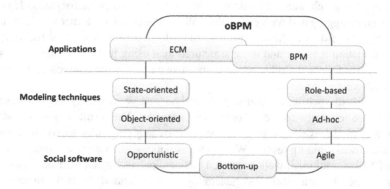

Fig. 6. oBPM and related applications and techniques (Figure adapted from [9])

Fleischmann et al. [21] coined the term subject-oriented BPM (S-BPM), describing a bottom-up process modeling approach that pursues similar aims as the bottom-up perspective introduced in this paper. The common goal is to involve the end-users in order to decrease the complexity of the models and design methodology while increasing the acceptance of the resulting automation solutions. However, using our approach, the model captures more details of the process artefacts including full object-oriented artefact specification and finite state machines. Furthermore, our approach not only provides a bottom-up design methodology but also increases the number of task execution paths and therefore provides end-users with more flexible automation solutions.

5   Conclusion

Although still in an early prototype phase, we clearly see the potential of oBPM to bring business process modeling and execution power to the business user without sacrificing on proven modeling techniques. Both software providers and end-user organizations could benefit from oBPM, since it opens up the space of business process automation from large-scale implementations and highly structured processes to a larger variety of solutions: On the one hand, oBPM potentially lowers the entry barrier to the world of process automation for small and medium enterprises. On the other hand, oBPM supports the user-centric IT enablement for unstructured processes that have so far been out of scope of traditional business process automation initiatives. It leverages social software without losing the advantages of structured models.

References

1. Christoph P, et al.: The alpha-flow use-case of breast cancer treatment - modeling inter-institutional healthcare workflows by active documents. In: Proceedings of the 8th International Workshop on Agent-based Computing for Enterprise Collaboration (ACEC), Larissa, Greece (2010)
2. Müller, D., Reichert, M., Herbst, J.: Data-driven modeling and coordination of large process structures. In: Meersman, R., Tari, Z. (eds.) OTM 2007, Part I. LNCS, vol. 4803, pp. 131–149. Springer, Heidelberg (2007)
3. Chiao, C.M., Künzle, V.: Manfred Reichert: Integrated modeling of process-and data-centric software systems with PHILharmonicFlows, pp. 1–10. CPSM@ICSM (2013)
4. COREPRO (Configuration-based Release Management Processes in the Automotive Sector) (2005–2007), University of Twente
5. PHILharmonic Flows - Process, Humans and Information Linkage for harmonic Business Flows, University of Ulm, Institute of Databases and Information Systems
6. Cohn, D., Hull, R.: Business artifacts: a data-centric approach to modeling business operations and processes. Bull. IEEE Comput. Soc. Tech. Comm. Data Eng. 32(3), 3–9 (2009)
7. Business Artifacts Research at IBM. http://researcher.watson.ibm.com/researcher/view_project.php?id=2501

8. Wikipedia article, Content-oriented workflow models. http://en.wikipedia.org/wiki/Content-oriented_workflow_models. Accessed 23 May 2014

9. Tanner, S.: Opportunistic BPM: Ein Prototyp, Masterarbeit an der ZHAW in Wirtschaftsinformatik, Juni 2014, Winterthur, Switzerland

10. Vom Brocke, J., Cleven, A., Simons, A.: Towards a business process-oriented approach to enterprice content management: the ECM-blueprinting framework. Inf. Syst. e-Bus. Manag. 9, S. 475–496 (2011). Berlin Heidelberg: Springer-Verlag

11. Benkler, Y.: The Wealth of Networks: How Social Production Transforms Markets and Freedom. Yale University Press, New Haven (2006)

12. Surowiecki, J.: The Wisdom of Crowds. Anchor, New York (2005)

13. Grünert, D., Keller, T.: Business process modeling using activity pattern. In: 12th International Conference on e-Society 2014, pp. 193–199. Madrid, Spain (2014)

14. Silver, B.: BPMN Method and Style: A Levels-Based Methodology for BPM Process Modeling and Improvement Using BPMN 2.0. Cody-Cassidy Press, Aptos (2009)

15. Mathiesen, P., et al.: Applying social technology to business process lifecycle management. In: Daniel, F., Barkaoui, K., Dustdar, S. (eds.) Business Process Management Workshops. Lecture Notes in Business Information Processing, pp. 231–241. Springer, Heidelberg (2012)

16. Martinho, D., Rito Silva, A.: Non-intrusive capture of business processes using social software. In: Daniel, F., Barkaoui, K., Dustdar, S. (eds.) Business Process Management Workshops. Lecture Notes in Business Information Processing, pp. 207–218. Springer, Heidelberg (2012)

17. Musser, J., O'Reilly, T.: Web 2.0 Principles and Best Practices. Harvard Law School, Boston (2006)

18. Koschmider, A., Song, M., Reijers, H.A.: Social software for modeling business processes. In: Ardagna, D., Mecella, M., Yang, J. (eds.) Business Process Management Workshops. Lecture Notes in Business Information Processing, vol. 17, pp. 666–677. Springer, Heidelberg (2009)

19. Johannesson, P., Andersson, B., Wohed, P.: Business process management with social software systems – a new paradigm for work organisation. In: Ardagna, D., Mecella, M., Yang, J. (eds.) Business Process Management Workshops. Lecture Notes in Business Information Processing, vol. 17, pp. 659–665. Springer, Heidelberg (2009)

20. Silva, A.R., Meziani, R., Magalhães, R., Martinho, D., Aguiar, A., Flores, N.: AGILIPO: Embedding Social Software Features into Business Process Tools. In: Rinderle-Ma, S., Sadiq, S., Leymann, F. (eds.) BPM 2009. LNBIP, vol. 43, pp. 219–230. Springer, Heidelberg (2010)

21. Fleischmann, A., et al.: Subject-oriented business process management. Springer Publishing, New york (2012)

22. Becker, K., Rosemann, M.: Business Process Lifecycle Management, White paper (2001)

DeMiMoP 2014

Constructing Probabilistic Process Models Based on Hidden Markov Models for Resource Allocation

Berny Carrera and Jae-Yoon Jung[(⊠)]

Department of Industrial and Management Systems Engineering,
Kyung Hee University, 1 Seochen-Dong, Giheung-Gu,
Yongin, Gyeonggi, Republic of Korea
{berny, jyjung}@khu.ac.kr

Abstract. A Hidden Markov Model (HMM) is a temporal statistical model which is widely utilized for various applications such as gene prediction, speech recognition and localization prediction. HMM represents the state of the process in a discrete variable, where the values are the possible observations of the world. For the purpose of process mining for resource allocation, HMM can be applied to discover a probabilistic workflow model from activities and identify the observations based on the resources utilized by each activity. In this paper, we introduce a process discovery method that combines an organizational perspective with a probabilistic approach to address the resource allocation and improve the productivity of resource management, maximizing the likelihood of the model using the Expectation-Maximization procedure.

Keywords: Probabilistic process discovery · Process mining · Resource allocation · Hidden markov models

1 Introduction

The basic idea of business process modeling is how enterprises can represent actual processes in the way that those processes can be analyzed and improved. Through this model, organizations can obtain a graphical representation of the process activities defining a workflow in order to reach and accomplish intended objectives of business processes [1].

Currently, existing process models do not consider a probabilistic analysis of resources. Consequently, this paper examines a probabilistic approach to resource allocation to represent the relationship between resources and their activities as well as analyze their transitions to indicate the importance of each resource in the related activity. Hence, based on the context of process mining and their perspectives [2], this study will emphasize a control-flow perspective combined with an organizational perspective to support resource allocation by constructing a stochastic model from an event log and reveal how the resources interact directly with the activities.

Meanwhile, machine learning and process mining techniques are closely related [3]. Some machine learning algorithms operate as a "black box" but are helpful for creating systems that can learn from data through poor control-flow discovery.

F. Fournier and J. Mendling (Eds.): BPM 2014 Workshops, LNBIP 202, pp. 477–488, 2015.
DOI: 10.1007/978-3-319-15895-2_41

Some machine learning techniques [4] are statistically based on the way that they have learned from data and are concerned with the collection, analysis, and interpretation of data, making these techniques the heart of quantitative reasoning which is necessary for making decisions and recommendations in systems. Hence, HMM is a technique that can deal precisely with noise, incompleteness and not over-fitting the model unlike other techniques e.g. decision trees, support vector machines, ANOVA, etc.

In general, HMM can be helpful in a specific form of the transition process and the process can be considered as a series of time slices. Basically, HMM is modeled after the process in different states for each activity, and the observations in HMM become the resources that interact with the activities. As a result, this research evaluates the possibility of discovering an extended probabilistic process model from a control-flow process with an organizational perspective by applying HMM for resource allocation, analyzing the resource attribute of each event and the activities flow, and estimating the parameters for each activity (state) and resource (observation).

Therefore, this paper investigates the contribution of the applicability of HMM for process mining based on previous premises by defining a probabilistic model that is likely to explain the observed behavior that considers the control-flow patterns, resources, and organization structure.

The remainder of the paper is organized as follows. First, the related work is discussed in more detail in Sect. 2. Section 3 introduces the event logs and HMM notations for the proposed model and explains HMM workflow discovery. Section 4 presents the estimation of the probabilities, resource allocation notations and applicability of the HMM Miner. Finally, Sect. 5 provides the conclusions and future work of the paper.

2 Related Work

There are a few research approaches of HMM in process mining. Rozinat et al. [5] propose a method that begins with a petri-net in order to construct a HMM for a quality evaluation of the model, taking into account different metrics like fitness and precision. Da Silva and Ferreira [6] apply HMM in sequence clustering, where all the elements of the sequence are related with each state in the model as well as propose five different topologies for the model. In [7, 8], the intension mining approach is proposed to identify the reasoning of processes that are behind of the activities.

A number of previous studies have focused on resource and actions or reactions in the business process execution. Rozinat and van der Aalst [3] propose a decision mining technique based on case perspective analysis. Song and van der Aalst [10] present social mining that has an organizational perspective which monitors the originators and relationships and focuses on how the originators interact between them, though not directly with the activities. Recently, Kim et al. [11] introduced a performer recommendation using a decision tree which focuses on time and organizational perspective, resulting in the length of the decision tree becoming too large and too difficult to analyze.

The proposed approach based on the probabilistic method differs from the existing studies from two perspectives: the control-flow perspective proposing a model based on the order of activities, and organizational perspective analyzing and proposing the best interaction between the activities and resources.

3   HMM-Based Process Mining

3.1   Resource-Oriented Event Log

An event log is used as input of process mining to construct models that explain and interpret some aspect of the behavior stored. The event log contains traces referring to the number of cases, activities and resources, as shown in Table 1. It should be noted that this study has not taken into account time stamps or other types of data. Instead, the formal models presented by van der Aalst [12] are extended for HMM miner which adds a limitation based on an event log and a footprint matrix, and it is defined as a resource-oriented event log which follows:

Definition 1. (Resource-Oriented Event Log) Let L be an event log. L is a tuple $< C, S, V >$, where C is the set of all possible cases, S of length N is the finite set of event labels $\{s_1, \ldots, s_N\}$ that has been performed over L, and $V \in L^*$ of length M is a set of originators $\{v_1, \ldots, v_M\}$ that specify the resource associated with the task.

The construction of HMM workflow is explained in Sects. 3.2 and 3.3. To calculate the initial parameters, the event log is needed to mine the frequency of the occurrence of the activities and resources. This is explained more in Sect. 4. Section 5 discusses how to find the maximum-likelihood estimation (MLE).

Table 1. Example of process log.

Case ID	Activity
1	$a_{Pete}, b_{Sue}, c_{Sean}, d_{Mike}$
2	$a_{Ellen}, b_{Sean}, c_{Sue}, d_{Pete}$
3	$a_{Mike}, b_{Sue}, c_{Sue}, d_{Mike}$
4	$a_{Pete}, c_{Sean}, b_{Sue}, d_{Mike}$
5	$a_{Pete}, c_{Sean}, b_{Sue}, d_{Ellen}$
6	$a_{Ellen}, e_{Sue}, d_{Pete}$

3.2   HMM Miner Algorithm

To accommodate the event log, process mining, and HMM in terms of resource allocation, the concepts of HMM workflow is introduced. The formal notation for the HMM workflow is as follows:

Definition 2. (HMM Workflow) Let L be a resource-oriented event log. A HMM workflow $\theta(L) = (s, V, Fs, Fv)$ is represented by:

- $s = \{s_1, \ldots, s_N, \varepsilon_{N+1}\} \in L$ where $\{s_1, \ldots, s_N\}$ are the states or activities of L and $\{\varepsilon_{N+1}\}$ a dummy end state.

- $V = \{v_1, \ldots, v_M, \varepsilon_{M+1}\} \in L$ where $\{v_1 \ldots v_M\}$ are the observations of resources and $\{\varepsilon_{M+1}\}$ a dummy observation of the dummy end state $\{\varepsilon_{N+1}\}$.
- Fs is an NxN matrix with footprint sequence and frequency of occurrence for transitions s_i to s_j.
- Fv is an NxM matrix with the frequency of occurrence for resources V in state s_i.

The procedure for constructing the HMM workflow is presented in Fig. 1. The HMM miner algorithm first investigates the control-flow perspective of a process model from an event log, and considers the order of the events within a case. The attributes such as case id, activity, and resource are utilized in the mining process.

1:	**Input:** event log L
2:	**Initialize**
3:	Find all activities S and all resources V in the traces in L.
4:	Find start activities S_s and end activities from S_e
5:	Create a footprint matrix with frequencies F_s from L
6:	Create a frequency matrix F_v from L
7:	Add the corresponding state s_i into the initial state set S_s with its starting probability π.
8:	Create dummy state $s_{N+1} = \varepsilon$ with an arc from ε to ε in S for refer the end of process
9:	Create dummy observation $v_{M+1} = \varepsilon$ to denote the end resource for state ε.
10:	All end activities given by S_e, the corresponding states s_i are end states; then create an arc from s_i to ε and calculate each frequency.
11:	**For** each pair (s_i, s_j) in S
12:	**If** fs_{ij} in Fs has a "direct follow" **then**
13:	Create an arc from s_i to s_j with its frequency (fs_{ij}).
14:	**End For**
15:	**For** each pair (s_i, v_j) in F_v
16:	**If** $fv_{ij} > 0$ **then**
17:	Create an arc from s_i to v_j with its frequency (fv_{ij}).
18:	**End For**
19:	HMM workflow $\theta(L) = (s, V, Fs, Fv)$
20:	Calculate probabilities for A in arcs and B for related activities of v_i in each s_i.
21:	**Output:** initial HMM: $\lambda = (N, M, A, B, \pi)$

Fig. 1. HMM miner algorithm.

3.3   Mining Markovian States

HMM workflow learns from the event log which is fully observed data where the states of the HMM can be represented based on the activities. It takes the notation of event logs to describe the example log in Table 1 where it observes the event sequences $L = < abcd, abcd, abcd, acbd, acbd, aed >$.

In order to discover a process model, the event log has to be analyzed while it is mining the causal dependencies by using the footprint notation for HMM Miner, and, when analyzed, different patterns of the states evaluate the precedence of each activity, and the frequency of the observed sequences. In order to satisfy these requirements the footprint matrix is introduced in Definition 3.

In process mining, α-algorithm [9] is considered one of the baseline techniques for analysis of patterns in event logs. In our approach, a footprint matrix is required to construct the state transitions of a HMM model analyzing the relations of a pair of activities. The footprint matrix is focused on a process perspective especially in analysis and differentiation of activities sequences. It can measure the frequency of activities and the sequences, helping to real situations where the data is not complete or has noise.

Definition 3. (Footprint Matrix for HMM Miner) Let L be an event log. Let $x_1, x_2 \in L$:

- $x_1 >_L x_2$ if and only if there is a trace $\sigma = <t_1, t_2, t_3,\ldots, t_n>$ and $i \in \{1,\ldots, n\text{-}1\}$ such that $\sigma \in L$ and $t_i = x_1$ and $t_{i+1} = x_2$ (Contains all pairs of activities in a "directly follows"). If is a directly follow, $fs = \sum_{\sigma \in L} L(\sigma)$
- $x_1 \rightarrow_L x_2$ if and only if $x_1 >_L x_2$ and $x_2 >_L x_1$ (Contains all pairs of activities in a "causality" relation
- $x_1 \#_L x_2$ if and only if $x_1 >_L x_2$ and $x_2 >_L x_1$
- $x_1 \|_L x_2$ of and only if $x_1 >_L x_2$ and $x_2 >_L x_1$

Table 2. Footprint matrix Fs for event log in Table 1.

	a	b	c	d	e
a	#	$\rightarrow$, 3	$\rightarrow$, 2	#	$\rightarrow$, 1
b	$\leftarrow$	#	$\|$, 3	$\rightarrow$, 2	#
c	$\leftarrow$	$\|$, 2	#	$\rightarrow$, 3	#
d	#	$\leftarrow$	$\leftarrow$	#	$\leftarrow$
e	$\leftarrow$	#	#	$\rightarrow$, 1	#

For our implementation activities x1, x2 … xn, are the states for the HMM, e.g. $a, b, \ldots, e$. After constructing the footprint matrix, the next step is to start with the construction of a Markov chain that simulates a dependency graph based on the states of HMM. The HMM diagram has states expressed by "oval shape and activity name," and transitions are represented by two different "arcs," one for transition activities and other for the resource relationships. The first one represents the successor states and in terms of resource mining, the relationship between the activities, and the second, the observations (resources) that correspond to that activity, e.g. activity a has a causality relation with activities b, c and e; so, it is creates a transition denoted by an "arc" from a to these activities. The initial states of the HMM workflow are denoted graphically by a double oval, and the probabilities of each initial state are assigned in the initial state distribution π. Figure 2 shows that all observations were represented with a "square shape and resource name" and assigned directly to each state, and, in turn, the resources are mined from the event log and related to specific activity.

To model the end of the process dummy state ε is added, which receives its input from the last activity in each sequence and from which no other state is reachable. Consequently, the transition probability from this state to itself should equal 1. Figure 2 describes a constructed HMM workflow and the interaction of the activities with the different resources show how after the state d is fired and reaches the state ε.

The next section describes how to estimate the probabilities in the mode which first, calculates the initial values for the state transition probability distribution A and for the observation symbol probability distribution B. After several steps, it is determined that the expectation maximization for these probabilities obtains the estimated $A*$ and $B*$.

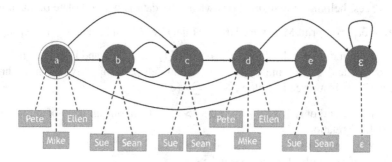

Fig. 2. HMM workflow constructed from the footprint matrix without probabilities of Table 2.

4 Resource Allocation with HMM Miner

4.1 Relating Resources to HMM

After obtaining the mined structure of HMM, including the number of states (activities) N, name of the different states s, count of observations (resources) M, label of each observation V and the initial states defined in π, the next step is to determine the initial state transition probability distribution A and the observation symbol probability distribution B. To begin analyzing both probability distributions, the frequency f of each activity and resource, is needed and with them, the weight of the arcs can be calculated, and it is possible to decide which elements should be kept for analysis, and which elements can be discarded to reduce the noise of the mined event log. Starting with the transition probabilities, the footprint matrix is needed to obtain the frequencies.

In order to start the analysis to get the probabilities for the HMM workflow the assumption is made that the data is from an event log $L = < C, S, V >$; and each event in L is given by a tuple (s, v) and the total events in L is K. Then $(s_k, v_k) = (s_1, v_1),...,$ (s_N, v_M) the probabilities can be computed and collected :

$$\prod_k P(s_K, v_K). \tag{1}$$

$$P(s, v) = \prod_i \pi_i^{f(i)} \cdot \prod_{i,j} a_{i,j}^{f(i,j)} \cdot \prod_{i,o} b_i(v_k)^{f(v_k)}. \tag{2}$$

Note in this equation, it is taken in account the frequency where $f(i)$ is the number of times i is the initial state in (s,v). In $f(i,j)$ the number of times j follows i in (s,v) this frequency is in the footprint matrix Fs and $f(v_k)$ the number of times i is paired with observation v is in matrix Fv.

According to these HMM parameters, the log probability can be easily calculated:

$$L(\lambda) = \sum_{l=1}^{k} log P(s_l, v_l). \tag{3}$$

$$Log(\lambda) = \sum_{l=1}^{k} \sum_{i} f(i) log(\pi_i) + \sum_{i,j} f(i,j) log(a_{i,j})$$
$$+ \sum_{i,v_k} f(v_k) log(b_i(v_k)). \tag{4}$$

In order to find λ that give us a maximum value for $L(\lambda)$ The following formula is needed: d $L(\lambda)/d\lambda = 0$

$$\pi_i = \frac{\sum_i f(i)}{\sum_i \sum_h f(h)}. \tag{5}$$

$$a_{i,j} = \frac{\sum_i f(i,j)}{\sum_i \sum_h f(i,h)}. \tag{6}$$

$$b_i(v_k) = \frac{\sum_i f(i)}{\sum_i \sum_{v'_k \in V} f(i, v'_k)} \tag{7}$$

Basically, a supervised learning from all mined activities and resources is taken, allowing for the calculation of the probability of each element independently.

4.2 Maximum Likelihood Estimation

Knowing the initial values $\lambda = (N, M, A, B, \pi)$; it would be possible to estimate the maximum likelihood in selecting the best values for the model parameters that make the observed data the most probable and obtain $\lambda^* = (N, M, A^*, B^*, \pi^*)$. As described in Fig. 3, EM procedure essentially calculates their values in 2 steps E and M can be calculated using forward and backward algorithms [4] for HMM.

In order to improve λ, the EM procedure uses α_i from the forward algorithm and β_i from the backward algorithm, which utilizes the variables γ and ξ as temporal variables [4] in order to estimate the values of A^*, B^*, and π^*.

$$\gamma_i(t) = \frac{\alpha_i(t) * \beta_i(t)}{\sum_{j=1}^{N} \alpha_j(t) * \beta_j(t)}. \tag{8}$$

$$\xi_{ij}(t) = \frac{\alpha_i(t) * a_{ij} * \beta_j(t+1) * b_j(v_{t+1})}{\sum_{p=1}^{N} \sum_{q=1}^{N} \alpha_p(t) * a_{pq} * \beta_q(t+1) * b_q(v_{t+1})}. \tag{9}$$

1:	**Inputs:** $\lambda = (N, M, A, B, \pi)$ and event log L
2:	**Initialize**
3:	**Repeat**
4:	Using forward algorithm calculate α_i for each trace in L
5:	Using backward algorithm calculate β_i for each trace in L
6:	Re-estimation of temporal variables
7:	Calculate γ and ξ based on $\sum \alpha_i$ and $\sum \beta_i$
8:	Calculate A^*, B^*, π^* from the temporal variables
9:	Updating λ
10:	**Until** A and B do not change
11:	**Output:** $\lambda^* = (N, M, A^*, B^*, \pi^*)$

Fig. 3. Expectation-Maximization procedure.

Given an observation sequence, $\gamma_i(t)$ is the probability of being in state i at time t and $\xi_{ij}(t)$ is the probability of being in state i at time t and being in state j at time $t + 1$. These temporal variables are useful in order to determine the maximum likelihood of the parameters, $\gamma_i(t)$ can be interpreted like the possibility to be in a specific activity on a determined time of the process and $\xi_{ij}(t)$ the probability of the following activities in a specified time.

$$\pi_i^* = \gamma_1. \tag{10}$$

where π_i^* is the expected initial state distribution at time 1 in state i. In other words, the expected probability is to begin the process in a specific activity.

$$a_{ij}^* = \frac{\sum_{t=1}^{T-1} \xi_{ij}(t)}{\sum_{t=1}^{T-1} \gamma_i(t)}. \tag{11}$$

where a_{ij}^* is the expected state transition probability distribution, and is the number of times that the transition i occurs in sequence from $t = 1$ to $T - 1$. Then, a_{ij}^* is the expected probability from being in activity i to j.

$$b_j^*(v_k) = \frac{\sum_{t=1; v_t = v_k}^{T-1} \gamma_j(t)}{\sum_{t=1}^{T-1} \gamma_j(t)}. \tag{12}$$

$b_j^*(v_k)$ is the expected observation symbol probability distribution, where is the expected number of times in state j and observing symbol v_k, divided by the expected number of times in j. In terms of this study, it is the predicted parameters of the resources assigned to a specified activity.

4.3   Example

The example is based on the event log from Table 1. It is used for the mining algorithm in Fig. 1 in order to construct the HMM workflow. In Table 2, a footprint matrix is created and Fig. 2 shows the mined HMM workflow without the frequencies. From this point, the next step is calculate the frequency matrix Fv for the analysis of resources, and calculates the initial parameters explained in Sect. 4.1, and the values for the maximum likelihood explained in Sect. 4.2.

First, the mined event log produces three different activity sequences and the algorithm estimate a percentage for $<$ abcdε $>$ with 0.5 %, $<$ acbdε $>$ with 0.33 % and $<$ aedε $>$ with 0.16 %, the number of states that identifies each activity are $N = 6$ with $s = \{$a, b, c, d, e, $\varepsilon\}$ and the number of resources that will be the observations $M = 6$ with $V = \{$Pete, Mike, Ellen, Sue, Sean, $\varepsilon\}$.

Table 3. Frequency matrix Fv for event log in Table 1.

	Pete	Mike	Ellen	Sue	Sean	ε
a	3	1	2	0	0	0
b	0	0	0	4	1	0
c	0	0	0	2	3	0
d	2	3	1	0	0	0
e	0	0	0	1	0	0
ε	0	0	0	0	0	1

Table 3 shows the frequency of resources s_i based on activities v_j and is used to create the observation symbol probability distribution $B = \{b_i(v_k)\}$. The initial state distribution is $\pi_i = [1, 0, 0, 0, 0, 0]^T$, where activity $\{$a$\}$ is the only one that starts all the process sequence.

Table 4. State transition probability distribution $A = \{a_{i,j}\}$

	a	b	c	d	e	ε
a	0	3/6	2/6	0	1/6	0
b	0	0	3/5	2/5	0	0
c	0	2/5	0	3/5	0	0
d	0	0	0	0	0	1
e	0	0	0	1.0	0	0
ε	0	0	0	0	0	1.0

Table 4 shows the probabilities for HMM workflow from Eq. 6 where it analyzes the transition from the state i corresponding to the current transition to all states j. For example to assign value probability from activity $\{$a$\}$ to $\{$b$\}$, after $\{$a$\}$ is fired $\{$b, c, e$\}$ can be the next state, the total frequency of sequences $\{$ab$\}$, $\{$ac$\}$ and $\{$ae$\}$ are 6, and evaluating just $\{$ab$\}$ the frequency is 3 showed in Table 2, the probability is 3/6. In the case of resources probabilities, Table 5 shows the observation probability distribution where it is analyzes the resources that interact with a specific activity. For example, in activity $\{$a$\}$ the resources used are $\{$Pete, Mike, Ellen$\}$ the total frequency is 6 and frequency observed for $\{$Mike$\}$ is 1 showed in Table 3, then applying Eq. 7 the probability is 1/6.

Table 5. Observation symbol probability distribution $B = \{b_i(v_k)\}$

	Pete	Mike	Ellen	Sue	Sean	ε
a	3/6	1/6	2/6	0	0	0
b	0	0	0	4/5	1/5	0
c	0	0	0	2/5	3/5	0
d	2/6	3/6	1/6	0	0	0
e	0	0	0	1.0	0	0
ε	0	0	0	0	0	1.0

With the initial values for the HMM workflow, the EM procedure is utilized to estimate the expected values for transition $A*$ and observation $B*$ distribution. Tables 6 and 7 are shown in graphical form in Fig. 3.

Table 6. Expected state transition probability distribution $A* = \{a_{ij}^*\}$

	a	b	c	d	e	ε
a	0	0.53298	0.3987	0	0.6832	0
b	0	0	0.51998	0.48002	0	0
c	0	0.42249	0	0.57751	0	0
d	0	0	0	0	0	1.0
e	0	0	0	1.0	0	0
ε	0	0	0	0	0	1.0

Table 7. Expected observation symbol probability distribution $B* = \{b_j^*(v_k)\}$

	Pete	Mike	Ellen	Sue	Sean	ε
a	0.5	0.16667	0.33333	0	0	0
b	0	0	0	0.79102	0.20898	0
c	0	0	0	0.44717	0.55283	0
d	0.33333	0.5	0.16667	0	0	0
e	0	0	0	1.0	0	0
ε	0	0	0	0	0	1.0

It should be noted that this study has been primarily concerned with the estimation of control flow probabilities and the analysis of work distributions between resources and activities. Our approach is helpful to answer related questions in resource allocation, such as: "How to determine the experience of resources in a specific activity?," "How to promote a resource effectively based on their experience?" and "What activity has to be scheduled and the resources required?."

We plan to conduct related experiments in the near future in order to compare and evaluate the proposed method using real-life event logs and implement it in a ProM framework (Fig. 4).

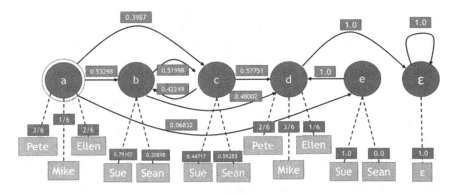

Fig. 4. Estimated HMM workflow constructed from the footprint matrix of Table 1.

5 Conclusions

This study presented designs a probabilistic discovery process from event log using HMM to support resource allocation. Specifically, the expectation maximization approach was adopted for estimating the model parameters. The proposed method is useful in real-world scenarios for managing standard errors and noise in real case event logs. Since determining the number of hidden states is very difficult, the following model was based on activities and resources in such a way that the comprehension of the model is enhanced. Also, the proposed technique is helpful to compare the performance of resources for activity executions. Future work includes the consideration of the time perspective to analyze if a resource is busy and the extension of the technique to other scenarios.

Acknowledgments. This research was supported by Basic Science Research Program through the National Research Foundation of Korea (NRF) funded by the Ministry of Science, ICT & Future Planning (No. 2012R1A1B4003505).

References

1. Aguilar-Saven, R.S.: Business process modelling: Review and framework. Int. J. Prod. Econ. **90**(2), 129–149 (2004)
2. van der Aalst, W., Adriansyah, A., de Medeiros, A.K.A., Arcieri, F., Baier, T., Blickle, T., Pontieri, L., et al.: Process mining manifesto. In: Florian, D., Kamel, B., Schahram, D. (eds.) BPM 2006. LNBIP, vol. 99, pp. 169–194. Springer, Heidelberg (2006)
3. Rozinat, A., van der Aalst, W.M.: Decision mining in ProM. In: Dustdar, S., Fiadeiro, J.L., Sheth, A.P. (eds.) BPM 2006. LNCS, vol. 4102, pp. 420–425. Springer, Heidelberg (2006)
4. Bishop, C.M.: Pattern Recognition and Machine Learning. Springer, New York (2006)
5. Rozinat, A., Veloso, M., van der Aalst, W.M.P.: Using hidden markov models to evaluate the quality of discovered process models. Extended Version. BPM Center Report BPM-08-10. BPMcenter.org (2008)

6. da Silva, G.A., Ferreira, D.R.: Applying hidden Markov models to process mining. In Sistemas e Tecnologias de Informação. AISTI/FEUP/UPF (2009)
7. Khodabandelou, G.: Supervised intentional process models discovery using hidden markov models. In: RCIS 2013, pp. 1–11. IEEE Press (2013)
8. Khodabandelou, G., Hug, C., Deneckère, R., Salinesi, C.: Process mining versus intention mining. In: Nurcan, S., Proper, H.A., Soffer, P., Krogstie, J., Schmidt, R., Halpin, T., Bider, I. (eds.) BPMDS 2013 and EMMSAD 2013. LNBIP, vol. 147, pp. 466–480. Springer, Heidelberg (2013)
9. van der Aalst, W.M.P., Weijters, T., Maruster, L.: Workflow mining: discovering process models from event logs. IEEE T. Knowl. Data En. 16(9), 1128–1142 (2004)
10. Song, M., van der Aalst, W.M.P.: Towards comprehensive support for organizational mining. Decis. Support Syst. 46(1), 300–317 (2008)
11. Kim, A., Obregon, J., Jung, J.-Y.: Constructing decision trees from process logs for performer recommendation. In: Lohmann, N., Song, M., Wohed, P. (eds.) BPM 2013 Workshops. LNBIP, vol. 171, pp. 224–236. Springer, Heidelberg (2014)
12. van der Aalst, W.M.P.: Process Mining: Discovery, Conformance and Enhancement of Business Processes. Springer, Heidelberg (2011)

Business Rules: From SBVR to Information Systems

Jandisson Soares de Jesus[✉] and Ana Cristina Vieira de Melo

Instituto de Matemática e Estatística, Universidade de São Paulo,
Rua do Matão 1010, Cidade Universitária, São Paulo, Brazil
{jandison,acvm}@ime.usp.br
http://www.ime.usp.br

Abstract. The ability to rapidly adapt to change is an important feature of any information system. Business rules play an important role in this dynamic as they have a high probability of being changed as time goes by. To closely follow these constant changes, the information system must be very flexible. The Semantic of Business Vocabularies and Business Rules (SBVR) is a model designed to be used by business people to communicate their business rules in a standard and formal way. SBVR and most of the business rules models do not define how to implement business rules in an information system in such a way that all flexibility needs are met. In this work we suggest an approach in with business rule implementations are confined to rules engines (independent systems designed to execute business rules) and kept separated from system executions. We will start explaining our method to identify which events in the SBVR model could lead to a violation of the defined business rules. Then we define a standard model to establish communication between business rule engines and all other information system elements. Our model uses the identified events of the first part to define when each business rule must be verified by the rule engines.

1 Introduction

Business rules are restrictions or guidelines adopted by, or imposed on an organization. They are defined by organizations to implement their enterprise strategies and policies, and to conform to external restrictions and laws. They are classified as vertical rules because, in general, they could affect various departments and processes in the organization. In other words, they are high-level restrictions applied to a large set of organizations' operations. Some examples of business rules are:

- "All projects estimated to run for at least six months have to be approved by a committee"
- "The client of a new gold account must be older than 24 years"
- "Special clients have 10 % discount on every order"

Organizations must be fast to adapt their systems to new business rules; otherwise they could suffer legal penalties or miss business opportunities. The ability of quickly adapting to new business rules must be included as a system feature at

© Springer International Publishing Switzerland 2015
F. Fournier and J. Mendling (Eds.): BPM 2014 Workshops, LNBIP 202, pp. 489–503, 2015.
DOI: 10.1007/978-3-319-15895-2_42

the design stage, enabling the system to evolve to new business rules. Together with this specified feature, the system architecture must be designed to encompass the evolutionary business rules. A good strategy to achieve this is the separation of business rules implementation (in the so called **rule engines**) from the other system elements implementation. This strategy helps manage business rules in a more independent and easy way because the impact of changing business rules becames more predictable.

Apart from the architectural strategy to accomplish with the evolutionary feature of business rules, one important aspect to consider when implementing business rules is how they are defined by business people. These rules need to be formally defined to avoid misunderstanding and be correctly implemented in information systems. SBVR (*Semantics model of Business Vocabularies and Business rules*) is an initiative created to represent business rules [1] with this purpose. This model is an OMG standard that provides an abstract language with a set of concepts and basic structures to formally and explicitly communicate the meaning of business rules. SBVR only describes how to represent business rules without giving directions on how to actually implement them in information systems or in rules engines.

The models used to represent business rules and the technologies to actually implement them are independent from each other. This leads to a gap between the specification and implementation of business rules. To overcome this gap our work provides two contributions. First, a standard abstract model is created to provide the communication behavior between rule engines and information systems, as suggested in our architecture; the business rules executions are separated from the system execution. Our standard model defines how this business rule execution and the other system elements must communicate with each other. The second contribution is a method to instantiate the abstract model by extracting from SBVR business rules definitions all events that may create rule violations and when they need to be checked. This approach smoothens business rules implementation since those models are used as guideline to correctly implement business rules and pointing out the time to check for rules violations.

The remainder of the paper is organized as follows: Sect. 2 describes the main concepts of SBVR and introduces its semantic formulations. We describe in Sect. 3 our approach to implement business rules in information systems. Section 4 describes our method to extract the relevant events from the SBVR semantic formulation. In Sect. 5 we describe our communication model between rule engines and information system. An example about how our approach can be used in a real scenario is given in Sect. 6. Some related works are described in Sect. 7. Finally, we present the conclusion of our work in Sect. 8.

2   Business Rules and SBVR

The *Semantic of Business Vocabulary and Business Rules* (SBVR) provides a set of concepts and abstract structures to allow organizations formally define the meaning of their business rules. This general specification can be used to create models to reduce (or remove) ambiguities and inconsistencies in business model definitions [2]. The SBVR rationale is based on the fact that business people tend to use their own language to express business rules. The language can be as informal as English, or based on predefined and more formal concepts like UML profiles [3]. Using SBVR, organizations can still use their own language to state business rules. However, along with these representations, they must have a formal statement on the meaning of the rules defined in SBVR. This formal statement is called a *semantic formulation* and it is based on first-order logic with a modal logic extension. As a result, rules become formally defined, opening the possibility of transferring business rules between organizations that use different representation models while still preserving the rule's meaning.

A SBVR semantic formulation of a given business rule is a logical definition of its meaning. In general, business people implicitly use these logical constructions such as quantifications, disjunctions, negation and implication when stating business rules in their own language. SBVR semantic formulation comes to express the same elements, but in an explicit and precise way. The semantic mapping provided in the semantic formulation will formally specify what the business rules mean. SBVR semantic formulations are represented as textual statements. Each row of these statements defines: a formulation element; some relationship between them; or some features related to elements in the formulation. For example, a description of what a quantification means together with information on its relationships and restrictions with other semantic elements in the system is part of a semantic formulation. It can also be recursive, re-usable and compositional, embedding other semantic formulations [1].

2.1 SBVR Formulation: Example

Here, we present a semantic formulation example generated from a business rule description written in English. Bajwa et al. [4] described a method to generate SBVR semantic formulations from business rules written in English. It is out of this paper's scope to explain the whole process since the focus is on the implementation models from SBVR formulations.

Business Rule Definition

> **BR0:** "Orders with total Value greater than $ 5000.00 must have 10 % discount."

SBVR Semantic Formulation of BR0

This proposition is meant by a universal quantification.
The universal quantification introduces a first variable.
The first variable ranges over the Order concept.
The universal quantification scopes over an implication formulation.
The antecedent of the implication formulation is a conjunction formulation.
The conjunction's operand 1 is an existential formulation.
The existential formulation introduces a second variable.
The second variable ranges over the Total Value concept.

The existential formulation scopes over an atomic formulation.
The atomic formulation is based on the fact type Order has Total Value.
The first role of the atomic formulation binds to the first variable.
The second role of the atomic formulation bounds to the second variable.
The conjunction's operand 2 is an atomic formulation.
The atomic formulation is based on the fact type number is greater than, or equal to number.
The first role of the atomic formulation bounds to the second variable.
The second role of the atomic formulation bounds to "5000".
The consequent of the implication formulation is an atomic formulation.
The atomic formulation is based on the fact type Order has Discount.
The first role is bounded to the first variable.
The second role is bounded to '10 %'.

The first lines define that the business rule starts with a quantification. This quantification is upon on a variable of the concept **Order** and the instances of this variable are constrained by an implication. This implication has a conjunction as antecedent that says that there is a **Total value** concept and this **Total value** is greater or equal to $5000,00. As the consequent of the implication, there is an atomic formulation connecting the **Order** concept with a 10 % discount. An atomic formulation is the simplest type of formulation to associate concepts. All these constructions together build up the meaning of the business rule.

3   Business Rules Implementation in Information Systems

The main idea of our approach is to separate rule engine execution from the overall system execution by modeling them as two independent processes running in parallel. Separating these elements is beneficial to software evolution because the system itself, and the business rules, can evolve independently. Business people can use tools to manage the business rules with lower impact to the information system. Besides that, as business rules execution is treated as an independent process, it can run in parallel with a set of other systems, allowing the use of business rules in a distributed architecture.

An important aspect of this separation is how to define the time each business rule needs to be checked by the rule engine. One option is to check all rules at each computational step of the information system. However, that would be very time consuming. A better approach, as illustrated in the Fig. 1, is checking for business rules violations when there is a real expectation of violation due to operations performed by the information system. In this case, the information system must have a mechanism that will communicate with the rule engine when it detects the occurrence of any event that could lead to a violation of a business rule. The rule engine, in turn, receives this notification and will be in charge of checking whether the business rule has been violated or not.

In order to achieve the implementation model depicted in Fig. 1, we need to consider two aspects. First, the information system must detect the occurrence of events that could lead to business rule violations. The second aspect is how

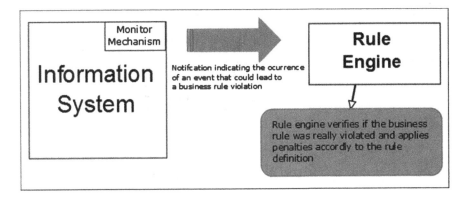

Fig. 1. Business rule verification and system execution running as two parallel processes.

the communication between the rule engine and the information system will be made. To satisfy these needs, we developed:

1. A **method to identify events**, from the SBVR model, that could lead to business rule violations. At the implementation level, whenever any of those events occur, the information system must invoke the business rule engine to apply inference algorithms to reason about rules satisfiability.
2. A **communication model** between the information system and the rule engine. The communication model must have a clear representation of which events need to be monitored in the system execution in order to request business rule validation. These events are those extracted from the SBVR model (previous item).

These aspects of our approach are detailed in Sects. 4 and 5.

4   Events Identification

During the use of an information system there is the occurrence of a lot of events generated by user interaction or some other external source. Examples of these events are the creation of a new product and the modification of a client record. Some of these events can lead to a business rule violation. The question is how to identify which events actually can represent a possible business rule violation and which do not. In order to identify these events, it is necessary to figure out which concepts are related to the observed business rule. For example, let us analyse the business rule **BR1**.

> **BR1:** All projects estimated to run for at least six months have to be approved by a committee.

In practice, **this rule could only be violated when a new project is created or the run-time of a project is modified**. The method for events

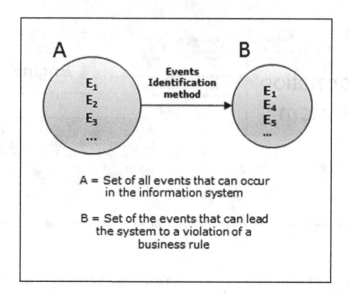

Fig. 2. Identification of the events that can lead the system to a violation of a business rule.

identification must systematically recognize those events from SBVR business rules specifications as depicted in the Fig. 2. The quantifications used in the semantic formulation of rules are the key point of this process.

As already shown in Sect. 2, SBVR semantic formulations use quantifications to introduce *variables*. Figure 3 illustrates how SBVR organizes concepts, variables and the corresponding instances. To recognize, from the SBVR semantic

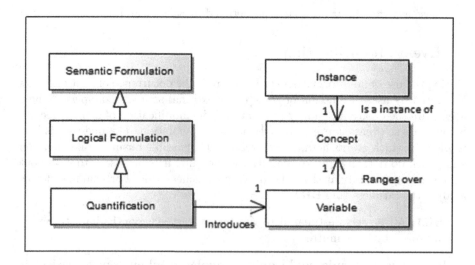

Fig. 3. Relation between SBVR variables, concepts and quantifications.

formulation, the events that can lead to a rule violation, we must first look at the quantifications to find out which *concepts* are related to that business rule. For example, the semantic formulation of the business rule.

BR2: All contracts must have at least one associated lawyer.

Must have two quantifications: a *universal* quantification to introduce the **contract** concept; and an *at-least-one* quantification to introduce the **lawyer** concept.

Analyzing the business rule **BR2**, we can see that if a lawyer retires or is fired, the rule engine must look at the contracts and lawyers databases to check if there is an orphan contract and then apply a corresponding operation to keep the system in a stable state. Note that the event "delete lawyer" could lead the system into a non-conformity state regarding the business rule **BR2**. This means that this event must be monitored and whenever it happens, the business rule satisfiability must be checked and an action to recover the system stability must be taken if the rule is violated. Similarly, the events of adding instances of contract must be monitored because the new contract must have at least one associated lawyer.

In a general way, the three abstract events that must be monitored in systems due to their capability of driving the system to non-conformity business rules states are: **creation, modification** and **removal** of any instance of the population of the concepts related to a business rule. For the sake of simplification, the work presented here addresses only the main types of SBVR rules, instead of covering rule types such as projections, objectifications and nominations.

5   Communication Model

The system architecture suggested in Fig. 1 requires two processes running in parallel: the system itself and the business rule engine, responsible for checking rules satisfiability. To make them running in parallel, a communication model to determine how these two processes will exchange information is needed. The information system will be responsible for monitoring events that could affect the business rules conformity state. Whenever certain events occur, the business rule engine takes control to check state conformity and pass the control back to the information system to recover from an unstable state, if necessary. The communication model is in between information system and rule engine to control their interaction.

In principle, we could check the business rule satisfiability whenever an event happens in the system. If so, the business rules engine would do this operation all the time, lessening the performance of the overall system. As observed in Sect. 4, the events that can affect the business rules conformity are restricted to creation, modification and removal of some concepts related to a business rule. Conformity checking can then be reduced to this restricted set of events, making the overall system more efficient.

Table 1. Main π-calculus syntax

Operator	Description
$P = Z\|Q$	Agents Z and Q running in parallel
$P = a.Q$	Execute action "a" and then behaves as Q
$P = (a + b).Q$	Execute action "a" or action "b" and then behave as Q
$P = a(x).Q$	Receive value "x" through channel "a" and then behave as Q
$P = \overline{a}\langle x \rangle.Q$	Send value "x" through channel "a" and then behaves as Q

5.1 Abstract Communication Model

The abstract communication model is a generic model which determines how the information will be passed to/from information systems and their rules engines counterparts. To describe our communication model, we use a formal language created to describe concurrent systems called π-calculus [5]. Table 1 shows the main syntax elements of the π-calculus.

Our abstract model is comprised of three main agents:

- *Listener* is in charge of monitoring events in the information system that could lead to business rules violation.
- *Notifier* notifies rules engine when the business rule satisfiability must be checked.
- Finally, *Integrator* puts the other two agents in parallel execution to control all events and their interaction.

Listener-#x = (

new**Var1**(Instance#u) +
alt**Var1**(Instance#u) +
del**Var1**Instance#u) +
. . .
new**Varn**(Instance#u) +
alt**Varn**(Instance#u) +
del**Varn**Instance#u)

). $\overline{notifyEngine}\langle\#x,\#u\rangle$. *Listener-#x*

Notifier-#x = notifyEngine(#x,#u) . τ . *Notifier-#x*

Integrator-#x = *Listener-#x* | *Notifier-#x*

The *Listener* process contains a sum of actions, representing exclusive choices because only a single event can be treated at a time. For each concept variable, detected in the identification step, a choice of the events of creation (new), modification (alt) or removal (del) over an instance of the variable is created. The *notifyEngine* action, in process *Notifier*, passes the control to the business rules engine when any of the events in the *Listener* is fired. This notification sends a #x parameter representing the identification of the business rule and a #u parameter to represent the concept variable. The behavior of agent *Integrator* is to perform the parallel composition of *Notifier* and *Listener*, giving the interaction control between the information system and the rules engine.

5.2   Model Instantiation

The model presented in the previous section is generic. For each particular system, it must be instantiated for each business rule specified in the system. To instantiate the abstract communication model, the main concepts (variables) recognized in the first step are used and applied to the communication model (Sect. 5.1).

Communication Model Instantiation. Given a system S with a set of business rules BRs formulated in SBVR, for each semantic formulation of a business rule $\#\ x \in BRs$:

1. Instantiate *Listener-#x*:
   For each variable introduced by a quantification in the formulation of business rule $\#\ u$ in SBVR: create an action within the process *Listener-#x* for each event related to this variable. This corresponds to instantiate the three events (new, alt and del) to each variable instance.
2. Instantiate *Notifier-#x*:
   For each variable introduced by a quantification in the formulation of business rule $\#\ u$ in SBVR: a notifyEngine(#x, #u) action must be created.
3. Instantiate the *Integrator-#x* process.

6   Application of the Approach

In order to use our approach in a real scenario we need to follow a set of steps:

1. Business people define the business rules that need to be enforced in the information system. The definition can be made using any language.
2. The semantics of these business rules are translated to SBVR semantic formulations (this translation is out of the scope of this work).
3. Each business rule semantic formulation is used to instantiate our abstract communication model.
4. The information system uses these communication model instances to inform the rule engine when there is a chance of a business rule violation.
5. The rule engine applies its algorithms to determine if the rule was actually violated.

Here, an application example is used to illustrate theses steps. We show how our approach can be used to facilitate business rule implementation in a real scenario. Suppose an e-commerce system allows customers to access a Website that offers a range of products, from different suppliers. Customers can choose and order products using this Website. Once a product is ordered, it is sent to a supplier who should deliver products directly to customers. The organization has several registered suppliers around the world and the choice of delivering a request to a particular supplier, instead of others, is based on a set of business rules. Two examples of possible business rules defined in this context are:

BR3: Old suppliers have priority over new suppliers.
BR4: Orders with a fraud rate greater than 10 % need to be manually approved.

Using the method described in Sect. 4 we identify, from the SBVR semantic formulation of **BR3**, the concepts which must be monitored.

SBVR Semantic Formulation of BR3

1. *This proposition is meant by a universal quantification*
2. *The universal quantification introduces a first variable*
3. *The first variable ranges over the concept **Old supplier***
4. *The universal quantification scopes over an existential quantification*
5. *The existential quantification introduces a second variable*
6. *The second variable ranges over the concept **New supplier***
7. *The existential quantification scopes over an implication formulation*
8. *The consequent of the implication formulation is an atomic formulation*
9 *The atomic formulation is based on the fact type supplier has priority over supplier*
10. *The first role is bounded to the first variable*
11. *The second role is bounded to the second variable*

For the **BR3**, we can recognize that **Old supplier** is a key-concept to be included in the communication model because it generates a variable (line 2.), quantified by a universal quantification (lines 1. and 2.). Similarly, **New supplier** is a key concept given by the existential quantification and introduced as a variable (lines 4. and 5.). In a similar way, we recognize **Order** and **Fraud rate** as key-concepts of **BR4** used in the instantiation of **BR4** communication model.

SBVR Semantic Formulation of BR4

1. *This proposition is meant by a universal quantification*
2. *The universal quantification introduces a first variable*
3. *The first variable ranges over the concept **Order***
4. *The universal quantification scopes over an implication formulation*
5. *The antecedent of the implication formulation is a conjunction formulation*
6. *The conjunction's operand 1 is an existential formulation*
7. *The existential formulation introduces a second variable*
8. *The second variable ranges over the concept **Fraud rate***
9. *The existential formulation scopes over an atomic formulation*

10. *The atomic formulation is based on the fact type Order has Fraud rate*
11. *The first role of the atomic formulation bounds to the first variable*
12. *The second role of the atomic formulation bounds to the second variable*
13. *The conjunction's operand 2 is an atomic formulation*
14. *The atomic formulation is based on the fact type number is greater than number*
15. *The first role of the atomic formulation bounds to the second variable*
16. *The second role of the atomic formulation bounds to "10 %"*
17. *The consequent of the implication formulation is an atomic formulation*
18. *The atomic formulation is based on the fact type Order need to be manually approved*
19. *The first role is bounded to the first variable*

Now, we can instantiate our abstract communication model for the business rules **BR3** and **BR4**.

BR-3 communication model instance.

Listener-#3 = (

new**OldSupplier**($\#u$) +
alt**OldSupplier**($\#u$) +
del**OldSupplier**($\#u$) +
new**NewSupplier**($\#u$) +
alt**NewSupplier**($\#u$) +
del**NewSupplier**($\#u$)

).$\overline{notifyEngine}\langle\#3,\#u\rangle$.*Listener-#3*

Notifier-#3 = notifyEngine($\#3,\#u$) . τ . *Notifier-#3*

Integrator-#3 = *Listener-#3* | *Notifier-#3*

Note that the communication model instance for **BR3** uses all its key-concepts from the SBVR formulation. For each of those concepts (**Old supplier** and **New supplier**) a corresponding creation (new), modification (alt) and removal (del) events are created. It means that all these events that could be signaled from the information system are monitored. Whenever one of them is observed, the control is passed to the rules engine, through action *notifyEngine*, to check **BR3** satisfiability. The **BR4** communication model is generated in the same way.

BR-4 communication model instance.

Listener-#4 $= ($

new**Order**$(\#u)$ +
alt**Order**$(\#u)$ +
del**Order**$(\#u)$ +
new**FraudRate**$(\#u)$ +
alt**FraudRate**$(\#u)$ +
del**FraudRate**$(\#u)$

$).\overline{notifyEngine}\langle\#4,\#u\rangle.Listener\text{-}\#4$

Notifier-#4 $=$ notifyEngine$(\#4,\#u)$. τ . *Notifier-#4*

Integrator-#4 $=$ *Listener-#4* | *Notifier-#4*

Finally, the behavior of the communication model (protocol) for the e-commerce application example shown is given by the parallel composition of the models for all its business rules.

Integrator-e-commerce $=$ *Integrator-#3* | *Integrator-#4*

6.1   System Architecture

The communication model composed by the identified events will be used in the information system to implement the business rules. As we can see in Fig. 4, an SOA based architecture is chosen. This architecture is concerned about a clear separation between the rule engines and the other information system elements. The communication model implementation uses events based on the SBVR semantic formulation to define when the rule engine must check a particular business rule. Some particular aspects must be regarded in order to actually implement this architecture. The first one is how the communication model implementation and the rule engines will be physically connected. We suggest the addition of an adapter between these two elements. This adapter will know how to communicate with the specific rule engine being used. Then if the rule engine being used needs to be replaced, only the adapter must be rewritten. The second aspect is related to the data that the rule engine needs to access in order to check the business rules satisfiability. As an example, we can use business rule **BR4**. The rule engine must have access to the orders database in order to check the fraud rate when a new order is created or modified. We can solve this problem by using a shared database between the rule engine and the information system. The notification of a possible violation includes an identification of the related instance. As a result, the rule engine can retrieve the information about this instance in the shared database and then check its satisfiability.

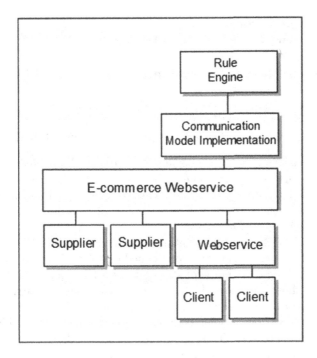

Fig. 4. System architecture

7   Related Work

A set of works have been found in literature related to our proposal. In [6], Cabot, Pau and Raventós provide an extensive mapping set from UML to SBVR elements. These mappings are used to do the transformation of UML models into SBVR models. This allows information inside UML models to be transmitted to business people in a more easy-to-understand language for those who do not have expertise in systems development. Another example of a SBVR-related transformation initiative is found at [7]. In this work, an approach to transform business rules written OCL into SBVR formulations is found. This transformation is given by identifying the main types that appear in the OCL language and mapping them to the corresponding representation in SBVR. One limitation of these works is that they only give another form of representation to the business rules defined in SBVR. They do not address the problem of implementing the business rules.

In [8], Roover and Vanthienen create a set of templates for the transformation of business rules defined in the SBVR structured English into an event-oriented representation. All of these templates have a general structure for a specific type of business rule and an indication of how this structure can be transformed into a general event description. Examples of templates proposed in their work are:

– **General integrity constraint**
   <Concept1> must be {less/larger/earlier/...}
   than <Concept2>
– **Translation to a event-based format**
   On IsCreated (<Concept1/2>) :
   if <Concept1> is no less than <Concept2> then notify (Rule #)
   On IsModified (<Concept1/2>) :
   if <Concept1> is no less than <Concept2>then notify (Rule #)

This event-based representation is made in order to allow the implementation of business rules in real systems. The authors expect that integrated mechanisms can be developed to receive these notifications and treat them appropriately. In [9] the same authors propose a prototype tool that implements the rules based on this technique of templates.

The proposal of Roover and Vanthienen differs from our proposal in some aspects. In their approach, there is a predefined template definition for each kind of business rule. People in charge of stating the business rules will be restricted to follow one of those templates. In our approach there are no restrictions for the way the business rule is defined. Another difference in their work is that there are no directions on how to effectively check the business rules. The checking mechanism is implicit in each rule template. It means that, for each new template, it is necessary to develop a new mechanism to check rules that follow the template. In our approach, we use rule engines which can check a large set of business rules.

8   Conclusions

The implementation of business rules in information systems is not an easy task. Models commonly used to represent them are limited in capturing the meaning of rules but do not provide means to effectively implement them in information systems. In this work we provided a method to extract information from SBVR semantic formulations that may affect business rules conformity, together with a standard communication model to help in implementing business rules systems. An abstract event-based communication model between business rule engines and other information system architecture is defined. It contains all events that must be monitored during systems execution in order to maintain the conformity with the business rules and can be instantiated to particular systems.

The major benefit of our approach is the separation between the rule engines and the overall information system elements in such a way that both elements can be managed independently. Another contribution of our approach is to facilitate business rules implementation by providing, in a standard way, the exact time a verification of business rules conformity is necessary and which events need to be observed. Besides that, with our approach the information system does not need to deal with all the details of the business rules definitions. Instead, the information system itself only needs to take care of a restricted set of events to ensure business rules conformity.

This approach can be extended in many ways. First, it is possible to extend its scope by increasing the number of compatible business rules types. Rules involving projections, objectifications and nominations were left aside in this work and could be included in a future work. Another form of improvement would be the creation of a business rules implementation reference model. This reference model would explain in detail how our communication model could be used as a basis for creating architectures that explicitly consider business rules and allow them to be implemented by rules engines. Also, a prototype to support the method of recognizing concepts and variables from SVBR formulations are of great help to automatize the instantiations process of the abstract communication model.

References

1. Team, S.: Semantics of business vocabulary and rules (sbvr), Technical Report dtc/06-03-02, Technical report (2006)
2. Chapin, D.: Sbvr: What is now possible and why. Bus. Rules J. **9**(3) (2008)
3. Cheesman, J., Daniels, J.: UML Components. Addison-Wesley, Reading (2001)
4. Bajwa, I.S., Lee, M.G., Bordbar, B.: Sbvr business rules generation from natural language specification. In: AAAI Spring Symposium: AI for Business Agility (2011)
5. Milner, R.: Communicating and mobile systems: the pi calculus. Cambridge University Press, Cambridge (1999)
6. Cabot, J., Pau, R., Raventós, R.: From uml/ocl to sbvr specifications: A challenging transformation. Inf. Syst. **35**(4), 417–440 (2010)
7. Pau, R., Cabot, J.: Paraphrasing OCL expressions with SBVR. In: Kapetanios, E., Sugumaran, V., Spiliopoulou, M. (eds.) NLDB 2008. LNCS, vol. 5039, pp. 311–316. Springer, Heidelberg (2008)
8. De Roover, W., Vanthienen, J.: Unified patterns to transform business rules into an event coordination mechanism. In: Proceedings of the 4th International Workshop on Event-Driven Business Process Management (edBPM'10), pp. 61–73 (2010)
9. De Roover, W., Caron, F., Vanthienen, J.: A prototype tool for the event-driven enforcement of SBVR business rules. In: Daniel, F., Barkaoui, K., Dustdar, S. (eds.) BPM Workshops 2011, Part I. LNBIP, vol. 99, pp. 446–457. Springer, Heidelberg (2012)

Integration of Business Processes with Visual Decision Modeling. Presentation of the HaDEs Toolchain

Krzysztof Kluza[✉], Krzysztof Kaczor, and Grzegorz J. Nalepa

AGH University of Science and Technology,
al. A. Mickiewicza 30, 30-059 Krakow, Poland
{kluza,kk,gjn}@agh.edu.pl

Abstract. Business Rules (BRs) allow for defining statements that determine or constrain some aspects of the business and precise what can be done in a specific situation. Together with Business Processes (BPs) they compose an efficient framework for business logic specification. In this paper, issues related to integration of the visual design of BRs with BPs modeling methods are considered. As a result of our previous research, the HaDEs framework for visual design of the rule bases was developed. The main goal of this paper is to present the HaDEs toolchain applications and show how they can be used for designing of decision process and effectively integrated with BPs modeling methods.

1 Introduction

Business Rules [1] allow for precise definition of the organization business policy, and this is why they play an important role in business applications. BRs can have a substantial impact on business operation from product development to marketing. Working on BR modeling, at least the following features of BR must be taken into account:

1. *Informal rule representation.* Informal methods are often used for BR representation where rules are commonly provided in a text-based format.
2. *Weak support for rule modeling.* Rules are usually designed not using dedicated tools but textual editors, spreadsheets, etc.
3. *Hard rule maintenance.* The nowadays applications provide the hard-coded business rules in the source code of the application, databases, spreadsheets and other hard to manage locations.
4. *Several rule types.* BR commonly provides three types of rules: derivation, constraint and invariant rules.
5. *Defined rule semantics.* It is important to have a precisely defined semantics of rules in order to use them in a proper way.

The paper is supported by the HiBuProBuRul Project funded from NCN (National Science Centre) resources for science (no. DEC-2011/03/N/ST6/00909).

F. Fournier and J. Mendling (Eds.): BPM 2014 Workshops, LNBIP 202, pp. 504–515, 2015.
DOI: 10.1007/978-3-319-15895-2_43

The result of our previous research is the SKE (*Semantic Knowledge Engineering*) [2] methodology. It aims at providing an integrated process for design, implementation, and analysis of rule based systems supported by the HADES [2] toolchain. The main features of this methodology are:

1. *Visual rule representation.* The provided formal rule language based on the Attributive Logic with Set of Values over Finite Domains [3] allows for visual representation of rules, what makes the design more transparent and clear.
2. *Supported rule modeling.* The HADES toolchain provides a set of dedicated tools, which facilitate the design process.
3. *Easy rule maintenance.* The HADES-based design process consists of three stages (see Fig. 1 with the steps of the stages and the tools taking part in particular steps). The transitions between stages are formally defined and automatically performed (modifications can be automatically propagated).
4. *One rule type.* As opposed to BRs, SKE provides only one type of rule – production rule. However, the methodology provides different inference strategies that correspond to different types of BRs, e.g. derivation rule type corresponds to backward chaining inference mode.
5. *Formal rule semantics.* As the SKE methodology provides a formal rule language, the semantics of the rules is precisely defined.

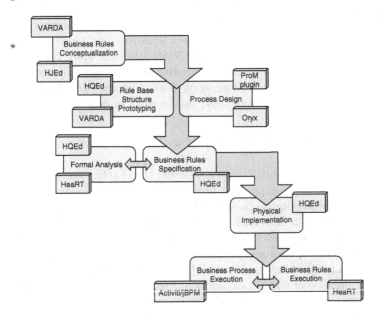

Fig. 1. Design process using the HADES toolchain

In this paper, we present the HADES toolchain[1] developed by the GEIST research group. We describe how it can be used for designing of decision process, and show how to integrate them with Business Process modeling methods.

---

[1] The tools of the HADES toolchain are available at the webpage: http://geist.agh.edu.pl/pub:software:start.

Among the existing implementations of rule based systems, one can distinguish tools providing similar features as the SKE methodology. One of such tools is DROOLS [4], a modern JAVA-based implementation of BR approach providing dedicated rule language, RETE-based inference engine and integrated visual modeling of decision processes based on BPMN (*Business Process Modeling Notation*) [5]. Nevertheless, DROOLS rule language does not have any underlying formal model what makes its semantics is not precisely defined and efficient formal verification and validation impossible. Another tool, PROLOGA [6], allows for modeling business rules, decision models, complex procedures, analysis specifications in the form of decision tables systems. The emphasis is on support for the construction of decision tables – visual representation, manipulations, and full verification and validation against completeness, consistency, redundancy, and correctness [7]. One of the important features supported by PROLOGA is modeling of structure of single decision tables as well as relations between them what determine structure of the whole decision process. Unfortunately, the separation of knowledge from the definition of decision process structure is not clear and thus application of Business Processes for representing this structure becomes impossible. There are also other tools for rule-based system modeling like OPENRULES[2] or IBM ILOG[3], but they are mainly intended to model and execute rule-based knowledge and do not provide features like verification and validation, modeling of advanced decision process structures.

This paper is organized as follows: Sect. 2 introduces a use case example designed in the BR-based manner. Section 3 describes the main concepts of the methodology. This section also introduces the HADEs tools by modeling our use case example as well as the integration with Business Processes. The paper is summarized with the conclusions and future work in Sect. 4.

2 Polish Liability Insurance Use Case

To demonstrate the rule modeling process using the HADEs tools, we use a Polish Liability Insurance example that presents a system of determining the price of the insurance protecting against third party insurance claims. The price can be determined based on data such as the driver's age, the period of holding the license, the number of accidents in the last year, etc. Other relevant factors in calculating insurance premium are data about the vehicle: the engine capacity, age, car seats, a technical examination. The insurance premium can be increased or decreased because of number of payment installments, other insurances, continuity of insurance or the number of cars insured.

For the compact representation, all rules are grouped within decision tables. The calculation proceeds in three steps. First, the basic rate is determined based on the engine capacity (see Table 1). Then, the discounts and increases are calculated based on accident-free driving (see Table 2). The last step takes into account other discounts or increases (see Table 3).

---

[2] See: http://openrules.com.

[3] See: http://www.ibm.com/software/info/ilog.

Table 1. Calculating the base rate

Car capacity [cm^3]	Base rate [PLN]
<900	537
1300	753
1600	1050
2000	1338
>2000	1536

Table 2. Bonus-Malus table

Customer class	Base rate percent	New customer class depending on number of accidents in the last year		
		1 accident	2 accidents	more than 2
M	260	M	M	M
0	160	M	M	M
1	100	0	M	M
2	90	0	M	M
3	80	1	0	M
4	70	2	1	M
5	60	3	1	M
6	60	3	2	M
7	50	4	3	M
8	50	6	3	M
9	40	7	4	0

3 Visual Business Rule Design Process with the HaDEs Toolchain

This section describes how the presented use case can be designed using the tools from the HaDEs toolchain. The toolchain aims at supporting the SKE approach [2], which is a result of our research motivated by a critical analysis of the state-of-the art of the rule based systems design. In this approach, the logic is expressed using forward-chaining decision rules. They form an intelligent rule-based controller or simply a business logic core. The logic controller is decomposed into multiple modules represented by decision tables.

HaDEs supports a complete hierarchical design process for the creation of knowledge bases. The whole process consists of three stages: conceptual, logical and physical design and is supported by a number of tools providing the visual design and automated implementation[4]. The tools overview for the consecutive stages with the files exchanged between tools can be observed in Fig. 2.

---

[4] See: https://ai.ia.agh.edu.pl/wiki/hekate:hades.

Table 3. Other discounts and rises

Discount/ Rise	Rule
−50 %	When the car is antique
−20 %	When the customer has other insurance
	When the car age do not exceed 1 year
−15 %	When the car age do not exceed 2 years
−10 %	When the car age do not exceed 3 years
	When single payment
	When the customer prolongates the insurance
	When the customer buys more than one insurance
	When the driver age is between 44 and 55 years
+10 %	In case of installments
+15 %	When the car age exceeds 10 years
+20 %	When the car has more than 5 seats
	When the car do not have a valid technical examination
+30 %	When the driver have the driver license shorter than 3 years
+50 %	When the driver age is younger than 25 years
+60 %	When the car do not have an insurance history

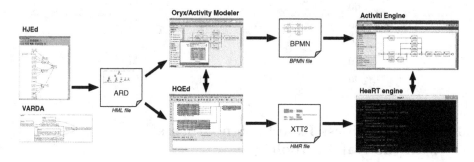

Fig. 2. An overview of the HADEs tools and how they interact with each other via their input/output formats

3.1   Conceptual Design

The conceptual design is the first stage of the process. During this step, the ARD+ (*Attribute Relationships Diagrams*) [2] method is used. This phase is optional during the whole design process and can be considered as a supportive phase for the rule modeling. The principal idea for this stage is to build a graph defining functional dependencies between attributes on which the rules are built. This stage is supported by three visual tools: VARDA [8], HJED [9] and HQED (see Sect. 3.2). The transition from this phase to the following one is automatic and based on generating the table headers connected by links which correspond to the dependencies between attributes. The transition algorithm is implemented in VARDA and HQED.

The HJED editor is a cross-platform tool implemented in Java. Its main features include the ARD+ diagram creation with on-line design history available. Once created, the ARD+ model can be saved in an XML-based HML file, which can be then imported by the HQED design tool supporting the logical design.

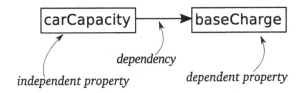

Fig. 3. An example of the ARD+ dependency

Considering the presented use case, the example of capturing the attributes as well as dependencies between them can be presented using Table 1. This table has two columns: *Car capacity* and *Base rate*, which identifies two attributes named *carCapacity* and *baseCharge*. It can be then marked that the attribute *baseCharge* depends on the *carCapacity* i.e. in order to determine a value of the attribute *baseCharge*, the value of the attribute *carCapacity* must be defined. Attributes and such relations can be introduced to the model using the HJED editor. As a result, the relation is depicted in the design diagram, see Fig. 3. The complete ARD+ diagram for the use case can be observed in Fig. 4.

VARDA [8] is a prototype semi-visual editor implemented in Prolog for modeling ARD+ diagrams. The tool provides an on-line model visualization using Graphviz. It also supports prototyping of the XTT2 model, where the connected table headers are created, see Fig. 5. The ARD+ design is encoded in Prolog, and the resulting model can be stored in the HML file.

Moreover, the algorithm for automatic generation of business process models from the ARD diagrams was presented in [10]. A ProM plugin for this translation is being developed.

3.2   Logical Design

The logical design is the second stage of the process. During this stage, rules are designed using the visual XTT2 (*Extended Tabular Trees version 2*) [11] method. This phase, supported by the HQED editor [12] can be performed as the first one in the design or as the second one, when the input is provided from the conceptual design.

HQED provides all the necessary mechanisms for rule visual modeling as well as for integration with external systems. It also provides all the necessary features that facilitate creation of a rule base using a user-friendly graphical interface (see Fig. 6). This tool allows for visual modeling of rule bases using the XTT2 tables.

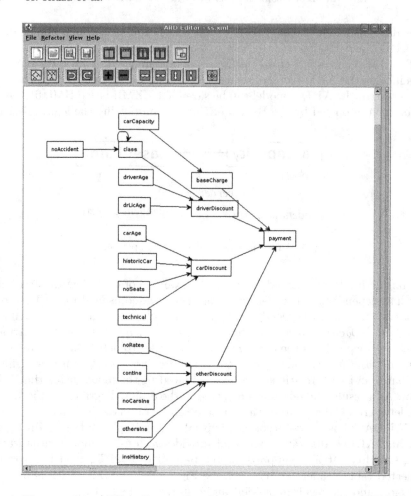

Fig. 4. The complete ARD+ diagram for the presented example in the HJEd editor

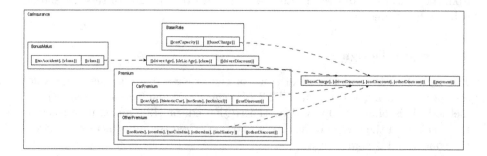

Fig. 5. The XTT2 model prototyping in VARDA

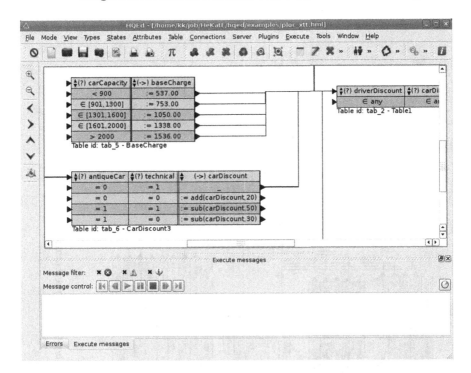

Fig. 6. HQED editing session

The HQED modeling is supported by two mechanisms that assure the high quality of a rule base:

- *Visual design* – the visual knowledge representation makes the design more transparent what allows for more effective finding and fixing errors and anomalies and makes the rules understandable for people.
- *Limited Quality Analysis* – the design is supported by two types of the verification that allows for discovering anomalies and errors omitted by a designer:
  - *Syntax Analysis* – The HQED internal representation of the model is continuously monitored against the syntax errors, e.g. out of domain values, inaccessible rules, orphan tables, etc.
  - *Logical Analysis* – Although HQED does not have a built-in logical analysis engine, the model is checked by HEART, an external tool working simultaneously with HQED as plug-in.

Having a complete XTT2-based model of our use case (see Fig. 7), the physical implementation can be automatically generated. HQED allows for generating the physical implementation in the HMR format, which can be directly read and interpreted by the HEART tool.

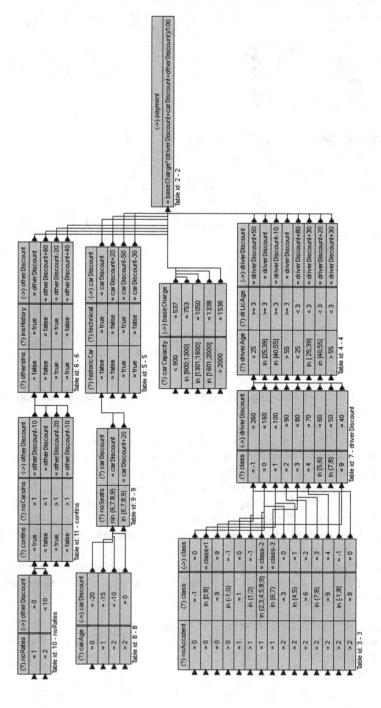

Fig. 7. The use case designed in the XTT2 representation

3.3 Physical Design

At this stage, a logical model is transformed into an algebraic syntax called HMR[5], which is a textual representation of the XTT2 logic having a human readable form, as opposed to the machine readable HML format.

HMR can be directly executed [13] by the dedicated HEART[6] inference engine tool. HEART is implemented in Prolog in order to directly interpret HMR. It allows for storing and exporting models in HMR files, and verifying HMR syntax and logic.

The HEART engine has also communication and integration facilities. It supports Java integration based on callback mechanism and Prolog JPL library. HEART provides direct interaction via Prolog console based on callback mechanism. The tool can operate in two modes: stand-alone and as a TCP/IP server, offering TCP/IP-based integration mechanism with other applications, e.g. Semantic Wiki [14,15] or Business Process Engine [16].

3.4 Integration of HADES with Business Processes

The HADES toolchain was integrated with the Oryx Business Process editor [17]. Figure 8 shows the integration of the BPMN Business Processes with the XTT2-based Business Rules for the presented use case. The *Calculate the base price* rule task triggers the proper XTT2 table. The connection between a BR task and a decision table can be either generated from the ARD+ model or selected during the BP design. The HQED provides a socket-based interface for its services, so the XTT2 rules can be edited in the HQED editor connected via network with the BPMN editor. The plugin for this connection was developed for the following process editors: Oryx, Activiti Modeler and Activiti Designer. In such a case, opening a rule task in the Oryx editor allows for XTT2 editing in HQED.

Then, the process model with the specified rules in BR tasks can be executed in the process engine, such as jBPM [18] or Activiti Engine [19], extended with our plugins [16,20]. In the case of BR tasks, the process engine delegates rule execution to the HEART engine.

4 Summary and Future Work

This paper presents the HADES toolchain. We propose using a hierarchical visual design method for Business Rules supported by the HADES framework. The main features of this method are visual rule representation, supported rule modeling, easy rule maintenance, and formal rule semantics.

We discuss an approach to business logic specification that takes advantage of HADES and involves Business Rules and Business Processes technologies. The paper describes how these tools can be used for designing of decision process, as well as present the integration with Business Process modeling methods.

---

[5] See https://ai.ia.agh.edu.pl/wiki/hekate:hmr.
[6] See https://ai.ia.agh.edu.pl/wiki/hekate:heart.

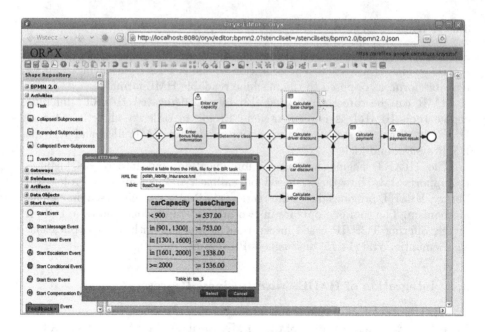

Fig. 8. Screenshot from the prototype Oryx GUI for XTT2 [17]

The main topic for the future work involves the extension of the presented methodology towards more comprehensive business logic modeling. This includes the extension of the XTT2 formalization aiming at providing more rule types as well as interoperability and integration of the representation with the DMN (*Decision Model and Notation*) [21] standard.

References

1. Ross, R.G.: Principles of the Business Rule Approach, 1st edn. Addison-Wesley Professional, Boston (2003)
2. Nalepa, G.J.: Semantic Knowledge Engineering. A Rule-Based Approach. Wydawnictwa AGH, Kraków (2011)
3. Ligęza, A.: Logical Foundations for Rule-Based Systems. Springer, Heidelberg (2006)
4. Browne, P.: JBoss Drools Business Rules. Packt Publishing, Birmingham (2009)
5. OMG: Business Process Model and Notation (BPMN): Version 2.0 specification. In: Object Management Group, Technical report formal/2011-01-03, January 2011
6. Vanthienen, J.: PROcedural LOgic Analyzer 5.1, September 2000
7. Vanthienen, J., Mues, C., Wets, G., Delaere, K.: A tool-supported approach to inter-tabular verification. Expert Syst. Appl. **15**(3), 277–285 (1998)
8. Nalepa, G.J., Wojnicki, I.: VARDA rule design and visualization tool-chain. In: Dengel, A.R., Berns, K., Breuel, T.M., Bomarius, F., Roth-Berghofer, T.R. (eds.) KI 2008. LNCS (LNAI), vol. 5243, pp. 395–396. Springer, Heidelberg (2008)

9. Kaczor, K., Nalepa, G.J.: HaDEs - presentation of the HeKatE design environment. In: Baumeister, J., Nalepa, G.J. (eds.) 5th Workshop on Knowledge Engineering and Software Engineering (KESE2009) at the 32nd German Conference on Artificial Intelligence: September 15, 2009, Paderborn, Germany, pp. 57–62 (2009)

10. Kluza, K., Nalepa, G.J.: Automatic generation of business process models based on attribute relationship diagrams. In: Lohmann, N., Song, M., Wohed, P. (eds.) BPM 2013 Workshops. LNBIP, vol. 171, pp. 185–197. Springer, Heidelberg (2014)

11. Nalepa, G.J., Ligęza, A., Kaczor, K.: Formalization and modeling of rules using the XTT2 method. Int. J. Artif. Intell. Tools **20**(6), 1107–1125 (2011)

12. Kaczor, K., Nalepa, G.J.: Design and implementation of HQEd, the visual editor for the XTT+ rule design method. In: AGH University of Science and Technology, Technical report CSLTR 02/2008, December 2008

13. Nalepa, G.J., Bobek, S., Ligęza, A., Kaczor, K.: Algorithms for rule inference in modularized rule bases. In: Bassiliades, N., Governatori, G., Paschke, A. (eds.) RuleML 2011 - Europe. LNCS, vol. 6826, pp. 305–312. Springer, Heidelberg (2011)

14. Adrian, W.T., Bobek, S., Nalepa, G.J., Kaczor, K., Kluza, K.: How to reason by HeaRT in a semantic knowledge-based wiki. In: Proceedings of the 23rd IEEE International Conference on Tools with Artificial Intelligence, ICTAI 2011, Boca Raton, Florida, USA, November 2011, pp. 438–441. http://ieeexplore.ieee.org/xpls/abs&tag=1

15. Nalepa, G.J., Bobek, S.: Embedding the HEART rule engine into a semantic wiki. In: Katarzyniak, R., Chiu, T.-F., Hong, C.-F., Nguyen, N.T. (eds.) Semantic Methods for Knowledge Management and Communication. SCI, vol. 381, pp. 265–275. Springer, Heidelberg (2011). http://www.springerlink.com/content/f39827272u6732h0/

16. Nalepa, G.J., Kluza, K., Kaczor, K.: Proposal of an inference engine architecture for business rules and processes. In: Rutkowski, L., Korytkowski, M., Scherer, R., Tadeusiewicz, R., Zadeh, L.A., Zurada, J.M. (eds.) ICAISC 2013, Part II. LNCS, vol. 7895, pp. 453–464. Springer, Heidelberg (2013). http://www.springer.com/computer/ai/book/978-3-642-38609-1

17. Kluza, K., Kaczor, K., Nalepa, G.J.: Enriching business processes with rules using the oryx BPMN editor. In: Rutkowski, L., Korytkowski, M., Scherer, R., Tadeusiewicz, R., Zadeh, L.A., Zurada, J.M. (eds.) ICAISC 2012, Part II. LNCS, vol. 7268, pp. 573–581. Springer, Heidelberg (2012). http://www.springerlink.com/content/u654r0m56882np77/

18. jBPM User Guide, 5th ed., The jBPM team of JBoss Community, Dec 2011. http://docs.jboss.org/jbpm/v5.2/userguide/

19. Rademakers, T., Baeyens, T., Barrez, J.: Activiti in Action: Executable Business Processes in BPMN 2.0, ser. Manning Pubs Co Series. Manning Publications Company (2012)

20. Kaczor, K., Kluza, K., Nalepa, G.J.: Towards rule interoperability: design of drools rule bases using the XTT2 method. In: Nguyen, N.T. (ed.) Transactions on Computational Collective Intelligence XI. LNCS, vol. 8065, pp. 155–175. Springer, Heidelberg (2013)

21. OMG: Decision model and notation beta1. Object Management Group, Technical report dtc/2014-02-01, Feb 2014

Generating Business Process Recommendations with a Population-Based Meta-Heuristic

Steven Mertens[✉], Frederik Gailly, and Geert Poels

Department of Business Informatics and Operations Management,
Faculty of Economics and Business Administration, Ghent University,
Tweekerkenstraat 2, 9000 Ghent, Belgium
{steven.mertens, frederik.gailly, geert.poels}@ugent.be

Abstract. In order to provide both guidance and flexibility to users during process execution, recommendation systems have been proposed. Existing recommendation systems mainly focus on offering recommendation according to the process optimization goals (time, cost...). In this paper we offer a new approach that primarily focuses on maximizing the flexibility during execution. This means that by following the recommendations, the user retains maximal flexibility to divert from them later on. This makes it possible to handle (possibly unknown) emerging constraints during execution. The main contribution of this paper is an algorithm that uses a declarative process model to generate a set of imperative process models that can be used to generate recommendations.

Keywords: Business processes · Recommender systems · Declarative process model · Run-time flexibility

1 Introduction

A business process is a set of one or more connected activities which collectively realize a particular business goal [1]. These processes can be formally represented by using one of numerous business process modelling languages (e.g., BPMN, UML, BPEL, Petri-net...). Business process engines (BPE) offer support for the implementation of business processes by enabling the execution based on the respective process model. They provide a software framework to handle human and non-human interaction and to ensure conformance with the specified process models.

In highly dynamic environments that need to offer high flexibility (e.g., hospitals and personalized customer service departments) it is hard to find a single fitting process model, and even more difficult to find an optimal one. There are many possible paths that should be allowed and many, often complex, restrictions to keep in mind. As example, consider the simplified case of a cancer treatment center for short stays (see Sect. 3 for more details). In this environment a set of rules (e.g., the process starts when the registration of the patient, a CT or MRI scan has to be directly followed by a doctor's visit...) and limitations (e.g., taking a strong painkiller means that a chemotherapy session is no longer possible in the remainder of the process instance) apply. The order

F. Fournier and J. Mendling (Eds.): BPM 2014 Workshops, LNBIP 202, pp. 516–528, 2015.
DOI: 10.1007/978-3-319-15895-2_44

of the activities for a certain process instance cannot be predetermined; instead it has to be personalized according to the additional emergent constraints (e.g., the patient is allergic to the painkiller) of the specific instance. For a doctor it can be difficult to correctly apply all these rules (although in the simplified example this is manageable) on specific variations of the process that possibly have been handled by other doctors up to that point.

The resulting question is: how can business process engines offer support and flexible assistance in this context? A differentiation has to be made between build-time flexibility and run-time flexibility. The first is intrinsic to the created model, the latter is the flexibility allowed by a process after being deployed [2].

An approach to add build-time flexibility to the process would be to create a model that entails all possible paths. A first issue arising here is that the model would be very big and complex making human understanding difficult. This is, however, not as much of a problem when using business process engines, since human understanding isn't strictly necessary once the model is deployed. In addition, the size of the model can also make the implementation of all paths significantly more time consuming. In static environments this is not that important, but this step would have to be repeated on regular basis in dynamic environments where the constraints change frequently. Finally, a problem concerning the decisions emerges when increasing the number of paths represented in the process model. It is one thing to allow many paths, another to choose one for a specific instance of the process. This responsibility is shifted to the process participants, because no information is offered on the advantages and/or disadvantages of choosing a certain option.

As stated in [3], there is an apparent paradox between providing guidance and flexibility in how to proceed during process execution. Guidance is often thought of as forcing the user in a certain direction. This can be countered by using a business process engine offering recommendations to the users. A recommendation entails a single activity or a set of parallel activities to be executed next based on a certain goal, considering previously executed activities (i.e., a process instance that was started but not completed yet) [4]. They are ordered based on criteria not necessarily visible to the user. The user is encouraged to choose the 'best' recommendation, but is free to choose another one based on the specific circumstances that apply (e.g., patient requests an additional CT-scan before consenting with an operation). In the cancer treatment center, it would be beneficial to have a system that makes these recommendations based on the details of the specific case, while making sure that the next step is also conformant with the process in general. The approach is similar to what a GPS-system offers users compared to a street map. The GPS-system shows the user step by step how to navigate to his destination. If the user chooses to diverge from the recommended path, the GPS-system will offer an alternative optimized path based on its current position, and thus based on the previous choices of the user. In the ideal situation it also will not propose paths that are not possible (e.g., wrong way in a one-directional street). This alleviates some of the responsibilities placed on the user, while offering flexibility in the form of run-time flexibility. Similar recommendation systems have already been proposed in [3–5]. In [3, 4] process mining techniques are used to calculate or estimate the criteria (e.g., shortest duration, lowest cost...) to sort the recommendations.

The approach of [5] uses constraint programming techniques to produce business enactment plans, which are used to generate recommendations.

A common starting point for the systems in [3] and [5] is a declarative process model (e.g., a Declare model [6]) as opposed to a specific imperative process model (e.g., BPMN), just like a GPS-system internally uses a map combined with additional information (e.g., on-way streets, traffic information...) and not one path. Declarative process models [6] comprise a specification of the environment, its limitations and its rules in terms of a set of constraints. This gives leeway to follow different paths and avoids over-specification. When changes to the environment occur, the set of constraints is all that needs to be adjusted in the system itself. Imperative process models on the other hand, represent the precise (often overspecified) control-flow of a business process. They can still be used internally to generate possible valid paths based on the declarative model, but they are not necessarily visible to users of the system (only recommendations for the next step are visible).

A limitation of all three mentioned recommendation systems is that they only focus on the direct optimization goals of the process. The systems are most suitable for processes that require limited flexibility and variability. They generally assume the top recommendation will be followed by the user. It is, however, possible that the choice to initially follow an optimal path limits the freedom to diverge to other paths further down the road. So in the context of a highly dynamic environment with high flexibility needs, these systems will not produce the results we are looking for. The path they are suggesting might be optimal at the time it is generated, but when the context changes during the execution of the activities in that path, it might lose its optimal position. Therefore, specifically for highly dynamic environments, we believe a technique to generate robust process models (i.e., in a sense immune against bounded uncertainty) is still missing.

The main contribution of this paper is thus to propose an alternative to the aforementioned systems: a robust process engine that can deal with changes to its very dynamic and complex environment at run-time. Hence, it has to try and find a balance between the optimization goals of the process according to the current context and maximizing the freedom to diverge from the recommended paths (e.g., because of emergent constraints or requirements). We will primarily focus on the latter, offering recommendations that allow the most flexibility in the later steps of the process. Also, this indirectly entails checking the feasibility of possible next actions.

The novel idea is to use a population-based meta-heuristic for the generation of a set of imperative process models based on a declarative model (e.g., Declare). In the context of a very dynamic and complex environment that requires high flexibility, this offers some interesting advantages. The most important advantage is that the technique allows us to incorporate a new measure for run-time flexibility based on the population kept. The measure provides an estimate of the run-time flexibility of a certain imperative process model relative to the set of models in the population.

The remainder of this paper will first discuss the idea behind the proposed algorithm as well as the actual implementation algorithm in Sect. 2. This is followed by a short demonstration using the example of the cancer treatment center in Sect. 3. In Sect. 4 we discuss an important optimization. Finally, a summary of the contribution of this paper and further research will be presented in Sect. 5.

2 Solution Design

The developed population-based meta-heuristic takes its inspiration from nature and more specific from the artificial immune system (AIS) [7], which in turn is based on the vertebrate immune system. It is tasked with the protection of the organism from malfunctioning cells in the body (e.g., cancers) and foreign diseases-causing elements, called antigens. Two major groups of immune cells, called B-cells and T-cells, are tasked with identifying and stopping antigens from going rampant through the body of the organism. While being generally similar, they differ in how they recognize antigens. The algorithm, described below, is based on the functioning of the B-cells.

The environment in which the AIS functions is very similar to the problem environment described in the introduction of this paper. The solution space is also very large and dynamic, which makes finding an optimal solution hard and one that stays optimal in a changing environment impossible. This makes the AIS approach a great fit for calculating recommendations in a very dynamic and complex environment that requires high flexibility. The fact that the solution could be a suboptimum is not a big problem in this context, as the focus is on providing a robust solution.

Figure 1 gives an overview of the proposed implementation. At the start a set of random unique imperative process models, called the random population, is generated. The only requirement for these models is that they are valid according to the set of constraints contained by the declarative model. The initial population is created with the best models (based on the fitness function discussed below) from the random population. This initial population is sorted (again based on the fitness function) and will then be used as input for the iterative steps of the algorithm: clonal selection, mutation and selection. The three iterative steps, described below, will be executed until the stop criteria are met (i.e., 100 iterations done or the average model fitness score rises less than 1 % and drops less than 0.5 % over the last 5 iterations).

As mentioned before, the output of the algorithm is a ranked set of models, called the result population. Initially, the result population is filled with the models from the random population, removing those that are contained by one or more other models in the result population. A model is contained by another model when the other model allows everything that the first model allows and more. For example, the left model is contained by the right in Fig. 2. New valid models generated in iterations are added to the result population continuously. Every time new models are added, the result population is sorted based on the fitness function. If the population gets bigger than its specified maximal size, than the bottom models are removed to make it fit again.

Note that the proposed population-based meta-heuristic does not use recombination. The target environment is very complex, so finding new valid models starting from the valid models in the random population is always going to be hard. However, the chances of finding such a model are arguably higher when using a sequence of mutations than by randomly combining two models. This is because mutations entail relatively small changes to the model, whereas recombination is more disruptive. It is thus a choice between incremental versus disruptive change. The disruptive character of recombination offers as advantage a high diversity of models found. This is why it is important to add random seeds from the random population to the edit population

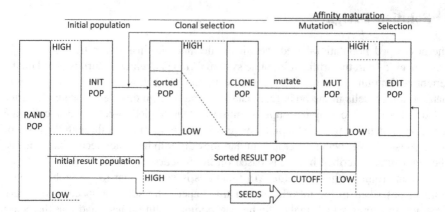

Fig. 1. Proposed artificial immune system implementation (based on Fig. 1 from [7])

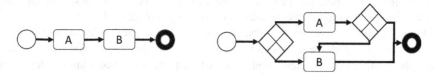

Fig. 2. Illustration of contained (left) and containing (right) imperative models

during iterations in the AIS technique. This ensures that new models are being searched in all search directions, which means that diversity is also ensured provided that the random population is in fact generated at random (special attention was paid to this in the implementation of the proof of concept).

Clonal selection. The B-cells of the vertebrate immune system use receptor molecules (i.e., antibodies), present on their surface, to bind with molecules covering the antigens (i.e., epitopes). They are cloned proportional to the degree to which the B-cell can recognize a certain antigen. The composition of the clone population (Fig. 1) tries to mimic this. The best p_{clone} percentage (e.g., 60 %) of models in the input population are cloned and put in the clone population. To make this population the same size as the input population, multiple clones of the same model are allowed. The fitness function of a model determines the chance that that model is chosen to be duplicated in the clone population (more than twice is possible).

Mutation (hypermutation). Random changes are made to the variable region of the receptor molecules of B-cells. The higher the degree to which the B-cell can recognize the target antigen, the lower the mutation rate and vice versa. Similarly, the models in the clone population are mutated (see Table 1) and then added to the mutation population (Fig. 1). The amount of mutations per model is determined by its fitness score. The models will be mutated at least once, possibly more. The chance that a model is mutated more is inversely proportional to its fitness score.

Note that models in the mutation population are not necessarily valid. This is not a problem because invalid models could become valid again after more mutations in

Table 1. The proposed set of mutations

	Original	Mutation
Activate empty transition	A B	A → B
Remove active transition	A → B	A B
Exclusive to parallel		
Parallel to exclusive		
Add exclusive to parallel		
Add parallel to exclusive		
Serial to exclusive		
Serial to parallel		

subsequent iterations or are filtered out since they are assigned the minimal fitness score of zero. All valid mutation found are also added to the result population. Like before, all doubles and contained models are removed from the result population. It is then sorted and the worst models are removed until the result population has again its intended size.

Selection (receptor editing). The mutations to the cloned B-cells cause many to become useless due to a bad combination of mutations. These non-functional B-cells are removed from the population by a programmed cell death (i.e., apoptosis). The last intermediate population, called the edit population (Fig. 1), does the same with the models in the mutation population. It is partially filled with the best p_{edit} percentage (e.g., 50 %) of models from the mutation population (again, invalid models are possible). The remainder of the edit population is filled with randomly selected seed models. Half of these seed models are taken from the random model, to keep searching in all directions, and the other half from the result population, to possibly optimize already found results.

Fitness function. The fitness function is used to estimate the value of an imperative process model multiple times during each iteration of the algorithm. The absolute fitness score of a model is not important; it is only of relative importance compared to scores of the other models in the population during one execution. It would thus be incorrect to directly compare the fitness scores of models from different executions of the algorithm (even if they start from exactly the same declarative process model). In this subsection we will discuss the three weighted components that are used: overall completion time, build-time flexibility and run-time flexibility. The actual weights used in the proof of concept (see Sect. 3) are based on our perceived importance of each subscore, respectively 20 % - 40 % - 40 %, but are still open for discussion based on the specific application environment.

- Overall completion time: the optimization goal we have pursued in our current implementation (but others can be used instead or in combination). It represents the time needed to complete the whole process using this model. If each activity is executed exactly once, then the overall completion time can easily be determined exactly. But when other existence-templates of the Declare model are used, we can only estimate how many times a certain activity will be executed. For example, 'Existence3(A)' specifies that activity A is executed at least 3 times with no upper bound. Combining this with the given estimates of the duration of an activity (e.g., 'Duration(A) = 5'), an estimate of the completion time of the model can be calculated. Since it is not always known exactly how many times an activity will be executed, the variable bound (e.g., the 3 in Existence3) of the template will be used as the number of times used in the estimation of the overall completion time. Machine learning algorithms will be used to offer a better estimation in the final system.

- Build-time flexibility: the inherent degree of flexibility of the model itself at build-time, also known as the looseness of the model [2]. Processes with a high degree of looseness are processes where the goal is known a priori, but a high degree of freedom is given on how to achieve it. The respective score is determined by counting the number of transitions from one activity to another allowed by the model, divided by the total number of transitions allowed by the input declarative model.

- As an example the left and right model from Fig. 2 will be scored in the context of a declarative model allowing six transitions (start-A, start-B, A-B, A-end, B-A and B-end). The left model has three transitions: start-A, A-B and B-end. This means that the build-time flexibility score is 3/6. The right model on the other hand has a build-time flexibility score of 5/6: start-A, start-B, A-B, A-end and B-end. This reflects that in the left model allows only one path (e.g., start-A-B-end), whereas in the right model three paths (e.g., also start-A-end and start-B-end) can be followed.

- Run-time flexibility: a property of a process instance according to [2]. In our case, the process instance is actually a recommendation system based on a declarative model. This is what is deployed, and thus, this is the context in which it has to be measured. The flexibility offered by the system depends on the result population, because only next steps contained by this population are sorted. The remaining steps are still selectable (requiring recalculation to check feasibility and generate a new result population), but not recommended. This means that run-time flexibility is not scored on an individual model level like the previous two scores, but rather relative to the models in the result population. Our proposition is to score the run-time flexibility with two conflicting scores, so that a balance has to be reached.

When scoring a model compared to a model from the population, the first score represents the number of activities at which one could switch to the other model, divided by the total number of activities (defined in the input declarative model). It is possible that for a certain activity some cases allow a switch and other cases don't. If 0 represents a no scenario where no switch is possible and 1 represents that a switch is always possible, then partial points represent the number of cases in which it is possible, relative to the all cases. The total aggregated score of a certain model compared to the population allows us to valuate if the model can be used when diverging from another model to this model, or when diverging from this model, there are other models in the set that can be used.

It is important for the correct calculation of the first score that models that are contained by other models are removed from the result population before evaluating them based on this component. If not, it causes the component to estimate the value of the models incorrectly. The scores of the containing and contained models will be higher than they should be, because of the similarity between them, but have no real value since switching between these models is pointless.

A limitation to the first score is that it has a preference for similar models with different endings, since this allows the maximal amount of switching between them. This means that certain variations at the beginning of the model will only have a small chance to be in the population. To counteract this tendency, the second part of the run-time flexibility score is inversely proportional to the frequency of transitions used in a model compared to the population. This tends to equalize the diversity and thus balances out the total run-time flexibility score.

3 Demonstration

In this section, a brief demonstration of the recommendation system will be given. The system itself has not been fully implemented yet, but the proposed algorithm[1] has. The demonstration will use the simplified cancer treatment center described in the introduction. Patients initiate the process by registering at the reception. The next activity is a doctor's visit to evaluate what has to happen next (e.g., order scans, operate...). The only other certainty is that the patient will have to unregister at the end. The example environment is represented by the Declare model, with the given estimates for the durations, described in Fig. 3. This model is complex enough to highlight the basic aspects of the proposed recommendation system. This model is used as input for the algorithm proposed in this paper. The result is a set of imperative models, 30 models in this case, that comply with the given declarative process model.

Based on the sorted set of models in the result population, a sorted set of recommendations is created (see Table 2). This possibly leaves the user with one or more possible next steps that are not present in any model in the result set (i.e., steps that severely limit the flexibility later on). These are placed below the lowest recommendation, as they are not really recommended, but could still be chosen in rare cases. Impossible next steps are of course disregarded. Parallel next steps are currently not supported by the recommendation system (but could possibly be in the result population), so they will not be included in this demonstration. The first column of Table 2 contains the activity trace that is followed during this demonstration. A row contains

---

[1] https://github.ugent.be/MIS/AIS_Population_RecommendationSystem/.

the enumeration of the possible next activities. The content of each box indicates if a certain next activity is a recommendation or not at that time. Initially, only the first row is given. The choice made then adds the chosen activity to the trace and a new row is added with recommendations for the next step. The numbers represent the ranking of the recommendations. A lower rank is preferred, while equal rank means that both next steps are allowed by the same model. Unranked recommendations are marked with a dash (-) and impossible next steps are marked with an X.

The process starts with two activities with no alternatives (and thus no other recommendations). The patient registers at the reception of the cancer treatment center and then he is examined by the doctor. The doctor decides that a CT-scan is needed. He thus follows one of the top recommendations. Right after the session, another examination is performed by the doctor to check if everything is in order. However, the

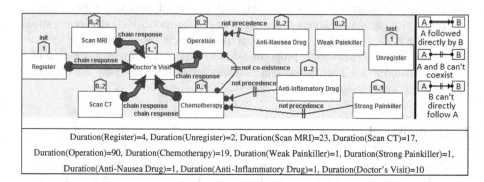

Duration(Register)=4, Duration(Unregister)=2, Duration(Scan MRI)=23, Duration(Scan CT)=17, Duration(Operation)=90, Duration(Chemotherapy)=19, Duration(Weak Painkiller)=1, Duration(Strong Painkiller)=1, Duration(Anti-Nausea Drug)=1, Duration(Anti-Inflammatory Drug)=1, Duration(Doctor's Visit)=10

Fig. 3. Example Declare model with given estimates of duration of each activity

Table 2. Example of an execution trace of the recommendation system.

	Register	Unregister	Scan MRI	Scan CT	Chemotherapy	Operation	Weak Painkiller	Strong Painkiller	Anti-Nausea Drug	Anti-Inflammatory Drug	Doctor's Visit
○	1	X	X	X	X	X	X	X	X	X	X
Register	X	X	X	X	X	X	X	X	X	X	1
Doctor's Visit	X	1	1	1	1	18	1	-	1	-	1
Chemotherapy	X	X	X	X	X	X	X	X	X	X	1
Doctor's Visit	X	1	1	1	1	18	1	-	1	-	1
Operation	X	X	X	X	X	X	X	X	X	X	1
Doctor's Visit	X	1	1	1	1	5	1	○	-	-	1
	RECALCULATION										
Strong Painkiller	X	1	1	1	X	2	1	X	1	1	1
Unregister											
○											

doctor notices that something is wrong and concludes that the patient needs instant surgery. Even though this is not the top recommendation, another model in the population (ranked 18th of the 30 original models) does allow the next activity to be an operation. The operation is successful and the doctor gives him a strong painkiller to ease the pain. At this point, there is no model left in the population (as models are removed that do not allow the current chosen activity trace) that allows the next activity to be the prescription of a strong painkiller. This means that the algorithm has to recalculate. After some time the patient feels ready to go home, so he goes back to the reception and unregisters himself from the cancer treatment center. The newly calculated result population has this last step now as one of the top recommendations. This step is also the end of the process.

4   Optimization Fitness Function

As was described before, the fitness function is an estimation of the value of a certain model that can be used to compare models during one execution of the proposed algorithm. It was also mentioned that models from the population contained by other models from the population are removed, because they negatively impact the valuation made by the fitness score. This, however, applies not only to containing models in the population, but also containing models that have not been discovered yet. Theoretically, this has no effect on the outcome of the algorithm since contained models will eventually be removed when the containing model is found. Nonetheless, in practice processing time is limited and thus it is possible that they are never discovered. This causes a systematic overestimation of the fitness score (as similarities between contained models are high). Also, when a containing model is found, one or more models are suddenly removed from the result population. This causes the average fitness score to possibly rise or drop significantly based on the composition of the result population as can be seen in Fig. 4 (between iteration 145 and 160 the population drops from 30 to 13, resulting in a big drop in the average fitness score). The other side effect is that previously disregarded models now suddenly could have become relevant. These models where however forgotten by the algorithm, so they have to be rediscovered, slowing down the convergence (as it takes about 40 iterations to get back to 30 models in the result population in Fig. 4).

An optimization step is proposed to handle the issue, which is executed before the fitness scores are calculated. In this step an attempt is made to combine each pair of models in the result population.[2] If there exists a valid model containing both models, it has to contain at least the union of both these models, since it is know that each model in the result population is valid. So if the union is valid, a containing model of both models has been found. This filters out all models contained by other models in the population (as there union will be equal to the containing model from the population), but it also discovers new models that contain one or more models in the population.

---

[2] This is not the same as recombination, as the result is not a composition of smaller parts of each model. The result is a model that contains both models fully.

By repeating this step each time models are added to the result population, no significant errors will be made during the valuation of the models. It also eliminates the drops in size of the population, giving the average fitness score of the result population a smoother progression during iterations (see Fig. 5).

Note that it is still possible that a certain model in the population is contained by another valid model not in the population. This is not a problem because the fitness scores will not be negatively influenced by this, since it concerns just one model in the population. The containing model can be found with a certain combination of mutations. At which point the containing model will just replace the contained model in the result population. So similarities between multiple containing/contained models do not come into play.

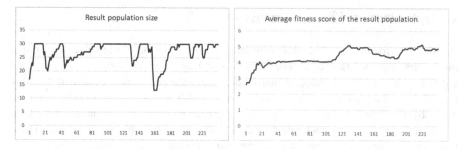

Fig. 4. The effects of the systematic removal of intrapopulation contained models on size and average fitness score (X-axis) of the result population during iterations (Y-axis).

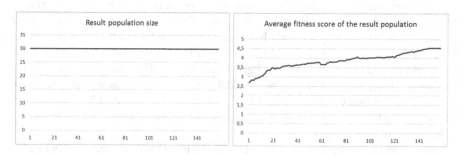

Fig. 5. The size and average fitness score (X-axis) of the result population with the optimized algorithm during iterations (Y-axis)

5   Conclusion

This paper presents a recommendation system based on an AIS algorithm to generate imperative process models from a declarative model. In contrast to existing recommendations systems, this one is made to thrive in dynamic and complex environments with high flexibility needs. This requires a focus on the flexibility of a process instead of just the optimization goals. This flexibility is divided along two dimensions:

build-time and run-time. Build-time flexibility is an intrinsic property of a model, which is measured by comparing the number of transitions allowed by the imperative model to the number of possible transitions allowed by the declarative model. Run-time flexibility is the flexibility allowed after deployment. A new measure of the run-time flexibility was introduced, suited for this context and made possible by the proposed algorithm. The proposed algorithm also has several other advantages:

- Instead of returning one optimal model to be used as recommendation, the proposed algorithm returns a ranked set of models. This reduces the need to recalculate when the user diverges from the top recommendation.
- The original result population will contain less valid models as execution progresses because some models will become invalid by the choices made. A threshold can be used to determine if the population has become too small relative to size of the road ahead. Recalculations can be faster than normal calculations when using the remaining valid (or even the invalid) models as start population (possibly supplemented with some newly generated models).
- Small changes to the environment (e.g., adjusting estimates for the duration of activities) can often be handled by re-sorting the set of models. If there are still enough valid models (based on a threshold mentioned above) in the set no recalculations are needed. When recalculations are needed, these will be faster depending on how many valid models remained from the previous population.

This paper is only the starting point of this research. The idea for the robust and recommendation-based process engine has been fully developed and its implementation has begun. An implementation of the algorithm has been made that proves its usefulness, whereas the implementation of the recommendation system in a whole is still a work in progress. But first off, a thorough evaluation of the implemented algorithm is needed. This should reveal the optimal parameter values for the algorithm (i.e., fitness function weights, population sizes…) generally or in specific cases. These parameter values are also needed to allow a correct evaluation of the performance of the algorithm. This can be combined with a theoretical comparison of the technique to other techniques to determine its performance and usability. Additionally, an evaluation in real life cases can provide clear guidelines for which situations tend to be most suitable for using this technique. Finally, further research can also be done in how to improve the technique by adding resource constraints and combining it with decision models, machine learning techniques and/or process mining techniques.

References

1. Weske, M.: Business Process Management: Concepts, Methods, Technology. Springer, Berlin (2007)
2. Reichert, M., Weber, B.: Enabling Flexibility in Process-Aware Information Systems. Springer, Heidelberg (2012)
3. Van der Aalst, W.M.P., Pesic, M., Schonenberg, H.: Declarative workflows: Balancing between flexibility and support. Comput. Sci. Dev. **23**, 99–113 (2009)

4. Schonenberg, H., Weber, B., van Dongen, B.F., van der Aalst, W.M.: Supporting flexible processes through recommendations based on history. In: Dumas, M., Reichert, M., Shan, M.-C. (eds.) BPM 2008. LNCS, vol. 5240, pp. 51–66. Springer, Heidelberg (2008)
5. Barba, I., Weber, B., Del Valle, C., Jiménez-Ramírez, A.: User recommendations for the optimized execution of business processes. Data Knowl. Eng. **86**, 61–84 (2013)
6. Goedertier, S., Vanthienen, J., Caron, F.: Declarative business process modelling: principles and modelling languages. Enterp. Inf. Syst. 1–25 (2013)
7. Van Peteghem, V., Vanhoucke, M.: An artificial immune system for the multi-mode resource-constrained project scheduling problem. In: Cotta, C., Cowling, P. (eds.) EvoCOP 2009. LNCS, vol. 5482, pp. 85–96. Springer, Heidelberg (2009)

Bidimensional Process Discovery for Mining BPMN Models

Jochen De Weerdt$^{(\boxtimes)}$, Seppe K.L.M. vanden Broucke, and Filip Caron

Department of Decision Sciences and Information Management, KU Leuven,
Naamsestraat 69, 3000 Leuven, Belgium
jochen.deweerdt@kuleuven.be

Abstract. This paper presents "BPMN Miner", a process discovery technique that uses BPMN as the representational language for the discovery result. The proposed approach is novel in the sense that it is able to represent control-flow with BPMN constructs, but also because it augments the control-flow perspective with an organizational dimension by discovering swimlanes that represent organizational roles in the business process. Additional advantages of the proposed mining approach can be summarized as follows: it provides intuitive and easy-to-use abstraction/specification functionality which makes it applicable to event logs with various complexity levels, it provides instant feedback about the conformance between the input log and the resulting model based on a dedicated fitness metric, it is robust to noise, and it can easily integrate with modeling and other BPM tools with exporting functionality through the XPDL-format. In this way, BPMN Miner will take process mining one step closer to the status of indispensable for business process reengineering as discovered models are immediately available in the preferred language of a majority of practitioners, educators and researchers.

Keywords: Process mining · Process discovery · Business Process Model and Notation · BPMN

1 Introduction

The research field of process mining deals with the extraction of knowledge from event logs—transactional data repositories containing historical information as stored by process aware information systems [1]. Process mining analysis tasks are commonly distributed over three, broad categories: process discovery (derive some sort of descriptive model from a given event log), conformance checking (match the behavior seen in a given event log with that of a process model), and process enhancement (improve and extend an existing model based on additional data). Without doubt, the process mining analysis task of process discovery has received the most attention in the research community. As such, a great deal of algorithms and techniques have been proposed to this end. In many cases, the representational language utilized by techniques to represent discovered models reflect the same semantics as common process modeling standards which are

F. Fournier and J. Mendling (Eds.): BPM 2014 Workshops, LNBIP 202, pp. 529–540, 2015.
DOI: 10.1007/978-3-319-15895-2_45

being used by practitioners and researchers. As such, popular output formats for discovered models include: Petri nets [2], Heuristic nets [3], Causal nets [4] and EPCs [5].

However, one particular process modeling standard which has been somewhat overlooked in the process mining community is the Business Process Model and Notation (BPMN) standard [6]. This is peculiar, as the majority of educators and researchers have adopted BPMN as the language of choice when working with business processes. The reason for this stems mainly from the fact that BPMN has, for a long time, lacked a formal definition of its execution semantics. The initial specifications [7] defined behavioral semantics using the notion of token flow, similar to Petri nets and UML activity diagrams, but solely described the execution semantics in narrative form. Although researchers have defined formalized definitions, ranging from attempts to define a formal semantics for a subset of BPMN [8,9] to more complete approaches [10–12], the fact remains that both BPMN's many visual objects and its weak semantic formalization have caused scholars to develop process discovery techniques based on more formalized modeling approaches.

Nevertheless, given BPMN's wide dissemination, we argue that the availability of a native BPMN-based process discovery technique could be of great benefit within process identification, optimization and re-engineering efforts. Therefore, this paper introduces a new process discovery technique—*BPMN Miner*—which represents discovered control-flow aspects using BPMN constructs. We select a subset of constructs, both because discovering some constructs is near-impossible using only historically recorded process execution "traces", as well as because scholars have indicated that only a small subset of BPMN's constructs are used by the majority of practitioners [13]. However, our proposed approach is unique in the sense that it combines the control-flow perspective with an organizational dimension by discovering swim lanes that represent organizational roles in the business process. In addition, our technique provides intuitive and easy-to-use abstraction/specification functionality which makes it applicable to event logs with various complexity levels, provides instant feedback about the conformance between the input log and the resulting model based on a dedicated fitness metric, is robust to noise, and can easily be integrated with modeling and other BPM tools by exporting the discovered model.

The remainder of this paper is structured as follows. Section 2 outlines the rationale behind our proposed approach. Section 3 presents a comparative study regarding currently available process discovery techniques. Section 4 provides a formalization of the developed technique. Section 5 outlines a case study, illustrating the benefits of the BPMN Miner using a concise example. Section 6 concludes the paper.

2   Rationale

In this section, it is argued why automated process discovery with BPMN as the underlying modeling language is of utmost relevance for practitioners, education, and researchers.

2.1   Relevance for Practitioners

BPMN is considered as the de facto standard for process modeling [14] and is widely adopted by both business and IT communities [15]. Practitioners from both communities use the notation standard mainly for documenting, improving, simulating and implementing business processes [16].

While the adoption of BPMN for the purpose of process modeling has been successful, the adoption of process mining as the most valuable tool for business process improvement initiatives is somehow lagging. It is argued that a core factor contributing to this effect consists of a lack of deep technical understanding from typical business practitioners involved in such improvement initiatives with regard to conventional languages used by process mining tools. Even despite the uptake of commercial and highly user-friendly process discovery tools, the mismatch in modeling notation and the subsequent translation effort required to go from the analysis phase to redesign brings about an unnecessary adoption barrier. Therefore, we contend that the mining of BPMN models from execution data will prove highly beneficial for the further adoption of process mining, along the following lines of reasoning:

Automated Process Identification. Practitioners involved in process identification and modeling, can be persuaded into using automated process discovery techniques if such techniques provide effortless integration with popular modeling tools. With the capability to discover BPMN models from event logs, actual time savings can be realized for practitioners who are now typically involved in a two-step process of first interpreting automated discovery results and then making use of the insights gained for designing or adapting process models. Note that the survey in [17] showed that process model editing functionality is amongst the most desired additional features for the ProM-framework. This clearly indicates that (automated) analysis and (re)design are tightly coupled and tools and techniques in both areas should be maximally aligned.

Facilitating the Process Re-engineering Cycle. In typical redesign scenarios, people observe the as-is state of a process or set of processes, take certain improvement decisions, analyze the outcomes, and subsequently take additional improvement measures if necessary. Currently available automated process discovery techniques require business (process) analysts to possess additional skills and knowledge about typical output modeling notations such as Petri nets, Heuristic nets, or Fuzzy models. In addition, next to interpretation, practitioners will also be required to compare the results of automated discovery with existing process models. Such a comparison is far from effortless requiring profound technical understanding often unavailable in organizations with lower BPM maturity. With discovered process models in native BPMN format, the mapping of discovered vs. existing models becomes significantly easier.

Improved Communication of Process Mining Results. Working with a unified process model notation throughout the entire BPM life cycle will enable improved communication between functional units as well as across organizational hierarchies. Due to the fact that many organizations heavily rely on process modeling for documentation and communication, investments in data collection and data analysis might be perceived more worthwhile because these investments should not be looked at in isolation, but can actually contribute to and improve existing BPM practices.

2.2 Relevance for Education

A second stakeholder group for which BPMN-based process discovery is of value is educators and students. Generally speaking, BPM courses and text books (e.g. [18]) kick off with a thorough discussion on process modeling, with BPMN often receiving a great deal of attention. In later stages or chapters, process mining is brought up as well. However, this often requires educators to introduce new modeling notations, most notably Petri nets, Heuristic nets, and Fuzzy models, given their popularity for process mining. Moreover, the introduction of such new paradigms quickly obfuscates the link with process modeling and execution topics. While several programs can already leverage upon previously acquired knowledge, a majority of students, e.g. in business/management-oriented studies, do not possess such background knowledge. For that reason, a high-quality process discovery tool which presents its results in BPMN is likely to lower the effort required by educators to incorporate process mining in their units. It is pointed out that, from a student perspective, a positive attitude towards the usability and ease of use has been observed with respect to BPMN and its tool support [19].

2.3 Relevance for Research

Key research contributions in the process mining field have traditionally been strongly technical in nature. While valuable application studies have been published as well, there exists a significant opportunity for research about topics such as usefulness, ease of use, user acceptance, etc. of process mining within organisations. A process discovery technique with BPMN as underlying modeling language will lower barriers to conducting such studies, which often involve technically lower skilled individuals. Ultimately, user-centered studies could provide valuable insights into how the full potential of process mining can be realized or in what directions future process mining research should develop.

3 Comparative Study

The quality of discovered process models is inherently determined by the implicit search space implied by the representational bias of a process discovery technique (and thus its associated representation language). In [20], the authors advocate for selecting the "right" representational bias when discovering process models from event logs. They argue that the representational bias should be based on essential properties of a process model and should not be driven by the desired graphical representation. The process mining manifesto also lists the aspect of representational bias as one of the key challenges in the process mining domain [21].

While we don't contest that the search for an optimal representational bias for process discovery in terms of the implicit search space is of interest, a more pragmatic stance is taken in this paper. This is because, from a knowledge discovery viewpoint [22], patterns discovered from data should adhere to several principles: validity, novelty, usefulness, and understandability. While the use of for instance Causal nets for process discovery is likely to produce rich and high quality results, such an approach suffers from a steep learning curve which often leads to problems of understandability. For this reason, we argue that a more pragmatic, user-centered stance with respect to the suitability of the representational bias is worth pursuing. This pragmatic approach is based upon an assessment of some key characteristics of process modeling notations for the purpose of process discovery, as detailed in Table 1. It is argued that there exist two contrasting effects that make it difficult to agree on one fit-for-all modeling notation for process discovery.

Table 1. Key characteristics of process modeling notations for the purpose of process discovery.

Modeling Notation	Ease of Interpretation	Suitability Rep. Bias Proc. Disc.	Popularity (Modeling)	Popularity (Mining)
Petri net	●●○○○	●●○○○	●○○○○	●●●●○
Heuristic net	●●●○○	●●●●○	○○○○○	●●●●●
Fuzzy model	●●●●○	●●●●○	○○○○○	●●●●●
Causal net	●○○○○	●●●●●	○○○○○	●●○○○
EPC	●●●●○	●○○○○	●●●●○	●●○○○
BPMN	●●●●●	●●○○○	●●●●●	○○○○○

Based on a comparative analysis of various modeling notations, it is observed that traditionally popular modeling notations used for process discovery (i.e. Heuristic nets, Fuzzy models, and Causal nets) put a strong emphasis on the suitability of the representational bias. Note that our judgment about the representational bias reflects how well these notations help process discovery techniques at expressing a large number of possible constructs, while at the same time avoiding syntactically incorrect models as much as possible. Therefore, Petri nets, another popular representation choice, are scored lower because it is actually non-trivial to avoid the construction of incorrect Petri nets. On the other hand, representation languages with a less steep learning curve such as EPC and BPMN make it more difficult for process discovery techniques in terms of representational bias because modeling constructs are difficult to map against recorded data and because of the broad set of available constructs in the case of BPMN. A second, even stronger, contrast exists in terms of the level of popularity for modeling vs. mining. Basically, there exists an important discrepancy in the BPM domain between languages used for modeling and languages used for mining. While some might argue that models can be translated from one language to another (for instance through the use of Petri nets as BPM's Esperanto), this often involves non-trivial procedures. With this paper, we opt to bridge the gap between modeling and mining by making use of BPMN as the representational language.

To conclude, we recognize that BPMN presents several drawbacks as a representational language for process discovery. Most importantly, many of its concepts are difficult or impossible to map with recorded event data. In addition, the broad range of concepts also leads to the absence of a clear and crisp definition of its execution semantics, which is a much desired characteristic for process discovery. However, given the rationale in Sect. 2 for a native BPMN miner, the next section details how these limitations can be dealt with.

4   Implementation

This section provides a formalization of the developed technique, together with an overview regarding its implementation as a ProM plugin[1].

4.1   Preliminaries

We define the following terms and notations. An *event log L* is defined as a multi set of traces. Each trace $\sigma \in L$ is a finite sequence of events with σ_i the event at position i in trace σ. Let T_L denote a set of activities occurring in the event log L. Let O_L denote a set of originators occurring in the event log L. $a : L \to T_L$ is the function returning the activity for a given event, $o : L \to O_L$ is the function returning the originator (i.e. the role, person, group, department...) having executed the event. A trace can simply be denoted in full based on the activities and originators of its event, e.g.: $\sigma = \langle start^{alice}, register^{bob}, \ldots \rangle$.

The *Business Process Model and Notation* (BPMN) is a well-known diagrammatic notation to support the specification of business processes. BPMN consists of a high amount of notational elements, classified into four types: flow objects, connecting objects, artifacts and swim lanes. Artifacts and swim lanes are unrelated to process flows and thus do not come into play for BPMN's token-based execution semantics. Due to space constraints, we do not provide a full description of BPMN, but instead refer the reader to [6].

4.2   Control-Flow Discovery

One of the novel contributions of our process discovery technique is that it directly applies BPMN as the representational language for discovering process models from event logs, thus not relying on a translation. As stated in the introduction, the discovery of BPMN models has been somewhat overlooked so far,

---

[1] In analogy with the WEKA toolkit for data mining, ProM is an extensible framework that supports a wide variety of process mining techniques in the form of plug-ins. See: http://www.processmining.org.

mainly due to fact that BPMN lacks a formal definition of its execution semantics and its many notational constructs pose a challenge for discovery techniques.
To overcome this issue, our proposed approach deliberately considers a subset
of BPMN's notational constructs in order to perform the control-flow discovery.
Other works have illustrated that only a small subset of BPMN is actually being
applied in real-life modeling practice [13], those being gateways (XOR and parallel), tasks, sequence flow, start and end event, and swim lanes. All of these
constructs are also supported by our approach. In addition, we highlight the
fact that discovered BPMN process models by our approach do provide an ideal
starting point which can easily be adapted, extended, and modified by modelers
and practitioners, as the discovered model lies much closer to the representational language practitioners are already applying, thus preventing conversion
steps (with potential loss of accuracy or behavioral representation) or having to
learn other modeling notations.

To perform the control-flow discovery, our technique applies an algorithm
which is similar to the one applied in Heuristics Miner [3]. The basic idea works
as follows. First: dependency information is derived between activities in the
event log to construct a so called dependency graph $D = \{(a,b)|a \in T_L \land b \in T_L \land \exists \sigma \in L : [\exists \sigma_i \in \sigma : [a(\sigma_i) = a \land a(\sigma_{i+1}) = b]]\}$. Next, the splits and joins in
the dependency graph need to be characterized by semantic information and con-
verted to BPMN constructs. For example, for the split $\{(a,b), (a,c), (a,d)\} \subset D$,
we aim to investigate whether b, c, and d all occur in parallel (AND split), independently (XOR split), or a mixture of both. This is done by iterating over the
traces in the event log and investigated succession and precedence relations for
the given split or join respectively, similar to the approach applied in Heuristics
Miner [23]. For example, for the split above, we investigate to see how many
times b alone occurred after a, c alone occurred after a, d alone occurred after
a, b and c occurred after a, b and d occurred after a, c and d occurred after a,
and how many times all three activities occurred after a (always before the next
occurrence of a). Based on these frequencies, we derive the semantics of the split
or join, and thus define $I : T_L \rightarrow \mathcal{P}(\mathcal{P}(T_L))$ and $O : T_L \rightarrow \mathcal{P}(\mathcal{P}(T_L))$ as the
functions returning the input and output patterns for each task. A pattern is
defined as a set of sets where each set of activities is interpreted as a disjunction
(XOR), and the activities within a set are interpreted as a conjunction (AND).

Based on this information, a BPMN model is constructed as follows. First,
start and end events are added. Second, the BPMN graph is constructed. Activities are added for each $a \in T_L$: A_a. Next, a XOR input and output gateway
is created for each activity A_a: XOR_a^i and XOR_a^o and connected to the activity with sequence flows (XOR_a^i, A_a) and (A_a, XOR_a^o). For each $a \in T_L$, AND
gateways are created for each set of activities in $I(a)$ and $O(a)$: $AND_a^{i,j}$ and
$AND_a^{o,k}$, which are connected to the input and output XOR gateways with
sequence flows $(AND_a^{i,j}, XOR_a^i)$ for $j = 1, \ldots, |I(a)|$ and $(XOR_a^o, AND_a^{o,k})$
for $k = 1, \ldots, |O(a)|$. Next, a set of XOR connecting gateways is constructed
for each $a_i \in \bigcup(I(a))$ with $a \in T_L | a \neq a_i$: $XOR_d^{a_i,a}$ and for each $a_o \in \bigcup(O(a))$ with $a \in T_L | a \neq a_o$: XOR_d^{a,a_o}. Sequence flows are added for each

$(AND_a^{o,k}, XOR_d^{a_i,a_o})$ so that $a_i \in T_L, a_o \in T_L, a \in T_L, k = 1, \ldots |O(a)|$ and with $a_i \in O(a)^{k2}$. Similarly, we add flows for each $(XOR_d^{a_i,a_o}, AND_a^{i,j})$ so that $a_i \in T_L, a_o \in T_L, a \in T_L, j = 1, \ldots |I(a)|$ and with $a_o \in I(a)^j$. Finally, the start and end event are connected with all the activities A_a for which $I(a) = \{\emptyset\}$ and $O(a) = \{\emptyset\}$ respectively. If no such activity can be found, the algorithm determines a single start/end activity based on the frequency of the activity occurring most commonly at the start/end of traces. On the other hand, if multiple start or ending activities can be identified, they are connected through a XOR gateway with the starting and ending event. The third phase of the control-flow discovery algorithm consists of simplification of the BPMN model. This simplification step consists of iterative removal of all gateways which only contain a single incoming and one outgoing sequence flow, merging all AND gateways with the same incoming activities and a single outgoing activity (using a XOR gateway to connect the merged outgoing activities to the AND gateway) and merging all AND gateways with the same outgoing activities and a single incoming activity (using a XOR gateway to connect the merged incoming activities to the AND gateway).

4.3   Filtering and Abstraction

Discovering process models containing a high amount of activities, dependencies and noise leads to spaghetti models with a high amount of variability. In this case, the value of the discovered process models decreases rapidly, as it is no longer possible to derive understandable insights on how the as-is process is behaving.

We have implemented a number of techniques to deal with the aspects of variability and noise. First of all, users have the option to configure a dependency threshold, similar as the dependency thresholds applied in Heuristics Miner, although here, only one dependency threshold is used. The dependency threshold affects which arcs will be taken into the account during the construction of the dependency graph D. Second, we also incorporate a split/join threshold, affecting which patterns will be considered to include in $I(a)$ and $O(a)$ (based on their frequency). Finally, in case event logs contain low-frequent activities, the implemented plugin also offers end users the option to first filter out these low-frequent activities from the log before continuing with the discovery.

4.4   Bidimensional Discovery

The majority of existing process discovery algorithms focus on discovering the control-flow perspective of an event log, meaning that they use the sequence and ordering of activities to derive a process model using a particular representational language. Other techniques exist which start from another event log perspective (social network extraction techniques [24], for instance). In BPMN

---

[2] We assume here that the input and output sets are ordered. $O(a)^k$ thus returns the jth subset of $O(a)$.

Miner, we apply a bidimensional approach, directly incorporating the social (i.e. originator) perspective in the discovered model, together with control-flow (i.e. the sequence flow between activities).

To model originator information, our technique makes use of the swimlane construct of BPMN, meaning that our technique attempts to create a number of swimlanes containing one or more activities. Each swimlane then represent a "worker pool" (or "role") which is responsible for executing its contained activities. The swimlanes are discovered as follows. Recall $o : L \rightarrow O_L$ as being the function returning the originator (i.e. the role, person, group, department...) having executed an event. Depending on the desired level of granularity, end-users can choose which originator attribute to use to construct the swimlanes. First, for each activity $a \in T_L$, a dedicated swimlane-representing set $S_i = \{a\}$ is constructed, containing this single activity, so that $S = \{S_1, \ldots, S_{|T_L|}\}$. Next, swimlanes S_i and S_j are merged iff $\exists o \in O_L, a_i \in S_i, a_j \in S_j, \sigma_i \in L, \sigma_j \in L :$ $[a(\sigma_i) = a_i \wedge a(\sigma_j) = a_j \wedge o(\sigma_i) = o(\sigma_j) = o]$. Ultimately, this leads to a set of merged swimlanes representing a grouping of activities which are to be contained in their swimlane. The grouping is performed such that each swimlane also represents a "role" (a distinct grouping of originators) responsible for this set of activities.

4.5   Conformance Analysis

Apart from discovering BPMN models using a bidimensional approach, we also incorporate conformance checking functionality in BPMN Miner. More precisely, we add the ability to replay an event log over a discovered BPMN model (using token-based execution semantics), to determine the fitness level of the BPMN model in respect to the given event log. An overall fitness metric is then defined as the number of events in the event log which could be correctly executed by the BPMN model over the total amount of events. In addition, since this fitness metric is defined in an event-granular manner, we can also, for each activity in the model, indicate its degree of conformance in a visual manner. The following section outlines an example illustrating this functionality.

4.6   Exporting

The final functional element of BPMN Miner we wish to emphasize is the ability to export and convert the discovered BPMN models. For exporting, we make use of ProM's built in exporting functionality to enable end-users to save discovered models to XPDL (XML Process Definition Language), which can then be read in by most existing modeling tools (ARIS, Bizagi, Signavio, Activiti, etc.). To accommodate the needs of researchers and scholars, functionality is also provided to convert the discovered BPMN models to Petri nets.

5   Illustrating Example

This section illustrates the developed BPMN Miner by means of a concise, fictitious example. To do so, we utilize the *driversLicenseLoop* event log (a commonly

used log in benchmarking setups, see [25]), and annotate this event log with originator information. Figure 1 depicts a number of screen captions illustrating the
features of the BPMN Miner plugin. Figure 1(a) shows the result of mining the
BPMN model from the *driversLicenseLoop* event log without creating swimlanes
or performing conformance analysis. This model can be exported to XPDL and
imported in third-party tools or converted in ProM to a Petri net and used for
further analysis. Figure 1(b) shows the discovered BPMN model with the bidimensional discovery and conformance analysis enabled. As shown, the model has
a perfect fitness level (all activities green). Each swimlane represents a pool of
originators responsible for the activities contained within the swimlane. Finally,
Fig. 1(c) shows the result of a conformance analysis of the mined BPMN diagram
(without swimlanes) against the event log in which a high amount of noise was
introduced and does thus not fit the discovered model. The coloring of activities
(green to red scale) indicate problematic areas with a high amount of deviations.

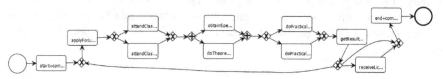

(a) Mined BPMN model without swimlanes or conformance visualization.

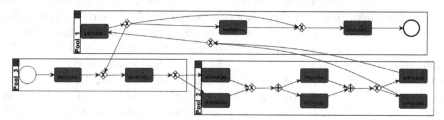

(b) Mined BPMN model with swimlanes and conformance visualization.

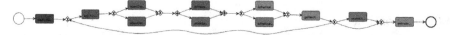

(c) Conformance analysis of mined BPMN diagram against noisy event log.

Fig. 1. Screen captions illustrating discovery features of BPMN Miner.

6   Conclusions

This paper describes BPMN Miner, a process discovery technique that directly
applies BPMN as its representational language for discovered models. The technique also provides functionality to discover resource-based swimlanes, thus

combining control-flow and resource information in one easily interpretable, bidimensional model. Moreover, BPMN Miner provides support for filtering and abstraction so as to deal with complex event logs presenting a wide variety of behavior. Finally, it provides the user with immediate feedback regarding the conformance between the input event log and the discovered model through an event-granular fitness metric and deviation visualization.

It is argued that BPMN Miner will lower the adoption barrier of process mining for practitioners, education, and researchers. In future work, we aim at further extending the set of supported BPMN constructs so as to ultimately develop a technique that can produce "rich" discovered process models, for instance with exception handling, sub-processes, data flows (discovery of data artifacts), or the discovery of external process participants based on interactions with the operating environment (this can be represented as collapsed pools with message flows). The discovery of hierarchical process structures with different invocation methods (subprocesses, call activities) is also put forward as future work.

Acknowledgements. We thank the KU Leuven research council for financial support under grant OT/10/010.

References

1. van der Aalst, W.M.P.: Process Mining - Discovery, Conformance and Enhancement of Business Processes. Springer, Heidelberg (2011)
2. Murata, T.: Petri nets:properties, analysis and applications. Proc. IEEE **77**(4), 541–580 (1989)
3. Weijters, A.J.M.M., van der Aalst, W.M.P.: Rediscovering workflow models from event-based data using little thumb. Integr. Comput.-Aided Eng. **10**(2), 151–162 (2003)
4. van der Aalst, W., Adriansyah, A., van Dongen, B.: Causal nets: a modeling language tailored towards process discovery. In: Katoen, J.-P., König, B. (eds.) CONCUR 2011. LNCS, vol. 6901, pp. 28–42. Springer, Heidelberg (2011)
5. Scheer, A.W., Thomas, O., Adam, O.: Process modeling using event-driven process chains. In: Dumas, M., van der Aalst, W.M.P., ter Hofstede, A.H.M. (eds.) Process-Aware Information Systems: Bridging People and Software Through Process Technology. Wiley, Hoboken (2005)
6. Object Management Group (OMG): Business Process Model and Notation (BPMN) Version 2.0. OMG Document - formal/2011-01-03 (2011)
7. Object Management Group (OMG): Business Process Model and Notation (BPMN) Version 1.2. OMG Document - formal/2009-01-03 (2009)
8. Dijkman, R.M.: Choreography-based design of business collaborations. Technical report, Eindhoven University of Technology (2006)
9. Dijkman, R.M., Dumas, M., Ouyang, C.: Formal semantics and automated analysis of BPMN process models. Technical report, Queensland University of Technology (2007)
10. Wong, P.Y.H., Gibbons, J.: A process semantics for BPMN. In: Liu, S., Araki, K. (eds.) ICFEM 2008. LNCS, vol. 5256, pp. 355–374. Springer, Heidelberg (2008)
11. Lam, V.S.: A precise execution semantics for BPMN. IAENG Int. J. Comput. Sci. **39**(1), 20–33 (2012)

12. Dijkman, R., Van Gorp, P.: BPMN 2.0 execution semantics formalized as graph rewrite rules. In: Mendling, J., Weidlich, M., Weske, M. (eds.) BPMN 2010. LNBIP, vol. 67, pp. 16–30. Springer, Heidelberg (2010)
13. zur Muehlen, M., Recker, J.: How much language is enough? theoretical and practical use of the business process modeling notation. In: Bubenko, J., Krogstie, J., Pastor, O., Pernici, B., Rolland, C., Sølvberg, A. (eds.) Seminal Contributions to Information Systems Engineering, pp. 429–443. Springer, Heidelberg (2013)
14. Recker, J.: Opportunities and constraints: the current struggle with BPMN. Bus. Proc. Manag. J. 16(1), 181–201 (2010)
15. Recker, J.C.: BPMN modeling-who, where, how and why. BPTrends 5(3), 1–8 (2008)
16. Chinosi, M., Trombetta, A.: BPMN: an introduction to the standard. Comput. Stand. Interfaces 34(1), 124–134 (2012)
17. Claes, J., Poels, G.: Process mining and the ProM framework: an exploratory survey. In: La Rosa, M., Soffer, P. (eds.) BPM 2012 Workshops. LNBIP, vol. 132, pp. 187–198. Springer, Heidelberg (2013)
18. Dumas, M., Rosa, M.L., Mendling, J., Reijers, H.A.: Fundamentals of Business Process Management. Springer, Heidelberg (2013)
19. Rozman, T., Horvat, R.V., Rozman, I.: Modeling the standard compliant software processes in the university environment. Bus. Process Manag. J. 14(1), 53–64 (2008)
20. van der Aalst, W.M.P.: On the representational bias in process mining. In: Reddy, S., Tata, S. (eds.): WETICE, pp. 2–7. IEEE Computer Society (2011)
21. van der Aalst, W., et al.: Process mining manifesto. In: Daniel, F., Barkaoui, K., Dustdar, S. (eds.) BPM 2011 Workshops, Part I. LNBIP, vol. 99, pp. 169–194. Springer, Heidelberg (2012)
22. Fayyad, U.M., Piatetsky-Shapiro, G., Smyth, P.: Knowledge discovery and data mining: Towards a unifying framework. In: KDD, pp. 82–88 (1996)
23. Weijters, A.J.M.M., van der Aalst, W.M.P., Alves de Medeiros, A.K.: Process mining with the heuristicsminer algorithm. BETA working paper series 166, TU Eindhoven (2006)
24. van der Aalst, W.M.P., Reijers, H.A., Song, M.: Discovering social networks from event logs. Comput. Support. Coop. Work 14(6), 549–593 (2005)
25. Alves de Medeiros, A., Weijters, A., van der Aalst, W.: Genetic process mining: an experimental evaluation. Data Min. Knowl. Discov. 14(2), 245–304 (2007)

Designing and Evaluating an Interpretable Predictive Modeling Technique for Business Processes

Dominic Breuker[(⊠)], Patrick Delfmann, Martin Matzner,
and Jörg Becker

Department for Information Systems,
Leonardo-Campus 3, 48149 Muenster, Germany
{breuker,delfmann,matzner,becker}@ercis.com

Abstract. Process mining is a field traditionally concerned with retrospective analysis of event logs, yet interest in applying it online to running process instances is increasing. In this paper, we design a predictive modeling technique that can be used to quantify probabilities of how a running process instance will behave based on the events that have been observed so far. To this end, we study the field of grammatical inference and identify suitable probabilistic modeling techniques for event log data. After tailoring one of these techniques to the domain of business process management, we derive a learning algorithm. By combining our predictive model with an established process discovery technique, we are able to visualize the significant parts of predictive models in form of Petri nets. A preliminary evaluation demonstrates the effectiveness of our approach.

Keywords: Data mining · Process mining · Grammatical inference · Predictive modeling

1 Motivation

In recent years, business analytics has emerged as one of the hottest topics in both research and practice. With stories praising the opportunities of data analysis being omnipresent, it is not surprising that scholars from diverse fields explore how data can be exploited to improve business understanding and decision making. In business process management (BPM), a research discipline called *process mining* has emerged that deals with analyzing historical data about instances of business processes [1]. The data usually comes in form of event logs, which are collections of sequences of events that have been collected while executing a business process. Events are of different types. The type describes the nature of an event. For instance, an event could represent an activity that was performed or a decision that was made.

Traditionally, process mining has been used mainly for retrospective analysis. The primary task of many process mining techniques is to discover the underlying process given an event log, with the goal of providing analysts with an objective view on an organization's collective behavior [2]. Further analyses can follow. One could verify

© Springer International Publishing Switzerland 2015
F. Fournier and J. Mendling (Eds.): BPM 2014 Workshops, LNBIP 202, pp. 541–553, 2015.
DOI: 10.1007/978-3-319-15895-2_46

that a process conforms to a given specification or improve the process based on the discovered insights [1].

In recent times, interest has been expressed into applying process mining no only ex post but also in an online setting. The idea is to apply insights gained from event logs to currently running process instances. The goals could be to predict properties of interest or recommend good decisions [3]. Techniques have been designed to predict the time at which a process instance will be completed [4] or to recommend performers for tasks such that performance is maximized [5].

In this paper, we consider a similar prediction problem. Interpreting events of an event log as outcomes of decisions, our goal is to build a predictive analytics model that accounts for the sequential nature of decision making in business processes. Provided with a partial sequence of events from an unfinished process instance, the model's task is quantifying the likelihood of the instance ending with certain future sequences. The model should be trained solemnly by means of event log data.

Such a predictive model could be useful in variety of situations. For instance, early warning systems could be built. Decision makers could be provided with a list of running process instances in which undesirable events will likely be observed in the future. A predictive model could also be used to estimate how many running instances will require a certain resource, again to warn decision makers if capacities will be exceeded. Moreover, anomaly detection approaches could be built to identify highly unlikely process instances. They could help pointing business analysts to unusual instances. It is also conceivable to use a predictive model to support other process mining endeavors, for instance by imputing missing values in incomplete event logs.

The first step in constructing a predictive modeling approach is defining a suitable representation of the data and the model structure. To find one, we tap into research from the field of grammatical inference, which is the study of learning structure from discrete sequential data [6], often by fitting probabilistic models [7]. After identifying a suitable model, we also discuss how to fit the model to data. Again, we draw on grammatical inference to identify a suitable technique. Subsequently, we adapt the probabilistic model to the BPM domain. As a consequence, we have to adapt the fitting technique too. By applying the predictive modeling approach to real-world event logs, we illustrate how it can be used and demonstrate its effectiveness.

The primary goal of our modifications is to define the probabilistic model such that its structure most closely resembles the structure of business processes. An advantage of that is that models with appropriate structure typically perform better when used in predictive analytics. The other goal is to keep the model interpretable. Whenever non-technical stakeholders are involved in predictive analytics endeavors, interpretability can be crucial to get them on board. For this reason, interpretable models may be preferred even if they perform worse than their black box counterparts [8]. By combining a technique from process mining [9] with our predictive modeling approach, we are able to visualize a predictive model's structure in form of process models. This puts domain experts in the position to judge the quality of a predictive model.

The remainder of this paper is structured as follows. In Sect. 2, we discuss probabilistic models and fitting techniques used in grammatical inference. Section 3 is devoted to the BPM-specific modifications we designed. In Sect. 4, we describe how process mining can be applied to create visualizations. The evaluation of our approach is documented in Sect. 5. In Sect. 6, we conclude and give an outlook to future research.

2 Grammatical Inference

2.1 Probabilistic Models of Discrete Sequential Data

The inductive learning problem tackled in grammatical inference [10] starts with a data set $X = \{x^{(1)}, \ldots, x^{(C)}\}$ with C strings. Each string $x^{(c)}$ is a sequence $(x_1^{(c)}, \ldots, x_{t_c}^{(c)})$ of symbols t_c, all of which are part of an alphabet: $x_t \in \{1, \ldots, E\}$. The number of different symbols shall be denoted E. When interpreting the data as an event log with C process instances, each of which consists of a sequence of events which, in turn, a part of the alphabet of event types, grammatical inference can be readily applied to event log data.

The task is to learn a formal representation of the language from which the sample strings in the data originate. These representations are either automata or grammars [6]. Instead of building automata and grammars that decide if strings belong to a language, it is often more useful to build probabilistic versions of these representations [10]. This allows further analyses such as finding the most probable string or predicting how likely certain symbols are given partial strings.

Since it is our goal to apply grammatical inference to the domain of BPM, we focus our discussion on automata. Automata consist of states and transitions between these states. By contrast, grammars consist of production rules that do not directly encode any states. A state-based representation appears most natural as modeling techniques used in BPM follow similar principles. Most importantly, explicit state modeling is one of the reasons for the popularity of Petri nets [11].

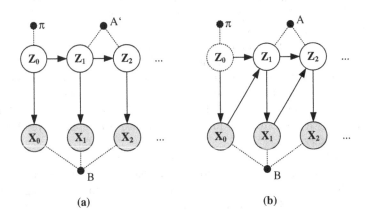

(a)   (b)

Fig. 1. Directed graphical models of an HMM (a) and a PFA (b). Circles represent random variables and are shaded grey if observations will be available. Directed arcs encode dependencies of random variables among each other. Conversely, missing arcs imply conditional independencies. Parameters are represented as solid black dots and are connected via dashed, undirected arcs to the random variables to whose distributions they belong [12]

There are many different variants of automata studied in the literature. Two of them are most popular [7]. One is the Hidden Markov Model (HMM), the other is the Probabilistic Finite Automaton (PFA). HMMs [13] are generative models of string distributions. They use an unobserved state space to explain how the strings have been generated. To that end, discrete time steps are defined and the model's state evolves in time. At each step, the HMM is in one state and emits a symbol. The probability of emitting a symbol depends only on the current state. Then, the HMM transitions to another state which it is in in the next time step. The transition probability also depends only on the current step's state. Figure 1 (a) illustrates the HMM.

Reflecting the HMM's model structure against the backdrop of the BPM domain unveils a problem. The process is driven mainly by the HMM's states and the transitions between them. The symbols however do not influence these transitions. In a typical business process though, we would expect the next state to depend on the event we have just observed. Consider the example of Petri nets, in which the state after firing a transition clearly depends on which transition is chosen. As the HMM assumes independence, we discard it is a probabilistic model for business processes.

This motivates considering the PFA [14]. We illustrated another graphical model in Fig. 1 (b). It is similar to that of the HMM, but with an additional arc from each symbol to the following state. Effectively, this arc removes the problematic assumption of independence. This model can now serve as the probabilistic equivalent of automata as applied in the BPM domain.

2.2 Learning Techniques

Approaches to learn probabilistic automata can be categorized broadly into three classes [7]. Those from the first class start with a very complex structure and iteratively merge states until the structure is simple enough. Approaches from the second class assume a standard structure and optimize parameters such that the likelihood of the data is maximal. The third class of approaches consists of sampling methods that rely not on estimating any model but on averaging over many possible models.

In a recent grammatical inference competition, different state-of-the-art learning approaches have been benchmarked against each other on a large collection of data sets [15]. The winning team [16] has designed a collapsed Gibbs sampler to estimate string probabilities, i.e., they applied a method from the third class. Second best scored a team [17] that used maximum likelihood (ML) estimation, i.e., the standard technique from the second class. Methods from the first class have also been applied, yet they scored worse than the others.

These results may indicate that sampling methods are the most promising learning techniques. However, they have an important drawback. While approaches from other categories deliver explicit representations of the analyzed processes along with interpretable parameters, the Gibbs sampling techniques draws randomly many such representations and averages over them when predicting. As a result, there is no way to compactly visualize the predictive model anymore. However, one of our design goals is to avoid creating a black box learning method. Hence, we design our approach not based on sampling techniques but instead based on parameter optimization, i.e., a technique from the second class.

3 PFA Learning with Event Logs

3.1 Adapting the PFA Model

In this section, we define two modifications of the PFA model of Sect. 2.1. The first addresses the problem of overfitting to small data sets. It is well-known that an ML estimator is at danger of delivering results that fit well to training data but perform badly on new data [18]. For process data, overfitting can be a severe problem. Process miners consider incompleteness of data as one of the major challenges their discipline has to tackle [19]. Consequently, we have to take precautions.

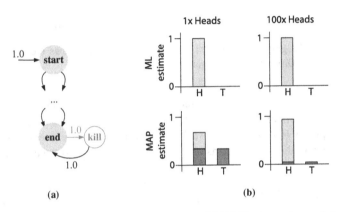

Fig. 2. Illustration of the modifications to the PFA model. (a) illustrates the predefined start and end states. (b) illustrates the effect of Bayesian regularization.

For our probabilistic model, we address this problem with Bayesian regularization [20]. This technique is best illustrated with the simple example of tossing a two-sided coin (cf. Fig. 2 (b) for the following explanation). Consider two data sets. In the first, heads was observed once, in the second, heads was observed 100 times. If the goal is to estimate p, the probability of heads, then for both data sets, the ML estimate will be $p = 1$. In the first scenario, we overfit to the small data set. This can be avoided by smoothing the estimates with artificial observations. In the example of Fig. 2 (b), we can add one artificial observation of both heads and tails, which would deliver an estimate of $p = 2/3$ in the first scenario and $p = 101/102$ in the second. This is achieved by interpreting p not as a parameter but also as a random variable with a distribution. When using the beta distribution in this example, the beta distribution's parameters can be used to specify the artificial observations [21]. Estimating p in such a setting is called Maximum a posteriori (MAP) estimation.

We can move to MAP estimation in our PFA model by treating the parameters as random variables and by defining their distributions to be Dirichlet distributions, which are conjugate priors for the discrete distributions used to define the other variables [21]. The parameters of the Dirichlet distributions can be interpreted as the artificial observations we want to add when estimating parameters of discrete distributions. See Fig. 3 (a) for the graphical model corresponding to the regularized PFA and Fig. 3 (b) for a formal definition of the model.

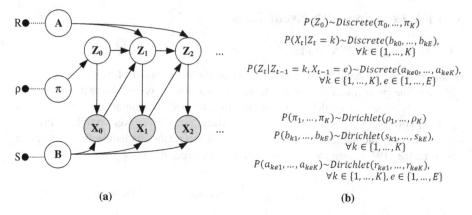

$$P(Z_0){\sim}Discrete(\pi_0,...,\pi_K)$$

$$P(X_t|Z_t=k){\sim}Discrete(b_{k0},...,b_{kE}),$$
$$\forall k \in \{1,...,K\}$$

$$P(Z_t|Z_{t-1}=k,X_{t-1}=e){\sim}Discrete(a_{ke0},...,a_{keK}),$$
$$\forall k \in \{1,...,K\}, e \in \{1,...,E\}$$

$$P(\pi_1,...,\pi_K){\sim}Dirichlet(\rho_1,...,\rho_K)$$

$$P(b_{k1},...,b_{kE}){\sim}Dirichlet(s_{k1},...,s_{kE}),$$
$$\forall k \in \{1,...,K\}$$

$$P(a_{ke1},...,a_{keK}){\sim}Dirichlet(r_{ke1},...,r_{keK}),$$
$$\forall k \in \{1,...,K\}, e \in \{1,...,E\}$$

(a)   **(b)**

Fig. 3. (a) shows the graphical model of the modified PFA. (b) shows the definition of the model's discrete and Dirichlet distributions.

The second modification is motivated by the notion of workflows nets, a special class of Petri nets well known in the BPM domain [11]. Workflow nets have designated start and end places (the *source* and *sink*) since well-designed process models should clearly show where the process starts and ends. We impose the same constraints on the PFA model.

To implement these constraints, we define a special starting state by keeping the vector π fixed at a value that allows the process to start only in that state. In the same way, a special ending state is defined in which only a designated termination event *"kill"* can be emitted. Also, the process is forced to stay in that state. *Kill* shall be an event that can only be emitted in the ending state. All other states have zero probability of emitting it. When processing he event log, the *Kill* must be appended to the end of each process instance. Figure 2 (a) illustrates the structural assumptions described above. They can all be enforced by keeping the corresponding parameters fixed at suitable values while executing the learning algorithm.

3.2 Learning Algorithm

MAP estimation aims at maximizing the posterior probability $P(\theta|X)$. θ denotes all parameters that must be estimated. This optimization can be implemented by optimizing the following expression: $\theta^* = \arg\max_{\theta}[P(X|\theta)P(\theta)]$ [22]. Direct optimization is computationally intractable in presence of unobserved variables such as our state variables. A solution is to apply the expectation maximization (EM) procedure [23]. Starting with (random) initial parameters, it iterates between computing the expectation of the hidden state variables Z with respect to current parameters θ^{old} (i.e., $\mathbb{E}_{Z|X,\theta^{old}}$ $\ln P(X,Z|\theta)$) and deriving updated parameters θ^{new} by optimizing them with respect to this expectation over states (i.e., $\theta^{new} = \arg\max_{\theta}\left[\mathbb{E}_{Z|X,\theta^{old}} \ln P(X,Z|\theta) + \ln P(\theta)\right]$). The algorithm stops once a local optimum is reached [24]. This optimum depends on the initial parameters, which is why it is advisable to run EM multiple times with different initial values to avoid bad local optima [25].

To apply EM to our probabilistic model, we must implement the four steps *initial parameter definition*, *E-step*, *M-step*, and the *check for convergence*. Our implementation generates initial parameters randomly, with the exception that we enforce a starting and ending state as described in Sect. 3.1. The corresponding parameters are fixed at 0 and 1 respectively. Convergence is also determined in the standard way, i.e., by defining a threshold and stopping the algorithm if the likelihood of the data does not improve enough after updating parameters.

To implement the E-step and M-step, we start with $\theta^{new} = \arg \max_{\theta} [\mathbb{E}_{Z|X,\theta^{old}} \ln P(X, Z|\theta) + \ln P(\theta)]$ and use Lagrangian multipliers to derive updating equations. These updating equations can be found in Eqs. 1–3. They all consist of a *data*-term, which is the contribution of the event log data, and a *prior*-term, which is the contribution of the corresponding Dirichlet distribution. In each M-step, these updating equations are used to compute updated parameter values.

$$\pi_k = \frac{data_k + prior_k}{\sum_{j=1}^{K}(data_k + prior_k)} \tag{1}$$

$$b_{ke} = \frac{data_{ke} + prior_{ke}}{\sum_{e=1}^{E}(data_{ke} + prior_{ke})} \tag{2}$$

$$a_{kej} = \frac{data_{kej} + prior_{kej}}{\sum_{j=1}^{K}(data_{kej} + prior_{kej})} \tag{3}$$

In each E-step, the *data*-terms are computed (the *prior*-terms are fixed and require no computations). All terms are shown in Eqs. 4–9. Within these equations, $T_e^{(c)}$ denotes the set of points in time at which an event of type e is observed in instance $x^{(c)}$. $T^{(c)}$ denotes all points in time regardless of the event types. All *data*-terms consist of sums over marginal distributions over the state variables. For our probabilistic model, they can be computed efficiently with a standard procedure called belief propagation [26], which we have implemented in our E-step.

$$data_k = \sum_{c=1}^{C} P\left(Z_0^{(c)} = k | X^{(c)}, \theta^{old}\right) \tag{4}$$

$$prior_k = \rho_k - 1 \tag{5}$$

$$data_{ke} = \sum_{c=1}^{C} \sum_{t \in T_e^{(c)}} P\left(Z_t^{(c)} = k | X^{(c)}, \theta^{old}\right) \tag{6}$$

$$prior_{ke} = s_{ke} - 1 \tag{7}$$

$$data_{kej} = \sum_{c=1}^{C} \sum_{t \in T_e^{(c)}, t \neq 0} P\left(Z_{t-1}^{(c)} = k, Z_t^{(c)} = j | X^{(c)}, \theta^{old}\right) \tag{8}$$

$$prior_{kej} = r_{kej} - 1 \tag{9}$$

3.3 Model Selection

The learning algorithm described in the previous section must be provided with some input parameters. To define the dimensions of the probabilistic model, the number of event types E and the number of states K must be given. The former is known, but the latter must be chosen arbitrarily. Hence, we use grid search to determine appropriate values for K. The same is necessary for ρ, S, and R, the parameters of the Dirichlet distributions. As we do not want to bias the model towards certain decisions, we use symmetric Dirichlet priors. However, the strength of these parameters must still be chosen arbitrarily, which again requires grid search.

In grid search, a range of possible values is defined for all parameters not directly optimized by EM. For each combination of values, EM is applied. The trained models from all these runs are subsequently compared to choose one that is best. Different criteria can be applied in this comparison. One solution is assigning a score based on likelihood penalized by the number of parameters, which favors small models. The Akaike Information Criterion (AIC) [27] is a popular criterion of this kind. One disadvantage of the AIC applied to probabilistic models of processes is that we would expect the models to be sparse, i.e., we expect that most transitions have very low probability. Hence, we also consider a less drastic criterion which we call the Heuristic Information Criterion (HIC). It penalizes the likelihood by the number of parameters exceeding a given threshold.

A different solution is to split the event log into a training set used for learning and a validation set used to score generalization performance. According to this criterion, the model performing best on the validation set is chosen.

4 Model Structure Visualization and Analysis

Since we carefully designed the probabilistic model to be interpretable, it is possible to derive meaningful visualizations from a learned model. Using the parameters, we could directly draw an automaton with K states and EK^2 transitions, i.e., a full graph. For all but the smallest examples though, the visualization would not be useful as it would be too complex. However, we can prune the automaton such that only sufficiently probable transitions are kept. For each transition, we delete it if its probability $b_{ke}a_{kej}$ is smaller than a given threshold. As there are KE transitions going out of each state, each transition would have a probability of $1/(KE)$ if all were equally probable. If they are not, then the probability mass will focus at the probable transitions, while probabilities of the improbable transitions will fall below this value. Hence, we define the pruning ratio *prune* relative to $1/(KE)$. Thresholds are defined as $1/(prune \cdot KE)$, such that a pruning ratio of *prune* $= 1.5$ means throwing away all transitions being 1.5 times as unlikely as if all transitions had probability $1/(KE)$.

As we effectively construct an automaton from an event log with this procedure, our technique has delivered not only a prediction approach but can also be used as a process discovery algorithm. To this end, we combine it with a technique that was used in the region miner algorithm [9]. In this algorithm, an automaton is constructed and then transformed into a Petri net using a tool called Petrify [28]. Hence, we can also apply Petrify to transform our pruned automata to Petri nets. We have implemented the entire approach as a process mining plugin for ProM.[1]

While discovering processes with our approach might have merits in itself, our primary motivation is to provide non-technical audiences with a visualization of a predictive model. If a stakeholder must be convinced that a certain predictive model should be implemented in his organization, the visualization approach could be used to build trust. Stakeholders can see in form of familiar process modeling notations what the most probable paths through the predictive model are.

5 Evaluation

Experimental Setup. To evaluate our approach as a predictive modeling technique, we apply it to a real-life event log from the business process intelligence challenge in 2012 [29]. It originates from a Dutch financial institute and contains about 262,000 events in 13,084 process instances. There are three subprocesses (called P_W, P_A, and P_O) and each event is uniquely assigned to one subprocess. Apart from the complete event log, we generated three additional event logs by splitting the complete log into these subprocesses. Each of the four event logs is split into a training set (50 %), a validation set (25 %) and a test set (25 %). The training set is used to run EM, the validation set is used during model selection, and the test set is used to assess final performance.

The EM algorithm was configured in the following way. Convergence was achieved when the log-likelihood increased less than 0.001 after the M-step. As a grid for K, we used $[2, 4, 8, 10, 12, 14, 16, 18, 20, 30, 40]$. The grid for the Dirichlet distributions' strength was defined relative to the sizes of the event logs. The overall number of artificial observations, distributed symmetrically over all Dirichlet distributions, was optimized over the grid $[0.0, 0.1, 0.2, 0.3, 0.4, 0.5, 0.75]$ and is expressed as a fraction of the total number of events in the logs. To compare different models in grid search, we separately tried all three methods described in Sect. 3.3, with the HIC applied with a threshold of 0.05.

One measure to estimate the quality is H, the cross entropy (as estimated w.r.t. the test set). We also consider a number of different prediction problems that could occur in practice. The most straightforward one is predicting what the next symbol will be. We report the average accuracy of our predictors. Accuracy is the fraction of predictions in which the correct event has been predicted. The other prediction problem is concerned

---

[1] http://goo.gl/FqzJwp.

Table 1. Accuracy, average sensitivity and average specitivity for different predictive models.

Event log	Predictor	Accuracy	Ø Sensitivity	Ø Specitivity	H
P_W	EM_HIC	0.685	0.558	0.950	12.810
	EM_AIC	0.719	0.578	0.955	11.183
	EM_Val	0.718	0.582	0.955	10.385
P_A	EM_HIC	0.801	0.723	0.980	3.093
	EM_AIC	0.769	0.658	0.977	3.393
	EM_Val	0.796	0.720	0.980	3.014
P_O	EM_HIC	0.809	0.646	0.973	4.588
	EM_AIC	0.811	0.647	0.973	4.513
	EM_Val	0.811	0.647	0.973	4.513
P_Complete	EM_HIC	0.735	0.508	0.988	17.273
	EM_AIC	0.694	0.460	0.986	17.726
	EM_Val	0.700	0.437	0.986	16.078

with specific types of events. After selecting an event type, the task is to predict whether or not the next event will be of this type. We measured the sensitivies (true positives) and specitivities (true negatives) for each predictor applied to the problem of deciding this for each event.

Note that our approach is not restricted to predicting the next event. Evaluating the distribution over an event arbitrarily far in the future is also feasible. However, our evaluation focusses on predicting the next event only.

Results. In Table 1, we list the results for all four event logs (*P_W*, *P_A*, *P_O*, and *P_Complete*). For each, we report performance statistics for the three different model selection criteria (EM_HIC, EM_AIC, and EM_Val). The sensitivies and specificities have been averaged over all symbols to keep the table compact.

A first observation is that accuracies do not rise up close to 1. However, accuracies that high cannot be expected, since there is inherent uncertainty in the decisions made in business processes. Thus, predicting the next event correctly must fail in some cases. Predicting events completely at random would deliver the correct event with probability $1/E$. For the three events logs, accuracies of random prediction would be below 0.10. Hence, our approach is significantly better than random guessing.

As for comparing the model selection criteria, the results demonstrate that using the validation set to assess performance delivered solid results if measured by cross entropy. For this metric, the validation set always delivered the best model, i.e., the one with the smallest cross entropy.

This is changing though if we turn to the actual prediction problems. The HIC performed best on *P_Complete* and *P_A*, yet bad on *P_W*, for which the AIC worked better. For event log *P_O*, all three methods deliver nearly the same performance. Hence, our preliminary results indicate that no model selection criterion can generally outperform the others.

In Fig. 4, an exemplary Petri net visualization is shown. It has been generated from a predictor for event log *P_A*, chosen by the HIC. An analyst could double-check this visualization with his domain knowledge. Alternatively, he could apply other process discovery techniques to verify that the predictive model is indeed a good model for the event log. Comparing this Petri net with results found during the challenge, we can see that the visualization of the predictor is almost identical to what has been discovered with other methods [30]. Hence, this visual comparison with other findings delivers further evidence for the appropriateness of the predictive model.

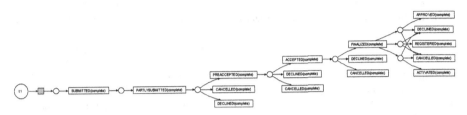

Fig. 4. Petri net visualization of predictor fitted with the HIC criterion, generated with the ProM plugin and a pruning ratio of 1.5.

6 Conclusion and Outlook

In this paper, we presented an approach to apply predictive modeling to event log data. We discussed different representations used in the literature of grammatical inference to model formal languages probabilistically. Against the backdrop of the BPM domain, we identified probabilistic versions of finite automata to be most appropriate. We also identified suitable learning techniques to fit these models to data. Starting with this theoretical background, we modified the probabilistic model to tailor it to the problem at hand. Subsequently, we derived an EM optimization algorithm, defined a grid search procedure to also optimize its inputs, and tested the approach on real-world event logs. Our preliminary results demonstrate the applicability of the approach. With the ProM plugin, in which we combined the predictive approach with ProM's Petri net synthesis capabilities, we provide a readily applicable process discovery tool.

In future research, we plan to conduct more extensive evaluations. In particular, we will systematically compare our model selection criteria to identify which work best under which circumstances. Adding experiments with synthetic data may also allow us to thoroughly investigate the performance of the predictive approach with respect to a known gold standard. For the real-life event log we used in the preliminary evaluation, the "true" probabilities are unknown, so that we cannot quantify the quality of the predictors generated with our approach in absolute terms.

References

1. van der Aalst, W.M.P.: Process Mining: Discovery, Conformance and Enhancement of Business Processes. Springer, Heidelberg (2011)
2. van der Aalst, W.M.P.: Process discovery: capturing the invisible. IEEE Comput. Intell. Mag. **5**(1), 28–41 (2010)

3. van der Aalst, W.M.P., Pesic, M., Song, M.: Beyond process mining: from the past to present and future. In: Pernici, B. (ed.) CAiSE 2010. LNCS, vol. 6051, pp. 38–52. Springer, Heidelberg (2010)
4. van der Aalst, W.M.P., Schonenberg, M.H., Song, M.: Time prediction based on process mining. Inf. Syst. J. **36**(2), 450–475 (2011)
5. Kim, A., Obregon, J., Jung, J.-Y.: Constructing Decision Trees from Process Logs for Performer Recommendation. In: Lohmann, N., Song, M., Wohed, P. (eds.) BPM 2013 Workshops. LNBIP, vol. 171, pp. 224–236. Springer, Heidelberg (2014)
6. de la Higuera, C.: A bibliographical study of grammatical inference. Pattern Recogn. **38**, 1332–1348 (2005)
7. Verwer, S., Eyraud, R., de la Higuera, C.: PAutomaC: a PFA/HMM learning competition. Mach. Learn. J. (2013)
8. Shmuelli, G., Koppius, O.R.: Predictive analytics in information systems research. Manag. Inf. Syst. Q. **35**(3), 553–572 (2011)
9. van der Aalst, W.M.P., Rubin, V., Verbeek, H.M.W., van Dongen, B.F., Kindler, E., Günther, C.W.: Process mining: a two-step approach to balance between underfitting and overfitting. Softw. Syst. Model. **9**(1), 87–111 (2010)
10. de la Higuera, C.: Grammatical Inference. Cambride University Press, Cambridge (2010)
11. van der Aalst, W.M.P.: The application of petri nets to workflow management. J. Circuits Syst. Comput. **8**(1), 21–66 (1998)
12. Koller, D., Friedman, N.: Probabilistic Graphical Models: Principles and Techniques. The MIT Press, Cambridge (2009)
13. Rabiner, L.R.: A tutorial on hidden markov models and selected applications in speech recognition. Proc. IEEE **77**(2), 257–286 (1989)
14. Vidal, E., Thollard, F., de la Higuera, C., Casacuberta, F., Carrasco, R.C.: Probabilistic finite-state machines - part I. IEEE Trans. Pattern Anal. Mach. Intell. **27**(7), 1013–1025 (2005)
15. Verwer, S., Eyraud, R., de la Higuera, C.: Results of the PAutomaC probabilistic automaton learning competition. In: 11th International Conference on Grammatical Inference, pp. 243–248 (2012)
16. Shibata, C., Yoshinaka, R.: Marginalizing out transition probabilities for several subclasses of Pfas. In: JMLR - Workshop Conference Proceedings, ICGI 2012, vol. 21, pp. 259–263 (2012)
17. Hulden, M.: Treba: efficient numerically stable EM for PFA. In: JMLR Workshop Conference Proceedings, vol. 21, pp. 249–253 (2012)
18. Hastie, T., Tibshirani, R., Friedman, J.: The Elements of Statistical Learning - Data Mining, Inference, and Prediction, 2nd edn. Springer, New York (2009)
19. van der Aalst, W.M.P., et al.: Process mining manifesto. In: Daniel, F., Barkaoui, K., Dustdar, S. (eds.) BPM Workshops 2011, Part I. LNBIP, vol. 99, pp. 169–194. Springer, Heidelberg (2012)
20. Steck, H., Jaakkola, T.: On the dirichlet prior and bayesian regularization. Neural Inf. Process. Syst. **15**, 1441–1448 (2002)
21. Barber, D.: Bayesian Reasoning and Machine Learning. Cambridge University Press, Cambridge (2011)
22. Bishop, C.M.: A new framework for machine learning. In: Zurada, J.M., Yen, G.G., Wang, J. (eds.) WCCI 2008, Plenary/Invited Lectures. LNCS, vol. 5050, pp. 1–24. Springer, Heidelberg (2008)
23. Dempster, A., Laird, N., Rubin, D.: Maximum likelihood from incomplete data via the EM algorithm. J. R. Stat. Soc. Ser. B **39**(1), 1–22 (1977)
24. Bishop, C.M.: Pattern Recognition and Machine Learning. Springer, New York (2006)

25. Moon, T.K.: The expectation-maximization algorithm. IEEE Signal Process. Mag. **13**(6), 47–60 (1996)
26. Murphy, K.: Machine Learning: A Probabilistic Perspective. The MIT Press, Cambridge (2012)
27. Akaike, H.: Information theory and an extension of the maximum likelihood principle. In: Second International Symposium on Information Theory, pp. 267–281 (1973)
28. Cortadella, J., Kishinevsky, M., Kondratyev, A., Lavagno, L., Yakovlev, A.: Petrify: a tool for manipulating concurrent specifications and synthesis of asynchronous controllers. IEICE Trans. Inf. Syst. **E80-D**(3), 315–325 (1997)
29. van Dongen, B.F.: BPI Challenge 2012 (2012). http://www.win.tue.nl/bpi/2012/challenge
30. Adriansyah, A., Buijs, J.: Mining Process Performance from Event Logs: The BPI Challenge 2012 Case Study. BPM Center Report BPM-12-15 (2012). BPMcenter.org

Doctoral Consortium at BPM 2014

Detecting, Assessing, and Mitigating Data Inaccuracy-Related Risks in Business Processes

Arava Tsoury[(⊠)], Soffer Pnina, and Iris Reinhartz-Berger

University of Haifa, Carmel Mountain, 31905 Haifa, Israel
{atsoury,spnina,iris}@is.haifa.ac.il

Abstract. Business process activities and their outcomes rely on data that is commonly stored in databases. If the stored data is not accurate, namely, it does not reflect the relevant real world values, the process execution might be disrupted and the process might not be able to reach its goal. Detection of such cases and analysis of their causes may help redesign processes to reduce the potential risks. In this research, we aim to develop a semi-automated method that will enable detection, assessment, and mitigation of risks related to data inaccuracy in business processes. The method will be built on and evaluated with real cases from the industry.

Keywords: Business processes · Data inaccuracy · Process design · Process mining · Risk assessment

1 The Research Problem Being Addressed

The management of business processes is commonly supported by process aware information systems (PAIS), storing, using and manipulating data. The process activities and their outcomes influence the state of the organization and its environment [6]. An underlying assumption is that the data truly reflects reality (real-world values). However, it is well known that the information which exists in PAIS is not always accurate [1].

As process activities rely on the existing (stored) data, incorrect values might harm decision-making and the resulting outcomes of the process. For understanding the impact of data inaccuracy on processes, we raise the following questions: how does inaccuracy of data affect the results of the process and the process ability to complete its execution? What are the risks associated with data inaccuracy? How can these risks be mitigated?

To illustrate, consider a conference management process through EasyChair. During papers bidding, the reviewers are asked to indicate whether they wish, don't mind, "resist", or have a conflict to review each paper. The resulting data might be inaccurate, not reflecting their "real" preferences and conflicts. This might happen due to lack of attention and using the default voting for some of the papers. As a result, paper assignment to reviewers might be harmed or might need corrections at a later phase, or the outcome of the review process might be negatively affected, e.g., by getting fewer reviews for certain papers.

F. Fournier and J. Mendling (Eds.): BPM 2014 Workshops, LNBIP 202, pp. 557–560, 2015.
DOI: 10.1007/978-3-319-15895-2_47

Data inaccuracy may never be discovered. Even if discovered, the consequences might depend on the time of discovery. This may occur after many actions have been performed based on the incorrect values. Discovery time has great impact on the severity of the risk (i.e., the amount of harm that can be expected due the use of inaccurate data). Therefore, data inaccuracy risks should be estimated with respect to time. Risk is defined as "the possibility that an event will occur and adversely affect the achievement of objectives" [2]. Metrics for assessing the criticality of data items and the robustness of the process design may support process redesign while also considering a cost benefit analysis of potential solutions.

The target of the proposed research is to provide a method that will enable the assessment of risks related to data inaccuracy in business processes. In particular, it will enable detecting situations of data inaccuracy in business processes and assessing data inaccuracy-related risks, leading to suggestions for redesign of the process to mitigate these risks. Note that our aim is not to fix and handle the inaccurate data when discovered, since the discovery time may be too late and the correction may be impossible or irrelevant (e.g., the review time has passed and the accepted papers need to be announced). Therefore, we concentrate on preventing such situations in the future by suggesting process redesign.

2   The Research Methodology and Techniques Being Applied

As a design science research, we aim to develop a method for detecting, assessing, and mitigating data inaccuracy-related risks. To this end, we first need to develop an understanding of how data inaccuracy is manifested in business processes. Then, patterns and guidelines will be developed to detect and address the associated risks. Finally, the method will be evaluated.

Explore patterns and impacts that reflect data inaccuracy situations: This activity will include performing a number of case studies in organizations of different sizes and market segments. Each case study will yield a list of specific data items, process paths suspected in creating inaccuracy situations, quantification of their frequency, and evaluation of the effect on performance indicators (e.g., cost, time).

Based on these findings, we will generalize the outcomes and the related risks and *develop* a method which will include patterns of errors and their associated risks, and guidelines for using these patterns. Moreover, the method will use a simulation tool that will support decision making in the context of the process redesign. It will help estimate the effort and the changes required in order to redesign a business process.

The method will be *evaluated* by reapplying it to the initial inputs of the case studies and by simulations. Final evaluation of the method will be made through an extensive new case study in an organization.

3   The Solution Proposed and Its Validity

As we mentioned above, the formed solution will be a semi-automated method which will include guidelines and patterns to detect inaccurate data-related situations in processes, patterns for assessing the severity of related risks, and a simulation tool which supports decision making in the context of process redesign. The potential users of this method are process experts, consultants, or any other employees that are involved in processes design. The method will be built based on case studies; each case study will include logs collection and mining to identify exceptional paths in the actual process, mining and manipulation of the actual databases, collection and analysis of process related artifacts such as models and documents, and performing interviews with employees involved in these processes. Data analysis will use automated tools such as relevant process mining algorithms, data base querying and filtering, data mining techniques (e.g., clustering and classifiers), and triangulation with qualitative analysis of the human interviews. For the propose of detecting data inaccuracies we intend to explore different existing techniques such as compliance checking, checking suitableness between the log file data and the actual system data, and searching abnormal data by preforming statistics on data with respect to the domain conventional values.

Currently, we are in the initial exploration phase. We performed a few small case studies in order to seek data inaccuracy-related situations that can be reflected in logs. As a guiding principle, we look for discrepancies in the process and between the log and the database. Unusual cases are further investigated by filtering, querying, and through interviews. For example, in one of the discovered process models, we found at a certain step 43 cases going back to the previous step (loop), as opposed to the "normal" flow taken by the rest of the cases. This finding raised our suspicion. Using the case ID for querying the database, we found that these records had null values for a specific attribute. They had to loop and be corrected for the process to continue.

4   The Relation of the Work to the State of Art in BPM

Considering data in processes, attempts have been made to ensure a correct process design in terms of its data flow [5, 7]. However, the underlying assumption of these studies is that the data is reliable and accurate at run time. As far as we know, data inaccuracy in business processes and reducing the related risks by process redesign have not been extensively addressed so far. Soffer [6] formalized data inaccuracy and discussed its potential consequences, introducing a basis for systematically addressing the possibility of runtime data deficiencies when designing processes. This is based on a formal representation of both real world and information system values. Recently, an extension of BPMN to address data quality issues has been proposed [3], but it mostly focuses on elicitation and definition of data quality requirements to be represented in a process model. These works address process design or redesign, but not based on real data analysis. Furthermore, it does not consider risk assessment.

5   The Expected Contribution of the Work of the Field of BPM

Until now, data inaccuracy has mainly been addressed in the area of business process management as a possible exception at runtime, to be resolved through exception handling mechanisms [4]. Note that exceptions are handled in some situations by terminating the case (namely, process failure). The proposed research will help detect data inaccuracy spots and assess and mitigate its consequences (the possible risks). Moreover, it will help estimate the efforts and the changes required in order to redesign a business process.

Acknowledgment. This research is partially supported by the Israel Science Foundation under grant 856/13.

References

1. Agmon, N., Ahituv, N.: Assessing data reliability in an information system. J. Manag. Inf. Syst. **4**(2), 34–44 (1987)
2. Committee of Sponsoring Organizations, "Enterprise Risk Management—Integrated Framework", p. 16 (2004)
3. Rodríguez, A., Caro, A., Cappiello, C., Caballero, I.: A BPMN extension for including data quality requirements in business process modeling. In: Mendling, J., Weidlich, M. (eds.) BPMN 2012. LNBIP, vol. 125, pp. 116–125. Springer, Heidelberg (2012)
4. Russell, N., van der Aalst, W.M., ter Hofstede, A.H.: Workflow exception patterns. In: Martinez, F.H., Pohl, K. (eds.) CAiSE 2006. LNCS, vol. 4001, pp. 288–302. Springer, Heidelberg (2006)
5. Sadiq, S., Orlowska, M., Sadiq, W., Foulger, C.: Data flow and validation in workflow modeling. In: Proceedings of the 15th Australasian Database Conference, ADC 2004, vol. 27, pp. 207–214 (2004)
6. Soffer, P.: Mirror, mirror on the wall, can I count on you at all? Exploring data inaccuracy in business processes. In: Bider, I., Halpin, T., Krogstie, J., Nurcan, S., Proper, E., Schmidt, R., Ukor, R. (eds.) BPMDS 2010 and EMMSAD 2010. LNBIP, vol. 50, pp. 14–25. Springer, Heidelberg (2010)
7. Trčka, N., van der Aalst, W.M., Sidorova, N.: Data-flow anti-patterns: discovering data-flow errors in workflows. In: van Eck, P., Gordijn, J., Wieringa, R. (eds.) CAiSE 2009. LNCS, vol. 5565, pp. 425–439. Springer, Heidelberg (2009)

Adaptation of Business Process Management to Requirements of Small and Medium-Sized Enterprises in the Context of Strategic Flexibility

Felix Reher[✉]

University of the West of Scotland, Paisley, UK
felix.reher@uws.ac.uk

Abstract. Business Process Management (BPM) has become a necessity for companies in a highly competitive business environment, as it is a powerful tool to enhance process and service performance. Unfortunately, BPM is primary linked to parameters in larger enterprises; no flexible and effective methods for a practical application are available for specific constraints of Small and Medium-sized Enterprises (SME). As a sequentially result, BPM for SMEs still remains largely atheoretical. Critical success factors in literature are often case-specific or of a generic kind and most of those papers fail to put their research within a theoretical grounded framework. This research focuses on maintaining the strategic flexibility and explores the situation in SMEs as well as the possibilities for an adaptation of an agile BPM within this type of companies. Aim is to propose a model that links business process management, organizational behavior and a framework for an adoption of BPM within this type of companies.

Keywords: BPM · SME · Adaptation · CSF · Agile · Model · Framework

1 Introduction

Companies' strategic agenda demands discipline and continuity instead of distraction and compromise [23]. Strategic continuity will make an organization's continual improvement more effective, but organizations must adopt new business models that rely on anticipation, speed and flexibility to create a competitive advantage. Their choice of re-positioning must be driven by the ability to find new trade-offs and leverage a new system of complementary activities into sustainable values. As a result, firms are in need "to reorganize their activities and realign their global strategies in order to provide the speed and flexibility necessary to respond to windows of market opportunity" [10, p. 8].

Business Process Management (BPM) is a systematic approach for improving an organization's existing business for delivering value-added products or services to "meet the objectives and business strategies of a company" [13, p. 1]. With the usage of BPM, "processes can be aligned with the business strategy, and so help to improve company performance as a whole thanks to the optimization of processes within

© Springer International Publishing Switzerland 2015
F. Fournier and J. Mendling (Eds.): BPM 2014 Workshops, LNBIP 202, pp. 561–566, 2015.
DOI: 10.1007/978-3-319-15895-2_48

business divisions or even beyond company borders" [1, p. 27]. Unfortunately, BPM as structured methodological approach, is primary linked to situations in larger enterprises.

2   Research Design

An increasing trend towards BPM consulting activities for SME can be found in recent years, but this trend is not yet visible in the scientific literature, however, still represent little [36]. A generic comprehensive methodology for a successful implementation is needed [8, 31].

2.1   Containment

Flexibility of the proposed approach is essential, a company must be able to fulfill "preplanned adjustments as well as spontaneous reactions to changes in the environment" [26]. Milberg [21, p. 26] defines the term 'changeability' as the sum of 'flexibility' and 'responsiveness', which are (1) the "ability of a system to change status within an existing configuration of pre-established parameters" and (2) the "propensity for purposeful and timely behavior change in the presence of modulating stimuli" [5, p. 41].

A requirement is understood as an inherent and mandatory "condition or capability that must be met" to achieve a specific objective or goal within an organization [16]. Both mentioned interpretations are utilized to limit the research within the broad domain of BPM.

2.2   Research Questions

This research explores the situation in SMEs as well as the possibilities for an agile solution for an adaptation and implementation of BPM within this type of companies. Due to the idiosyncrasies of SMEs, namely "existing organizational and structural heterogeneity, dynamism and complexity of characteristics" [29, p. 64], the focus shifts to management and organizational perspectives. Success of a realization and an implementation of changes depend on organizational behavior and given structures. For this purpose three primary research questions (RQ1-3) are being addressed, namely

- "What are specific Requirements for SMEs",
- "What aspects of BPM cause difficulties in SMEs"; and
- "How can a successful implementation of BPM in SMEs be ensured?"

Desired result is the elaboration of an applicable framework for adaptation of BPM within a defined cluster of SMEs.

2.3   Methodology

Literature Review. The currently carried out literature review is focused on three different topics, namely (1) Business Process Management, (2) Strategic Flexibility;

and (3) Critical Success Factors (CSF). An attempt is made, to structure the problem area through analysis of existing theories and thereof to answer the aforementioned research questions RQ1, RQ2 and RQ3.

Delphi Study and Triangulation. A model as well as an applicable framework for an adaptation will be developed and, for the validation of the theory, a structured mixed-method Delphi study will be conducted. The retrieved results will be triangulated with another qualitative research method in a later research phase (currently planned are either interviews or Focus Groups).

This method of triangulation will enable an extensive analysis of BPM issues across different stakeholders in SMEs, leading to a better understanding of overall issues. Necessary adaptations and modifications of the framework after the validation by experts will be reflected in a revision of the model and framework.

3 Current Status

The concept of BPM and the whole research topic has not yet been theoretically grounded well [24, 34]. Existing theories in addition to implementations have not been able to map the reality [32], only a few of current scientific contributions establish a concrete practice relationship or supply hints for the practical use of specific strategies [35]. Available papers still primarily describe what BPM actually 'does' or 'means' [24, p. 493] and recent papers on practical experiences during the last years have documented a large number of failed or unsuccessful BPM initiatives.

However, a number of papers [6, 20, 25, 32] raise the questions of whether BPM is generally applicable to SMEs but there has been quite little empirical research of CSFs and their post hoc evaluation of success [3]. Coherent to this, several papers try to identify CSFs but the research domain has several challenges over many categories and this has lead into difficulties of "clearly categorizing and making critical BPM factors general" [22, p. 1] and "identifying both generic and case-specific" CSFs [34, p. 125]. General CSFs are often either case-specific or dependent to parameters like industry, region or country [18]. The applicability on other firms is rarely confirmed. On the other hand, considered CSFs are often not linked up and their influences on each other are not clear. Moreover, many papers fail to put their research within a theoretical grounded framework.

What are the limits of a practical implementation are presented by the operational parameters or resources and do factors exists that prevent the holistically introduction? Is it possible to define a clear, delineable class or groups of entities that might promote these barriers – e.g. predominant ad hoc-structures within the company or nuisance influence by single individuals? Different sources identified major guidelines to BPM project success [8, 24, 28], namely (1) limited scope, (2) high value, (3) clear alignment to goals, (4) the right metrics, (5) goal agreement, (6) enthusiastic business sponsor, (7) business user engagement, (8) communication, (9) stakeholder involvement, and (10) governance. Existence of a (11) common language and semantic vocabulary for stakeholders has been recognized as inevitable. The dependence of such logical interconnected factors of 'human behavior' and 'technological parts' is found in various papers on BPM, especially in the last few years [3, 7, 24, 33]. Importance of organizational change in connection with a BPM implementation is discussed multiple [8, 19, 28]. An understanding and acceptance of process restructuring is crucial for success of a change.

4 Conclusion

We can identify a couple of guidelines to BPM project success in literature, which are particularly challenging in the specific surrounding of SMEs. A BPM initiative must be aligned to the organizational strategy and goals [27, 28]. What if, is there is no single but a multitude of influencing or even conflicting company's goals? Management of an organization based on its core processes is not possible, if indistinct strategies, goal setting and controlling of measures are contradictory.

Especially family-owned SMEs seem to have 'hidden' core processes, based on peculiarities compared to their larger competitors, i.e.: (1) closely held and owner-managed [4]; (2) conservative behavior, risk aversion and lack of willingness for Organizational Change [2, 11, 15, 17, 30]; management is focused on daily activities [14]; and an opportunistic information processing in SMEs [9, 12].

4.1   Implication and Limitations

To create a functional model of an affected problem area, an adopter requires (1) knowledge of the scientific discipline that deals with the nature of the problem, (2) a mutual understanding of domain itself and (3) how to represent this knowledge. As part of a working group with focus on interrelation between Requirement Engineering and BPM, approaches for requirement elicitation in non-BPM familiar target groups are considered. The outcome might be incorporated into the framework later.

The number of planed cases for validation is quite small and only random sample, the limited number of cases and interviews might not allow generalizable conclusions. Furthermore, the retrospective assessment of the situation prior to a BPM initiative limits the reliability of the findings.

4.2   Future Work

The perspective raised by this paper cannot deliver a full-fledged theoretical framework at this time, but it triggers a set of questions. Nevertheless, mentioned RQs and the results of the survey will form an understanding on the main issues in BPM for SMEs. The literature review constitutes groundwork for further obstacle identification by a survey and later interviews with practitioners as well as with academic experts. Through this multi-method approach, we will be able to identify three distinct sets of outcomes, namely (1) able to identify the generic requirements for BPM in SMEs; (2) gain insights into organizational behavior in SMEs; and (3) obtain an understanding of organizations' CSFs as well.

4.3   Expected Contribution of the Work to the Field of BPM

This paper provides a targeted discussion of the issues and challenges related to BPM adoption in SMEs. The focus of the research is to analyze business and organizational issues, to extract a set of key success factors for an implementation of BPM in context of the defined strategic flexibility.

Based on the conversion of theoretical results into an approach that enables organizations to follow a standard way of implementing BPM, the usability of management by process is worked out for SMEs and potential benefits are made tangible. This includes decreasing investment risk and increasing planning reliability, whereby a practical added value is generated.

References

1. ABPMP: ABPMP Guide to the BPM CBOK Version 3.0, 1st edn. CreateSpace Independent Publishing Platform (2013)
2. Aronoff, C.E., Ward, J.L.: Preparing Your Family Business for Strategic Change. Family Business Leadership Series, p. 9. Business Owner Resources, Marietta, Georgia (1997)
3. Bandara, W., Gable, G.G., Rosemann, M.: Factors and measures of business process modelling: model building through a multiple case study. EJIS **14**, 347–360 (2005)
4. Bennedzen, M., Wolfenzon, D.: The balance of power in closely held corporations. JFE. **58**, 113–139 (1999)
5. Bernardes, E.S., Hanna, M.D.: A theoretical review of flexibility, agility and responsiveness in the operations management literature: toward a conceptual definition of customer responsiveness. IJOPM **29**(1), 30–53 (2009)
6. Blyke, Y.: BPM and the discipline of execution. BPTrends, pp. 1–2 (2012). http://www.bptrends.com/publicationfiles/04-03-2012-ART-BPM%20and%20the%20Discipline%20of%20Execution-Yuri%20Blyke-Final.pdf
7. vom Brocke, J.: Culture in business process management: a literature review. BPMJ **17**(2), 357–378 (2011)
8. Burlton, R.: BPM critical success factors: lessons learned from successful BPM organizations. Bus. Rules J. http://www.brcommunity.com/a2011/b619.html
9. Ciborra, C.: Improvisation and information technology in organizations. In: Proceedings of the ICIS 1996, Paper 26 (1996)
10. Dekkers, R., van Luttervelt, C.A.: Industrial networks: capturing changeability? IJNVO **3**(1), 1–24 (2006)
11. Eisenhardt, K.M.: Agency theory: an assessment and review. Acad. Manag. Rev. **14**(1), 57–74 (1989)
12. Feldman, M.S., March, J.G.: Information in organizations as signal and symbol. Adm. Sci. Q. **26**(2), 171–186 (1981)
13. Freund, J., Rücker, B.: Real-Life BPMN - Using BPMN 2.0 to Analyze, Improve, and Automate Processes in Your Company, vol. 5. CreateSpace Independent Publishing Platform (2012)
14. Frieling, E.: Schriftenreihe Personal- und Organisationsentwicklung, vol. 5. Universität Kassel Institut für Arbeitswissenschaft, Kassel (2007)
15. George, G., Wiklund, J., Zahra, S.A.: Ownership and the internationalization of the small firm. JOM **31**(2), 210–233 (2005)

16. Institute of Electrical and Electronic Engineers: IEEE Standard Glossary of Software Engineering Terminology (IEEE Std 610.12-1990). Institute of Electrical and Electronics Engineers, New York, NY (1990)

17. Keasey, K., Thompson, S., Wright, M.: Corporate Governance: Accountability, Enterprise and International Comparisons. Wiley, London (2005)

18. Lu, X.-H., Huang, L.-H., Heng, M.S.H.: Critical success factors of inter-organizational information systems—a case study of Cisco and Xiao Tong in China. IM **43**(3), 395–408 (2006)

19. Mertens, W., Van den Bergh, J., Viaene, S., Schroder-Pander, F.: How BPM impacts jobs: an exploratory field study. In: 44th HICSS. Kauai, HI (2011)

20. Miers, D.: The Keys to BPM Project Success. BPTrends, pp. 1–10 (2006). http://www.bptrends.com/publicationfiles/01-06-ART-KeysToBPMProjSuccess-Miers.pdf

21. Milberg, J.: Eine treibende Kraft für unsere Volkswirtschaft. In: Reinhart, G., Milberg, J. (eds.) Mit Schwung zum Aufschwung. Münchener Kolloquium 1997, pp. 19–39. Moderne Industrie, Landsberg/Lech (1997)

22. Ohtonen, J., Lainema, T.: Critical success factors in business process management – a literature review. In: Leino, T. (ed.) Proceedings of IRIS 2011. TUCS Lecture Notes, No. 15, pp. 572–585. Turku Centre for Computer Science, Turku (2011)

23. Porter, M.E.: What is Strategy? Harvard Bus. Rev. **11, 98**, 61–78 (1996). HBS Publishing, Boston

24. Ravesteyn, P., Batenburg, R.: Surveying the critical success factors of BPM-systems implementation. BPMJ **16**(3), 492–507 (2010)

25. Reijers, H.A.: Implementing BPM systems: the role of process orientation. BPMJ **12**(4), 389–409 (2006)

26. Reinhart, G., Dürrschmidt, S.: Planning methodology for changeable logistics systems. In: Proceedings of the 34th CIRP International Seminar on Manufacturing Systems, 16–18 May 2001, Athens, Greece (2001)

27. Rosemann, M., vom Brocke, J.: The six core elements of business process management. In: vom Brocke, J., Rosemann, M. (eds.) International Handbooks on Information Systems, pp. 107–122. Springer, Heidelberg (2010)

28. Rosser, B.: Seven Key Guidelines to BPM Project Success; Research Paper, Gartner Research. Gartner Inc., Stamford (2009)

29. Rudolph, S.: Anwendungskontext mittelständische Unternehmen; Service-basierte Planung und Steuerung der IT-Infrastruktur im Mittelstand. Gabler Verlag, Wiesbaden, pp. 63–78 (2009)

30. Sharma, P., Chrisman, J.J., Chua, J.H.: Strategic management of the family business: past research and future challenges. Fam. Bus. Rev **10**(1), 1–35 (1997)

31. Singer, R., Zinser, E.: S-BPM ONE – Setting the Stage for Subject-Oriented Business Process Management, vol. 85, pp. 48–70. Springer, Heidelberg (2009)

32. Smith, H., Fingar, P.: Business Process Management: The Third Wave. Meghan-Kiffer Press, Tampa (2003)

33. Thiault, D.: Managing Performance Through Business Processes: From BPM to the Practice of Process Management. CreateSpace Independent Publishing, North Charleston (2012)

34. Trkman, P.: The critical success factors of business process management. IJIM **30**(2), 125–134 (2010)

35. Vöpel, N., Schulz, A.: Strategien von kleinen und mittleren Unternehmen – State of the Art; Jahrbuch der KMU-Forschung und Praxis 2010, pp. 562–599. Josef Eul Verlag, Köln (2010)

36. Wolters, W., Kaschny, M.: Geschäftsprozessmanagement in KMU: Dargestellt anhand der Auftragsabwicklung in der Gebäudetechnik. Josef Eul Verlag, Köln (2010)

A Language for Process Map Design

Monika Malinova[(⊠)]

WU Vienna, Welthandelsplatz 1, 1020 Vienna, Austria
monika.malinova@wu.ac.at

Abstract. Organizations are leaning towards becoming more process-oriented in order to better serve their customers. An approach that enables achieving such process orientation is business process management (BPM). In this context business process modeling is used to graphically represent business processes. As a result organizations are faced with large collections of process models. The process models are typically organized in a process architecture which comprises a number of levels. The most top level is commonly the process map where all processes of one organization and the relations between them are depicted in a very abstract manner. Whereas there are well-defined languages for modelling the details of singular processes (e.g. BPMN, EPC), such a language for supporting the design of process maps is still missing. As a result, we are faced with a vast variety of process map designs from practice, as practitioners typically rely on their own creativity when undertaking this task. This study addresses this gap by using various methods to develop a language for process map design which will support practitioners to design their process maps in a standardized manner.

Keywords: Process map · Process architecture · Process category

1 Introduction

Organizations are complex entities which consist of units and people that work together in order to satisfy the needs of customers. Many organizations are inclined towards vertical-thinking i.e. placing the focus on functional and hierarchical structures. However, as organizations today require flexibility and reactiveness to address emerging business challenges, they often transition to process orientation. In other words, they shift towards horizontal-thinking through better understanding of their business processes [1]. Business process management (BPM) is widely used as a method to increase such awareness and knowledge of processes. In this context, business process modeling is used to graphically represent business processes in form of process models. It has been recognized that having a process described visually instead of textually aids in easier and faster understanding, performance and control of processes [2]. Thus, BPM has proven to bring many benefits, such as a direct effect on customer satisfaction [3], business performance, cross-functional thinking and interaction among employees [4].

© Springer International Publishing Switzerland 2015
F. Fournier and J. Mendling (Eds.): BPM 2014 Workshops, LNBIP 202, pp. 567–572, 2015.
DOI: 10.1007/978-3-319-15895-2_49

The number of organizations adopting BPM is quickly increasing. By this means, so is the number of process models as result of a BPM initiative. Within a single organization this number often ranges from hundreds to even thousands of process models. In this context, companies organize their process models in terms of a process architecture. A process architecture defines how the set of process models of one company can be systematically organized [5]. It comprises of a process map which is considered as the top-view of the corresponding process architecture where the organization's processes and the relations between them are abstractly depicted, whereas the details of each process shown in the process map are stored in the lower levels of the process architecture. The purpose of a process map is to show a holistic view of all processes of one organization and aims to provide an overview of how the company operates as a whole, without necessarily going into process details [6]. Therefore, the way a process map is designed is important not only for enabling easier understanding of the company's processes, but also for the subsequent steps of the BPM implementation. This is because a process map is typically designed at the beginning of BPM initiatives and is thus used as a foundation for the detailed process modeling. Hence, all processes shown in the process map are those that will undergo the stages of the BPM lifecycle (process identification, process discovery, process analysis, process redesign, process implementation, and process monitoring & controlling) [2]. Moreover, the relations shown on a process map level should also be reflected in the detailed process modeling [7].

Whereas managing process model collections has recently been a focal point for research [8], aligning the process models in terms of a process architecture has still not received much attention. Furthermore, while there exist well-defined standardized languages for modeling singular processes (e.g. BPMN, EPC, etc.), to the best of our knowledge there is no such language for extensively supporting the design of process maps.

This study addresses this gap by using various methods to get insights of organization's business processes and process map design. Our focus is on the development of a language for supporting the design of process maps. The rest of this paper presents our research question and the methods we use to reach it. This position paper is structured as follows. In Sect. 2 we present a short background of BPM and process maps. Section 3 introduces our research question and the methods we use to answer it, while Sect. 4 concludes the paper.

2 Background

In this section we briefly discuss the concept of BPM, then we give insights into the current state of the art of process maps and highlight the motivation for our study.

2.1 Business Process Management

Business process management (BPM) is an approach used by many organizations in order to manage their vast amount of business processes. A business process consists of activities performed in a particular order in order to satisfy the needs of end-users [9,10]. An organization that adopts BPM starts depicting their business processes in form of business process models. A business process model is a graphical representation of a business process and is known to be more intuitive than, for instance, a textual description of the same, as it eliminates the ambiguity of natural language. The management activities related to BPM are often described as a lifecycle model, starting with process identification where all necessary processes to reach a particular goal are been identified [2]. Next, the current state of the processes is being discovered and captured in form of process models (as-is state). The resulting process models are being analyzed for process weaknesses. The weaknesses are addressed and the corresponding processes redesigned (to-be state). The redesigned processes are implemented throughout the organization, monitored for performance and periodically controlled [2]. Such a BPM initiative typically ends up with a large number of process models in both as-is and to-be states. Accordingly, these need to be systematically organized in terms of a process architecture in order to be continuously utilized, monitored and controlled.

2.2 Process Maps

One of the most commonly used techniques by practitioners for dealing with the complexity of large process model collections is the use of process maps. A process map is an abstract depiction of all processes of one organization [6,7]. The processes in a process map are typically clustered in three main categories, namely management, core and support process categories [2,6,7,11]. Each category holds processes that serve a similar purpose. For example, the core processes are those that bring in the revenue for a company (e.g. sales), while the support processes support the execution of the core processes (e.g. accounting). The processes in the core process category are commonly represented as a value-chain, which is a concept introduced in the 1990 s by Porter [12]. The value-chain model represents core processes of one organization as a chain, thus when the processes are executed in a certain order they create value for the customer [12].

Beyond process categories, in process maps nowadays we also observe additional concepts, such as process relations, inputs/outputs, actors, resources, etc. A process map uses a combination of all these concepts in order to show how a company operates without necessarily going into process details. The most common relation is the sequential relation which is used between the core processes to represent a value-chain. Also, many process maps from practice implicitly depict a relation between the different process categories, such as the manage relation, which is a relation between the management and the core processes and shows that the management processes manage the execution of the core processes. In other words, all that is done during a core process should comply to the rules defined by the management processes [7]. Inputs and outputs are used to show what triggers a core process to start, and what is the main outcome of a value-chain. An example of input/output is a customer request/customer satisfaction. In some process maps we can also identify the main actors for each process (e.g. process manager). This enables employees to immediately recognize the persons to talk to when interested in a particular process. Some examples of process maps can be found in literature [2,11,13–15]; nonetheless all refer to process maps coming from practice.

Despite their apparent importance in practice, very little research has been focused on process maps. Due to the lack of a language for process map design, we are faced with a vast amount of differently looking process maps from practice, although they all serve a similar purpose. Therefore, in this study we acknowledge the need for a standardized language for process map design. Accordingly, we address this gap by using various methods to get insights into business processes and process maps from practice and literature. As a result, we develop a language that will support practitioners in designing process maps in a standardized manner.

3   Research Question and Methods Used

This study aims in answering the following research question: *What are the components of a modeling language that provides extensive support for designing process maps?*

To develop a language for process map design we follow the design science research methodology [16] and comply to the design science guidelines [17]. We consider this methodology suitable for this purpose, especially because of the apparent necessity of such a standard language. Hence, this is a problem-centered entry point, therefore we develop an artifact i.e. the language, demonstrate the language's usability by applying it in a suitable context and evaluate it's performance [16].

When developing a process modeling language four aspects are typically considered: syntax, semantics, notation and pragmatics [18–20]. In terms of process map's, the language should provide symbols for the different process map concepts (notation), each symbol should be mapped to its appropriate semantics, and the language's syntax should support designing process maps such that their interpretation is pragmatic. Thus, the resultant process map should be able to convey its message among all employees within one organization. To develop such a language, as a first step, (1) we analyze process maps from practice for the concepts being used within a single process map and any means by which the identified concepts are related to each other. As a result, we generate a process map meta-model [7]. Next, (2) we conduct a systematic literature review on guidelines, principles, and quality criteria for designing modeling languages. A guideline is a rule that provides guidance to appropriate modeling. A principle is a standard that is accepted as true and used to improve the quality of languages, thus it helps designers meet their goals. A quality criteria is a standard in terms of which a language can be judged. For the literature review we follow the guidelines proposed by Kitchenham et al. [21]. As a result we derive an extensive list of guidelines, principles and quality criteria we use and follow when developing the process map language.

Furthermore, (3) we assess the extent to which existing process map's from practice are cognitively effective. A cognitively effective process map is one that is self-explanatory i.e. it enables a basic understanding of how an organization operates without going into process details [6]. We employ the Physics of Notations and its nine principles proposed by Moody [20]. These principles provide the basis of discussing visual notations from the perspective of cognitive effectiveness [20] and are based on the extent to which the eight visual variables proposed by Bertin [22] are used. As a result we derive a list of symbols used in process maps from practice, which we will assimilate in the language we develop for process map design. As step (4) we make a list of all symbols used by existing process modeling languages (e.g. BPMN, UML, EPC), and semantically match those symbols with the concepts seen in process maps from practice. We do this in order to reuse existing symbols which are already familiar to practitioners. Based on steps (1), (2), (3) and (4) we develop a language for designing process maps in a standardized manner.

For the evaluation phase we validate the appropriateness of the language for designing process maps by utilizing the Norman's theory of action [23]. This theory is used to ensure that the viewer of the produced process map has interpreted the correct domain that the designer of the process map has communicated. For this, we first conduct interviews with one of our industry partners in order to get insights into the processes shown in their existing process map. We analyze the interview transcripts in order to identify all those concepts that could be represented on a process map level. Accordingly, we redesign their existing process map by using the newly developed process map language. We conduct an experiment with the employees of the organization to be able to evaluate the extent to which the redesigned process map is easier to correctly interpret than the old process map.

4   Conclusion

In this paper we position our research on developing a language for designing process maps. As this is a problem-driven research, we use the design science research methodology in order to develop an artifact that will extensively support practitioners when designing process maps. We use various methods for the development of the language. We evaluate the language by redesigning the existing process map of one of our industry partners and conducting an experiment with the organization's employees in order to ensure that the redesigned process map is cognitively effective.

References

1. Reijers, H.A.: Implementing bpm systems: the role of process orientation. Bus. Process. Manage. J. **12**(4), 389–409 (2006)
2. Dumas, M., Rosa, M., Mendling, J., Reijers, H.: Fundamentals of Business Process Management. Springer, New York (2013)

3. Frei, F.X., Kalakota, R., Leone, A.J., Marx, L.M.: Process variation as a determinant of bank performance: evidence from the retail banking study. Manage. Sci. **45**(9), 1210–1220 (1999)

4. McCormack, K.: Business process orientation: do you have it? Qual. Prog. **34**(1), 51–60 (2001)

5. Malinova, M., Leopold, H., Mendling, J.: An empirical investigation on the design of process architectures. Wirtschaftsinformatik **75** (2013)

6. Malinova, M., Mendling, J.: The effect of process map design quality on process management success. In: Proceedings of the 21st European Conference on Information Systems (2013)

7. Malinova, M., Leopold, H., Mendling, J.: A meta-model for process map design. In: CAiSE Forum (2014)

8. Dijkman, R.M., La Rosa, M., Reijers, H.A.: Managing large collections of business process models-current techniques and challenges. Comput. Ind. **63**(2), 91–97 (2012)

9. Kettinger, W.J., Grover, V.: Special section: toward a theory of business process change management. J. Manage. Inf. Syst. **12**, 9–30 (1995)

10. Kiraka, R.N., Manning, K.: Managing organisations through a process-based perspective: its challenges and benefits. Knowl. Process. Manage. **12**(4), 288–298 (2005)

11. Weske, M.: Business Process Management: Concepts, Languages, Architectures, 2nd edn. Springer, New York (2012)

12. Porter, M.E.: Competitive advantage: Creating and sustaining superior performance (2008). SimonandSchuster.com

13. Harmon, P.: Business Process Change: A Guide for Business Managers and BPM and Six Sigma Professionals. Morgan Kaufmann, San Francisco (2010)

14. Jeston, J., Nelis, J.: Business Process Management: Practical Guidelines to Successful Implementations. Routledge, London (2008)

15. Becker, J., Kugeler, M., Rosemann, M.: Process Management: A Guide for the Design of Business Processes: with 83 Figures and 34 Tables. Springer, Heidelberg (2003)

16. Peffers, K., Tuunanen, T., Rothenberger, M., Chatterjee, S.: A design science research methodology for information systems research. J. Manage. Inf. Syst. **24**(3), 45–77 (2007)

17. Hevner, A., March, S., Park, J., Ram, S.: Design science in information systems research. MIS Q. **28**(1), 75–105 (2004)

18. Lindland, O.I., Sindre, G., Solvberg, A.: Understanding quality in conceptual modeling. IEEE Softw. **11**(2), 42–49 (1994)

19. Krogstie, J., Sindre, G., Jørgensen, H.: Process models representing knowledge for action: a revised quality framework. Eur. J. Inf. Syst. **15**(1), 91–102 (2006)

20. Moody, D.L.: The "physics" of notations: toward a scientific basis for constructing visual notations in software engineering. IEEE Trans. Softw. Eng. **35**(6), 756–779 (2009)

21. Kitchenham, B., Pearl Brereton, O., Budgen, D., Turner, M., Bailey, J., Linkman, S.: Systematic literature reviews in software engineering-a systematic literature review. Inf. Softw. Technol. **51**(1), 7–15 (2009)

22. Bertin, J.: Semiology of Graphics: Diagrams, Networks, Maps. The University of Wisconsin Press, Madison (1983)

23. Norman, D.A., Draper, S.W.: User Centered System Design: New Perspectives on Human-Computer Interaction. L. Erlbaum Associates Inc., Hillsdale (1986)

Graph-Based Process Model Matching

Christina Tsagkani[(✉)]

Department of Informatics and Telecommunications,
National and Kapodistrian University of Athens (NKUA),
Panepistimiopolis, 157 84 Ilisia, Greece
tsagkani@di.uoa.gr

Abstract. Nowadays organizations acquire multiple repositories with process specifications. Organization stakeholders such as business analysts and process designers need to have access and retrieve such information as it is proven that adapting existing business processes in order to meet current business needs is more effective and less error-prone than developing them from scratch. This thesis concentrates on process retrieval and will propose a business process searching mechanism, taking advantage and extending existing graph based matching techniques, with the aim to exploit the knowledge that already exists within an organization.

Keywords: Process model matching · Process model similarity · Graph matching

1 Introduction

The growing orientation in processes of contemporary information systems and service-oriented architectures has led to the existence of repositories with hundreds of process models that are a great source of knowledge. The process retrieval according to user's needs of such repositories has become crucial as it may have multiple applications (e.g. model: reuse, design, merge and conformance).

The problem with traditional search engines is that in most cases they are based on keyword search and text similarity and it is unclear how far search engines are appropriate for process model similarity queries [5]. Thus the aim of this thesis is to propose a technique for process matching that will address both label syntactic and structural metrics.

2 The Research Methodology and Existing Techniques

The proposed mechanism and the related research is driven by the followings: 1. The most natural representation of a business process is to view it as a directed and labeled (attributed) graph where each node represents an activity and each edge a control link between activities. 2. Process discovery uses graph matching techniques in order to identify similar process models.

The similarity aspects as defined in [5] are: Node similarity (similarity of labels and attributes), Structural similarity (e.g. Graph Edit Distance) and Behavioral similarity

© Springer International Publishing Switzerland 2015
F. Fournier and J. Mendling (Eds.): BPM 2014 Workshops, LNBIP 202, pp. 573–577, 2015.
DOI: 10.1007/978-3-319-15895-2_50

(e.g. casual relations between tasks or trace-based semantics). These similarity aspects are aided by the followings: Syntactic similarity, Semantic similarity, Attribute similarity, Type similarity and Contextual similarity.

The Graph matching algorithms used by different techniques can be subdivided into two broad categories based on their output:

- exact matching: defines if two graphs are identical or partially identical.
- inexact matching: determines if two graphs are identical or similar.

Inexact graph matching algorithms can be further distinguished by either finding optimal or sub-optimal (approximate) solutions. More specifically with the former algorithms it is guaranteed to find a solution that matches exactly to the query graph, if it exists. The later algorithms find a solution that is the local minimum of the matching cost and it is not guaranteed to find a solution that matches exactly to the query graph.

The current research is focused on Graph Edit Distance (GED) which is a graph matching paradigm that have been emerged and successfully used in diverse research areas (eg. pattern recognition and data mining). Due to its flexibility it may be applied to all graph types. The idea behind the GED is to define the minimum amount of distortion (using edit operations: insertion, deletion, substitution, join and split) required to transform one graph into another [19].

Reviewing the literature related to graph matching algorithms and GED approaches, algorithms that guarantee optimal result can be found such as [2] that uses the A* algorithm and algorithms that guarantee suboptimal result such as: [17] that suggests a greedy iterative algorithm based on local search that adds a sequence of edit operations calculated on the neighborhood graph matching to the global edit path, [18] that proposes two sub-optimal algorithms (A*beamsearch, A*pathlength), [16] that is based on a quadratic assignment formulation to solve the GED problem, [19] that is based on a linear assignment problem, [8] that uses a linear formulation method to derive lower and upper distance bounds in polynomial time and [20] that is based on local search by optimizing local criteria instead of global.

Besides, there have been many research efforts to address the problem of correspondence between activities of different process models such as: [9] that focuses on process model matching quality, by applying word stemming to labels prior to calculating the similarity scores using, the syntactical technique of Levenshtein [10] and semantically technique of Lin [12, 24] that proposes a framework composed of four types of components (Searchers, Boosters, Selectors and Evaluators), [3] the Triple-S matching technique combines similarity scores of three independent levels: Syntactic level, Semantic level and structural level, [3] the RefMod-Mine/NSCM - N-Ary Semantic Cluster Matching that is based on clustering process model nodes, [3] the RefMod-Mine/ESGM - Extended Semantic Greedy Matching that performs preprocessing to data by using a heuristic filter, semantic word matching using dictionary lookups, a syntactic similarity measure (Levenshtein edit distance [10]) and heuristic grouping based on a set of rules, [4, 5] that considers syntactic and semantic metrics for label similarity and follows a greedy algorithm to search the space of mappings and A* heuristics, [14] that identifies the structural similarity of activities and edges, [11] that identifies Graph Edit Distance by using high level change operations, [6] that focuses on activity labels similarity (syntactic and semantic) and then structural similarity is measured only when previously there was no perfect match, [13] that uses graph reduction rules and a selective reduce algorithm, while only considers structural similarity (order of activities), [21] that uses features (labels and position of a node into the process structure) in order to find related not similar models, [25] that concentrates on model matching prediction while taking into consideration syntactic, semantic, structural and behavioral aspects and [1] that provides visual queries to return process model matches through label and control-flow matching. Finally some process matching approaches that are based on behavioural similarity are indicatively mentioned in [7, 15, 22, 23].

3 The Proposed Solution

This thesis tackles process matching as a graph matching problem. Taking into consideration that large repositories of business processes are searched against a given query, it is obvious that the perfect match is very rare due to graph variability. Therefore users are well satisfied with results that seem similar to their graph query. Thus the thesis will concentrate on inexact Graph matching algorithms where the challenge is to compute how much two graphs differ or share by transforming process nodes to establish a total mapping using a Graph Edit Distance approach.

More precisely the proposed graph matching technique is going to contribute to the followings:

1. **Similarity metrics used to evaluate mapping distance.** The open research problem related to cost function determination of each edit operation that can be either known a priori or can be defined in a way that favors edit operations that are more likely to take place than others that are infrequent, will be tackled. The basic idea is to use the different similarity aspects as were identified previously in order to define the edit cost functions of operations. It is worthwhile mentioning that most of the existing approaches consider some kind of label matching (syntactic and semantic) in order to judge the similarity of model elements. Thus this thesis is going to estimate edit costs based, not only on label matching but structural matching as well, by taking into consideration aspects such as context, events, data input/output, roles and pre/post conditions.

2. **The algorithm that is used to explore the space of possible mappings.** As process repositories consist of large process models it has been decided to concentrate on providing ways of reducing the search space during the application of the algorithm by applying heuristics, while it will be investigated how the searching mechanism may be aided through the use of graph indexing techniques. As a first step to the current research the Business Process Execution Language (BPEL) has been studied in order to understand how its structural elements are used to describe business processes. It is identified that the type of process elements has a key role in the process matching. Thus it is proposed to use the type accompanied to each node to minimize the search space and instead of comparing each node of the query graph with all nodes of a graph under study, to examine only nodes that are of the same type (e.g. Interaction activities, structured activities, basic activities etc.). Also it is

proposed that the algorithm will follow a prioritization process with hierarchies of types of activities and start pairing/edit-cost measurement of nodes expressing for example interaction activities (because they are considered as a prerequisite and should be included in the result of the algorithm) and if the matching cost does not exceed a given threshold then to continue with other types of activities.

4 Conclusion

A problem that this thesis addresses is how to avail the knowledge from a diversity of process variants that exist in large business process model repositories, as an information resource and use it while creating new processes or optimizing existing ones.

Towards this direction, the current research, while aiming at identifying business process mappings, contributes on proposing a graph-based process matching approach that improves search space complexity and considers aspects that have not been addressed by existing approaches such as context, events, data input/output, and roles.

References

1. Awad, A., Sakr, S., Kunze, M., Weske, M.: Design by selection: A reuse-based approach for business process modeling. In: Jeusfeld, M., Delcambre, L., Ling, T.-W. (eds.) ER 2011. LNCS, vol. 6998, pp. 332–345. Springer, Heidelberg (2011)
2. Bunke, H., Allermann, G.: Inexact graph matching for structural pattern recognition. Pattern Recogn. Lett. **1**(4), 245–253 (1983)
3. Cayoglu, U., et al.: Report: The process model matching contest 2013. In: Lohmann, N., Song, M., Wohed, P. (eds.) BPM 2013 Workshops. LNBIP, vol. 171, pp. 442–464. Springer, Heidelberg (2014)
4. Dijkman, R., Dumas, M., García-Bañuelos, L.: Graph matching algorithms for business process model similarity search. In: Dayal, U., Eder, J., Koehler, J., Reijers, H.A. (eds.) BPM 2009. LNCS, vol. 5701, pp. 48–63. Springer, Heidelberg (2009)
5. Dijkman, R., et al.: Similarity of business process models: Metrics and evaluation. Inf. Syst. **36**(2), 498–516 (2011)
6. Ehrig, M., et al.: Measuring similarity between semantic business process models. In: 4th Asia-Pacific Conference on Conceptual Modelling, vol. 67, pp. 71–80. Australian Computer Society Inc. (2007)
7. Eshuis, R., Grefen, P.W.P.J.: Structural matching of BPEL processes. In: Fifth European Conference on Web Services, 2007, ECOWS 2007, pp. 171–180. IEEE (2007)
8. Justice, D., et al.: A binary linear programming formulation of the graph edit distance. IEEE Trans. Pattern Anal. Mach. Intell. **28**(8), 1200–1214 (2006)
9. Klinkmüller, C., Weber, I., Mendling, J., Leopold, H., Ludwig, A.: Increasing recall of process model matching by improved activity label matching. In: Daniel, F., Wang, J., Weber, B. (eds.) BPM 2013. LNCS, vol. 8094, pp. 211–218. Springer, Heidelberg (2013)
10. Levenshtein, V.I.: Binary codes capable of correcting deletions, insertions and reversals. In: Soviet physics doklady, vol. 10, p. 707 (1966)

11. Li, C., Reichert, M., Wombacher, A.: On measuring process model similarity based on high-level change operations. In: Li, Q., Spaccapietra, S., Yu, E., Olivé, A. (eds.) ER 2008. LNCS, vol. 5231, pp. 248–264. Springer, Heidelberg (2008)

12. Lin, D.: An information-theoretic definition of similarity. In: ICML 1998, Vol. 98, pp. 296–304 (1998)

13. Lu, R., Sadiq, S.K.: On the discovery of preferred work practice through business process variants. In: Parent, C., Schewe, K.-D., Storey, V.C., Thalheim, B. (eds.) ER 2007. LNCS, vol. 4801, pp. 165–180. Springer, Heidelberg (2007)

14. Minor, M., Tartakovski, A., Bergmann, R.: Representation and structure-based similarity assessment for agile workflows. In: Weber, R.O., Richter, M.M. (eds.) ICCBR 2007. LNCS (LNAI), vol. 4626, pp. 224–238. Springer, Heidelberg (2007)

15. Nejati, S., et al.: Matching and merging of state-charts specifications. In: 29th International Conference on Software Engineering, pp. 54–64. IEEE Computer Society (2007)

16. Neuhaus, M., Bunke, H.: A quadratic programming approach to the graph edit distance problem. In: Escolano, F., Vento, M. (eds.) GbRPR. LNCS, vol. 4538, pp. 92–102. Springer, Heidelberg (2007)

17. Neuhaus, M., Bunke, H.: Bridging the Gap Between Graph Edit Distance and Kernel Machines. World Scientific Publishing Co. Inc, River Edge (2007)

18. Neuhaus, M., Riesen, K., Bunke, H.: Fast suboptimal algorithms for the computation of graph edit distance. In: Yeung, D.-Y., Kwok, J.T., Fred, A., Roli, F., de Ridder, D. (eds.) SSPR 2006 and SPR 2006. LNCS, vol. 4109, pp. 163–172. Springer, Heidelberg (2006)

19. Riesen, K., Bunke, H.: Approximate graph edit distance computation by means of bipartite graph matching. Image Vis. Comput. 27(7), 950–959 (2009)

20. Sorlin, S., Solnon, C.: Reactive tabu search for measuring graph similarity. In: Brun, L., Vento, M. (eds.) GbRPR 2005. LNCS, vol. 3434, pp. 172–182. Springer, Heidelberg (2005)

21. Yan, Z., Dijkman, R., Grefen, P.: Fast business process similarity search with feature-based similarity estimation. In: Meersman, R., Dillon, T.S., Herrero, P. (eds.) OTM 2010. LNCS, vol. 6426, pp. 60–77. Springer, Heidelberg (2010)

22. van der Aalst, W.M., de Medeiros, A.K.A., Weijters, A.: Process equivalence: Comparing two process models based on observed behavior. In: Dustdar, S., Fiadeiro, J.L., Sheth, A.P. (eds.) BPM 2006. LNCS, vol. 4102, pp. 129–144. Springer, Heidelberg (2006)

23. van Dongen, B.F., Dijkman, R., Mendling, J.: Measuring similarity between business process models. In: Bellahsène, Z., Léonard, M. (eds.) CAiSE 2008. LNCS, vol. 5074, pp. 450–464. Springer, Heidelberg (2008)

24. Weidlich, M., Dijkman, R., Mendling, J.: The ICoP framework: Identification of correspondences between process models. In: Pernici, B. (ed.) CAiSE 2010. LNCS, vol. 6051, pp. 483–498. Springer, Heidelberg (2010)

25. Weidlich, M., Sagi, T., Leopold, H., Gal, A., Mendling, J.: Predicting the quality of process model matching. In: Daniel, F., Wang, J., Weber, B. (eds.) BPM 2013. LNCS, vol. 8094, pp. 203–210. Springer, Heidelberg (2013)

Service Analysis and Simulation in Process Mining

Arik Senderovich[✉]

Technion – Israel Institute of Technology, Haifa, Israel
sariks@tx.technion.ac.il

Modern business processes are supported by information systems that record process-related events into event logs. *Process mining* is a maturing research field that aims at discovering useful information about the business process from its corresponding event logs [1]. Recently, several works considered process mining in an operational setting; specifically, performance-oriented models were discovered from event data and later applied to operational analysis and support.

A central argument in our research claims that service operations must be modeled and analyzed via custom-tailored techniques, due to their unique characteristics. For instance, the main concern in service operations is the balance between quality-of-service and resource efficiency (utilization). Consequently, a natural theoretical framework for service modeling and analysis is Queueing Theory, since it accommodates the quality-efficiency trade-off. To date, studies on operational process mining did not consider queueing models as candidates for process discovery.

The primary goal of the proposed research is to bridge the gap between operational process mining and service analysis; concretely, the research aims at discovering queueing models from event logs and applying them to operational problems. The secondary objective of this research is to provide (data-based) validity for established theoretical results in Queueing Theory. This step is achieved by validating the discovered queueing models against their originating event logs.

A preliminary study serves as a proof-of-concept for the proposed approach. As a first step, the work introduces the *queueing perspective* for process mining and defines *queue mining* as the set of techniques that extracts queueing models from event logs. Then, two queue mining techniques are used to obtain solutions to a specific operational problem, which is *online delay prediction*. The queue mining predictors are compared to state-of-the-art benchmark techniques from process mining with respect to well-established prediction measures. Empirical evaluation against real-life event logs provides evidence that queue mining predictors are superior to other prediction techniques. Moreover, theoretical results that were (so far) well-known in Queueing Theory gain validity through these experiments. We shall now provide a brief overview of the techniques and results that we considered in our preliminary work [2].

© Springer International Publishing Switzerland 2015
F. Fournier and J. Mendling (Eds.): BPM 2014 Workshops, LNBIP 202, pp. 578–581, 2015.
DOI: 10.1007/978-3-319-15895-2_51

Preliminary Work

To demonstrate the value of queue mining, we formulate the operational problem of *online delay prediction*, then we specify our models and provide corresponding discovery techniques. Consequently, we validate the models against the corresponding event log and conclude the section with a discussion on our empirical insights into queue mining and future research directions.

Problem 1 (Online delay prediction). *Let W be a random variable that measures the delay time of a customer. Denote by $\widehat{W}$ the predictor for W. Then, the* online delay prediction *problem aims at identifying an accurate predictor $\widehat{W}$.*

In our empirical evaluation, we use, as concrete measures, root average squared error (RASE) for accuracy.

In order to solve the delay prediction problem, we propose two queue mining techniques that have grounds in Queueing Theory: one is based on an exact analysis of queueing models, while the other is based on a result from heavy-traffic approximations.

Predictors based on queueing models. We define two delay predictors based on the $G/M/n$ and the $G/M/n + M$ models, respectively. We refer to the first predictor as queue-length (based) predictor (QLP) and to the second as queue-length (based) Markovian (abandonments) Predictor (QLMP) [3]. As their names imply, these predictors use the queue length (in front of the customer) to predict its expected delay. We define the queue-length, $L(t)$, to be a random variable that quantifies the number of cases that are delayed at time t. The QLP for a customer arriving at time t is:

$$\widehat{W}_{QLP}(L(t)) = \frac{(L(t) + 1)}{n\mu} \tag{1}$$

with n being the number of agents and μ being the service rate of an individual agent. The QLMP predictor assumes finite patience and is defined as:

$$\widehat{W}_{QLMP}(L(t)) = \sum_{i=0}^{L(t)} \frac{1}{n\mu + i\theta}. \tag{2}$$

Intuitively, when a customer arrives, it may progress in queue only if customers that are ahead of him enter service (when an agent becomes available, at rate $n\mu$) or abandon (at rate $i\theta$ with i being the number of customers in queue). For the QLP, $\theta = 0$ and thus the QLMP predictor (Eq. 2) reduces to the QLP predictor (1).

Snapshot Predictors. An important result in queueing theory is the *(heavy-traffic) snapshot principle* (see [4], p. 187). A heavy-traffic approximation refers to the behaviour of a queue model under limits of its parameters, as the workload converges to capacity. In the context of Problem 1, the snapshot principle implies that under the heavy-traffic approximation, delay times (of other customers) tend to change negligibly during the waiting time of a single customer [3]. We define two snapshot predictors: Last-customer-to-Enter-Service (LES or $\widehat{W}_{LES}$) and Head-Of-Line (HOL or $\widehat{W}_{HOL}$). The LES predictor is the delay of the most recent service entrant, while the HOL is the delay of the first customer in line.

Model Validation. To test the operational validity of our delay predictors we ran a set of experiments on a real-life event log that comes from a call center process of a large Israeli bank. We compared the results of our predictors against two benchmark predictors that were based on the transition system method proposed by van der Aalst et al. [5]; first, we considered the plain transition system predictor (PTS), which performed poorly, in relation to our predictors. Then, we enhanced the state-space of the PTS with queueing information (queue length), to make the transition system method comparable to our queue mining techniques. We used the K-means algorithm to cluster the queue length into K classes and hence named the algorithm as K transition system, or KTS.

Our experiments show that the snapshot predictors outperform other predictors, in virtually every experimental setting considered. For the predictors based on transition systems we observe that the KTS leads to a significant improvement over the PTS. Both queueing predictors, in turn, performed worse than the snapshot predictors, since the queueing model assumptions suffered from low conceptual validity.

Figure 1 presents the root of the average squared error (RASE) in seconds. Snapshot predictors are superior across all scenarios, improving over the PTS by 34 %–46 %. Note that both snapshot predictors perform identically in terms of

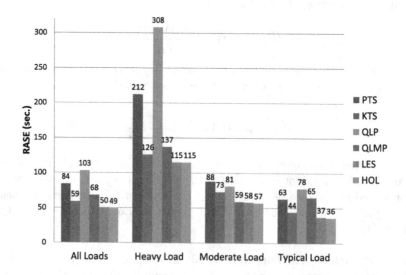

Fig. 1. Root-average squared error in seconds

RASE. This empirical proximity between the LES and the HOL, under certain assumptions, has a theoretical background in [3] (Theorem 4.4).

The QLP performed worse than PTS across scenarios, except the moderate load scenario, while the QLMP outperformed the PTS in all scenarios except the typical load scenario. In the moderate load scenario, the QLMP performs almost as well as the snapshot predictors. The KTS outperforms both the PTS and queueing model predictors, in all scenarios, except the moderate load scenario.

Future Work

The success of queue mining techniques motivates several directions for future research. First, we aim at relaxing some of the model assumptions for the queueing predictors, e.g. exponential distribution of individual service times and (im)patience. This relaxation can cause the models to be intractable for exact analysis. Therefore, the analysis of these models often resorts to simulation or approximation methods in the spirit of the *snapshot principle*.

Most business processes actually consist of multiple service stations. Therefore, another research direction involves the extension of single-station models to queueing networks. Once discovered from data, queueing networks, similarly to single-station queues, can be then validated via exact analysis (e.g. product-form solutions), approximations (e.g. in heavy-traffic) and simulation. For example, in theory, the snapshot principle was shown to work in queueing networks [4]. Therefore, investigating the use of this principle to queueing networks with a complex underlying process may provide competent delay prediction.

Lastly, we aim at developing an algorithm that, given several candidate queueing models, would search for the one that is most fitting. This research direction can be viewed as a special type of *model selection* in statistical learning [6, Ch. 7].

References

1. van der Aalst, W.M.P.: Process Mining - Discovery Conformance and Enhancement of Business Processes. Springer, Heidelberg (2011)
2. Senderovich, A., Weidlich, M., Gal, A., Mandelbaum, A.: Queue mining – predicting delays in service processes. In: Jarke, M., Mylopoulos, J., Quix, C., Rolland, C., Manolopoulos, Y., Mouratidis, H., Horkoff, J. (eds.) CAiSE 2014. LNCS, vol. 8484, pp. 42–57. Springer, Heidelberg (2014)
3. Ibrahim, R., Whitt, W.: Real-time delay estimation based on delay history. Manuf. Serv. Oper. Manage. **11**, 397–415 (2009)
4. Whitt, W.: Stochastic-Process Limits: An Introduction to Stochastic-Process Limits and Their Application to Queues. Springer, Heidelberg (2002)
5. van der Aalst, W.M.P., Schonenberg, M., Song, M.: Time prediction based on process mining. Inf. Syst. **36**, 450–475 (2011)
6. Hastie, T., Tibshirani, R., Friedman, J.: The Elements of Statistical Learning. Springer Series in Statistics. Springer New York Inc., New York (2001)

Process Discovery and Exploration

Sander J.J. Leemans[✉]

Eindhoven University of Technology, Eindhoven, The Netherlands
s.j.j.leemans@tue.nl

1 Introduction

Process mining, and in particular process discovery, have gained traction as a technique for analysing actual process executions from event data recorded in event logs. Process discovery aims to automatically derive a model of the process. Current process discovery techniques either do not provide executable semantics, do not guarantee to return models without deadlocks, or do not achieve a right balance between quality criteria.

A process model can be used in for instance automatic enactment of models in systems [10], in automatic prediction [13] and in compliance checking [11]. For all these purposes, the model needs to have executable semantics and must be sound, i.e. must be free of deadlocks and other anomalies.

Process Discovery. Figure 1 shows the context of process discovery. Traditionally, models have been evaluated using the event log, by means of fitness, precision and generalisation [4]: *fitness* measures what part of the event log is described by the model, *precision* measures what part of the model is present in the event log, and *generalisation* 'measures' what part of future behaviour is present in the model. Although fitness, precision, and generalisation are intuitively clear, different formal definitions are possible [5]. Measuring the quality of a discovered model with respect to its event log might be useful, but whether the best model for the event log is the best model for the system is not captured by these measures, while ultimately, process mining aims to learn information about the system and how it is used in practise by its users (we summarise this to just *system*). Therefore, we propose to (continue) study rediscoverability; if a process discovery technique has *rediscoverability*, it is able to discover models that have the same language as the system by which the log was produced [1,2,6], given some assumptions on the event log and model.

Several process discovery techniques have been proposed; for instance the α algorithm [1], the Integer Linear Programming miner (ILP) [12], and the Evolutionary Tree Miner (ETM) [3]. All these discovery techniques return process models having executable semantics. Of all process discovery techniques we encountered, only ETM guarantees to return sound models, which it achieves by using a hierarchical abstract view of block-structured workflow nets, called *process trees*. Rediscoverability has been proven for α [2], and likely ILP also provides some form of it. However, there is no process discovery technique available that both guarantees sound models and provides rediscoverability. Part of the project is to *introduce techniques that fulfil these basic requirements.*

F. Fournier and J. Mendling (Eds.): BPM 2014 Workshops, LNBIP 202, pp. 582–585, 2015.
DOI: 10.1007/978-3-319-15895-2_52

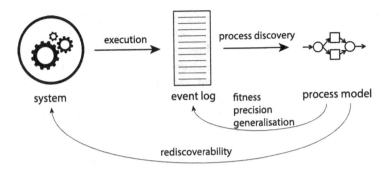

Fig. 1. Process discovery and quality metrics.

Process Exploration. As fitness, precision and generalisation compete [4], there is usually no model that is perfect according to these and other quality criteria. Thus, no discovery algorithm can be expected to result in the best model in all circumstances. That means that, unless a user knows the ins and outs of the event log and the parameters of the discovery technique, obtaining the best model for the job is a repetitive process of choosing a discovery technique, setting its parameters and evaluating the resulting model, until a satisfying model is found (for a reliable evaluation, the model should have executable semantics and be sound as well [9]). Academic tools usually provide executable semantics, but the repetitive nature of process exploration makes them tedious to use and most tools lack features like animation and seamless zooming. Commercial tools produce models that lack semantics, thereby disabling reliable evaluation and further automated use. Part of the project is to provide a methodology that allows process exploration tools to use sophisticated process mining and process discovery techniques, as these are currently used only in academic prototypes, while academic tools use simpler techniques with less extensibility.

2   Inductive Miner Family

The solution we propose to process discovery starts with process trees. This guarantees that the models returned have executable semantics and are sound. ETM uses a genetic approach to search for a process tree that is optimal with respect to several quality criteria, but is slow [7] and cannot guarantee rediscoverability.

Given the hierarchical nature of process trees, we have shown that can be exploited in a divide-and-conquer strategy to process discovery. The *Inductive Miner* (IM) applies such a strategy and performs three steps: (1) it searches for a partition of the process activities, (2) splits the event log and (3) recurses until it hits a base case. In [6], we have formally proven that IM provides rediscoverability and guarantees perfect fitness, i.e. the model describes all behaviour that is in the event log.

However, as process exploration requires a trade-off between quality criteria, perfect fitness is not always desired, for instance if the event log contains noise or infrequent behaviour and the user wants a global overview of the process. Therefore, we introduced the *Inductive Miner - infrequent* (IMi) [7], that closely resembles IM but applies log filtering in all three steps of IM. A case study showed that IMi trades fitness for precision, and discovers sound process models fast.

Both IM and IMi require the event log to contain a minimum amount of information, in particular in presence of concurrency. The *Inductive Miner - incompleteness* (IMin) [8] focuses on rediscoverability when facing logs containing incomplete information. It keeps the divide-and-conquer strategy of IM and IMi, but replaces the activity partitioning (1) step with an optimisation problem to find the best partition. A formal proof showed rediscoverability, a case study showed that IMin needs less information for rediscoverability than IM and therefore generalises better.

Using the members of the IM family, it became possible to introduce a process exploration tool that combines the executable semantics and guarantees of academic tools with the ease-of-use and features of commercial tools. The *Inductive visual Miner* (IvM) [9] uses a variant of IMi to discover a process model. It shows that to the user, extended with a visualisation of the deviations between log and model. A user can change some parameters and immediately gets a new model, enabling the repetitive nature of process exploration. Moreover, it animates the event log on the process model and provides several filtering options (although not as extensive as some commercial tools). IvM is the first process exploration tool of which users can verify the outcome and use the discovered model in automated use cases.

3   Future Research

First, work on the IM family has not finished yet: IMin is able to handle incompleteness and even a bit of noise, at the expense of run time. Moreover, several restrictions apply, such as that each process activity can only be present once and that so-called short loops cannot occur. Without these restrictions, rediscoverability cannot be guaranteed without making unrealistic assumptions about the information in the log: rediscovering arbitrary process trees requires infinite event logs. We would like to know what restrictions could be dropped without stretching the assumptions on the information in the log too far.

Second, we would like to further improve on noise filtering. Ideally, these new approaches would be evaluated using real-life event logs with known systems. In case of absence of these systems, approaches should be (and have been) compared to one another using fitness, precision and generalisation. Automated comparisons are challenging: reliable evaluation requires sound process models, which other approaches usually do not guarantee. These established criteria measure properties of the model with respect to the event log, while the more interesting (but not always answerable) question is how the models relate to the system. In particular, generalisation intuitively describes the probability that future behaviour will be included in the model. As the future is unknown, in the current practise in which the model is evaluated using training data, *any measure of generalisation is nothing more than a wild guess* (note that generalisation is still useful and valid to steer genetic algorithms). We would like to take steps towards an evaluation framework that circumvents these concerns, for instance using *k*-fold cross validation.

References

1. van der Aalst, W.M.P., Weijters, A., Maruster, L.: Workflow mining: discovering process models from event logs. IEEE Trans. Knowl. Data Eng. **16**(9), 1128–1142 (2004)
2. Badouel, E.: On the α-reconstructibility of workflow nets. In: Haddad, S., Pomello, L. (eds.) PETRI NETS 2012. LNCS, vol. 7347, pp. 128–147. Springer, Heidelberg (2012)
3. Buijs, J.C.A.M., van Dongen, B.F., van der Aalst, W.M.P.: A genetic algorithm for discovering process trees. In: IEEE Congress on Evolutionary Computation, pp. 1–8. IEEE (2012)
4. Buijs, J.C.A.M., van Dongen, B.F., van der Aalst, W.M.P.: On the role of fitness, precision, generalization and simplicity in process discovery. In: Meersman, R., et al. (eds.) OTM 2012, Part I. LNCS, vol. 7565, pp. 305–322. Springer, Heidelberg (2012)
5. De Weerdt, J., De Backer, M., Vanthienen, J., Baesens, B.: A multi-dimensional quality assessment of state-of-the-art process discovery algorithms using real-life event logs. Inf. Syst. **37**, 654–676 (2012)
6. Leemans, S.J.J., Fahland, D., van der Aalst, W.M.P.: Discovering block-structured process models from event logs - a constructive approach. In: Colom, J.-M., Desel, J. (eds.) PETRI NETS 2013. LNCS, vol. 7927, pp. 311–329. Springer, Heidelberg (2013)
7. Leemans, S.J.J., Fahland, D., van der Aalst, W.M.P.: Discovering block-structured process models from event logs containing infrequent behaviour. In: Lohmann, N., Song, M., Wohed, P. (eds.) BPM 2013 Workshops. LNBIP, vol. 171, pp. 66–78. Springer, Heidelberg (2014)
8. Leemans, S.J.J., Fahland, D., van der Aalst, W.M.P.: Discovering block-structured process models from incomplete event logs. In: Ciardo, G., Kindler, E. (eds.) PETRI NETS 2014. LNCS, vol. 8489, pp. 91–110. Springer, Heidelberg (2014)
9. Leemans, S.J.J., Fahland, D., van der Aalst, W.M.P.: Exploring processes and deviations. In: Fournier, F., Mendling, J. (eds.) BPM 2014 Workshops. LNBIP, vol. 202, pp. 302–314. Springer, Heidelberg (2015)
10. Meyer, A., Pufahl, L., Fahland, D., Weske, M.: Modeling and enacting complex data dependencies in business processes. In: Daniel, F., Wang, J., Weber, B. (eds.) BPM 2013. LNCS, vol. 8094, pp. 171–186. Springer, Heidelberg (2013)
11. Ramezani, E., Fahland, D., van der Aalst, W.M.P.: Where did I misbehave? Diagnostic information in compliance checking. In: Barros, A., Gal, A., Kindler, E. (eds.) BPM 2012. LNCS, vol. 7481, pp. 262–278. Springer, Heidelberg (2012)
12. van der Werf, J., van Dongen, B., Hurkens, C., Serebrenik, A.: Process discovery using integer linear programming. Fundam. Inform. **94**(3–4), 387–412 (2009)
13. Wynn, M., Rozinat, A., van der Aalst, W.M.P., ter Hofstede, A., Fidge, C.: Process mining and simulation. In: Hofstede, A.H.M., van der Aalst, W.M.P., Adams, M., Russell, N. (eds.) Modern Business Process Automation, pp. 437–457. Springer, Heidelberg (2010)

Author Index

Akkiraju, Rama   158
Amyot, Daniel   40
Andreev, Pavel   40
Andrikopoulos, Vasilios   165
Appelrath, Hans-Jürgen   383
Ariel, Elior   53
Astaraky, Davood   40

Bach, Thomas   165
Baesens, Bart   186
Bär, Florian   440, 452
Barros, Alistair   446
Bazhenova, Ekaterina   277
Becker, Jörg   541
Botezatu, Mirela   251
Breuker, Dominic   541
Broens, Tom   53
Brucker-Kley, Elke   463
Buijs, J.C.A.M.   291
Burattin, Andrea   408

Cagnin, Maria Istela   130
Caron, Filip   529
Carrera, Berny   477
Cimitile, Marta   408
Cognini, Riccardo   210
Cordes, Carsten   383
Corradini, Flavio   210

de Jesus, Jandisson Soares   489
de Leoni, Massimiliano   235
de Melo, Ana Cristina Vieira   489
De Smedt, Johannes   198
De Weerdt, Jochen   529
Delfmann, Patrick   541
Depaire, Benoît   342
Desel, Jörg   353
Dijkman, Remco   251
Dustdar, Schahram   145

Fahland, Dirk   75, 304
Fleuriot, Jacques   28
Fournier, Fabiana   222
Fung, Nick   53

Gailly, Frederik   516
García-Sáez, Gema   53
Goldstein, Ayelet   53
Grünert, David   463
Guanciale, Roberto   96
Gulden, Jens   420
Gurov, Dilian   96

Härting, Ralf-Christian   440
Henis, Ealan   59
Hernando, Elena   53
Herzberg, Nico   3
Hewelt, Marcin   16
Hipp, Markus   395
Hull, Richard   175

Jones, Valerie   53
Jugel, Dierk   452
Jung, Jae-Yoon   477

Kaczor, Krzysztof   504
Karni, Reuven   429
Keller, Thomas   463
Kirchner, Kathrin   3
Kluza, Krzysztof   504
Kunde, Aaron   16
Kuziemsky, Craig   40

Landre, Geraldo   130
Leemans, Sander J.J.   304, 582
Leopold, Henrik   105, 118
Levy, Meira   429
Li, Runzhuo   40
Limonad, Lior   222
Lu, Xixi   75

Maggi, Fabrizio Maria   408
Malinova, Monika   567
Mannhardt, Felix   235
Marberg, John   59
Matzner, Martin   541
Meinel, Christoph   16
Mendling, Jan   118
Mertens, Steven   516

Michalowski, Wojtek   40
Michelberger, Bernd   395
Möhring, Michael   440, 452
Motahari Nezhad, Hamid R.   158
Mutschler, Bela   395

Nagin, Kenneth   59
Nakagawa, Elisa Yumi   130
Nalepa, Grzegorz J.   504

Paiva, Débora Maria   130
Palma, Edilson   130
Papapanagiotou, Petros   28
Pittke, Fabian   118
Pizarro, Gustavo   317
Pnina, Soffer   557
Poels, Geert   516
Polini, Andrea   210
Pufahl, Luise   277

Quaglini, Silvana   53

Rabinovici-Cohen, Simona   59
Raichelson, Lihi   330
Re, Barbara   210
Reher, Felix   561
Reichert, Manfred   395
Reijers, Hajo A.   105, 235, 367
Reinhartz-Berger, Iris   557
Russell, Nick   446

Sacchi, Lucia   53
Sáez, Santiago Gómez   165
Schäfer, David Richard   165
Schmidt, Rainer   440, 452
Schunselaar, D.M.M.   105, 367

Schweda, Christian M.   452
Senderovich, Arik   578
Sepúlveda, Marcos   317
Serral, Estefanía   198
Shahar, Yuval   53
Shalom, Erez   53
Soffer, Pnina   330
Strauss, Achim   395

Tariq, Muhammad Adnan   165
(Terry) Heath III, Fenno F.   175
Truong, Hong-Linh   145
Tsagkani, Christina   573
Tsoury, Arava   557

van der Aalst, Wil M.P.   75, 105, 264, 304, 367
van der Werf, J.M.E.M.   89
van Dongen, B.F.   291
van Eck, M.L.   291
vanden Broucke, Seppe K.L.M.   186, 529
Vanthienen, Jan   186, 198
Verbeek, H.M.W.   89, 105, 264, 367
Vogelgesang, Thomas   383
Völzer, Hagen   251

Wakup, Christian   353
Weske, Mathias   3, 16, 277
Wilk, Szymon   40

Zhu, Guobin   186
Zhu, Xinwei   186
Zimmermann, Alfred   440, 452